Q&A | Course Review | NCLEX-Prep

Davis's SUCCESS SERIES

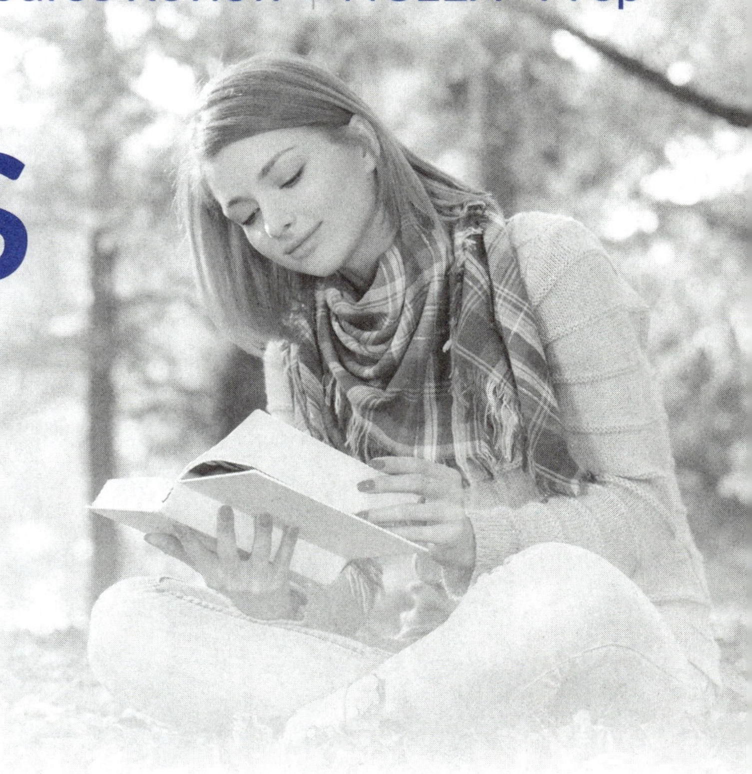

- Fundamentals
- Test Prep
- Pharmacology
- Maternal & Newborn
- Pediatric
- Med-Surg
- Psychiatric Mental Health Nursing

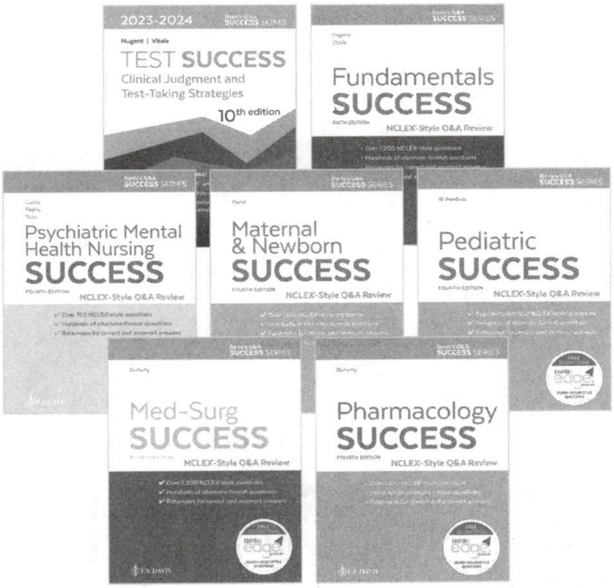

★★★★★

"My test scores definitely went up after I found these books."

—Sakin M.

★★★★★

"My #1 go-to the week before ANY exam!"

—Andrea A.

★★★★★

"The rationales are the reason I love the books in the Davis Success series."

—Lynn C.

Test **Success**

Clinical Judgment and Test-Taking Strategies

TENTH EDITION

Patricia M. Nugent, RN, MA, MS, EdD
Professor Emeritus
Adjunct Professor
Nassau Community College
Garden City, New York
Private Practice—President of Nugent Books, Inc.

Barbara A. Vitale, RN, MA
Professor Emeritus
Nassau Community College
Garden City, New York
Private Practice—Professional Resources for Nursing

F.A. DAVIS
Philadelphia

F. A. Davis Company
1915 Arch Street
Philadelphia, PA 19103
www.fadavis.com

Printed in the United States of America

Last digit indicates print number: 10 9 8 7 6 5 4 3 2 1

Acquisitions Editor: Jacalyn Sharp
Content Project Manager: Veronica Neff
Design and Illustrations Manager: Carolyn O'Brien

As new scientific information becomes available through basic and clinical research, recommended treatments and drug therapies undergo changes. The author(s) and publisher have done everything possible to make this book accurate, up to date, and in accord with accepted standards at the time of publication. The author(s), editors, and publisher are not responsible for errors or omissions or for consequences from application of the book and make no warranty, expressed or implied, in regard to the contents of the book. Any practice described in this book should be applied by the reader in accordance with professional standards of care used in regard to the unique circumstances that may apply in each situation. The reader is advised always to check product information (package inserts) for changes and new information regarding dose and contraindications before administering any drug. Caution is especially urged when using new or infrequently ordered drugs.

ISBN: 978-1-7196-4724-3

Preface

WHY THIS BOOK IS NECESSARY

- Nursing information and technology are accelerating at a breathtaking rate. Student nurses must learn how to function successfully within nursing programs that have strenuous academic demands.
- The role of the nurse is evolving as the delivery of health care is changing. Student nurses must develop critical thinking skills and become empowered.
- Multiple factors affect the education of beginning nursing students (e.g., students who work full- or part-time, who have been out of secondary education for several years, who are single parents juggling numerous roles within the family, and who speak English as a second language). Student nurses must learn how to study, manage their time effectively, and develop a positive mental attitude.
- Society requires higher educational standards within the professions that provide health-care services. Student nurses must maximize their acquisition of information in the affective, cognitive, and psychomotor domains to increase their success on standardized nursing examinations that require not only the regurgitation of information but also the comprehension, application, or analysis of information.

WHO SHOULD USE THIS BOOK

- Students entering a nursing program
- Students who are preparing to take tests at the end of a unit of instruction in nursing or at the completion of a course on the fundamentals of nursing
- Students in licensed practical nurse programs who are preparing for class tests, the NCLEX-PN®, or advanced-standing examinations for entry into a registered nurse program
- Students preparing for the NCLEX-RN® for licensure
- Licensed professional nurses preparing for a certification examination
- Nursing faculty members who are helping beginning nursing students achieve success in a nursing program
- Nursing faculty members who are designing a test-taking workshop for student nurses

CONTENT IN *TEST SUCCESS* THAT HELPS STUDENTS MAXIMIZE SUCCESS

Chapters 1 through 10 contain information designed to maximize success by helping students to do the following:

- Develop a positive mental attitude
- Understand how critical thinking supports clinical reasoning
- Be introduced to clinical judgment and the Next Generation NCLEX®
- Manage their time
- Study and learn more effectively
- Become test wise by using the nursing process and test-taking techniques
- Explore all testing formats, specifically multiple-choice and alternate question formats (e.g., multiple-response, hot spot, graphic illustration, exhibit, fill-in-the-blank, drag-and-drop [also called ordered response], audio, and video items)
- Appreciate computer applications in nursing education and evaluation

Chapter 11 contains approximately 525 questions divided into 15 content areas common to nursing practice. The questions in each content area can be answered by a student at the completion of equivalent content in a nursing program. Also included in Chapter 11 are new Clinical Judgment Case Studies that test the six cognitive skills of the National Council of State Boards of Nursing's (NCSBN's) Clinical Judgment Measurement Model. This includes recognizing cues, analyzing cues, prioritizing hypotheses, generating solutions, taking actions, and evaluating outcomes. Practicing with these unfolding case studies and understanding these steps are important in developing strong clinical judgment skills and preparing for the Next Generation NCLEX®.

Chapter 12 contains a 100-question Comprehensive Final Book Examination. This examination contains 50 multiple-choice questions and 50 alternate question format items reflective of NCLEX® examinations. It includes information from all 15 content areas addressed in Chapter 11. This test can be taken at the completion of a course in fundamentals of nursing or when preparing for an NCLEX® examination.

Every question in the book has rationales for the correct and incorrect options. These rationales should help the learner review some of the basic content in nursing theory as well as practice answering and mastering questions. In addition, when appropriate, the questions include a Test-Taking Tip that emphasizes one or more of the techniques presented in Chapter 7.

Students can access two 75-item unique Comprehensive Course Examinations online. These examinations incorporate information from the 15 content areas in Chapter 11. Each 75-item examination contains more than 35 alternate question format items reflective of NCLEX® examinations. Every question is accompanied by rationales for the correct answer and the incorrect options to reinforce fundamentals of nursing theory and principles. Most questions have Test-Taking Tips identical to the tips presented in Chapter 7.

TERMINOLOGY USED IN THE TEXT

- *Client* is used throughout the book to indicate the consumer of health care.
- *Nurse* is used consistently to indicate a licensed nurse. This individual may be referred to by other titles, such as "nursing care coordinator" or "nurse manager."
- *Nurse's aide* and *nursing assistant* are used consistently to indicate credentialed or noncredentialed supportive nursing staff members.
- *Primary health-care provider* indicates health-care professionals with prescriptive privileges (e.g., physicians, nurse practitioners, physician assistants, podiatrists, and dentists).

SELF-ASSESSMENT TOOLS TO EXPLORE PERSONAL PERFORMANCE

Many tools are included to allow the student to perform self-assessments and ultimately improve time management, studying, and testing performance.

Chapter 3 presents three tools and an individualized corrective action plan to maximize productivity:

- Assessment of Inconsistencies Between Values and Behavior
- Personal Time/Activity Journal
- Self-Assessment of Barriers to Productivity
- Corrective Action Plan to Maximize Your Productivity

Chapter 10 presents two tools and two individualized corrective action guides:

- Information-Processing Analysis Tool
- Corrective Action Guide for Information-Processing Analysis Tool
- Knowledge Analysis Tool
- Corrective Action Guide for Knowledge Analysis Tool

Contributors

Nancy Beck Irland, DNP, MSN, RN
Certified Nurse Midwife (retired)
Policy Analyst for Nursing Education and Assessment
Oregon State Board of Nursing
Portland, Oregon (retired)

Contents

How to Use This Book to Maximize Success

It is amazing what **you** can achieve when **you** are tenacious, organized, and determined to attain a goal! By purchasing this book, **you** have demonstrated a beginning commitment to do what **you** have to do to improve your success in nursing examinations. This book is designed to introduce **you** to various techniques that can contribute to a positive mental attitude, promote the development of critical thinking skills, and help **you** become test wise. If you are beginning to get the feeling that **you** is an important word, **"you"** are right! Learning requires you to be an active participant in your educational activities. Your ultimate success can be maximized if you progress through this book in a planned and organized fashion and are willing to practice the techniques suggested. Effort is directly correlated with the benefits you will derive from this book. After you have determined that you are eager and motivated to learn, you are ready to begin.

Chapter content is organized in a specific order to provide you with skills that will contribute to your success when taking a nursing examination.

Chapter 1: Empowerment—Develop a positive mental attitude.

Chapter 2: Critical Thinking—Maximize your critical thinking abilities.

Chapter 3: Time Management—Use self-assessment tools to maximize your use of time.

- Assessment of Inconsistencies Between Values and Behavior
- Personal Time/Activity Journal
- Self-Assessment of Barriers to Productivity
- Corrective Action Plan to Maximize Your Productivity

Chapter 4: Study Techniques—Use general and specific study techniques to increase your ability to recall, understand, apply, and analyze information when answering nursing examination questions.

Chapter 5: The Multiple-Choice Question—Improve your understanding of the components of a multiple-choice question: the first part that asks a question (stem) and the second part that presents potential answers (options).

Chapter 6: The Nursing Process—Expand your ability to identify the focus of a nursing examination question within the framework of the nursing process to better understand what the question is asking.

Chapter 7: Test-Taking Techniques—Learn to use specific test-taking techniques to critically analyze the stem and options in a question.

Chapter 8: Testing Formats Other Than Multiple-Choice Questions—Increase your ability to analyze and answer alternate question format items (fill-in-the-blank calculation, hot spot, graphic, drag-and-drop/ordered response, multiple-response, exhibit, and multimedia in multiple-choice and alternate question format items) that appear on the NCLEX® examinations. Learn about the new Next Generation NCLEX® cases and item types and the key steps of the NCSBN's Clinical Judgment Measurement Model.

Chapter 9: Computer Applications in Education and Evaluation—Understand that you must be an active participant in the use of computers in education, evaluation, and the clinical setting.

Chapter 10: Analyze Your Test Performance—Use self-assessment tools to identify what you know, and what you need to know.

- Information-Processing Analysis Tool
- Corrective Action Guide for the Information-Processing Tool
  - Corrective Action Guide for Processing Errors
  - Corrective Action Guide for Personal Performance Trends
- Knowledge Analysis Tool

- Corrective Action Guide for the Knowledge Analysis Tool
  - Corrective Action Guide for Knowledge Categories
  - Corrective Action Guide for the Nursing Process

Chapter 11: Practice Questions With Answers and Rationales—Practice answering 525 nursing questions, almost 50% of which are alternate question format items reflective of the NCLEX-RN®. The questions are divided into 15 content areas common to the fundamentals of nursing practice. Every question has the rationales for the correct answer(s) and the incorrect options to reinforce fundamentals of nursing theory and principles. Most questions have one or more Test-Taking Tips identical to the tips presented in Chapter 7. Practice your clinical judgment skills and prepare for the Next Generation NCLEX® with unfolding case studies that test the six cognitive skills of the NCSBN's Clinical Judgment Measurement Model. This includes recognizing cues, analyzing cues, prioritizing hypotheses, generating solutions, taking actions, and evaluating outcomes.

Chapter 12: Comprehensive Final Book Examination—Practice taking a comprehensive 100-item test, 50% (50 items) of which are alternate question format items reflective of the NCLEX-RN®. This test incorporates information from the 15 content areas in Chapter 11. Every question has the rationales for the correct answer(s) and the incorrect options to reinforce fundamentals of nursing theory and principles. Most questions have one or more Test-Taking Tips identical to the tips presented in Chapter 7.

Access the 75-item unique Comprehensive Course Examinations online. These exams incorporate information from the 15 content areas in Chapter 11. Each 75-item exam contains more than 35 alternate question format items reflective of NCLEX® examinations. Every question has the rationales for the correct answer and the incorrect options to reinforce fundamentals of nursing theory and principles. Most questions have Test-Taking Tips identical to the tips presented in Chapter 7.

TIPS TO USE THIS TEXT TO ITS BEST ADVANTAGE

Read Chapters 1 through 10. Then answer the questions in Chapter 11. Be sure to study the rationales, because this information will review and reinforce the material you are learning in your fundamentals of nursing course. To maximize learning, it is suggested that you answer the questions in the specific categories in Chapter 11 after you have learned the content in class. Evaluate your performance after completing each section by using the tools presented in Chapter 10. This analysis will help you identify information-processing errors, personal performance trends, and knowledge deficits and will provide suggestions for corrective action. In addition, a review of the rationales should expand your knowledge, and your performance should improve as you progress through Chapter 11. Finally, take the Comprehensive Final Book Examination in Chapter 12 and the two 75-item comprehensive examinations online. Again, evaluate your performance using the self-assessment tools in Chapter 10, and use the corrective action plans to focus your study. The self-assessment tools should be used not only in conjunction with this book but also to analyze your performance after every test you take in your nursing courses. To become familiar with answering nursing questions on a computer, you can access additional questions online.

You should be commended for your efforts to achieve success. It is hard work to take responsibility for your own learning. The magnitude of your learning will be in direct proportion to the amount of energy you are willing to expend in the effort to improve your knowledge and skills. You will become a more successful test taker when you:

- Function from a position of strength
- Think critically
- Manage your time
- Study more effectively
- Become test wise
- Are able to apply the nursing process to determine what a question is asking
- Practice test taking
- Analyze your test performance

WE WISH YOU MUCH SUCCESS ON YOUR NURSING EXAMINATIONS!

1

Empowerment

DEVELOP A POSITIVE MENTAL ATTITUDE

A positive mental attitude can help you control test anxiety. This positive attitude limits anxious responses and makes you a more successful test taker. A positive mental attitude requires you to function from a position of strength. This does not imply that you have to be powerful, manipulative, or dominant. What it does require is that you develop techniques that put you in control of your own thoughts and behavior. To be in control of yourself, you should operate from a position of positive self-worth with a feeling of empowerment. This begins with self-assessment.

You have both strengths and weaknesses. Both should be identified to maximize your potential. Strengths are easy to focus on because they are safe and nonthreatening. Weaknesses are more difficult to focus on because they may make you feel inadequate and uncomfortable. When performing a self-assessment, be honest with yourself. You must separate your ego from your assessment. Only you will know the result. Remember, few people are perfect! Have the courage to be honest with yourself and to identify your imperfections. You can have weaknesses and imperfections and still have a positive self-concept.

To develop a positive self-concept, you must be willing to look within yourself and appreciate that you are valuable. Acting from a position of strength requires you to start saying and believing that you are worthwhile. A positive self-concept increases when you believe, down to your very core, that you are important.

A feeling of empowerment increases when you are able to use all your available resources and learned strategies to achieve your goals. To achieve empowerment, you must develop techniques and skills that not only make you feel in control but also actually put you in control. When you are in control, you function from a position of strength.

To achieve a sense of self-worth and a feeling of empowerment that will help you succeed in test taking, you must learn various techniques and practice them before taking the test. These techniques will help you control stressful situations, reduce anxious responses, and enhance concentration. This improves your analytical and problem-solving abilities and strengthens your test performance. By learning and practicing the following techniques, you will have a foundation of strength.

Establish a Positive Internal Locus of Control

Henry Ford once said, "Whether you think you can, or you think you can't . . . you're right." In other words, what you *think* can be a self-fulfilling prophecy. The way you talk to yourself influences the way you think about yourself. What you say indicates how you feel about your control of your behavior and your life. "I was lucky to pass that test." "I could not help failing because the teacher is hard." "I got anxious, and I just became paralyzed during the test." Each of these internal monologues indicates that you see yourself as powerless. When you say these things, you fail to take control.

Identify your pattern of talking to yourself. Do you blame others, attribute failure to external causes, and use the phrases "I couldn't," "I should," "I need to," or "I have to"? If you do, you are using language that places you in a position of impotence, dependence, vulnerability, and hopelessness. YOU MUST ESTABLISH A POSITIVE INTERNAL LOCUS OF CONTROL. You do this by replacing this language with language that reflects control and strength. You must say "I want," "I can," and "I will." When you use these words, you imply that you are committed to a task until you succeed. Place index cards stating "I WANT," "I CAN," and "I WILL" around your environment to cue you into a positive pattern of talking to yourself.

Challenge Negative Thoughts

Your value as an individual should not be linked to how well you do on an examination. Your self-worth and your test score are distinctly isolated entities. If you believe that you are good when you do well on a test and bad when you do poorly, you must alter your thinking. You need to work on recognizing that this is illogical thinking. Illogical or negative thinking is self-destructive. Negative thoughts must be changed into positive thoughts to build confidence and self-worth. As confidence and self-worth increase, anxiety can be controlled and minimized.

Positive thinking focuses your attention on your desired outcomes. If you think you can do well on a test, you are more likely to fulfill this prophecy. It is critical that you control negative thoughts by developing a positive mental attitude. When you say to yourself, "This is going to be a hard test. I'll never pass," CHALLENGE THIS STATEMENT. Say to yourself, "This is a ridiculous statement. Of course I can pass this test. All I have to do is study hard!" It is crucial that you challenge negative thoughts with optimistic thoughts. Optimistic thoughts are valuable because they can be converted into positive actions and feelings, thus placing you in a position of control.

For this technique to work, you must first stop negative thoughts. Use the technique called ARREST NEGATIVE THOUGHTS to identity the pattern of negative thinking that you use to defend yourself. After you identify a negative thought, envision a police car with flashing lights that signifies ARREST NEGATIVE THOUGHTS. You can even place pictures of police cars around your environment to cue you to ARREST NEGATIVE THOUGHTS. After you identify negative thoughts, handcuff them and lock them away so they are no longer a threat. Actually envision negative thoughts locked up in a cell with bars and yourself throwing away the key.

After you stop a negative thought, replace it with a POSITIVE THOUGHT. If you have difficulty identifying a positive thought, praise yourself or give yourself a compliment. Tell yourself, "Wow! I am really working hard to pass this test." "Congratulations! I was able to arrest that negative thought and be in control." To increase control, take an inventory of the things you can do, the things you want to achieve, and the feelings you want to feel that contribute to a positive mental attitude. Throughout the day, take an "attitude inventory." Identify the status of your mental attitude. If it is not consistent with your list of the feelings you want to feel or the positive image you have of yourself, CHALLENGE YOUR ATTITUDE. Compose statements that support the feelings you want to feel, and read them over and over. Such statements may include "I can pass this test!" or "I am in control of my attitudes, and my attitudes are positive!" "I am becoming a nurse!" Make sure that you end the day with a positive thought, and even identify something that you want to accomplish the next day. Forecasting positive events establishes a positive direction in which you can focus your attention.

Use Diaphragmatic Breathing

An excellent way to reduce anxiety is to use the technique of diaphragmatic breathing. On inspiration, diaphragmatic breathing causes the diaphragm to flatten and the abdomen to expand outward. On exhalation, the abdominal muscles contract. As you slowly let out this deep breath, the other muscles of the body tend to "let go," promoting relaxation. You probably do this now unconsciously. Most people take a deep breath and exhale, or sigh, several times an hour. When you "sigh," you are using a form of diaphragmatic breathing. You can break the pattern of shallow short breaths associated with anxious feelings when you perform this type of breathing. Anxious responses tend to occur at the beginning of a test, when you are stumped by a tough question, or when you are nearing the end of a test. Using diaphragmatic breathing during these critical times can induce the relaxation response.

When practicing diaphragmatic breathing, place your hands lightly over the front of the lower ribs and upper abdomen so that you can monitor the movement you are trying to achieve. As you become accomplished in this technique, you will not need to position your hands on your body. Practice the following steps:

1. Gently position your hands over the front of your lower ribs and upper abdomen.
2. Exhale gently and fully. Feel your ribs and abdomen sink inward toward the middle of your body.
3. Slowly inhale, taking a deep breath through your nose and expanding your abdomen first and then your chest. Do this as you slowly count to four.
4. Hold your breath at the height of inhalation as you count to four.
5. Exhale fully by contracting your abdominal muscles and then your chest. Let out all the air slowly and smoothly through your mouth as you count to eight.

Monitor the pace of your breathing. Notice how your muscles relax each time you exhale. You may feel warm, tingly, and relaxed. Enjoy the feeling as you breathe deeply and evenly. You should practice this technique so that controlled breathing automatically induces the relaxation response after several breaths. After you are able to induce the relaxation response with controlled breathing, you can effectively draw on this strategy when you need to be in control.

It is important not to do this exercise too forcefully or too rapidly because it can cause you to hyperventilate. Hyperventilation may cause dizziness and light-headedness. These symptoms should subside if you continue this exercise less vigorously. Always monitor your responses throughout the exercise.

Desensitize Yourself to the Fear Response

Individuals generally connect a certain feeling with a specific situation. To learn to control your feelings, you must first recognize how you consider and visualize events. It is not uncommon to connect a feeling of fear with an examination. In a testing situation, the examination is the event, and fear may be the response/feeling. If you experience a fear response during an examination you must interrupt this response. You have the ability to control how you respond to fear. When you are able to separate the event from the feeling, you establish control and become empowered. However, establishing control does not happen automatically. You have to desensitize yourself to the event to control the fear response.

Desensitization involves repeatedly exposing yourself to the identified emotionally distressing event in a limited and/or controlled setting until the event no longer precipitates the feeling of fear. Desensitization depends on associating relaxation with the fear response. To achieve this response, you should practice the following routine.

First, you must practice the relaxation response. Controlled breathing, an excellent relaxation technique, has already been described. After you are comfortable with the technique of controlled breathing, you can use it in the desensitization routine.

Second, you should make a list of five events associated with a testing situation that cause fear and rank them, starting with the one that causes the most anxiety and progressing to the one that causes the least anxiety. A sample list follows.

1. Taking an important examination on difficult material
2. Taking an important examination on material you know well
3. Taking a small quiz on difficult material
4. Taking a small quiz on material you know well
5. Taking a practice test that does not count

Event number 5 should evoke the least amount of fear.

Third, you should practice the following routine:

1. Practice controlled breathing and become relaxed.
2. Now imagine event number 5. If you feel fearful, turn off the scene and go back to controlled breathing for about 30 seconds.

3. After you are relaxed, again imagine scene number 5. Try to visualize the event for 30 seconds without becoming uncomfortable.
4. After you have accomplished the previous step, move up the list of events until you are able to imagine event number 1 without feeling uncomfortable.

When you are successful in controlling the fear response in an imagined situation, you can attempt the same success in simulated tests at home. After you are successful in controlling the fear response in simulated tests at home, you can take some simulated tests in a classroom setting. Continue practicing desensitization until you have a feeling of control in an actual testing situation. This may take practice. It will not be accomplished in one practice session.

Another way you can use the concept of desensitization is to practice positive dialogue within yourself. For example, imagine the following internal dialogue within yourself:

Questions	Responses
"How am I feeling about the examination today?"	"A little uncomfortable and fearful."
"Do I want to feel this way?"	"Absolutely not!"
"How do I want to feel?"	"I want to feel calm, in control, and effective."
"What am I going to do to achieve that feeling?"	"I am going to practice relaxation and controlled breathing."

You might say to yourself, "I don't see myself doing this. This is silly." However, the resilient and tenacious individual who is willing to try new techniques is in a position of control. If your goal is to be empowered, then you have only to be open and willing to learn. In the same way that laboring women practice breathing techniques for labor pain, the astute student can practice these techniques to control test anxiety.

Perform Muscle Relaxation

The muscle relaxation technique involves learning how to tense and relax each muscle group of your body until all of your muscle groups are relaxed. This technique requires practice. Initially, you must assume a comfortable position and then sequentially contract and relax each muscle group in your body from your head to your toes. When a muscle group is tensed and then released, the muscles relax. This technique cannot be quickly described in a short paragraph. However, the following brief exercise is included as an example.

Find a comfortable chair in a quiet place. Close your eyes and use diaphragmatic breathing, taking several deep breaths to relax. You are now ready to begin progressive muscle relaxation. Sequentially, move from one muscle group in the body to another, contracting and relaxing each for 10 seconds. After each muscle group is tensed and then relaxed, take a slow, deep breath using diaphragmatic breathing. As you are relaxing, observe how you feel. Experience the sensation. You may want to reinforce the feeling of relaxation by saying, "My muscles are relaxing. I can feel the tension flowing out of my muscles." Visualize the tension like a mist leaving your body through the ends of your fingers and toes. Remember not to breathe too forcefully to avoid hyperventilation.

The following is a sample of muscle groups that should be included in a progressive muscle relaxation routine:

1. Bend your head and try to rest your right ear as close as you can to your right shoulder. Count to 10. Assume normal alignment, relax, and take a slow, deep breath. Release.
2. Bend your head and try to rest your left ear as close as you can to your left shoulder. Count to 10. Assume normal alignment, relax, and take a slow, deep breath. Release.
3. Flex your head and try to touch your chin to your chest. Count to 10. Assume normal alignment, relax, and take a slow, deep breath. Release.

4. Make a fist and tense your right forearm. Count to 10. Relax and take a slow, deep breath. Release.
5. Make a fist and tense your left forearm. Count to 10. Relax and take a slow, deep breath. Release.
6. Tense your right biceps by tightly bending (flexing) the right arm at the elbow. Count to 10. Relax and take a slow, deep breath. Release.

Continue moving from the head and arms to the trunk and legs by contracting and relaxing each of the muscle groups within these areas of your body. You can understand and master this technique by obtaining an audiotape or video that is designed to direct and instruct you through the entire routine of tensing and relaxing each muscle group. The muscle relaxation technique should be practiced every day until it becomes natural. After you have mastered this technique, you can use a shortened version of progressive relaxation along with controlled breathing at critical times during a test.

Use Imagery

Using imagery can help you to establish a state of relaxation. When you remember a fearful event, your heart and respiratory rates increase just as they did when the event occurred. Similarly, when you recall a happy, relaxing event, you can recreate the atmosphere and feeling that you had during that pleasant period. Using imagery is not a difficult technique to master. Just let go and enjoy the experience.

Position yourself in a comfortable chair, close your eyes, and construct an image in your mind of a place that makes you feel calm, happy, and relaxed. It may be at the seashore or in a field of wildflowers. Let your mind picture what is happening. Observe the colors of the landscape. Notice the soothing sounds of the environment. Notice the smells in the air, the shapes of objects, and movement about you. Recall the positive feelings that flowed over you when you were in that scene, and relax. You can now open your eyes relaxed, refreshed, and calm.

At critical times during a test, you can take a few minutes to use imagery to induce the relaxation response. To reduce stress successfully, you must position yourself in control. Some students use the mantra, "I've got this!" from the moment they begin a test. When you are in control, your test performance generally improves.

Overprepare for a Test

One of the best ways to reduce text anxiety is to be overprepared. The more prepared you are to take the test, the more confident you will be. The more confident you are, the more able you are to challenge the fear of being unprepared. Study the textbook, read your notes, take practice tests, and prepare with other students in a study group. Even when you think you know the information, study the same information again to reinforce your learning. For this technique to be successful, you should schedule a significant amount of time for studying. Although this is time-consuming, it does build confidence and reduce anxiety. No one has said that learning is easy. Any worthwhile goal deserves the effort necessary to achieve success. Being overprepared is the BEST way to place yourself in a position of strength.

Consider the following scenario. A student is not doing well in school and asks what she can do to improve her performance. The concept of being overprepared is discussed, and she works out a study schedule of 2 hours a day for 2 weeks before the next test. After the test, the student says she thinks she did well because the test was easy. It is pointed out that she perceived the test as easy because she attained the knowledge that enabled her to answer the questions correctly. Her eyes light up as if someone has turned on a light bulb over her head!

When you recognize that you have the opportunity to be in control and take responsibility for your own learning, you become all that you can be. Recognize that the purpose of your learning is to be the best nurse you can be.

Exercise Regularly

Exercising regularly helps you to expend nervous energy. Walking, doing aerobic exercise, swimming, bike riding, or running at least three times a week for 20 minutes is an effective way to maintain or improve your physical and mental status. The most important thing to remember about regular exercise is to slowly increase the degree and duration of the exercise. Your exercise program should not be so rigorous that it leaves you exhausted. It should serve to clear your mind and make you mentally alert and better able to cope with the challenge of a test. Also, exercise should not be performed just before going to bed because it can interfere with sleep.

Regular exercise should become a routine activity in your weekly schedule, not just a response to the tension of an upcoming test. After you establish a regular exercise program, you should experience physical and psychological benefits.

ESTABLISH CONTROL BEFORE AND DURING THE TEST

It is important to maximize your opportunities to feel in control in a testing situation. Additional techniques you can use to establish a tranquil and composed atmosphere require taking control of your testing equipment, your activities before and during a test, and your immediate physical space. Techniques to create this atmosphere are reinforced in Chapter 7, "Test-Taking Techniques." However, they also are discussed here because they can be used to reduce anxiety and promote empowerment.

Manage Your Daily Routine Before the Test

It is important to maintain your usual daily routine the day of the test. Eat what you usually eat, but avoid food and beverages with caffeine. Caffeine can lessen your attention span and reduce your concentration by overstimulating your metabolism. Avoid the urge to stay up late the night before a test. If you are tired when taking a test, your ability to concentrate and solve problems may be limited. Go to bed at your regular time. Following your usual routines can be relaxing and can contribute to a feeling of control.

Manage Your Study Habits Before the Test

Do not stay up late studying the night before a big test. Squeezing in last-minute studying may increase anxiety and contribute to feelings of powerlessness and helplessness. DO NOT CRAM. If you have implemented a study routine in preparation for the test, then you should have confidence in what you have learned. Establish control by saying to yourself, "I have studied hard for this test, and I am well prepared. I can relax tonight because I know the material for the test tomorrow, and I will do well." Avoid giving in to the desire to cram. Instead, use the various techniques discussed earlier in this chapter to maintain a positive mental attitude.

Manage Your Travel the Day of the Test

Plan to arrive early the day of the test. It is important to plan for potential events that could delay you, such as traffic jams or a flat tire. The more important the test is, the more time you should schedule for travel. If you live a substantial distance from the testing site, you might ask another student who lives closer to allow you to sleep over the night before the test. The midterm or final examination for a course may be held in a different location than the regularly scheduled classroom used for the lectures. If you are unfamiliar with the examination room, make a practice run to locate where it is, and note how long it takes to get there. Nothing produces more anxiety than rushing to a test or arriving after the start of a test. A feeling of control reduces tension and the fear response. You can be in control if you manage your travel time with time to spare.

Manage the Supplies You Need for the Test

The more variables you have control over, the more calm and relaxed you will feel. Compose a list of items to bring with you to the test. Sometimes the supplies that can be used are stipulated by the institution giving the test. They may include pencils, pens, scrap paper, erasers, a ruler, a watch, and even a lucky charm. It is suggested that you collect the items the day before the test. This eliminates last-minute rushing to gather needed supplies on the day of the test and contributes to your sense of control. Some testing sites do not permit the presence of any personal items. These sites include venues for nurse licensure examinations.

Manage Your Personal Comfort

Maslow's hierarchy of needs specifies that basic physiological needs must be met before you attempt to meet higher-level needs. Be aware of your basic needs relating to factors such as nutrition, elimination, and physical comfort. Meet these basic needs before the test because unfulfilled needs will compete for your attention. For example, arrive early so that you can visit the restroom; wear layers of clothing so you can adjust to various environmental temperatures; and eat a light, balanced meal to maintain your blood glucose level. Once these basic needs are met, then you can progress up the ladder of needs to self-actualization.

Manage the Test Environment

When you arrive early, you generally have a choice of where to sit in the room. This contributes to a feeling of control because you are able to sit where you are most comfortable. You may prefer to sit by a window, near a heat source, or in the back of the room. Generally, it helps to sit near the administrator of the test. Directions may be heard more clearly, and the administrator's attention may be gained more easily if you have a question. It is wise to avoid sitting by a door. The commotion made by people entering or exiting the room can be a distraction and can interfere with your ability to concentrate. Take every opportunity to control your environment. Measures that help you feel in control contribute to a positive mental attitude.

Maintain a Positive Mental Attitude

Remind yourself of how hard you have worked and how well prepared you are to take this test. ESTABLISH CONTROL by arresting negative thoughts and focusing on the positive. Say to yourself, "I am ready for this test! I will do well on this test! I can get an 'A' on this test!" These statements support a positive mental attitude and enhance a feeling of control.

Manage Your Physical and Emotional Responses

At critical times during the test, you may feel nervous, your breathing may become rapid and shallow, or you may draw a blank on a question. Stop and take a mini-break. Use controlled breathing to induce the relaxation response. You may also use a shortened version of progressive relaxation exercises to induce the relaxation response. Daily practice of breathing and relaxation exercises will enable you to induce the relaxation response quickly during times of stress. After these techniques are implemented, you should feel in control and empowered.

SUMMARY

The techniques described in this chapter are designed to increase your mastery over the stress of the testing situation. When you feel positive about yourself and have a strong self-image and a feeling of self-worth, you will develop a sense of control. When you are able to draw on various techniques that empower you to respond to the testing situation with a sense of calm, you will improve your effectiveness. Use these techniques along with the other skills suggested in this book, practice the questions, and take the comprehensive final book exam as instructed in the section "How to Use This Book to Maximize Success" at the beginning of this text. These activities will support a positive mental attitude, provide you with a feeling of control, and increase your effectiveness in the testing situation.

2 Critical Thinking, Clinical Judgment, and the Next Generation NCLEX®

If your ultimate goal is to become a competent nurse, you have to first identify what knowledge base and skills are required to achieve this goal. Study skills, critical thinking skills, and problem-solving skills are essential in achieving success as a learner. Your immediate objective should be to develop skills that support your ability to use reasoning and not just react by rote (a fixed, routine, mechanical way of doing something). Several chapters in this book are designed to assist you in the journey toward this goal. General and specific study skills are addressed in Chapter 4; the nursing process as a problem-solving process is addressed in Chapter 6; and critical thinking skills are addressed in this chapter.

No one can argue with the statement that a nurse must be a safe, qualified, and technically proficient practitioner. Consumers of nursing care are most aware of the actions (psychomotor skills) that nurses engage in and generally rate the quality of nursing care according to how well their expectations have been met. However, the quality of nursing care is based on more than just what the nurse does. It also is based on how the nurse thinks (cognitive skills) in relation to how conclusions are drawn, decisions are made, and problems are resolved.

Thinking is the hardest work there is, which is the probable reason why so few engage in it.

—Henry Ford

Thinking skills that are rarely recognized by the consumer, such as reflecting, clarifying, analyzing, and reasoning, are crucial to the development of a competent nurse. Historically, critical thinking in nursing was associated with just the nursing process (assessment, analysis, planning, implementation, and evaluation). This theoretical framework, which is used to identify and attain solutions to complex problems, is the foundation for nursing education, practice, and research. It is a systematic, orderly, step-by-step progression with a beginning and an end (a linear format). Clinical decision making in relation to the nursing process produces a plan of care or "product." In Chapter 6, the steps in the nursing process are addressed, and many sample test questions are provided that demonstrate application of information within the context of the nursing process. Nursing entails more than just solving problems. The concept of critical thinking as a "process" has been receiving increasing attention in nursing because of the complexity of medical treatments, advanced technology, and reengineering of the health-care workforce. Various researchers believe that critical thinking in nursing is more than just a behavioral, task-oriented, linear approach demonstrated in problem solving and that critical thinking should be based on an emancipatory model. Emancipatory models embrace the concept of empowerment and autonomous action stemming from critical insights. These models stress critical thinking as a process rather than just a method of producing a product or solution.

DEFINITION OF CRITICAL THINKING

Leaders in the field of nursing do not agree on any one definition of critical thinking. However, the following excerpts may enhance your understanding of the concept. Chaffee (2018) explains that "the process of thinking critically involves thinking for ourselves by carefully examining the way that we make sense of the world." He further explained that as humans we have an ability to reflect back on what we are thinking, doing, or feeling; this reflection makes us more effective thinkers.

In contrast, Alfaro-LeFevre (2009) stated that critical thinking:

- Entails purposeful, goal-directed thinking.
- Aims to base clinical judgments on evidence (facts) rather than conjecture (guesswork).
- Is based on principles of science and the scientific method.
- Requires strategies that maximize *human potential* and compensate for problems caused by *human nature*. Alfaro-LeFevre (2017) further indicated that the word *reasoning* could be used as a synonym for critical thinking because it implies careful, deliberate thought.

The Delphi Research Project characterized the ideal critical thinker as one who is habitually inquisitive, well informed, trustful of reason, open-minded in evaluation, honest in facing personal biases, prudent in making judgments, willing to reconsider, clear about issues, orderly in complex matters, diligent in seeking relevant information, reasonable in the selection of criteria, focused in inquiry, and persistent in seeking results that are as precise as the subject and the circumstances of inquiry permit (American Philosophical Association, 1990).

Brookfield (1991) described four components of critical thinking: identifying and challenging assumptions, becoming aware of the importance of context in creating meaning, imagining and exploring alternatives, and cultivating a reflective skepticism.

Pless and Clayton (1993) identified these cognitive skills and subskills as essential for critical thinking:

- Interpretation—categorizing, decoding significance, and clarifying meaning.
- Analysis—examining ideas, identifying arguments, and analyzing arguments.
- Evaluation—assessing claims and assessing arguments.
- Inference—querying evidence, conjecturing alternatives, and drawing conclusions.
- Explanation—stating results, justifying procedures, and presenting arguments.
- Self-regulation—self-examination and self-correction.

CRITICAL THINKING IN NURSING

Nursing requires not only the learning of facts and procedures but also the ability to evaluate each unique client situation. In Chapter 4, "Study Techniques," a section titled "Specific Study Techniques Related to Cognitive Levels of Nursing Questions" addresses the variety of thinking processes—knowledge, comprehension, application, and analysis—that the nurse uses when managing data and identifying and meeting a client's needs.

Because these thinking processes are important to both the process and the product inherent in nursing care, Chapter 4 presents multiple-choice questions that are designed to test your knowledge base, comprehension of information, application of theory and principles, and analytical ability. In all but knowledge-type questions, intellectual skills that involve more than just the recall of information are required. In comprehension-type questions, you are required to translate, interpret, and determine the implications, consequences, and corollaries of the effects of information. In application-type questions, you are required to use information in a new situation. In analysis-type questions, you must interpret a variety of data and recognize the commonalities, differences, and interrelationships among the ideas presented. Numerous sample items in Chapter 4 also challenge your analytical abilities, address the cognitive domains, and demonstrate the concepts being presented. Beginning in 2023, the licensing examination for registered nurses will include questions that allow the nurse to demonstrate clinical judgment. This will be in addition to the current, traditional question formats. The new format, called "Next Generation NCLEX" (NGN), uses a case study and six questions that build on each other to assess the test taker's clinical judgment (https://www.ncsbn.org/ngn-resources.htm). Samples of these questions are given in Chapter 8.

An understanding of the nursing process and the cognitive domains is important; however, critical thinking and clinical judgment skills must be developed if you are going to be a successful thinker and, ultimately, an expert nurse. The first step is to build a foundation of knowledge and information that eventually can be applied in clinical situations.

Both minds and fountain pens will work when filled. But minds, like fountain pens, must first be filled.

—Arthur Guiterman

Before you can apply knowledge, you need to know what needs to be known and how that knowledge can be applied. Therefore, you must ask yourself serious questions, such as "What do I know?" "What do I need to know?" "What do I have to do to know it?" "What do I already know that links to this information?" This is a new activity for some students. It can be threatening and even anxiety producing. It is not easy to acknowledge the degree of your own lack of knowledge or ignorance, and it can be a sobering experience.

The more I know I know, I know the less.

—John Owen

Therefore, to fill voids in your knowledge, you need to study. Avoid the pitfall of being a superficial thinker. This type of thinker devotes excessive time to memorization and rote learning. Become a deep thinker.

Many brings the rake, but few the shovel.

—Scottish Proverb

A deep thinker develops a thorough understanding of the material studied. In Chapter 4, "Study Techniques," strategies are discussed that will help you study more effectively and efficiently and answer some of the Sample Items included in this chapter.

After you know basic information, you are better able to recognize the significance of cue data. Nursing questions are carefully designed to test your knowledge and comprehension of information regarding key concepts and your ability to analyze and apply this information in various situations. As you move from being a neophyte to a more experienced student, you will be better able to identify the significance of cues and respond readily in all situations, whether in a laboratory setting, in a computer simulation, in a clinical setting, or in a testing environment. As an experienced student, you will be able to recognize the key words and concepts being tested with nursing questions. This requires that you ask, "What is happening?" and "What should I do?" In addition, clinical judgment requires that you ask, "What is most important to do, what should I *not* do, and what should I do first?" Before you can answer these questions, however, it is helpful to identify the information processing style you use when confronted with a situation that requires a response.

Left-Hemisphere and Right-Hemisphere Brain Information Processing

Taggart and Torrance (1984) explored left- and right-hemisphere information processing and found that individuals who used **left-hemisphere information processing functions** used rational problem-solving strategies and logical sequencing. Rational learners broke down situations into components and looked for universal rules and approaches that could be applied in all situations. Individuals who used **right-hemisphere information processing functions** looked for main ideas to establish relationships that could be abstracted as the foundation for intuitive problem solving. The intuitive learner first learned from context and experience and then applied and analyzed principles. Additional research in this area has demonstrated that although both the novice and the expert use logical and rational problem-solving strategies, the expert used a broad range of thinking skills that integrated both logical and intuitive thinking to address facts and feelings and achieve accurate decision making.

Clinical Judgments

Clinical judgments are conclusions or enlightened opinions arrived at via reasoning or critical thinking. The ability to build a foundation of data, inferences, and hypotheses for nursing decision making is based on the use of several types of clinical judgments. **Perceptual judgments** are judgments you make regarding the data you need to collect and validation of the importance of the data you have collected within the context of the situation. **Inferential judgments** are judgments you make when you determine which data are significant, eliminate data that are insignificant, and identify the relationships that exist among the data collected. **Diagnostic judgments** are judgments that you make when you link clusters of data with patterns affiliated with a specific hypothesis or conclusion.

The National Council of State Boards of Nursing (NCSBN), which develops the National Council Licensure Examination (NCLEX) examination, has found that 65% of nursing errors are the result of errors in clinical judgment, and 50% of those involve novice nurses (https://www.ncsbn.org/ngn-resources.htm). The NCSBN's research showed that although knowledge is certainly necessary, a nurse who earned the highest scores on knowledge tests didn't always provide the safest care. Often, the clinical judgment piece was missing (Muntean et al, 2016).

The NCSBN developed and rigorously tested the NCSBN Clinical Judgment Measurement Model (NCJMM) to measure clinical judgment. The NCJMM format is given primarily in a case study format, with six questions related to the same case study that reveal the six steps of clinical judgment.

1. Recognize cues—what matters most?
2. Analyze cues—what could it mean?
3. Prioritize hypotheses—where do I start?
4. Generate solutions—what can I do?
5. Take action—what will I do?
6. Evaluate outcomes—did it help?

Step number five is where the results of the nurse's clinical judgment are revealed, when the nurse takes action.

Levels of Critical Thinking

As your knowledge of theory and your experience increase, you will be constructing a scientific foundation to support critical thinking and clinical decision making. When developing critical thinking skills, you will advance through three levels of competence: basic, complex, and expert. As a student, you are a basic-level critical thinker. As a **basic-level critical thinker,** you are building a novice's database of information and experiential knowledge. When you are confronted with a situation, initially your response is based on recall and rote memory. You tend to guide your responses by rules and procedures and seek concrete actions. You reduce situations to their distinct and independent parts. For example, when applying a simple dry, sterile dressing for an abdominal wound with approximated edges (healing by primary intention), you may use a procedure book and follow each step as outlined.

As you acquire more knowledge and experience, you advance from a basic-level thinker to a complex-level thinker. As a **complex-level thinker,** you are guided by the need to explore options based on principles and patterns and an understanding of commonalities and differences. You will begin to identify cue data, analyze clustered information, sort and choose the most appropriate action, and evaluate the client's response. For example, when performing a sterile dressing for an open wound with no readily approximated edges (healing by secondary intention), you may need to modify the procedure. Depending on the situation, you may reposition the client, use additional sterile equipment, or irrigate the wound. The more knowledge and experience you gain, the more solid the connections between your knowledge base and the application of that knowledge will become. You are now becoming an expert critical thinker.

As an **expert critical thinker,** you develop reasoning based on models, patterns, and standards associated with the "uniqueness" and "wholeness" of each situation. For example, when you perform a sterile dressing on a large, gaping wound that is purposely being left open (healing by tertiary intention), critical thinking will require a higher level of sophistication. You will need to consider concepts such as dehiscence, evisceration, fistula formation, sinus tracking, undermining, presence of infection, necrosis, factors that impair or facilitate wound healing, and dressing alternatives. The expert views the situation from an entire perspective that can be accomplished only with a broad and deep knowledge base and experience.

All critical thinkers should begin by asking "What is wrong?" These are the cues, step 1 in the clinical judgment process described earlier. Ask, "What's not normal?" Then ask, "Why?" Analyze the cues (step 2) and determine a list of ideas (hypotheses) of what is likely going on. Next, determine "How should I proceed?" This is step 3, when you prioritize the hypotheses by the most serious one first, to determine where you should start helping. Having identified the issue, consider "What can I do?" (Step 4). This may include asking "What should I NOT do?" Take action (step 5), and then evaluate the outcomes (step 6). If things have not improved, or are worsening, go back to the start of the process and ask, "What else is going on?" "What did I miss?" and even "So what!" "What could happen?"

These questions should be asked when studying, when faced with a clinical situation (whether simulated or real), and when challenged by a test question. However, at each successive level of critical thinking, the degree of sophistication required to explore these questions increases. As a beginning nursing student, you are a novice, not an expert! Nursing school is several years long for a purpose. Be realistic with your self-expectations. It takes time to acquire and integrate the knowledge and experience necessary to be an expert critical thinker. Your license will be a "license to learn"—you won't be expected to know everything and be an expert simply because you are licensed.

PRACTICE CRITICAL THINKING

You first learned how to turn over, crawl, stand, walk, and then run by practicing balance and building strength and endurance. You must also learn and practice critical thinking and problem-solving skills until you are proficient in using them and can respond accurately and achieve your goal of being an expert critical thinker. For you to be able to tap these critical thinking skills when taking an examination, they must be well entrenched in your approach to all professional endeavors. Critical thinking is the process of stacking information together into a reasonable whole, noting where the pieces do not fit. Keep asking, "Where does that conclusion or hypothesis not make sense?"

Strategies to Employ in Critical Thinking

When challenged by any client situation, you should employ these strategies:

- Identify assumptions.
- Use a method to collect and organize information.
- Validate the accuracy and reliability of collected information.
- Determine the significance of collected information.
- Determine inconsistencies in collected information.
- Identify commonalities and differences.
- Identify patterns of client responses.

- Identify stressors and common responses to stressors.
- Identify discrepancies or gaps in information.
- Cluster information to determine relationships.
- Make inferences based on collected information.
- Identify actual problems and clients who may be at risk for problems.
- Establish priorities (Maslow's hierarchy of needs is an excellent model to use to achieve this goal).
- Formulate specific, client-centered, realistic, measurable goals with time frames.
- Identify appropriate nursing actions.
- Evaluate outcomes.
- Evaluate and modify critical thinking activities.

This list of strategies reflects sophisticated, deep thinking. Critical thinking is a type of highly developed thinking that links information. It must be learned. The learner must be actively involved in the learning process. Critical thinking cannot be memorized; it must be practiced.

Knowledge is a treasure, but practice is the key to it.

—Thomas Fuller

Specific Activities to Improve Critical Thinking

To develop or refine your thinking, try engaging in the activities that follow while incorporating the strategies listed in the previous section.

Thinking Aloud

The proficient thinker expresses thought processes and rationales. Expressing thoughts in words helps to clarify and solidify thinking. You can think aloud while you are engaged in an activity that does not involve a client or later when you review your performance. Likewise, clinical post-conferences and individual mentoring experiences in which information is exchanged promote critical thinking.

Review of Client Scenarios

When performed in a group, chart reviews, grand rounds, and case study approaches provide interdisciplinary exchanges, a variety of different thinking perspectives, and opportunities to learn from role models. These approaches require verbal exchange that includes reasoning, interpreting, identifying evidence, deducing, and concluding. In these situations, you can examine your viewpoint in relation to the viewpoints of others. This exchange promotes learning and stimulates critical thinking.

Written Assignments

Written assignments are not just "busy work." Journal writing is an activity that requires you to log and respond to important and meaningful situations. Faculty review of your journal (with comments) and your own periodic study and review of it will enable you to identify your progress and growth, and point out where your conclusions might not make sense. Journal writing involves you in the process of learning. It encourages you to use abstract thinking and to conceptualize, elaborate, generalize, and interpret, all of which promote critical thinking. A term paper is a written assignment that involves you not only in the process of writing but also in the development of a product. When this product is reviewed by the instructor, conclusions can be drawn regarding your command of the information and your ability to convey your knowledge to others. Written assignments require organizing, prioritizing, integrating, persuading, proving, and summarizing, all of which require *critical thinking*.

COMPUTER-ASSISTED LEARNING

Computers provide an environment that enhances and challenges critical thinking skills. Software offers a variety of critical thinking programs, from a simple lesson presenting content using an interactive linear approach to a program that challenges the learner to seek solutions to complex problems following a branching design. Computers allow for thinking and learning in a nonthreatening and safe environment. Refer to Chapter 9, "Computer Applications in Education and Evaluation," for more details regarding the valuable use of computers to increase learning.

VIDEOTAPING

Videotaping can be used to record role-playing scenarios or the performance of a skill. Videotaping allows you to engage in an activity and then review your performance. During this review, you as well as others can examine, analyze, rationalize, justify, and correct your performance, a process that can support critical thinking.

CLINICAL PROCESS RECORDS

A clinical process record is a focused writing assignment that, similar to a case study, centers on a simulated or specific client experience. It requires you to use the problem-solving process, examine the scientific reasons for health-care interventions, assess outcomes, and evaluate and modify a plan of care, all of which contribute to critical thinking.

EXAMINATIONS

Examinations should be approached as learning opportunities. Small groups of four or five students should review and discuss each question in practice and actual examinations. Group members help one another to identify the key concepts being tested and how to best answer the questions "What is happening?" and "What should I do?" When reviewing examination questions, be willing to listen to other people's interpretation of them. If all of your energy is spent defending your response, then your mind is not open to different perspectives, and this limits your learning. Reviewing examinations requires you to integrate information, apply theory and principles, analyze content, compare and contrast information, and rationalize your response, all of which contribute to critical thinking.

APPLY CRITICAL THINKING TO MULTIPLE-CHOICE QUESTIONS

Case (1994) explored the concept of critical thinking as a journey, not a destination. Case stated, "We cannot stand in the same river twice, because water rushes away as new water takes its place and the rushing water changes the river bed. The decisions we make today may not fit circumstances that change tomorrow." This concept applies to clinical situations as well as nursing test questions. Just as no clinical situation will be exactly like a previous experience, no test question will be exactly like a previous question. Altering a single factor in a situation can change the entire landscape of that situation. One different word in a question can change what the question is asking. Practicing critical thinking when answering questions will improve your ability to think critically and be more successful when taking a test.

Identify the Key Concept Being Tested

Each question scenario is different and requires you to identify the key concept being tested and to answer the questions "What is happening?" and "What should I do?" Reframe, critique, and evaluate the stem of each question. Then, try to construct the correct answer before looking at the options. When assessing the options in a multiple-choice question, manipulate the information by using cognitive activities such as organizing, correlating, differentiating, reasoning, and evaluating against standards of practice, criteria, and critical elements. Review Sample Item 2-1.

SAMPLE ITEM 2-1

A client is transferred from the operating room to the postanesthesia care unit. The client has a urinary retention (Foley) catheter, an IV line, and an oral airway and is unresponsive. Which nursing assessment should be made first?

1. Check the surgical dressing to ensure that it is intact.
2. Confirm the placement of the oral airway.
3. Observe the Foley catheter for drainage.
4. Examine the IV site for infiltration.

First, you need to identify the key concept being tested in the question. The key concept in this question is **priority care for the unresponsive postoperative client.** Second, identify the key words in the question that address "What is happening?" These are: **client is transferred from the operating room to the postanesthesia care unit, oral airway,** and **unresponsive.** Third, identify the key words in the question that address "What should I do?" These are: **assessment** and **should be made first.** The question being asked is **What assessment takes priority when caring for an unresponsive postoperative client with an oral airway?** Although the IV line, the retention catheter, and the surgical dressing are important and must be assessed, ensuring the correct placement of the oral airway takes priority.

To answer this question, you must know the normal anatomy and physiology associated with the respiratory system and the body's essential need for a continuous exchange of oxygen and carbon dioxide; that a patent airway is essential to the exchange of oxygen and carbon dioxide; the ABCs of life support, which refer to Airway, Breathing, and Circulation, and that maintaining an airway takes priority; that a common response to anesthesia is lack of a gag reflex; and that a correctly placed oral airway will help maintain an open airway.

Another critical thinking technique to use when answering multiple-choice questions is exploring the consequences of each nursing action presented in the alternatives. You can ask many different questions: "Is the action safe or unsafe?" "Is the statement true or false?" "Is it fact or an inference?"

Avoid Reading Into the Question

Highly discriminating questions are questions that are answered correctly by the test taker who scored in the top percent of the class versus the test taker who answered the question incorrectly and scored in the bottom percent of the class on the same examination. The student who correctly answers a highly discriminating question is generally responding to subtle cues using more highly developed critical thinking skills. However, students who come to the testing situation with an in-depth perspective sometimes will "read into" the meaning of the question because of the "context" they bring to it. It is often frustrating for students who are sophisticated, deep thinkers to accept lost points on an examination because they "read into" the question.

You should ask yourself the following questions when analyzing test items you answered incorrectly. "Did I add information to the stem?" "Did I have difficulty deciding among the options presented because I would have done something completely different?" "Did I delete an option because my experience was different from the client situation presented?" "Did I view the question at a more sophisticated level of curricular content than that being tested?" "Did I view the client scenario in more depth and breadth than was necessary?"

Multiple-choice items provide all the information necessary to answer the questions. Your job is to use critical thinking to answer the question, not rewrite it. For additional information, see Chapter 10, "Analyze Your Test Performance."

Study the Rationales for the Right and Wrong Answers

Every nursing action is based on a standard of practice that has a scientific foundation. When practicing test taking, identify in your own words the reason why the option you chose is correct and why the options you consider incorrect are wrong. Now compare your rationales with the rationales presented. When you answer a question correctly, review the rationales several times to reinforce your knowledge. When you answer a question incorrectly, identify your faulty thinking by comparing your rationale with the presented rationale. When you identify content that you did not know or cannot apply, review this content in your nursing textbook. An excellent study technique associated with principles is to identify other situations in which the same principle applies and situations in which it is different. See Chapter 10, "Analyze Your Test Performance," to design a corrective action plan.

Change the Focus of the Question

A great way to explore additional situations using multiple-choice questions is to change one of the key facts in the stem of a question to alter its focus (see Sample Items 2-2 and 2-3). Also, when a question requires you to set a priority, you can eliminate the option that is the correct answer (see Sample Items 2-4 and 2-5). This requires you to identify the next best option that answers the question. When the context of the question is altered even slightly, the contour or territory around it changes, and that may significantly rearrange the internal structure of the entire question. When a question is altered, the meaning of the situation may require a distinctly different nursing assessment or action.

SAMPLE ITEM 2-2

Which is a priority physiological need of a client with a colostomy?

1. Disturbance in body image
2. Inadequate nutrition
3. Lack of knowledge
4. Skin breakdown

The correct answer is option 4. The word *physiological* modifies the word need and is a clue in the stem. For study purposes, you can change the focus of this question by changing the word *physiological* in the stem to *psychological*. Now answer this question from this new perspective.

SAMPLE ITEM 2-3

Which is associated with a psychological need of a client with a colostomy?

1. Disturbance in body image
2. Inadequate nutrition
3. Lack of knowledge
4. Skin breakdown

The correct answer is option 1. The entire focus of this question has changed. The focus has moved from "physiological" to "psychological." Now the clue in the stem is the word *psychological*. By using this technique, you can apply critical thinking to multiple-choice questions and maximize opportunities for learning. This is an effective strategy either when working alone or when working with a study group.

SAMPLE ITEM 2-4

A preoperative client talks about being afraid of pain because of a previous experience with painful surgery. What should the nurse do *first* to help the client cope with this fear?

1. Encourage the client to not be afraid
2. Teach the client relaxation techniques
3. Listen to the client's concerns about pain
4. Inform the client that medication is available

The correct answer is option 3. The word *first* is asking you to set a priority. For study purposes, you can change the focus of the question by eliminating the correct answer as a choice and then attempting to answer the question with the remaining three options. Now answer the question from this new perspective.

Sample Item 2-5 is the same item as Sample Item 2-4 with the correct answer (option 3) removed. When this option is removed, the context of the question is altered, requiring you to select the next best option from among the three remaining options. This strategy can be used when practicing multiple-choice items that ask you to identify the option that is the priority.

SAMPLE ITEM 2-5

A preoperative client talks about being afraid of pain because of a previous experience with painful surgery. What should the nurse do *first* to help the client cope with this fear?

1. Encourage the client to not be afraid
2. Teach the client relaxation techniques
3. Inform the client that medication is available

The correct answer is option 2. The technique of eliminating the correct answer and attempting to select the next best action requires you to rank the options presented in order of importance. This strategy works only with questions that require you to set a priority. Key words such as *initially, first, best, priority,* and *most* should alert you that the question is a priority question. By using this strategy, you increase opportunities to sharpen your critical thinking skills.

Study in a Small Group

When a study group jointly seeks a solution to a highly discriminating question, members build a body of knowledge that increases their perspective and context. This technique is particularly helpful because different people bring different perspectives and thinking styles that enrich the group learning experience. More perspectives produce a variety of views of a problem and generate more approaches to the most accurate response. However, small groups are most effective when limited to three to five people. Larger groups tend to have inherent problems (e.g., some members may not provide input, one member may monopolize the discussion, or the activity may progress to a social gathering rather than a focused work group).

Where all think alike, no one thinks very much.

—Walter Lippmann

SUMMARY

In our informational society, there is no way you can know or experience everything. With the explosion of knowledge and technology and changes in the role of the nurse within a fluid health-care delivery environment, what is learned today may be obsolete tomorrow. Consequently, an integral part of your continuing education consists of the development and refinement of critical thinking skills. To be a critical thinker, you must be intellectually humble, able to listen, dissatisfied with the status quo, creative, flexible, self-confident but aware of your limitations, and willing to change. Take time to cultivate your critical thinking skills because they are the ultimate tool you will bring to client-care situations—*the therapeutic use of self*. When you can think critically, you are empowered to maximize your abilities to meet client needs.

ANSWERS AND RATIONALES FOR SAMPLE ITEMS IN CHAPTER 2

2-1 1. Although checking the surgical dressing is important, it does not involve a life-threatening situation.

2. Confirming the placement of the oral airway ensures a patent air passage. An oral airway displaces the tongue and prevents obstruction of the trachea, thus permitting free passage of air to and from the lungs. Oxygen is essential for life, and this action takes priority.

3. Although observing the Foley catheter for drainage is important, urinary output at this time is less critical than assessing airway, breathing, and circulation.

4. Although examination of the IV site is important, an infiltration can be tolerated for a few minutes while higher-priority assessments are made.

2-2 1. Concern about body image is a psychological, not a physiological, concern.

2. Although inadequate nutrition is a physiological problem, it is not the priority need of a client with a colostomy.

3. A knowledge deficit is a cognitive/perceptual problem, not a physiological problem.

4. Skin breakdown is a common physiological problem associated with the presence of a colostomy because of the digestive enzymes present in feces.

2-3 **1. Concern about body image is a psychological problem often encountered when a person has surgery that alters the body's structure or function.**

2. Nutrition is a physiological, not a psychological, problem.

3. Knowledge deficit is a cognitive/perceptual problem, not a psychological problem.

4. Skin breakdown is a physiological, not a psychological, problem.

2-4 1. Encouraging the client to not be afraid denies his or her fears.

2. Although relaxation techniques may be taught eventually, they are not the priority at this time.

3. Listening to the client's concerns about pain supports his or her need to express fears.

4. Although medication may be available, this is false reassurance and cuts off communication.

2-5 1. Encouraging the client to not be afraid denies his or her fears.

2. Depending on the relaxation technique used, it can reduce muscle tension, distract the person from the stimulus, and/or limit the physiological response to *fight or flight*, thus reducing pain.

3. Although medication may be available, this statement is false reassurance and cuts off communication.

3 Time Management

TIME MANAGEMENT EQUALS SELF-MANAGEMENT

Time is an elusive concept that is reflected in countless wise sayings. Time is of the essence! Where did the time go? It's now or never! Never put off until tomorrow what you can do today! Time flies when you're having fun! Time is money! A stitch in time saves nine! Time is on your side! And finally, the most significant saying: You are the only one who can waste your time!

To achieve your goal of being a nurse, you must progress from being a beginning nursing student (HERE) to graduating and passing a licensing examination (THERE). **The major difference between HERE and THERE is the letter T. This T represents Time Management,** which equals self-management. How you use your time will reflect directly on how successfully you manage the efforts that will ultimately help you attain your goal. The purpose of this chapter is to help you identify personal values and behaviors that relate to time management and learn ways to maximize your productivity through time-management strategies.

TAKE THE TIME TO ASSESS YOUR TIME-MANAGEMENT ABILITIES

Today many people, particularly students, are attempting to function in a society that stresses the concept of "24/7." They are not running out of time—they are running into it! They are like horses on a merry-go-round that is going faster and faster, and they cannot get off. If you can relate to these people, it is time to take the time to think about time management! The first step in developing a time-management program is to know yourself. It is important to identify how you actually spend your time, identify your personal values, and identify your personal barriers to productivity. Take the time to implement the following self-assessment tools:

1. Assessment of Inconsistencies Between Values and Behavior
2. Personal Time/Activity Journal
3. Self-Assessment of Barriers to Productivity

Assessment of Inconsistencies Between Values and Behavior

Values are enduring beliefs or attitudes about the worth of a person, object, idea, or action. A **value system** is an organized set of values that is internalized by a person. **Value clarification** is a complex process in which you identify, examine, and develop your own individual values. It is impossible to attempt this process here. However, a simple method is presented for you to identify inconsistencies (i.e., disagreement) between what you consider important and how you behave in relation to the delegation of your time.

Make a list of areas in your life that you value, and then next to each one identify the total percentage of time (including travel time) you believe you should allocate to it on a daily basis. After you have completed your Personal Time/Activity Journal, compare the amount of time you actually devoted to activities related to these areas with the percentage of time you allocated to them on your list. Evaluate whether your behavior reflects what you stated you believe is important. When your behavior reflects your values (attitudes and beliefs), you are in harmony. When your behavior does not reflect your values, you are in "value imbalance," and eventually you will experience emotional and physical consequences.

Often, when people have a value imbalance, they are reluctant to create change; however, change is necessary to promote harmony intrapersonally (within yourself) and interpersonally (with others). Seeking balance is a challenge. However, the challenge can be manageable because it does not have to be outside your value system, nor does it have to be permanent. Adjustments may be necessary only during an academic semester. A colleague of ours used to say, "You can do anything for 16 weeks!" The following is an example of an assessment tool to identify inconsistencies between values and behavior. Modify the areas in your life that you value accordingly to meet your needs.

ASSESSMENT OF INCONSISTENCIES BETWEEN VALUES AND BEHAVIOR TOOL

Areas in My Life That I Value	Desired Percentage of Time	Actual Percentage of Time
Self-care (eating, sleeping, grooming)		
Work		
Leisure		
Relationships (family, friends)		
School/studying		
Community activities		
Religion/spiritual		

Personal Time/Activity Journal

Financial consultants who advise on money management recommend that, for 1 week, their clients write down every penny they spend. At the end of the week, the information is examined to determine where all the money went. **The big difference between time and money is that money can be saved but time cannot.** How you spend your minutes and hours can make a difference. Therefore, keep track of what you are doing every hour in a journal. At the end of the week, review what you did, and next to each entry identify whether it was something you had to do, wanted to do, or did not need to do. The contents of this personal time/activity journal should be compared with the areas you identified as being important in your life. Activities that are not necessary functions of daily living or are not your priorities in life should be curtailed, delegated, or eliminated.

The following is an example of an activity journal. Modify it to meet your needs.

Personal Time/Activity Journal Tool

Time	Activity	Had to Do	Wanted to Do	Did Not Need to Do
6–7 a.m.				
7–8 a.m.				
8–9 a.m.				
9–10 a.m.				
10–11 a.m.				
11–12 a.m.				
12–1 p.m.				
1–2 p.m.				
2–3 p.m.				
3–4 p.m.				
4–5 p.m.				
5–6 p.m.				
6–7 p.m.				
7–8 p.m.				
8–9 p.m.				
9–10 p.m.				
10–11 p.m.				

Self-Assessment of Barriers to Productivity

Productivity reflects the amount and quality of outcomes that result from labor. Inherent in this definition are two concepts: amount of outcomes and effectiveness of outcomes. These concepts can be related to studying nursing content in a textbook. If you spend 1 hour studying a chapter in a nursing textbook and at the end of the hour you can define all the significant words, you have numerous concrete results from your studying. If you spend 1 hour studying arterial blood gases and at the end of the hour you are able to understand the interrelationship of the components of acid-base balance, you understand a limited concept. However, you have a quality outcome because this topic is complex. Your effort has been constructive and valuable!

Many internal and external factors can affect your productivity. However, they are not as overwhelming as you may think because most people are creatures of habit, and there is a pattern to their behavioral responses and performance. With a little honesty and soul searching, you should be able to identify some barriers to your productivity by using the Self-Assessment of Barriers to Productivity tool that follows. Read each self-assessment statement in relation to yourself, and check either the Yes or No column. After you have completed the self-assessment tool, compare your results with the Corrective Action Plan to Maximize Your Productivity.

SELF-ASSESSMENT OF BARRIERS TO PRODUCTIVITY TOOL

Self-Assessment Statement	Yes	No
1. I tend to procrastinate.		
2. I expect little help from members of my family.		
3. I lack organization.		
4. I flutter from one task to another.		
5. I tend to be obsessive/compulsive.		
6. I tend to socialize when I should be studying.		
7. I fall behind in my responsibilities.		
8. I have difficulty delegating tasks.		
9. I tend to feel overwhelmed.		
10. I have too many conflicting deadlines.		
11. I set high standards for myself.		
12. I attempt to do too much.		

You have just completed the Self-Assessment of Barriers to Productivity tool. Now look at how you answered each question in the tool. Match each number with a "Yes" answer to its corresponding number in the Corrective Action Plan to Maximize Your Productivity tool. If your response to one or more of the related questions is a "Yes," review the strategies related to the factors that may be interfering with or limiting your productivity.

Corrective Action Plan to Maximize Your Productivity

Question Number*	Self-Assessment Statement	Corrective Action Plan
1	I tend to procrastinate.	Overcome Procrastination, page 34
2	I expect little help from members of my family.	Delegate, page 33
8	I have difficulty delegating tasks.	
11	I set high standards for myself.	
3	I lack organization.	Get Organized, page 27
9	I tend to feel overwhelmed.	
4	I flutter from one task to another.	Identify Goals, page 25
5	I tend to be obsessive/compulsive.	Achieve a Personal Balance, page 32
6	I tend to socialize when I should be studying.	Develop Self-Discipline, page 28
7	I fall behind in my responsibilities.	
10	I have too many conflicting. deadlines.	Set Priorities, page 26
12	I attempt to do too much.	

*From Self-Assessment of Barriers to Productivity at the top of this page.

Maximize Your Productivity

Now that you have given some thought to what is important to you, how you spend your time, and your barriers to productivity, you must devise a proactive plan to achieve your goals. To maximize productivity and achieve your goals, you need to manage your attitudes and behaviors so your time is used constructively.

Identify Goals

A goal is an object or aim you want to attain. Goals can be long term, intermediate, or short term.

Long-term goals are related to lifelong journeys that frequently include career aspirations or ambitions. Long-term goals generally address desired outcomes 5 or more years in the future. Two examples of long-term goals are "I will earn a bachelor's degree in nursing by the time my children enter high school" and "I will be a nurse manager in an acute-care setting within 10 years after graduation from nursing school."

Intermediate goals are related to aims you want to achieve within 1 to 5 years. Appropriately set intermediate goals are the keys to successfully reaching long-term goals. Two examples of intermediate goals are "I will complete my science prerequisites for the nursing program within 2 years" and "I will attend all of my child's soccer games this year."

Short-term goals address desired results that take hours, days, weeks, or months to attain. Some people consider them objectives that must be met to reach intermediate and long-term goals. When short-term goals reflect immediate outcomes, they may end up being just a "to-do" list. Examples of short-term goals are "I will earn a minimum grade of B in my Fundamentals of Nursing course this semester" and "I will read two chapters in my textbook this weekend."

When setting goals, remember that they must contain certain elements to be effective. They must be specific, measurable, and realistic and must have a time frame. A goal that is **specific** identifies precisely what is to be attained. A goal that is **measurable** sets a minimum satisfactory level of performance. A goal that is realistic has a reasonable chance of being attained. A goal with a **time frame** states the length of time it will take to attain it. Compare these criteria with the goals just stated and with each goal that you write in the future. Work tends to expand in length when there are no guidelines for its performance. Goals are a major way to prevent wasting time in this manner because you know your destination before you begin and you have a time frame in which to get there. There is an old saying that goes something like this: *"If you want to get something done, give it to the busiest person you know."* Effective, busy people understand the need to set specific, measurable, realistic goals that can be achieved within a specific time frame.

Most students understand the importance of goals but do not understand how to set them because of the complexity of their lives. One way to begin goal setting is to identify your roles in life. How you identify your roles depends on your frame of reference. For example, you may decide you want to look at your roles in relation to how you relate to people (individual, spouse, parent, friend, coworker), or you may decide you want to look at your roles in relation to what you do (housekeeper, cook, family support person, nurse's aide, Girl Scout leader, Sunday School teacher). After you have defined your roles, identify one or more goals that you want to achieve in each role. They can be short-term, intermediate, or long-term goals, depending on what is important to you. When setting goals, ensure that you take into account the various areas in your life that you considered important when you completed the Assessment of Inconsistencies Between Values and Behavior tool. Your goals should be in harmony with your values (attitudes and beliefs).

Involve your family members when writing a goal. They will have a vested interest in you attaining your goal when they understand the rationales for it. For example, when you earn your license as a registered nurse, you can quit your second job, earn more money for vacations, or work the night shift, all of which will allow you to spend more time with them. These are the rewards for attaining your goal. Family-centered goals should be like a pebble dropped in a lake—the ripples of pleasurable rewards should affect all members of the family. Put your goals in writing. It makes them more tangible, and you can review them routinely to remain focused. Share your goals with everyone who will listen. A goal that exists only in your mind is a dream or fantasy and is less likely to become reality. Telling people your goals can be motivating because you create additional emphasis on the need to perform. When you attain goals, reward yourself and family members when appropriate. This will motivate you to recognize the significant others in your life who are helping you to attain your goals.

Goals should be revisited. In our fast-paced society, our roles, responsibilities, and relationships change over time. You must be flexible enough to revise, eliminate, or reset a goal, depending on the factors that change in your life. For example, after taking 12 college credits in one academic semester while working full-time, you realize that you are overwhelmed. You may revise your goal of attaining a bachelor's degree in nursing by prolonging the time frame in which to attain it. If you have twins while in school, you may decide that taking one course a semester is more realistic than taking three courses a semester. Revising your goals is not a sign of failure, but rather a mature recognition of reasonable expectations that require you to reset your goals accordingly.

Set Priorities

After students identify their goals, they often ask, "Now what?" Well, now is the time to set priorities! **Setting priorities** is the process of identifying the preferential order of doing things. In other words, what requires your attention first? It is helpful to have criteria for classifying activities so you can prioritize with less difficulty. For example, you can classify things to do into four categories:

1. **Pressing/Important Tasks**—Tasks that are pressing and important relate to activities you consider vital or valuable and that require your immediate attention. Important activities relate to your values and your stated goals. Pressing activities relate to tasks that have to be accomplished in the short term, such as hours or days. These activities must be tackled first. Examples are reviewing class notes for an examination the next day, taking care of a sick child, and finishing a written assignment that has to be submitted tomorrow. We all have urgent or unexpected activities that must be addressed, but this should not become a standard method of functioning. If you put most of your activities in this category, you are in a crisis management mode because you are dealing with emergencies, problems, or last-minute deadlines. When you constantly function in this mode, you will be anxious, overworked, overwhelmed, and speeding toward burnout.
2. **Not Pressing/Important Tasks**—Tasks that are not pressing but are important also relate to activities that you consider vital and valuable. However, they do not have to be completed for several days or weeks. Although you have the luxury of time, you must be self-directed and proactive and take the initiative to complete them. Most activities in your life, including academically related tasks such as reading a textbook for an examination in 2 weeks, can be placed in this category. Other examples are paying monthly bills and playing with your children. If you put most of your activities in this category, you are probably self-directed and are effectively managing your time. However, if you delay or ignore activities in this category, the pressure to accomplish the task increases until it must be reclassified into the pressing/important category. In this category, paying attention to details is like doing preventive maintenance on a car. Tasks get accomplished before the situation breaks down and becomes a crisis. When you function in this category, you are in control and anxiety is kept to a minimum.
3. **Pressing/Not Important Tasks**—Tasks that are pressing but are not important compete for your immediate attention, but they relate to activities you do not consider vital or important. Examples are listening to a telephone call from a telemarketer, watching a specific program on television, and doing something that someone else thinks you should do. When setting priorities, you should limit activities in the pressing/not important category because they are categorized as such—not important. If most of your activities are in this category, reacting and responding are your modes of action rather than being proactive. You are responding to urgent stimuli; however, more often

than not the urgency and importance of the activity are based on the expectations of others. You are meeting other people's needs, not your own.

4. **Not Pressing/Not Important Tasks**—Tasks that are not urgent and not important are small, minor, insignificant activities. They are not competing for your immediate attention, and you do not consider them important. Examples are cleaning the sock drawer, sharpening all the pencils in your desk, and socializing with uninvited visitors. When setting priorities, you should limit or eliminate activities in the not pressing/not important category. Why get involved with tasks that are insignificant and unimportant? Why waste your time? If you put most of your activities into this category, you may be overwhelmed and trying to escape from the urgent problems or activities in the pressing/important category. Escape may be your only way to obtain relief.

The examples provided may not reflect your values. Obviously, you need to identify the activities that are important and pressing to you. When setting priorities, you are the only person who can decide whether something is important. You can make choices that are in harmony with your values and goals. Unfortunately, you may or may not have control over time frames. Emergencies arise that require immediate attention, due dates for school assignments may be indicated weeks in advance, and some deadlines are self-imposed. Some deadlines cannot be altered, but others may be extended without giving up your goals. The ability to set priorities puts you in a position of control because you are the one making the decisions.

Get Organized

When you look at your life, do you feel like a juggler attempting to keep multiple balls aloft while walking on a bed of fire? If so, you are on overload. You may be a mother, daughter, father, son, brother, sister, wife, husband, friend, employee, student, social advocate, and so on. Each role has its related responsibilities and stresses. As a result, you may have *multiple-role overload!* In our world, and especially in nursing, the volume of new information is expanding dramatically. Years ago, a nursing fundamentals textbook was several hundred pages long. Today, a fundamentals textbook is more than a thousand pages long. As a result, you may have *information overload!* Today, corporations are focusing on increasing productivity. Your place of business may be reorganizing to maximize your work effort. As a result, you may have *work overload!* The explosion in technology has produced voice mail, call forwarding, e-mail, text messaging, cell phones, Twitter, and Facebook. You are connected and accessible "24/7." As a result, you may have *access overload!* When overloaded for any length of time, you can spiral toward an overload crisis. You must be organized to regain control of the situation.

Being on overload is a problem, and time management may be the solution. There are many ways to manage time, but a simple, concrete method is the use of calendars. If your goal is to graduate from a nursing program, you should make a master calendar listing the courses you must take each semester to meet the curriculum requirements for graduation. Next, you may need more detailed calendars, such as monthly, weekly, or daily schedules, to provide additional structure. Also, calendars facilitate planning for short- and long-range assignments, provide consistency with a regular schedule, identify priorities, and reduce anxiety.

Monthly calendars help control mental clutter. Make monthly calendars for every month within a semester and insert important personal events (e.g., social engagements, doctor's appointments) and school-related requirements (e.g., first and last days of the semester, examination days, due dates for written assignments or special projects). Also, insert school holidays and vacation periods. These reminders provide a broad overview of your monthly activities. After you insert important events in the calendar, do not use mental energy to keep that information in the forefront of your mind. You just have to check your calendar to verify when an event will take place.

Weekly calendars present an overview of the week and provide consistency concerning your day-to-day schedule. They should be constructed just before beginning a new week. Block in all of your required commitments on your weekly calendar. Include time for activities of daily living (e.g., sleeping, grooming, food preparation, eating, doing laundry), child-related activities, work, scheduled classes, religious services, and so on. Allocate additional time to commitments that require travel.

After all your required tasks are inserted into the calendar, you can decide how to carve up the remaining time. Factors that must be considered include setting consistent times to study each day, scheduling breaks within study periods, ensuring recreational activities, determining the time of day when you are most productive, deciding how much time you need to study, and so on. An old formula states that you should study 1 to 2 hours a week for every hour you are in class. For example, if you are in school 12 hours a week, you should be studying 12 to 24 hours a week outside of class. Although this is often true, it is a generality. Only you can decide from your past and present performance how much time you need for studying or preparing written assignments outside of class to be successful. In addition, when developing a weekly calendar, it is essential to establish consistency in activities from one day to the next; this creates a routine that is familiar, and familiarity reduces anxiety. Also, it reduces the need to expend energy to make decisions. You made the decision once at the beginning of the week to study from 7 to 9 p.m. Monday through Friday. Your job now is to implement the plan without using energy to explore the pros and cons of studying or overcome your own objections to studying. You made a commitment to yourself to study, and you must have the integrity to keep your commitment.

Daily calendars organize your activities so that you can achieve your daily goals efficiently and effectively. In the evening, design the calendar for the next day. This helps to reduce anxiety because you have organized your thoughts, identified your goals, and planned a time to accomplish them. Plan a calendar that is simple. Start by slotting in all the personal and school-related special events for the day that appear on your weekly calendar. Do not include routine tasks such as class time, work, or personal activities (e.g., eating or sleeping). Now make a list of all the academic and nonacademic activities that you want to accomplish. Be as specific as you can. Many people call this a "to-do list." Rank each activity on the list in order of priority, that is, items that must get done first, then those that should get done, and finally those you would like to get done. Plot these activities (particularly the tasks that must get done) around your standard tasks, and coordinate the scheduling of activities to take advantage of blocks of available time that are appropriate for the tasks. Also, combine activities so you can accomplish more than one task at a time. For example, shop at stores that have multiple departments so that school supplies and food for dinner can be bought with one stop; study flash cards while performing a chore; or use a similar topic for assignments in two different courses so that one search of the literature can be used for both assignments. Welcome to "multitasking," a necessity when maintaining a busy schedule!

Although you may have a full schedule, every minute of every day does not have to be accounted for. Tasks may take longer than planned, and unexpected situations may occur. Some tasks—preferably the lower-priority activities—may not be accomplished by the end of the day. If you have tasks left over, you may have to revise your future daily lists with a more realistic attitude, move an uncompleted task to the next day, delegate the task, or eliminate it entirely.

Obviously, everyone's calendar will be different, depending on family-, school-, and work-related commitments. Although individualized, all calendars should be simple, realistic, and flexible. They should not be so complex that they become an additional chore. The course of study to become a nurse is demanding and takes time and energy. Energy can be conserved if time is used efficiently. Many people say they do not have the time to design calendars, but a well-thought-out plan that is followed promotes the efficient use of time, resulting in more available time. **You need to spend time to save time!**

Develop Self-Discipline

When you feel overwhelmed, have you ever said to yourself, "If only there were 25 hours in a day, I would get all my work done." If the truth be told, you probably still would not get your work done if you had 26 hours in a day. The reality is there are only 24 hours in a day and only 168 hours in a week. How you manage yourself in relation to that time is the key to feeling in control rather than feeling overwhelmed.

Start by setting your goals and priorities. If you are to be successful and graduate from nursing school, school must be a priority. If you work full-time or several days a week, manage a home with children, and are involved in community activities, the demands on your time and energy may be excessive. Only you can decide what you are capable of doing. Setting realistic demands on your time and energy is difficult. You may be able to do anything you want, but you may not be able to do everything you want. Rarely in life can you have it all. Therefore, to manage your time and responsibilities efficiently and fairly, you may have to make hard decisions. Reducing work hours, sharing household chores, hiring a babysitter, or limiting your social life may be necessary strategies to help you manage your responsibilities in relation to your schoolwork. You may even decide to delay your goal by taking fewer credits per semester or deciding that this is not the best time to be going to school. Sacrifices in and of themselves should not be viewed negatively. Often, these sacrifices promote growth in you and your family.

After you and your family have set your goals and priorities, you must get their help in establishing your weekly calendar. This calendar should set "firm boundaries" for your future behavior, recognizing that it should be flexible enough to "bend" with emerging or unexpected priorities. With this calendar, you have made a commitment to yourself and others to achieve certain goals within a time frame. In other words, you have made a promise. Now you must keep it! Keeping promises expands your basic habits of personal effectiveness and builds character, but it requires self-discipline.

Self-discipline is orderly conduct in relation to self-imposed constraints. Self-discipline is an internal factor that is influenced only by what you bring to a situation. Self-discipline involves three important abilities: the ability to say "No," the ability to avoid time traps, and the ability to self-motivate.

Saying "No"

No is a small word that can have a big impact on your ability to manage your life. If you are similar to others who enter the helping professions, you usually use the word *Yes* more often than you use the word *No*. You want to help and give of yourself and thus put the needs of others before your own. However, when you are going to school, it is time to make your needs a priority. Learn to say *No*. When asked to do something by someone else, you have to ask yourself questions such as the following:

- Is this consistent with my identified goal/priorities?
- Is this something I have to do?
- Is this something I want to do?
- Is this something I do not need to do?
- Is this person able to do this by himself or herself?
- Is there anyone else who can do this task?
- Why is it important for me to do this task now?

Depending on your responses to these self-directed questions, you can say "Yes" or "No" to the person who is asking you to do something. If you are undecided, buy yourself some time with a response such as "That sounds interesting, but let me think about it overnight, and I will get back to you tomorrow." This response allows you an opportunity to consider how much time the activity will demand and to make a decision that is within your value system. If your answer is "No," it gives you time to construct a response.

The most common consequence of saying "No" is the feeling of guilt. Guilt is a self-imposed feeling that occurs when your conscience indicates that something you have done or not done is unacceptable; only you can make yourself feel guilty. You waste energy when you feel guilty; therefore, use the energy of guilt to prevent guilty feelings. You can cope with guilt in several ways:

- Recognize that you may never eliminate feelings of guilt because you are human. However, you can *limit* feelings of guilt.

- Understand that there is "good guilt" and "bad guilt." **Good guilt** is feeling bad about something you have done or not done according to what you identify as ethically or morally important. Use the energy of good guilt to reestablish your goals, priorities, and calendars (e.g., "I will schedule time in my calendar to spend an hour a day in the evening playing with my children."). **Bad guilt** is feeling bad about something over which you have no control. Do not waste energy on bad guilt because it is irrational and physically and emotionally draining (e.g., "I am a single parent, and I must work to put food on the table and a roof over our heads. I am going to school so that I will be able to reach my goals of being a nurse and earning a better living. While I am in school, I must spend more time with my studies and less time with my children.").
- You can change the belief on which your guilty feelings are based (e.g., "It is appropriate for me to meet my needs before someone else's needs; I am not a bad person if I decide not to do what someone else expects of me.").
- You can make a weekly calendar that respects your goals and priorities. When studying, you should not feel guilty about not spending time with the family because you have scheduled time to address family needs.
- You can compensate for your behavior. Compensation is repaying yourself or someone else when something is done or not done as expected. It is used when unexpected priorities arise. However, if you are constantly using compensation, you need to revisit your goals, priorities, and calendars (e.g., "I want to watch the ball game on TV tonight, so I will study 2 hours more on the weekend." "We had fast food three times this week, so tonight I will make a great home-cooked meal.").

Use feelings of guilt to your advantage. This is an opportunity for personal change and growth.

Avoiding Time Traps

Time traps are interruptions that interfere with your ability to use your time productively. Earlier in this chapter, you were advised to complete a Personal Time/Activity Journal. A review of your journal should reveal to you how you spent your time and whether you were productive or you got caught in time traps. You were also asked to perform a self-assessment to identify your barriers to productivity, which included procrastination, difficulty with delegation, lack of organization, an inability to set goals and priorities, perfectionism, and lack of self-discipline. Each of these barriers to productivity has time-trap elements, and corrective actions for each are addressed in this chapter. This section will help you identify seemingly unavoidable events that interfere with your use of time. Do not dribble away time when you are out of control or when others control you. Some time traps cannot be completely avoided. However, an awareness of how events are interfering with your use of time followed by effective management can help you address most of these events. First, you must identify when you are caught in a time trap and realize how much time is being wasted. Second, you need to set limits on yourself and others and regain control of your time.

Events over which you may believe you have little control include the following:

- Unwanted phone calls or phone calls that involve unimportant conversations (small talk)
- Long-winded conversations that do not get to the point
- The arrival of unwanted guests
- A crowded library or store
- Waiting for others
- Rush-hour traffic
- Excessively researching a topic
- Too much socializing
- Unnecessary meetings
- Assuming the role of listener or counselor to meet the emotional needs of friends

Many of these events occur because you are unaware of how much time they waste, you have not organized your day, or you have not set limits on yourself or others. You are not powerless to control these events. However, to limit or eliminate time traps, you must be proactive. Suggested solutions are as follows:

Manage accessibility:

- Turn off your cell phone or use it only for outgoing calls.
- Indicate on your voice mail that you are available only during certain times.
- Make your home phone unlisted.
- Give your e-mail address only to selected individuals.
- Use caller ID to screen phone calls.
- Turn off the ringer or unplug the phone when studying.
- Set a timer for ending the activities with friends or family when you are not studying, so you remain aware of the passing of time.
- Block out time for studying when you absolutely cannot be interrupted.
- Learn to say, "It's nice to hear from you, but I really can't talk right now. I'll catch up with you next week." This generally works. If the other person is persistent, say, "I'm sorry. I really have to go." And then close the door or hang up.
- Put a "Do Not Disturb" sign on your door. (I used this approach when I had a newborn, and I put a picture of a sleeping baby on the sign.)
- When you are studying, give family members instructions to interrupt you only if there is an emergency.

Manage waiting time:

- Set limits on the amount of time you are willing to wait. Your time is as valuable as the other person's time.
- Capture moments of free time by studying flash cards or class notes.
- Use captured moments of time to get small tasks accomplished. For example, while waiting for an appointment, write a thank-you note for a gift, write a grocery list, review your schedule for the next day, write a check and prepare a bill for mailing, or brainstorm how you are going to tackle an upcoming assignment.
- Make appointments with primary health-care providers the first or last appointment of the day. Call to ensure that the primary health-care provider is on schedule.

Avoid wasting time:

- Keep a list of what is done and what still needs to be done; then, if you stop in the middle of a project, you can pick up where you left off.
- Multitask your errands. Go one-stop shopping, and use stores that carry food, hardware, clothes, and so forth.
- Simplify shopping. Reduce trips to the store, follow a shopping list, and maintain a full pantry.
- Simplify meals. Cook one-dish meals. Cook double the amount, and freeze half for another day.
- Eat out or buy ready-made food when short on time.
- Avoid travel during rush hour. Leave earlier or later, and use the saved time to your best advantage. Truck stops are filled with trucks during rush hour. Professional drivers use this time to eat and sleep rather than spend time in "gridlock." Do the same.
- Simplify gift giving. For example, books are a great gift, and all your holiday shopping can be done in one store. Each book can be personalized by topic, and a personal message can be inscribed on the inside cover.
- Avoid meetings unless they are absolutely necessary, such as a parent/teacher conference. If a meeting is necessary, set a time limit on each subject to be discussed and the amount of time each person can speak, and stick to it. This requires participants to be concise and focused.
- Shop for food when stores open in the morning or late at night, preferably midweek, because these are the least-crowded times.
- Avoid using the library just before midterms and finals. Using the library at these times is generally the sign of a procrastinator.

Manage your own emotions:

- Lower your expectations. For example, you do not have to research every topic beyond what is necessary to meet the criteria of an assignment, or you do not have to prepare a four-course meal every day. Perfection is not necessary to pass a nursing course or to be a "good" person.
- Recognize when you are experiencing "good guilt" versus "bad guilt" and act accordingly. For more information, see the section on self-discipline earlier in this chapter.
- Avoid accepting the role of counselor for your friends. Listening to other people's problems is a time-consuming and emotionally exhausting process. Listen for a few minutes and then say, "I'm not a counselor. I think you need to talk to someone who is trained to help you with this problem."

Motivating Yourself

Motivation is the driving force that encourages you to do something. It is an incentive or bribe that induces you to action. Motivation can come from within. Learning something new, attaining a goal, and being impressed with your performance are examples of internal motivation. You have to be future oriented to use internal motivation to stimulate yourself toward the achievement of a long-term goal. For example, visualize yourself walking up to receive your diploma, wearing your nurse's uniform, or receiving your first paycheck for being a nurse. This can be difficult because you have to delay gratification in the present for an abstract future goal.

Motivation can also come from without. Earning a high grade, obtaining respect from others, and receiving a reward are examples of external motivations. Additional examples of external motivators include a break from studying, a candy bar, a walk around the block, or a cold drink.

Each person's motivator is individual. Think about the tasks that you accomplish every day. What payoff do you receive for completing them? When you are able to identify what really spurs you to action, you can use these same incentives for accomplishing school-related activities. For further discussion about motivation, see "Balance Sacrifices and Rewards" in Chapter 4, "Study Techniques."

Achieve a Personal Balance

Do you write and rewrite an assignment until it is perfect? Do you always have to get an "A" on every test? Do you think that no one can do as good a job on a particular project as you can? Do you like others to have an image of you as superman or superwoman? Do you study constantly to the detriment of other personal needs? Do you think that you can be all things to all people? Do you think that the office/committee/family will collapse without you? If you answered "Yes" to several of these questions, you may be a perfectionist.

A **perfectionist** is a person who compulsively strives to attain a degree of excellence according to a given standard. In other words, you think you are perfect. Also, a perfectionist tends to have an idealized self-image. That is, he or she displays to the world a self that is expected to be admired, respected, and loved by others. Unfortunately, if you are a perfectionist, then you are striving for the impossible. It is humanly impossible to be perfect, and attempting to maintain an idealized image is irrational, impractical, and self-destructive.

Perfectionism can be physically and emotionally debilitating. Because you can never really achieve perfection, you set yourself up for not performing according to your imaginary standard of perfection. When this happens, emotionally you shatter your self-image, an event that at best can be demoralizing and unmotivating and at worst can promote feelings of failure. Also, attempting to complete every role (e.g., spouse, parent, worker, and student) to perfection can take its toll on your body. A little stress keeps you alert, motivated, and focused. However, excessive stress taxes the endocrine, neurological, and cardiovascular systems and eventually results in physical depletion and exhaustion. Perfectionism, although considered a noble trait by some, can be emotionally and physically self-destructive and should be brought under control.

To conquer obsessive/compulsive, perfectionistic thinking, you must achieve a sense of personal balance. There is a big difference between expecting perfection and striving for excellence! First, you should recognize that no one, including you, is perfect. Then you must alter your frame of reference. To alter your frame of reference you should ask yourself the following questions.

- Will I still graduate if I earn less than an "A" in my nursing courses?
- Is a grade of "A" on a written assignment worth not going to a child's sporting event?
- Will doing what it takes to earn an "A" in a nursing course negatively affect the other things I think are important in my life?
- Does this task require perfect effort?
- Does dinner really have to be on the table at 6 p.m.?
- Can I afford to have my lawn cut by someone else rather than cut it myself?
- Does dust provide a protective barrier for the surfaces of furniture?

Individualize the questions you ask yourself to reflect your personal and family responsibilities. We are not suggesting that you lower your standards on those things that are most important to you. However, if you are adding a huge commitment to your life (e.g., nursing school), something else in your life has to give. A student once told us that although she picked up around the house every day, she dusted only every other week. One day, she saw the following note from her husband written in the dust on a tabletop: "I love you!" Underneath the note, she wrote back "Ditto!" She said they had a good laugh over the exchange, but she also demonstrated to him that the dust was not one of her priorities and she was not going to be pressured into dusting. Another student indicated that he never studied on Saturday night. He and his girlfriend always had a standing date so they could spend time together. Likewise, at graduation, several graduates may have an opportunity to talk at the convocation. Usually, at least one graduate will make reference to the fact that there will be more home-cooked meals and less pizza and Chinese food now that they have graduated. One of these examples reflects a behavior that addresses an important value (i.e., spending time with a significant other). The other examples demonstrate a relaxation of standards of perfection (a dust-free house and home-cooked meals).

Controlling perfectionism and relaxing an idealized self-image are not easy tasks. However, you must remain true to yourself in light of your values and goals. Strive for growth and development, not perfection, as you seek balance in your personal life.

Delegate

If you look up the word *delegate* in a dictionary, you will find words such as *surrender, relinquish, renounce,* and *give up* used to explain its meaning. Unfortunately, this is why many people have difficulty delegating tasks to others. They look at delegation as a loss, as giving something up or yielding control. Delegation does the exact opposite. When you delegate, you transfer a task to another person and you gain, not lose, something. You gain more time and experience less stress! For delegation to achieve desired results and positive feelings for both people involved, you must adhere to the guidelines in the following paragraphs.

Identify the personal qualities of the people to whom you can delegate. Before you delegate a task to another person, you must identify, alone or in conjunction with the other person, whether he or she has the capacity to complete the task. Does the person have the appropriate intellectual, physical, and/or attitudinal ability to be successful at the task? The focus here is not on whether this person has ever done this task before but on whether the person has the potential to do the task and is the appropriate person for the task. For example, it is inappropriate to expect 5-year-old children to clean a house, but it is appropriate to expect them to pick up their own toys.

Identify the outcomes of the task to be accomplished. Explore with the other person the expected result. You should both have a clear, concise, mutual understanding of what is to be accomplished. The focus here is not on how the task will be done but rather on the product or conclusion. For example, if you delegate doing the laundry, the outcome may be that clothing will be clean, dried, and folded (or at least sorted) every 3 days. You are not focusing on how the clothing got washed or what cleaning products were used.

Identify the resources that are necessary to accomplish the task. For a task to be successfully delegated, you must consider the human, economic, technical, and organizational resources that may be needed. Information or skills may need to be practiced before the person becomes successful in performing a new task. The focus here is not on excessive detail but rather on flexibility in the extent of support. For example, to cook dinner, one person may draw on past experiences, another may need a cookbook, and another may require a demonstration with supervised practice.

Relinquish accountability for the task. Accountability exists when a person assumes responsibility for something. When you delegate in your personal life, you transfer the responsibility for the task to another person, and that person assumes ownership of his or her actions and the results of those actions. You will not feel free from the burden of a task unless you relinquish accountability for it. The focus here is not on authoritarian supervision or consequences for tasks not accomplished but rather on the concept of trust. For example, you cannot hover over, breathe down the neck of, or micromanage another person when he or she is working on a delegated task. You must allow the person room to explore, practice, and grow. Occasionally, you may have to wear pink underwear, tolerate dusty baseboards, or eat tasteless meals. Initially, less-than-perfect outcomes go with the territory of delegation.

Delegation does not occur in isolation. Communicate your needs to family and friends. Have a family meeting, and explore what tasks must be done, what people would like to do, and what skills need to be learned. When family members are involved in the decision-making process, there is "ownership," which increases the probability of success. This is an opportunity for both you and family members to grow. You will learn the art of delegation, share your needs, recognize that you are interdependent, and reinforce that you must trust in others. Family members, even children, will learn new skills, feel important, develop confidence, and gain independence.

Finally, routinely review the plan and evaluate how it is working. Ask questions such as "Are people accountable? Should tasks be rotated? Do people need additional resources? Is someone ready to learn a new skill? Are priorities being met?" Change the plan as necessary. Delegation plans must be flexible to meet the needs of both the family as a whole and the individuals within it.

Overcome Procrastination

Procrastination is putting off or postponing something until a later time. It is a protective mechanism to delay having to deal with something that we would rather not deal with. We procrastinate because in the short term it reduces anxiety. However, in the long term, procrastination wastes time and increases anxiety. We all procrastinate to some degree; however, when taken to an extreme, it can interfere with our ability to complete tasks for which we are responsible.

When delaying a project, have you ever said the following to yourself?

- This is boring.
- This is too hard.
- I do not know where to begin.
- I am not in the mood.
- I am too tired.
- I am angry/annoyed/frustrated that I have to do this.
- I have more important things to do.
- I can do it tomorrow.
- I have plenty of time.
- I work better under pressure.

These are just a few of the ways in which we rationalize our behavior. **Rationalization** is giving socially acceptable reasons or explanations for our behaviors. When rationalization is used to explain why we did not do something we were expected to do, it usually is an excuse! Sometimes our excuses are so believable that we convince ourselves. To overcome procrastination, you must first realize that you are procrastinating, stop the procrastinating behavior, and then take constructive action to overcome the procrastination.

Breaking the cycle of procrastination requires a new mindset. When we delay tasks, it is often because we look at them as "chores," routine activities, or responsibilities that we may consider demanding or unpleasant. The word *chores* has a negative undertone. Therefore, tasks associated with schoolwork must never be viewed as chores but should be placed within a positive frame of reference. They are tasks that must be accomplished to reach your goal of becoming a nurse.

For example, take your explanation for why something should be postponed and challenge it with logic or motivating strategies:

- This is boring. "This is not dull and unexciting, because it will help prepare me to be a nurse. It has to get done sooner or later, and it might as well be now."
- This is too hard. "I can do this! It may be difficult, but I did not get this far in my education without being able to do what I have to do to pass a course."
- I do not know where to begin. "Yes, I do! I need to review the requirements related to this assignment. I will make an outline showing how I should move forward. I will focus on just a small part of the assignment. I will discuss what I finish today with my instructor tomorrow."
- I am not in the mood. "I will never be in the mood to do this assignment. I can divide the assignment into several parts and reward myself when I finish each part."
- I am too tired. "I am always tired. I will break down the job into sections, and I can do at least one section today."
- I am angry/annoyed/frustrated that I have to do this. "I am feeling this way because..., but my feelings are standing in the way of my completing this task. I need to *get a grip*. I will deal with my feelings in more depth after finishing what I have to do now. I have chosen to be a nurse, and this task is moving me forward."
- I have more important things to do. "Oh, really! Let me list the other things I have to do, and I will put them in order of importance. Which of these things can I eliminate or delegate? This is the most important thing I have to do now."
- I can do it tomorrow. "No, I will think about it right now. I should not put off until tomorrow what I can do today!"
- I have plenty of time. "I never have plenty of time. There is no time like the present!"
- I work better under pressure. "Who am I kidding? When I leave it to the last minute, I get it done because I have no other choice. I will do a much better job now if I give myself enough time to do it right."

These sample self-challenge statements are not universal responses. Make your own statements. However, each statement should follow these simple guidelines: Identify that you are procrastinating; challenge the procrastination with a direct, opposing thought; and justify your challenging statement with a logical explanation. Sometimes the explanations that challenge procrastination involve larger changes, such as modifying your priorities or restructuring your activities of daily living. However, more often than not, they involve smaller changes, such as using strategies of motivation. You can motivate yourself by setting short-term goals, providing rewards for finished tasks, using positive self-talk, and being a firm self-taskmaster. Procrastination is a behavior initiated from within. When you know and manage yourself, you are in control of your learning instead of the other way around.

SUMMARY

Controlling the use of time to your best advantage depends on your desire and efforts to identify and correct negative patterns that waste time. You should be proactive in the control of your time. To be proactive, you should implement the tools presented in this chapter to identify barriers to productivity, identify common time traps, and implement suggested corrective actions. If successful, you will have more time to tackle the tasks that are not pressing but are important. When addressing tasks in this category, you will feel more in control, more productive, and less overwhelmed and anxious. With a little effort and a desire to change, you can be a master of your own time! Using your time productively can maximize the time you have for studying for nursing examinations.

4 Study Techniques

Learning is the activity by which knowledge, attitudes, and/or skills are acquired. Learning is a complex activity that is influenced by various factors such as genetic endowment, level of maturation, experiential background, effectiveness of formal instruction, self-image, readiness to learn, and level of motivation. Although you cannot change some of these factors, you can control others.

Learning is an active process that takes place within the learner. Therefore, the role of the learner is to participate in or initiate activities that promote learning. Like test taking, learning is an acquired skill. This chapter presents both general and specific study techniques that should increase your ability to learn. The general study techniques presented include skills that facilitate learning regardless of the topic being studied. Specific study techniques are presented in relation to levels of thinking process that are required to answer questions in nursing: knowledge, comprehension, application, and analysis. Using these techniques when studying will help you comprehend more of what you have studied and retain the information for a longer period. This information should increase your success in answering test questions.

GENERAL STUDY TECHNIQUES

General techniques to improve study skills can be applied to any subject, whereas a few specific techniques are particularly applicable to studying for nursing examinations. Both types are discussed here.

Establish a Routine

Set aside a regular time to study. Learning requires consistency, repetition, and practice. Deciding to sit down to study is the most difficult part of the process. We tend to procrastinate and think of a variety of things we should do instead of studying. By committing yourself to a regular routine, you eliminate the need to repetitively decide to study. If you decide that every evening from 7:00 to 8:30 you are going to study, you are using your internal locus of control and establishing an internal readiness to learn. You must be motivated to learn.

Your study schedule must be reasonable and realistic. More frequent short study periods are more effective than long study periods. For most people, 1- to 3-hour study periods with a 10-minute break each hour are most effective. Periods of learning must be balanced with adequate rest periods because energy, attention, and endurance decrease over time and limit efficiency of learning. Physical and emotional rest makes you more alert and receptive to new information.

When planning a schedule, involve significant family members in the decision making. Because a family is an open system, the action of one member influences the other members. When family members are involved in the decision making, they have a vested interest in it and will probably be more supportive of your need to study.

Set Short-Term and Long-Term Goals

A goal is an outcome that a person attempts to attain; it may be long term or short term. A long-term goal is the eventual desired outcome. A short-term goal is a desired outcome that can be achieved along the path leading to the long-term goal. In other words, a long-term goal is your destination, whereas each short-term goal is an objective that must be attained to help you eventually reach your destination. Each long-term goal may have one or more short-term goals.

Goals to promote learning should be purposeful, should serve as guides for planning action, and should establish standards so that learning can be evaluated. Goals must be specific, measurable, and realistic and must have a time frame. A specific goal states exactly what is to be accomplished. A measurable goal sets a minimum acceptable level of performance. A realistic goal must be potentially achievable. A goal with a time frame states the time parameters in which it will be achieved.

When studying, a typical long-term goal is "I will read and study the content in Chapter 1 in my *Fundamentals of Nursing* textbook within 7 hours." Typical short-term goals may be to read the first 10 pages of Chapter 1 in the next half hour, or to highlight important information in Chapter 1 within 2 hours, to list the principles presented in Chapter 1 within 1 hour, and to compare and contrast information in your class notes with information in the textbook within 2 hours. It may also be to complete the creation of flash cards for 10 or 20 medications you're studying. Each of these short-term goals can be achieved as a step toward attaining the long-term goal. It is wise to break a big task into small, manageable tasks because it is easier to learn small bits of information than large blocks of information. The most effective learning is goal-directed learning. In other words, planned learning with a purpose. In addition, attainment of goals increases self-esteem and motivation.

Simulate a Testing Environment

There are vast differences in learning styles, and many students are unconventional learners. This discussion does not imply that there is only one way to learn. However, this textbook presents information that will help promote success on an examination. Therefore, to desensitize yourself to the testing environment, it is helpful to simulate that environment when studying. When studying for a test, your posture, surroundings, and equipment should be similar to those in the testing environment. Study at a desk or table and chair and ensure adequate lighting. Avoid the temptation to study in a reclining chair, on the couch, or in bed. Keep pets in another room, avoid eating, and mute the ringer on your phone. Remember, the familiar generally is less stressful than the unfamiliar.

Control External and Internal Distractors

Stimuli, both external and internal, must be controlled to eliminate distractions. External stimuli are environmental happenings that interrupt your thinking and should be limited. Select a place to study where you will not be interrupted by family members, phone calls, the doorbell, or family pets. These stimuli compete for your attention when you should be focusing on your work. Internal stimuli are inner thoughts, feelings, or concerns that interfere with your ability to study. Internal stimuli often are more difficult to control than external stimuli because they involve attitudes. Review the techniques in Chapter 1 that promote a positive mental attitude. By limiting or eliminating external and internal distractors, you should improve your ability to concentrate.

Prepare for Class

To prepare adequately for class, you need to know the content that will be addressed. Look at the course outline or ask your instructor (i.e., "If you don't know where you're going, you can't get there!"). After you know the topic, identify the appropriate content in your textbook. To "pre-*pare*" for class you must *pare* down the written information in your textbook. To *pare* means to trim, clip, or cut back. When reviewing textbook material before class, it is not always necessary to read every word.

- **First,** read the chapter headings. This will give you an overview of the topic presented.
- **Second,** look at tables and figures and read their captions. These provide visual cues.
- **Third,** skim the chapter content but read information that is CAPITALIZED, *italicized,* or **boldfaced.** These formats indicate important information; use highlighting to accentuate these terms and other areas of meaningful content.
- **Fourth,** list the questions you may want to ask in class. You are now minimally prepared for class. Finally, to be well prepared, read the chapter thoroughly to gain an in-depth understanding of the content.

Take Class Notes

Taking notes in class is critical. Class notes are valuable because they provide you with a blueprint for study when preparing for an examination. Writing things down helps you make sense of the material and remember it. The following are note-taking tips:

- **Stay focused on the topic being presented.** Generally, instructors present material that they believe is important. Compare this information with the material you highlighted in your textbook.
- **Use your notebook creatively.** Open your notebook so that you have facing sheets. Use the page on the left side for class notes. Save the page on the right side for adding information from the textbook or other sources that clarify the class notes.
- **Use an outline format and abbreviations.** There is no way you can write down every word that comes out of your instructor's mouth. Focus on concepts because you can expand on the content later. For example, if an instructor is talking about abnormal respiratory rates such as apnea, bradypnea, and tachypnea, write these words down and listen to the instructor's presentation. The definitions can be added to the page on the right side of your notebook at a later time.
- **Ask questions to clarify information.** Your goal is not to be a stenographer. Your goal is to understand the information. Ask questions that you have prepared before class or that you may have as a result of the discussion in class. If you have a question, other students probably have the same question. Have the courage to ask questions. Two of the roles of an instructor are to make the information more understandable and to clarify misconceptions. Your tuition pays the instructor's salary, so get your money's worth!
- **Review your notes after class.** You should review your notes within 48 hours after class. Reviewing, reorganizing, and rewriting class notes are techniques of reinforcement. Repetition helps commit information to memory. Retell the information to yourself out loud. By explaining it (teaching it) to yourself, you are more likely to remember it. Some instructors allow you to use a recorder in class. Reviewing class recordings is particularly helpful for students who are auditory learners, those who have difficulty grasping complex material the first time, and those for whom English is a second language.

Identify Learning Domains

Learning styles are never identical for any two people, and they can even vary for one person depending on the situation. Over the years, you have developed a learning style that you feel comfortable with and that has proven to be successful. It is in your best interest, however, to be open to a variety of learning approaches. These approaches vary according to the purpose/goal of the activity: to attain new information (cognitive domain), acquire new physical skills (psychomotor domain), or form new attitudes (affective domain).

Cognitive Domain

Cognitive learning is concerned with understanding information acquired through exploring thoughts, ideas, and concepts. It advances from the simple to the complex and progresses from knowing and comprehending information to applying and analyzing it.

New information usually is learned through symbols such as words or pictures. We read them, see them, or hear them. Use all of your senses to acquire new information. The more routes information takes to travel to your brain, the greater the chances that you will learn the information. For example, when information about positioning clients is read, learning is reinforced by viewing pictures of people in various positions.

Psychomotor Domain

Psychomotor learning is concerned with the development of skills. It involves perceptual abilities as well as physical abilities related to endurance, strength, and dexterity. Integrated body movements progress from reflexive movements, to basic fundamental movements, to skilled movements.

New skills involve the physical application of information. It is possible for a person to understand all the goals and steps of a procedure and yet not be able to perform that procedure. For information to get from the head to the hands, the learner must do more than read a book, look at pictures, view a video, or watch other people. The learner must become actively involved. Physical skills are not learned by osmosis or diffusion; they are learned by doing. For example, when learning how to change a sterile dressing, the learner can read a book and look at a video; however, it is essential that the learner actually practice changing a sterile dressing.

Affective Domain

Affective learning is concerned with the development of attitudes, which include interests, appreciation, feelings, and values; it progresses from awareness to increasing internalization of or commitment to the attitude.

Learning new attitudes is the most difficult domain in which to make change, because attitudes result from lifelong experiences and tend to be well entrenched. For example, a student may know and understand the theory concerning why a person should be nonjudgmental and yet still be judgmental toward a client in a clinical situation. The development of new attitudes is best learned in an atmosphere of acceptance by exploring feelings, becoming involved in group discussions, and observing appropriate role models. For example, before providing physical hygiene for a client for the first time, it is beneficial to explore your own feelings about invading a client's personal space.

Capture Moments of Time

Using spare moments to review information is a method of maximizing your time for constructive study. We all have periods during the day that are less productive than others, such as time spent waiting for an appointment or standing in line at a store. There are also times when you engage in repetitive tasks, such as vacuuming a rug or raking leaves. Capture these moments and use them to study. Carry flash cards, a vocabulary list, or categories of information that you can review when you have unexpected time. These captured moments should be in addition to, rather than a replacement for, your regularly scheduled study periods. An old saying states that "Time is on your side." Capture spare moments of time and use them to your advantage. For additional information about time management, review Chapter 3.

Use Appropriate Resources

The theories and principles of nursing practice are complex. They draw from a variety of disciplines (e.g., psychology, sociology, anatomy and physiology, microbiology), use new terminology, and require unique applications to clinical practice. When you study, you will find that your learning does not proceed in a straight line, moving progressively forward. You may experience plateaus, remissions, and/or periods of confusion when dealing with complex material. When your forward progress is slowed, identify your needs and immediately seek help. Your instructor, another student, a study group, or a tutor may be beneficial. When studying with another student, make sure that the person is a source of correct information. When studying in groups, three to five students are ideal because a group of more than five people becomes a "party." The group should be heterogeneous; that is, there should be a variety of academic abilities, attitudes, skills, and perspectives among the members. This variety should enrich the learning experience and provide checks and balances for the sharing of correct information. Remember, you learn not only from the instructor but also from your classmates.

Generally, people do not like to admit that they have learning difficulties because they think it makes them look inadequate in the eyes of others. For this reason, people may be embarrassed to ask for help. This can be self-destructive because it denies them the opportunity to use resources that support growth. Be careful that you do not fall into this trap! To obtain access to the appropriate resources, you must be willing to be open to yourself and others. Resources (e.g., extra help sessions; computer labs; reading, writing, and math centers; psychological counseling; and availability of faculty during office hours) are there to be used. Have the courage to acknowledge to yourself and others that you need help. Seeking help is a sign of maturity rather than a sign of weakness. When you ask for help, you are in control because you are solving problems to meet your own needs.

Balance Sacrifices and Rewards

When you decided to enter nursing school, no one promised you a rose garden. Your commitment to becoming a nurse requires sacrifice. Your time and energy are being diverted from usual activities related to your job, family members, friends, and pleasurable pastimes. Rigorous activity, whether physical or mental, requires concentration and endurance. However, too much work hinders productivity. You must establish a balance between energy expenditure and rewards for your efforts.

Rewards can be internal or external. Internal rewards are stimulated from within the learner and relate to feelings associated with meaningful achievement. Learning something new, achieving a goal, and increasing self-respect are examples of internal rewards. External rewards come from outside the learner. A grade of 100%, respect and appreciation from others, and a present for achieving a goal are examples of external rewards.

Unfortunately, the rewards for studying are usually not immediate but appear in the extended future. Graduating from nursing school, passing an NCLEX® examination, earning a paycheck, and enjoying the prestige of being a nurse are future-oriented rewards. Therefore, you should be the one to provide immediate rewards for yourself for studying. During study breaks or at the completion of studying, reward yourself by thinking about how much you have learned, reflecting on the good feelings you have about your accomplishments, relaxing with a significant other, having a beverage, watching a favorite television show, texting a friend, or taking a weekend off. Short-term rewards promote a positive mental attitude, reinforce motivation, and provide a respite from studying.

SPECIFIC STUDY TECHNIQUES RELATED TO COGNITIVE LEVELS OF NURSING QUESTIONS

The nurse uses a variety of thinking processes when caring for clients. Therefore, examinations must reflect these thinking processes to effectively evaluate the safe practice of nursing. Four thinking processes may be required to answer questions concerning the delivery of nursing care: **knowledge, comprehension, application,** and **analysis** (for this discussion, analysis includes synthesis and evaluation). These thinking processes are within the cognitive domain and are ordered according to complexity; that is, a knowledge question requires the lowest level of thinking (recalling information), whereas an analysis question requires the highest level of thinking (comparing and contrasting information).

In this section of the book, each cognitive level is discussed, and sample multiple-choice items are presented to illustrate the thinking processes involved in answering the item. In addition, specific study techniques are presented to help you strengthen your critical thinking abilities.

The correct answers for the sample items in this chapter and the rationales for all the options are presented at the end of the chapter.

Knowledge Questions

Knowledge questions require you to recall or remember information. To answer a knowledge question, you need to commit facts to memory. To answer knowledge questions correctly, you must know terminology, specific facts, trends, classifications, categories, criteria, structures, principles, generalizations, and theories. This basic information is the foundation for thinking critically. This type of information is best learned by using flash cards.

SAMPLE ITEM 4-1

Which level of prevention is hospice care?
1. Secondary prevention
2. Morbidity prevention
3. Primary prevention
4. Tertiary prevention

To answer this question, you need to know the definitions of the various types of prevention as well as what services hospice provides.

SAMPLE ITEM 4-2

A nurse must make an unoccupied bed. Which is the first step of the procedure for making the bed?
1. Cleaning hands
2. Pulling the curtain
3. Collecting clean linen
4. Placing the bottom sheet

To answer this question correctly, you need to know the sequence of steps in making an unoccupied bed or the basic principle that your hands must be cleaned before all procedures.

SAMPLE ITEM 4-3

Which is within the expected range of a radial pulse for an adult?
1. 50 to 65 beats per minute
2. 70 to 85 beats per minute
3. 90 to 105 beats per minute
4. 110 to 125 beats per minute

To answer this question correctly, you need to know the expected range of a radial pulse for an adult.

STUDY TECHNIQUES TO INCREASE YOUR KNOWLEDGE

The techniques in this area will help retain information on a short-term basis because the information is learned by rote without any in-depth understanding. Learning via these techniques is helpful, but the information may be forgotten unless reinforced through additional study techniques or application in your nursing practice.

REPETITION/MEMORIZATION: Through repetition, information is committed to the brain for recall at a later date. Repeatedly studying information by reciting it out loud, reviewing it in your mind, or writing it down increases your chances of remembering the material because a variety of senses are used. Memorization can be facilitated by using lists of related facts, flash cards, or learning wheels:

- On an index card, you can list the steps of a procedure or use a portable electronic device that displays the steps. This can be carried with you to study when you capture moments of time.
- You can write a word on the front of an index card and define the word on the back. An entire deck of cards can be developed for the terminology within a unit of study. Use flash cards when you have unexpected time to study.
- To make a learning wheel, cut a piece of cardboard into a circle and draw pie-shaped wedges on the front and back. On a front wedge, write a unit of measure, such as 30 mL, and on the corresponding back wedge, write its conversion to another unit of measure, such as 1 ounce. Then, on individual spring clothespins, write each of the units of measure that appear on the back of the wheel. When you want to study approximate equivalents, mix up the clothespins and attempt to match each one to its corresponding unit of measure. You can turn the wheel over and evaluate your success by determining whether the clothespin you attached to the wheel matches the unit of measure on the back of the wheel.

ALPHABET CUES: Memorization can be facilitated when the information is associated with letters of the alphabet. Each letter serves as a cue that stimulates the recall of information. The most effective alphabet cues are those you make up yourself. They meet a self-identified need, and you have to review the information before you can design the alphabet cue. You can use any combination of letters as long as it has meaning for you and your learning. Examples of alphabet cues include the following:

- Identify people at risk for injury through the letters **A, B, C, D, E, F,** and **G: A**ge—the young and very old; **B**lindness—lack of visual perception; **C**onsciousness—decreased level of consciousness; **D**eafness—lack of auditory perception; **E**motional state—reduced psychological status; **F**requency of accidents—history of accidents; and **G**ait—impaired mobility.
- The **Three Ps** for the cardinal signs of diabetes mellitus are **P**olyuria, **P**olydipsia, and **P**olyphagia.

ACRONYMS: The use of acronyms is a technique to retrieve previously learned information. An acronym is a word formed from the first letters of a series of terms or a phrase. Each letter of the acronym relates to the information it represents. It is useful for learning because each letter of the word jolts the recall of information. Examples of acronyms include the following:

- The American Cancer Society teaches the early warning signs of cancer by using the word **CAUTION:**

  Change in bowel and bladder habits

  A sore that does not heal

  Unusual bleeding or discharge

  Thickening or a lump

  Indigestion or difficulty in swallowing

  Obvious change in a wart or mole

  Nagging cough or hoarseness

- When assessing a person for indicators of infection, remember the word **INFECT:**

  Increased pulse, respirations, and white blood cell count

  Nodes enlarged

  Function impaired

  Erythema, **E**dema, **E**xudate

Comments reporting discomfort or pain

Temperature increase—local and/or systemic

ACROSTICS: An acrostic is a phrase, motto, or verse in which a letter of each word (usually the first letter) prompts the memory to retrieve information. Memorizing information can be difficult and boring. This technique is a creative way to make learning more effective and fun. Examples of acrostics include the following:

- When studying the fat-soluble vitamins, recall this motto: "**A**ll **D**ieters **E**at **K**ilocalories." This should help you remember that **A, D, E,** and **K** are the fat-soluble vitamins. "ADEK."
- When studying the cranial nerves, recall this acrostic: "**On O**ld **O**lympus's **T**owering **T**ops, **A F**inn and a **S**wedish **G**irl **V**iewed **S**ome **H**ops," which stands for **O**lfactory, **O**ptic, **O**culomotor, **T**rochlear, **T**rigeminal, **A**bducens, **F**acial, **S**ensorimotor (vestibulocochlear), **G**lossopharyngeal, **V**agus, **S**pinal accessory, and **H**ypoglossal nerves. These are the cranial nerves.

MNEMONICS: A mnemonic is a variation of an acrostic. It is a phrase, motto, or verse that jogs the memory. It differs from an acrostic in that not every word is related to a specific piece of content. Mnemonics promote retention by connecting new or difficult information to known or less difficult information using mental associations or visual pictures.

- When studying apothecary and metric equivalents, remember this verse, "There are **15 grains** of sugar in **1 graham (gram)** cracker." This sentence should help you remember that **15 grains** are equivalent to **1 gram.**
- When trying to remember the difference between low-density lipoproteins (LDLs) and high-density lipoproteins (HDLs), refer to this mnemonic: **LDL** is **L**ousy cholesterol and **HDL** is **H**appy cholesterol. This sentence should help you remember that increased LDL levels are associated with plaque deposits in arteries and are undesirable (lousy cholesterol) and that HDL promotes excretion of cholesterol from the body (happy cholesterol).

Comprehension Questions

Comprehension questions require you to understand information. To answer a comprehension question, you must commit facts to memory as well as translate, interpret, and determine the implications of that information. You demonstrate understanding when you paraphrase information; interpret or summarize information; or determine the implications, consequences, corollaries, or effects of information. To answer comprehension questions correctly, you must know as well as understand the information being tested. After you understand basic information, you can identify its significance, which is an initial step in critical thinking.

SAMPLE ITEM 4-4

The nurse administers a cathartic. Which therapeutic outcome should the nurse expect when assessing the client's response to this medication?

1. Increased urinary output
2. Decreased anxiety
3. Bowel movement
4. Pain relief

To answer this question, you need to know not only that a cathartic is a potent laxative that stimulates the bowel (knowledge) but also that the increase in peristalsis will result in a bowel movement (comprehension).

SAMPLE ITEM 4-5

A nurse uses the interviewing technique of clarification when interviewing a client. What is the nurse doing when this communication technique is used?

1. Paraphrasing the client's message
2. Restating what the client has said
3. Verifying what the client is implying
4. Reviewing the client's communication

To answer this question, you need to know that clarification is a therapeutic tool that promotes communication between the client and nurse (knowledge), and you also must explain why or how this technique facilitates communication (comprehension).

SAMPLE ITEM 4-6

A nurse administers an intramuscular injection and then massages the insertion site after the needle has been withdrawn. Which is the purpose of massaging the insertion site at the completion of the procedure?

1. Limit infection
2. Prevent bleeding
3. Reduce discomfort
4. Promote absorption

To answer this question, you need to know that massage is one step of the procedure for an intramuscular injection (knowledge), and you must understand the consequence of massaging the needle insertion site after the needle has been withdrawn (comprehension).

STUDY TECHNIQUES TO INCREASE YOUR COMPREHENSION OF INFORMATION

EXPLORE THE "WHYS" AND "HOWS": The difference between knowledge questions and comprehension questions is that you must know facts to answer knowledge questions, but you must understand the significance of the facts to answer comprehension questions. Facts can be understood and retained longer if they are relevant and meaningful to the learner. When studying information, ask yourself why or how the information is important. For example, when learning that immobility causes pressure ulcers, explore *why* they occur. Pressure compresses the capillary beds, which interferes with the transport of oxygen and nutrients to tissues, resulting in ischemia and necrosis. When studying a skill such as bathing, explore how soap cleans the skin. Soap reduces the surface tension of water and helps remove accumulated oils, perspiration, dead cells, and microorganisms. If you interpret information and identify why or how the information is relevant and useful, then the information has value. When information increases in value, it is less readily forgotten.

STUDY IN SMALL GROUPS: After you have studied by yourself, it is usually valuable to study the same information with another person or in a small group. The sharing process promotes your comprehension of information because you listen to the impressions and opinions of others, learn new information from a peer tutor, and reinforce your own learning by teaching others. In addition, the members of the group reinforce your interpretation of information and correct your misunderstanding of information. The value of group work is in the exchange process. Group members must listen, share, evaluate, help, support, reinforce, discuss, and debate to promote learning. There is truth in the saying "One hand washes the other." Not only do you help the other person when you study together, but you also help yourself.

Application Questions

The application of information demonstrates a higher level of understanding than just knowing or comprehending data because it requires the learner to show, solve, modify, change, use, or manipulate information in a real situation or presented scenario.

To answer an application question, you must apply concepts you learned previously to a specific situation. The concepts may be theories, technical principles, rules of procedures, generalizations, or ideas that have to be applied in a presented scenario. Application questions test your ability to use information. The making of rational and reflective judgments, which is part of the critical thinking process, results in a course of action.

SAMPLE ITEM 4-7

An older adult's skin looks dry, thin, and fragile. Which should the nurse do when providing back care to this client?

1. Apply a moisturizing body lotion
2. Massage using short, kneading strokes
3. Use soap when washing the client's back
4. Leave excess lubricant on the client's skin

To answer this question, you need to know that dry, thin, fragile skin is common in older adults (knowledge) and that moisturizing lotion helps the skin to retain water and become more supple (comprehension). When presented with this client scenario, you have to apply your knowledge concerning developmental changes in older adults and the consequences of the use of moisturizing lotion (application).

SAMPLE ITEM 4-8

A nurse is caring for several clients on bladder-retraining programs, and a variety of toileting time frames are employed. Which time frame for toileting is always included in a toileting schedule?

1. Every 2 hours when awake
2. When going to bed at night
3. At 8 a.m., 2 p.m., 8 p.m., and 2 a.m.
4. Every few hours including through the night

To answer this question, you need to know the principle that nursing care should be individualized (knowledge). You also must understand the commonalities within the procedure of bladder retraining (comprehension). When presented with this concrete situation, you have to apply your knowledge about client-centered care and the theoretical components of bladder-retraining programs (application).

SAMPLE ITEM 4-9

A client asks the nurse for help in moving higher in bed. Which should the nurse do to prevent self-injury?

1. Keep the knees and ankles straight
2. Straighten the knees while bending at the waist
3. Place the feet together and keep the knees bent
4. Position the feet apart with one foot placed forward

To answer this question, you need to know (knowledge) and understand (comprehension) the principles of body mechanics. You also need to apply these principles in a particular client-care situation, moving a client higher in bed (application).

STUDY TECHNIQUES TO INCREASE YOUR ABILITY TO APPLY INFORMATION

RELATE NEW INFORMATION TO PRIOR LEARNING: Learning is easier when the information to be learned is associated with what you already know. Therefore, relate new information to your foundation of knowledge, experience, attitudes, and feelings. For example, when studying the principles of body mechanics, review which principles are used when you carry a heavy package, move from a reclining to a standing position, or assist an older person in walking up a flight of stairs. When studying the principles of surgical asepsis, recall and review various situations when you performed sterile technique, and identify the principles that were the foundation of your actions. Applying concepts, such as principles and theories, in actual situations reinforces your ability to use them in future circumstances.

Make it simple. Make it visible. Consider that blood vessels are flexible tubes that can constrict in response to chemical releases from inside or outside (hormones such as adrenaline from inside, medications from outside). This will increase the pressure inside (hypertension) as if you were running water through a small hose, instead of through a large one. The pressure inside can also be increased by adding to the volume of fluids within the tubes (IV fluid bolus). In addition, any injury to the tube (a bleeding wound) will release some of the fluid and reduce the pressure at which the fluid flows inside the tube.

IDENTIFY COMMONALITIES: A commonality exists when two different situations require the application of the same or similar principles. For example, when studying the principle of gravity, you must understand that it is the force that draws all mass in the earth's sphere toward the center of the earth. Now try to identify situations that employ this principle. As a nurse, you apply this principle when you place a urine collection bag below the level of the bladder, hang an IV bag higher than the IV insertion site, raise the head of the bed for a person with dyspnea, and elevate the legs of a person with edema of the feet. This study technique is particularly effective when working in small groups because it involves brainstorming. Others in the group may identify situations that you have not considered. Identifying commonalities reinforces information and maximizes the application of information in client-care situations.

Analysis Questions

Analysis questions require you to interpret a variety of data and recognize the commonalities, differences, and interrelationships among presented ideas. To answer an analysis question, you must identify, examine, dissect, evaluate, or investigate the organization or structure of the information presented in the question. Analysis questions are based on the assumption that you know, understand, and can apply information. They then require the ability to examine information, which is a higher thought process than knowing, understanding, or applying information. For example, when studying blood pressure, you first memorize the parameters of a normal blood pressure level (knowledge). Next, you develop an understanding of what factors influence and produce a normal blood pressure reading (comprehension). Then you identify a particular situation that necessitates obtaining a blood pressure reading (application). Finally, you differentiate among a variety of situations and determine which has the highest priority for assessing the blood pressure (analysis). Analysis questions are difficult because they demand scrutiny of a variety of complex data presented in the stem and options and require a higher-level critical thinking process. For each possible response, ask yourself, "Where does this not make sense?"

SAMPLE ITEM 4-10

A client with obesity has dependent edema of the ankles and feet. Which diet should the nurse expect the primary health-care provider to prescribe?

1. Low in sodium and high in fat
2. Low in sodium and low in calories
3. High in sodium and high in protein
4. High in sodium and low in carbohydrates

To answer this question, you need to know and understand the relationships between salt in the diet and fluid retention and between obesity and caloric intake (comprehension). You must also understand the impact of carbohydrates, proteins, and fats in a diet for a client with edema and obesity (comprehension). When you answer this question, you must examine the information presented, identify the interrelationships among the elements, and arrive at a conclusion (analysis).

SAMPLE ITEM 4-11

A client who is undergoing cancer chemotherapy says to the nurse, "This is no way to live." Which response uses the reflective technique?
1. "Tell me more about what you are thinking."
2. "You sound discouraged today."
3. "Life is not worth living?"
4. "What are you saying?"

To answer this question, you need to know and understand the communication techniques of reflection, clarification, and paraphrasing (knowledge and comprehension). Also, you must analyze each statement and identify the communication technique being used. This question requires you to differentiate information presented in the four options to arrive at the correct answer.

SAMPLE ITEM 4-12

A nurse is assessing a client who reports being incontinent. Which question should the nurse ask to elicit information related to urge incontinence?
1. "Does urination occur immediately after coughing?"
2. "Do you urinate small amounts of urine frequently?"
3. "Do you begin urinating immediately after feeling the need to urinate?"
4. "Does urination occur at predictable intervals without feeling the need to urinate?"

To answer this question, you must recall and understand the characteristics associated with the various types of incontinence (e.g., stress, functional, urge, and reflex). This step uses the thinking processes of knowledge and comprehension. Next, you must identify which type of incontinence is related to the information that is elicited by each question indicated in the options 1 through 4. This step uses the thinking process of application. Finally, you must differentiate among the questions in the four options to identify the one that relates to urge incontinence and arrive at the correct answer. This last step uses the thinking process of analysis.

STUDY TECHNIQUES TO INCREASE YOUR ABILITY TO ANALYZE INFORMATION

IDENTIFY DIFFERENCES: To study for complex questions, you cannot just memorize and understand facts or identify the commonalities among them; you must also learn to discriminate. Analysis questions often require you to use differentiation to determine the significance of information. When studying about increased blood pressure levels, identify the different causes and why they may increase blood pressure. Blood pressure can increase for a variety of reasons: Infection increases metabolic rate; fluid retention causes hypervolemia; and anxiety causes an autonomic nervous system response that constricts blood vessels. In each situation, blood pressure increases, but for a different reason. Identifying differences is an effective study technique to broaden the interrelationship and significance of learned information.

PRACTICE TEST TAKING: Taking practice tests is an excellent way to improve the effectiveness of your learning. Reviewing rationales for the right and wrong answers serves as an effective study technique. It reinforces learning, and it can help you identify areas that require additional study.

As you practice test taking, not only do you increase your knowledge, but you also become more emotionally and physically comfortable in a simulated testing situation. This practice is most effective if you gradually increase the time you spend taking tests to 2 to 3 hours. This will help build stamina, enabling you to concentrate more effectively during both short-term and long-term tests. Marathon runners have long recognized the value of building stamina and the need for practice to achieve a "groove" that enhances performance. Marathon runners also manage their practice so that they "peak" on the day of the big event. The same principles can be applied to the nursing student preparing for an important test. You are at your peak and can achieve a groove when you feel physically, emotionally, and intellectually ready for the important test.

Practicing test taking can assist you in the following areas:

- Acquiring new knowledge
- Comprehending information
- Understanding concepts
- Identifying rationales for nursing interventions
- Applying theories and principles
- Identifying commonalities and differences in situations
- Analyzing information
- Reinforcing previous learning
- Applying critical thinking

In addition, practicing test taking should assist you in the following:

- Using test-taking techniques
- Effectively managing time during a test
- Controlling your environment
- Controlling physical and emotional responses
- Feeling empowered and in control
- Developing a positive mental attitude

SUMMARY

Learning takes place in the learner. However, this does not occur without work. General study techniques and specific study techniques related to the cognitive levels of nursing practice should be employed routinely before taking a nursing examination. Use of these techniques will help you to learn, retain, and apply more information when confronted with a nursing test item. When you increase your depth and breadth of nursing information, you will increase your score on nursing examinations.

ANSWERS AND RATIONALES FOR SAMPLE ITEMS IN CHAPTER 4

4-1 1. Secondary prevention refers to strategies for the care of people in whom disease is present. The goal is to halt or reverse the disease process.
2. There is no category called morbidity prevention. The word *morbidity* refers to illness; *mortality* refers to death.
3. Primary prevention refers to strategies used to prevent illness in people who are considered free from disease.
4. Tertiary prevention uses strategies to help people adapt physically, psychologically, and socially to permanent disabilities.

4-2 **1. Cleaning the hands removes microorganisms that can contaminate clean linen. Washing the hands or using a hand sanitizer is referred to as *hand hygiene*.**
2. Pulling the curtain is unnecessary when making an unoccupied bed; this is required to provide privacy when making an occupied bed.
3. Collecting clean linen is done after the hands are cleaned to prevent contamination of the linen.
4. Placement of the bottom sheet is done after the hands have been cleaned and the clean sheets have been collected.

4-3 1. 50 to 65 beats per minute is less than the expected range for the pulse of an adult.
2. 70 to 85 beats per minute is within the expected range of 60 to 100 beats per minute for the pulse of an adult.
3. Although 90 beats per minute is at the high end of the expected range for the pulse of an adult, 105 beats per minute is above the expected range.
4. 110 to 125 beats per minute is above the expected range for the pulse of an adult.

4-4 1. Diuretics, not cathartics, produce an increase in urinary output.
2. Antianxiety agents (anxiolytics) reduce anxiety.
3. Cathartics stimulate bowel evacuation; therefore, the client should be assessed for a bowel movement.
4. Analgesics, not cathartics, alter the perception and interpretation of pain.

4-5 1. Paraphrasing, also called *restating*, is an interviewing skill that repeats the client's basic message in similar words to encourage additional communication.
2. Restating, also called *paraphrasing*, is a technique that repeats the client's basic message in similar words to promote further communication.
3. Clarification is a method of verifying that the client's message is understood as intended; it is an attempt to obtain more information without interpreting the original statement.
4. Reviewing involves summarizing the main points in a discussion; this is useful at the end of an interview or teaching session.

4-6 1. Using sterile equipment and sterile technique, not massaging the needle insertion site, limits infection.
2. Removing the needle along the line of insertion limits trauma, which prevents bleeding.
3. Instilling the solution slowly and removing the needle along the line of insertion reduce discomfort.
4. Massage disperses the medication in the tissues and facilitates its absorption.

4-7 **1. Moisturizing lotion limits dryness and reduces the friction of the hands against the skin, which prevents skin trauma.**
2. Massaging with short, kneading strokes can injure delicate, thin skin; light, long strokes should be used.
3. Soap should be avoided because it can further dry the skin.
4. Excess lubricant on the skin may promote skin maceration and also provides a warm, moist environment for the growth of microorganisms that should be avoided.

4-8 1. Toileting a client every 2 hours when awake may not be appropriate for everyone; some clients may need to be toileted every hour, and others may require toileting every 3 hours. The schedule should be individualized.
2. All clients, regardless of the specifics of each individual's bladder-retraining program, will be toileted before going to bed at night and after awakening in the morning.
3. Toileting four times a day is too infrequent when implementing a bladder-retraining program.
4. Every few hours is a nonspecific time frame. It may not be necessary to awaken the client every few hours during the night because this may interfere with the client's sleep.

4-9
1. Keeping the knees and ankles straight causes strain on the muscles of the back and should be avoided.
2. When clients are moved, the nurse's knees should be flexed, not straight, and the knees and hips should be flexed, not the waist; these actions use the large muscles of the legs rather than the back.
3. Keeping the feet together produces a narrow base of support that can result in a fall.
4. **Both actions provide a wide base of support that promotes stability; placing one foot in front of the other facilitates bending at the knees, which permits the muscles of the legs, rather than the back, to bear the client's weight.**

4-10
1. Although a low-sodium diet is appropriate to limit edema, a diet high in fat should be avoided by an obese individual because fats are high in calories.
2. **Sodium promotes fluid retention, and increased calories add to body weight; therefore, both should be avoided by a client with obesity and edema.**
3. Sodium promotes fluid retention and should be avoided by a client with edema; protein may or may not be related to this client's problem.
4. Although carbohydrates may be restricted in an obese individual to facilitate weight loss, a high-sodium diet promotes fluid retention and should be avoided.

4-11
1. This response uses the technique of clarification and asks the client to expand on the message so that it becomes more understandable.
2. **This response uses a reflective technique because it attempts to identify feelings in the client's message.**
3. This response uses the technique of paraphrasing; it restates the client's basic message in similar words.
4. This response uses the communication technique of clarification. When this technique is used, the nurse is attempting to better understand what the client is saying.

4-12
1. This option is related to stress incontinence. Stress incontinence occurs when intra-abdominal pressure increases (e.g., with coughing, laughing).
2. This option is related to overflow incontinence. Overflow incontinence occurs when there is an involuntary passage of urine related to an overdistended bladder.
3. **Urge incontinence is associated with a sudden desire to void. Urge incontinence is related to decreased bladder capacity and bladder irritation.**
4. This option is related to reflex incontinence. Reflex incontinence is the involuntary passage of urine at somewhat predictable intervals. It is associated with an inability to sense the urge to void or that the bladder is full.

5 The Multiple-Choice Question

In our society, success is generally measured in relation to levels of achievement. Before you entered a formal institution of learning, your achievement was subjectively appraised by your family and friends. Success was rewarded by smiles, positive statements, and perhaps favors or gifts. Lack of achievement or failure was acknowledged by omission of recognition, verbal corrections, and possibly punishment or scorn. When you entered school, your performance was directly measured against acceptable standards. In an effort to eliminate subjectivity, you were exposed to objective testing. These tests included true/false questions, matching columns, and multiple-choice questions. Achievement was reflected by numerical or letter grades. By themselves, these grades provided rewards and punishments.

In nursing education, achievement can be assessed in a variety of ways: a client's physiological response (Did the client's condition improve?), a client's verbal response (Did the client express improvement?), student nurses' clinical performance (Did the students do what they were supposed to do?), and student nurses' levels of cognitive competency (Did the students know what they were supposed to know?). You must pass the National Council Licensure Examination known as NCLEX-PN® to work legally as a licensed practical nurse or the NCLEX-RN® to work legally as a registered nurse. These examinations consist of multiple-choice and alternate-format items. Consequently, both types of questions frequently are used in schools of nursing to evaluate students' progress throughout the curriculum and to familiarize the students with these formats. They also are used because they are objective, are time efficient, and can comprehensively assess understanding of curriculum content that has depth and breadth. Therefore, it is important for you to understand the components and dynamics of multiple-choice and alternate-format items early in your nursing education. Only multiple-choice questions are addressed in this chapter.

In the spring of 2003, alternate-format items were introduced in nursing licensure examinations. **Alternate-format items** require the test taker to select multiple answers to a multiple-choice question, perform a calculation and fill in the blank, place options in priority order, or respond to a question in relation to an exhibit. As noted in Chapter 8, another new innovation in test question formats will be included in the NCLEX® test, beginning in 2023. These will be questions that allow the test taker to demonstrate clinical judgment. For more information, refer to the National Council of State Boards of Nursing (NCSBN) Web site (https://www.ncsbn.org/ngn-resources.htm). Chapter 8 includes examples of clinical judgment questions. For these and other examples of alternate-format items, review Chapter 8, "Testing Formats Other Than Multiple-Choice Questions."

COMPONENTS OF A MULTIPLE-CHOICE QUESTION

A multiple-choice question is an objective test item. It asks a question and presents three or more potential answers. The test taker must pay careful attention to the instructions at the end of the question. In bold font, the instructions may say, **Select two,** or **Select all that apply.** If neither of these additional instructions is present, the test taker will select just one answer. The entire multiple-choice question is called an ***item***. Each item consists of two parts. The first part is known as the ***stem***. The stem is the statement that asks the question. The second part contains the possible responses, which are called ***options***. One (and sometimes more than one, as previously noted) of the options answers the question posed in the stem and is the **correct answer** or **answers.** The remaining options are the incorrect answers and are called ***distractors***. They are referred to as *distractors* because they are designed to distract you from the correct answer.

For all sample items presented in this chapter, the correct answers and the rationales for all the options appear at the end of the chapter. Test yourself and see whether you can correctly answer the sample items.

SAMPLE ITEM 5-1

Which should the nurse do immediately before performing any procedure? (STEM)
1. Shut the door (DISTRACTOR)
2. Wash the hands (CORRECT ANSWER)
3. Close the curtain (DISTRACTOR)
4. Drape the client (DISTRACTOR)

SAMPLE ITEM 5-2

A nurse is assessing placement of a nasogastric tube. Where should the distal end of the tube be within the body? (STEM)
1. Trachea (DISTRACTOR)
2. Bronchi (DISTRACTOR)
3. Stomach (CORRECT ANSWER)
4. Duodenum (DISTRACTOR)

SAMPLE ITEM 5-3

A parent says to the nurse, "My kid is difficult to get along with and is only concerned about the opinions of friends." How old is the child? (STEM)
1. 3 years old (DISTRACTOR)
2. 7 years old (DISTRACTOR)
3. 14 years old (CORRECT ANSWER)
4. 22 years old (DISTRACTOR)

SAMPLE ITEM 5-4

When providing contraceptive counseling to a woman, which of the following factors should the nurse consider? **Select all that apply.** (STEM)
1. Age (CORRECT ANSWER)
2. Obstetric history (CORRECT ANSWER)
3. Religious beliefs (CORRECT ANSWER)
4. Employment (DISTRACTOR)
5. Body structure (DISTRACTOR)

Adapted from Irland, 2021.

THE STEM

The stem is the initial part of a multiple-choice item. The purpose of the stem is to present the problem in a clear and concise manner. The stem should contain all the details necessary to answer the question.

The stem of an item can be a complete sentence that asks a question. It also can be an incomplete sentence that becomes a complete sentence when it is combined with one of the options of the item.

In addition to sentence structure, a characteristic of a stem that must be considered is its polarity. The polarity of the stem can have either a positive or negative context. A stem with positive polarity asks the question in relation to what is true, whereas a stem with negative polarity asks the question in relation to what is false.

The Stem That Is a Complete Sentence

A complete sentence is a group of words that can stand independently. When a stem is a complete sentence, it asks a question and ends with a question mark (?). It should clearly and concisely formulate a problem that can be answered before you read the options.

SAMPLE ITEM 5-5

Which should be the first action of the nurse when a fire alarm rings in a health-care facility?
1. Determine if it is a fire drill or a real fire
2. Move clients laterally toward the stairs
3. Take an extinguisher to the fire scene
4. Close doors on the unit

SAMPLE ITEM 5-6

Which is the most common reason why older adults become incontinent of urine?
1. They use incontinence to manipulate others.
2. Their muscles that control urination become weak.
3. They tend to drink less fluid than younger clients.
4. Their increase in weight places pressure on the bladder.

SAMPLE ITEM 5-7

Which part of the body requires special hygiene when a client has a nasogastric feeding tube?
1. Rectum
2. Abdomen
3. Oral cavity
4. Perineal area

The Stem That Is an Incomplete Sentence

When a stem is an incomplete sentence, it is a group of words that forms the beginning portion of a sentence. The sentence becomes complete when it is combined with any of the options in the item. Some items will have a colon at the end of the stem, and others will not. Some options will end with a period, and others will not. Whether there is a colon or period or not, each option should complete the sentence with grammatical accuracy. However, the answer is the only option (or options) that correctly completes the sentence in relation to the informational content. When the stem is an incomplete sentence, you must read the options before you can answer the question. The items that follow are included here in case you are challenged with a question that has an incomplete sentence for a stem.

SAMPLE ITEM 5-8

To best understand what a client is saying, the nurse should:
1. listen carefully.
2. employ touch.
3. show interest.
4. remain silent.

SAMPLE ITEM 5-09

The most important reason why nurses should teach people not to smoke in bed is because it can:
1. upset a family member.
2. precipitate lung cancer.
3. trigger a smoke alarm.
4. result in a fire.

SAMPLE ITEM 5-10

When helping a client with dementia to groom the hair, the nurse should:
1. alternate using a brush and a comb.
2. set time aside for a long teaching session.
3. offer constant support and encouragement.
4. teach how to apply a moisturizer before brushing.

The Stem With Positive Polarity

A stem with positive polarity is concerned with the truth. It asks a question with a positive statement. The correct answer is accurately related to the statement. It is in accord with a fact or principle, or it is an action that should be implemented. A positively worded stem determines whether you can understand, apply, or differentiate correct information.

SAMPLE ITEM 5-11

An older adult who is dying starts to cry and says, "I was always concerned about myself first, and I hurt many people during my life." Which is the underlying feeling being expressed by the client?
1. Ambivalence
2. Sadness
3. Anger
4. Guilt

SAMPLE ITEM 5-12

Which intervention **most** accurately supports the concept of informed consent for a surgical procedure?
1. Explaining what is being done and why
2. Involving the family in the teaching plan
3. Obtaining the client's signature on the document
4. Teaching preoperative deep breathing and coughing

SAMPLE ITEM 5-13

Which should the nurse do when a client appears to be asleep but does not react when called by name?
1. Loudly say, "Are you awake?"
2. Say to the client, "Can you squeeze my hand?"
3. Inform the nurse manager in charge immediately.
4. Gently touch the client's arm while saying the client's name.

The Stem With Negative Polarity

A stem with negative polarity is concerned with what is false. The question is posed as a negative statement. The stem usually incorporates words such as *except*, *not*, or *never*. These words are obvious. However, sometimes the words used are more obscure, for example, *contraindicated*, *further*, *unacceptable*, *least*, and *avoid*. When a negative term is used, it may be emphasized by an underline (e.g., except), italic font (e.g., *least*), boldface type (e.g., **not**), or capitals (e.g., NEVER). A negatively worded stem requires you to recognize exceptions, detect errors, or identify interventions that are unacceptable or contraindicated. Many nursing examinations do not have questions with negative polarity or do not emphasize negative words used in a stem. However, this information is included here in the event you are challenged by questions with negative polarity.

SAMPLE ITEM 5-14

On what part of the body should the nurse avoid using soap when bathing a client?
1. Eyes
2. Back
3. Under the breasts
4. Glans of the penis

SAMPLE ITEM 5-15

The nurse determines that range-of-motion (ROM) exercises should NOT be done:
1. for comatose clients.
2. on limbs that are paralyzed.
3. beyond the point of resistance.
4. for clients with chronic joint disease.

SAMPLE ITEM 5-16

Which suggestion by the nurse is not therapeutic when teaching the client about promoting personal energy?
1. Eat breakfast every day.
2. Exercise three times a week.
3. Get adequate sleep each night.
4. Drink a cup of coffee each morning.

SAMPLE ITEM 5-17

Which position is contraindicated for a client who has dyspnea?
1. Fowler
2. Supine
3. Contour
4. Orthopneic

A question with negative polarity might also be worded as follows:

SAMPLE ITEM 5-18

The nurse is orienting a certified nursing assistant (CNA) and observes the CNA bathing a client. Which of the following actions by the CNA requires follow-up?
1. Uncovering the area being washed
2. Using long, firm strokes toward the heart
3. Washing from the rectum toward the pubis
4. Replacing the top sheets with a cotton blanket

THE OPTIONS

As noted previously, all of the answers presented within an item are called *options*. When just one option is expected, just one of the options is the *best* response and is therefore the correct answer. Obviously, a question that asks the test taker to **Select two,** or **Select all that apply,** will include more than one correct option. The other options are incorrect and distract you from selecting the correct answer. Incorrect options are called *distractors*. These options may seem like they could apply, or could apply in specific situations. The test taker must not overthink the stem, however, and unless a unique situation is given, select the most generally appropriate response. A multiple-choice item must have a minimum of three options, but the actual number varies among tests. The typical number of options is four, which reduces the probability of guessing the correct answer while limiting the amount of reading to a sensible level. Options usually are listed by numbers (1, 2, 3, and 4), lowercase letters (a, b, c, and d), or uppercase letters (A, B, C, and D). The options appear in four grammatical formats. An option can be a sentence, it can complete the sentence begun in the stem, it can be an incomplete sentence, or it can be a single word.

The Option That Is a Sentence

A sentence is a unit of language that contains a stated or implied subject and verb. It is a statement that contains an entire thought and stands alone. Options can appear as complete sentences. Some tests have a period at the end of these options, and others do not. Whether there is a period or not, each option should be grammatically correct. When the option is a verbal response, it should incorporate the appropriate punctuation, such as quotation marks (“ ”), a comma (,), an exclamation point (!), a question mark (?), or a period (.).

SAMPLE ITEM 5-19

Which should the nurse do first before performing a procedure?
1. Raise the bed to its highest position for the procedure
2. Collect the equipment for the procedure
3. Position the client for the procedure
4. Explain the reason for the procedure

SAMPLE ITEM 5-20

A client who is Catholic tells the nurse, "Before being hospitalized, I went to mass and received Communion every morning." Which should the nurse do to meet this client's spiritual needs?
1. Encourage the client to say the rosary every day
2. Make arrangements for the client to receive Communion
3. Transfer the client to a room with another client who is Catholic
4. Have a priest administer the sacrament of Anointing of the Sick to the client

SAMPLE ITEM 5-21

A male client is crying, and the only word the nurse understands is "wife." Which should the nurse say?
1. "I'm sure that your wife is fine."
2. "You are concerned about your wife?"
3. "What did your wife do to upset you?"
4. "Your wife will be visiting later today."

The Option That Completes the Sentence Begun in the Stem

When an option completes the sentence begun in the stem, the stem and the option together should form a sentence. Some tests have correct punctuation at the end of these options, and others do not. Regardless of whether there is a period, each option should complete the stem in a manner that is grammatically accurate.

SAMPLE ITEM 5-22

A nurse understands that the primary etiology of obesity is a:
1. lack of balance in the variety of nutrients.
2. glandular disorder that prevents weight loss.
3. caloric intake that exceeds metabolic needs.
4. psychological problem that causes overeating.

SAMPLE ITEM 5-23

A nurse can best prevent the client from getting a chill during a bed bath by:
1. exposing only the area being washed.
2. giving a hot drink before the bath.
3. pulling the curtain around the bed.
4. rubbing the skin briskly.

SAMPLE ITEM 5-24

A nurse offers to assist a client with a bed bath. However, the client has just returned from a diagnostic test, is in pain, and refuses the bath. The nurse should:
1. encourage a shower instead.
2. give a partial bath quickly.
3. cancel the bath for today.
4. delay the bath until later.

The Option That Is an Incomplete Sentence

When an option is an incomplete sentence, it does not contain all the parts of speech (i.e., subject and verb) necessary to construct a complete, autonomous statement. The option that is an incomplete sentence usually is a phrase or group of related words. Although not a complete sentence, it conveys a unit of thought, an idea, or a concept.

SAMPLE ITEM 5-25

Which nursing intervention is common when caring for all clients with infections?
1. Donning a mask
2. Wearing a gown
3. Washing the hands
4. Discouraging visitors

SAMPLE ITEM 5-26

When should the nurse administer mouth care to an unconscious client?
1. Whenever necessary
2. Every four hours
3. Once a shift
4. Twice a day

SAMPLE ITEM 5-27

Which action by the nurse helps meet a client's basic need for security and safety?
1. Addressing a client by name
2. Accepting a client's angry behavior
3. Ensuring a client gets adequate nutrition
4. Explaining to a client what is going to be done

The Option That Is a Word

A word is a series of letters that form a term. It is the most basic unit of language and is capable of communicating a message. The option that is a single word can be almost any part of speech (e.g., noun, pronoun, verb, or adverb) as long as it conveys information.

SAMPLE ITEM 5-28

Which is a primary source for obtaining information related to the independent functions of a nurse?
1. Chart
2. Client
3. Nurse
4. Surgeon

SAMPLE ITEM 5-29

A hospitalized client is told that a significant other has died. The client reacts with loud crying and anguished verbal responses. Which approach should be used by the nurse when caring for this grieving client?

1. Confronting
2. Supporting
3. Avoiding
4. Limiting

SAMPLE ITEM 5-30

What is the nurse doing when coming to a conclusion based on a cluster of data that are significant?

1. Planning
2. Assessing
3. Analyzing
4. Implementing

SAMPLE ITEM 5-31

A nurse is performing passive range of motion for a client whose right upper and lower extremities are paralyzed. Which range-of-motion exercise is being used when the nurse moves the client's arm so that the forearm almost touches the upper arm?

1. Flexion
2. Extension
3. Supination
4. Abduction

SUMMARY

Multiple-choice questions generally make up many of the questions on nursing examinations. A multiple-choice question consists of a statement that asks a question (stem) and gives a minimum of three potential answers (options). Of these options, unless the instructions after the stem indicate **Select two, Select all that apply,** or any other number, only one option answers the question raised in the stem (correct answer) and the other options are incorrect answers (distractors). In multiple-choice items, stems and options can be presented in a variety of ways. Being familiar with these variations before taking a test will allow you to focus on the content of the test item rather than its format, increasing your test-taking ability.

ANSWERS AND RATIONALES FOR SAMPLE ITEMS IN CHAPTER 5

5-1 1. Shutting the door should be done before washing the hands. The hands become contaminated when the door is touched.
2. **Before touching the client, the nurse should wash his or her hands to remove microorganisms.**
3. Closing the curtain should be done before washing the hands. Curtains are considered contaminated.
4. Draping the client is done after washing the hands.

5-2 1. The trachea is a passage between the posterior nasopharynx and the bronchi and is part of the respiratory system.
2. The bronchi are passages between the trachea and the bronchioles and are part of the respiratory system.
3. **The tube enters the nose, passes through the posterior nasopharynx and esophagus, and enters the stomach through the cardiac sphincter.**
4. The duodenum is distal to the stomach and is the first portion of the small intestine; a nasogastric tube is designed to be advanced into the stomach, not the duodenum.

5-3 1. Toddlers are concerned about themselves and their autonomy, not others.
2. School-age children are easy to get along with and are concerned about performing and achieving.
3. **Adolescents are concerned about their identity, independence, and peer relationships; this causes tension between them and their parents.**
4. Young adults are developing intimate relationships and becoming socially responsible.

5-4 1. **Age must be considered in the recommendation for contraception. Birth control pills containing estrogen should not be recommended to women 35 years of age and older, as ongoing exposure to estrogen may increase the risk of stroke and thrombosis in this age group.**
2. **If a client states that she feels she has completed her family, she may be interested in a permanent family planning method.**
3. **A client's religious beliefs may rule out any method other than a natural family planning method.**
4. A client's employment has nothing to do with contraception.
5. A client's body structure does not affect recommendations for contraception.

5-5 1. Whenever the fire alarm rings, it should be considered an indication of a real fire.
2. Clients should be moved only if they are in danger.
3. The location of the fire must be identified before an extinguisher can be taken to the scene.
4. **Of the options provided, closing the doors on the unit should be the initial action. A closed door provides safety because it is a barrier that impedes the spread of the fire.**

5-6 1. This is untrue; most people want to be independent and in control of their bodily functions.
2. **Muscles, particularly the perineal muscles, tend to lose strength as people age.**
3. Incontinence is unrelated to fluid intake.
4. Older adults do not necessarily gain weight; many lose weight because of the loss of subcutaneous fat associated with aging. Body weight does not influence incontinence.

5-7 1. A nasogastric tube is unrelated to the rectum. Special care of this area of the body is unnecessary; care provided during a routine bed bath is adequate.
2. A nasogastric tube enters the body through the nose, not the abdomen. Cleansing of the abdomen during a routine bed bath is adequate.
3. **A nasogastric tube feeding generally negates the need to chew; with lack of chewing, salivation decreases, which causes the mucous membranes to become dry.**
4. The perineal area is unrelated to a nasogastric tube. Bathing of the perineal area during a routine bed bath is adequate.

5-8 1. **Attentive listening is important so that the nurse can pick up key words and identify emotional themes within the message.**
2. Touch is used to communicate a message of caring, not to receive, understand, or interpret a message from another person.
3. Although showing interest may indicate acceptance and encourage expression of feelings, it does nothing to promote understanding by the nurse.

4. Although remaining silent may encourage further communication, it will not by itself promote understanding of the client's message.

5-9
1. Although smoking can physically and emotionally disturb a family member, this is not the priority.
2. Although smoking may precipitate lung cancer, this is not the reason for not smoking in bed.
3. Smoke from a cigarette will not trigger a smoke alarm.
4. **Sleepy, confused, weak, or lethargic individuals may drop lighted cigarettes or ashes, which can ignite bed linens.**

5-10
1. Alternating a brush and a comb may promote confusion; people with dementia need consistency.
2. People with dementia cannot concentrate long enough for a prolonged teaching session; learning occurs best with short, frequent teaching sessions.
3. **People with dementia become confused easily and need support and encouragement to stay focused and motivated.**
4. Learning involves cognitive and psychomotor skills that a person with dementia probably does not possess.

5-11
1. Ambivalence demonstrates two simultaneous conflicting feelings. The client is expressing one feeling, not two.
2. Although the client may be unhappy about past behaviors, it is the underlying thoughts about hurting others that precipitated the client's statement.
3. Anger is a feeling of displeasure caused by opposition or mistreatment; it is demonstrated when a client uses words or gestures in an attempt to fight back at the cause of the feeling.
4. **Guilt is a painful feeling of self-reproach resulting from the belief that one has done something wrong.**

5-12
1. **It is the surgeon's responsibility to explain what is going to be done and the potential negative and positive consequences (risks and benefits). This ensures that the client is making a decision based on accurate information.**
2. Although the family may be involved, it is the client who must sign the informed consent form.
3. Although the client's signature on the informed consent form gives the surgeon permission to do the surgery, the signature alone does not indicate that the client understands what will be done and why. Some clients waive the right to know details about the surgery.
4. Preoperative teaching is necessary only when the client consents to surgery. Signing an informed consent form is not necessary to perform client teaching.

5-13
1. Speaking loudly may frighten the client; one of the other senses should be stimulated because there was no client response to a previous verbal intervention.
2. The nurse must get the client's attention before giving a direction.
3. The nurse should assess the client further before informing the nurse in charge.
4. **These actions are necessary. These actions are part of the first step to further assess this client. Touch and sound stimulate two senses, and using the client's name is individualizing care.**

5-14
1. **Soaps usually contain sodium or potassium salts of fatty acids, which are irritating and can injure the sensitive tissues of the eyes.**
2. The back needs soap and water to remove perspiration that collects on the skin.
3. Body surface areas that touch are dark, warm, and moist and must be washed with soap and water to limit the growth of microorganisms.
4. The glans of the penis needs soap and water to remove perspiration, urine, and smegma.

5-15
1. Range of motion should be performed for unconscious clients because they usually are immobile and are at risk for developing contractures.
2. Paralyzed limbs must be moved through the full range of motion by the nurse to prevent loss of range secondary to inactivity.
3. **Resistance indicates that there is strain on the muscles or joints; continuing range of motion beyond the point of resistance can cause injury and should be avoided.**

4. People with chronic joint disease usually need gentle range-of-motion exercises to keep the joints mobile.

5-16 1. Food contains nutrients and calories, which provide energy.
2. Exercise promotes muscle tone and energy.
3. Sleep is restful and restorative.
4. **Caffeine, although a stimulant, can be harmful to the body.**

5-17 1. When in a Fowler position, the diaphragm moves toward the abdominal cavity during inspiration with minimal pressure of the abdominal organs against the diaphragm; this allows for maximal thoracic expansion.
2. **When in the supine position the abdominal contents press against the diaphragm, which impedes expansion of the thoracic cavity and subsequently the lungs.**
3. The contour position is desirable because the abdominal contents drop by gravity, permitting efficient contraction of the diaphragm and expansion of the thoracic cavity.
4. An upright position with the head higher than the hips (orthopneic position) allows the diaphragm to move toward the abdominal cavity during inspiration with minimal pressure of the abdominal organs against the diaphragm.

5-18 1. Only the area being washed should be exposed to permit adequate bathing and inspection.
2. Using long, firm strokes toward the heart is desirable because it promotes venous return.
3. **This may contaminate the urinary meatus with microorganisms from the perianal area. The preceptor should "follow up" with the CNA and remind him or her kindly, in the moment, of this risk.**
4. Using a cotton blanket is desirable; it absorbs moisture, provides warmth, and promotes privacy.

5-19 1. This may be frightening if the client does not know why the action is being done; also, not every procedure requires that the bed be raised to its highest position.
2. Equipment should be gathered after the client agrees to the procedure.
3. Positioning the client is done immediately before the procedure is performed.
4. **Explaining the procedure meets the client's right to know why and how care will be provided. It should be done before initiating any step of the procedure.**

5-20 1. This focuses on a different ritual and denies the client's concerns about missing mass and not receiving Communion.
2. **This helps to meet the client's spiritual needs and is easily accomplished in a hospital setting.**
3. The nurse should assist the client in meeting spiritual needs. The nurse should not expect another client who is Catholic to assume this role.
4. The sacrament of Anointing of the Sick is a different ritual than attending mass and receiving Communion.

5-21 1. This statement offers false reassurance and draws a conclusion based on insufficient information.
2. **This response encourages further communication, which is necessary to obtain more information about what is upsetting the client.**
3. This is a judgmental statement that is not based on fact.
4. This is not an open-ended question that allows the client to express concerns; this is a statement that may or may not be true.

5-22 1. A lack of balance in nutrients can result in malnutrition, not necessarily obesity; it also can result in weight loss.
2. Although glandular disorders such as hypothyroidism may result in obesity, they are not the primary causes of obesity.
3. **If more calories are ingested than the body requires for energy, they will be converted to adipose tissue, which causes weight gain.**
4. A psychological problem is just one of many factors that influence overeating; it is not the primary cause of obesity.

5-23 1. **Exposing only the area being washed limits the evaporation of fluids on the skin and radiation of heat from the body, which prevents the client from getting a chill.**
2. A hot drink will not prevent a chill.
3. Although this may prevent drafts, it will not prevent the client's getting a chill from the environmental temperature, excessive exposure, or evaporation of water from the skin.

4. Rubbing the skin briskly causes vasodilation, which promotes heat loss.

5-24 1. A shower may be an unsafe activity when a client is in pain. The client has a right to refuse care.
2. This ignores the client's right to refuse care and the fact that the client is in pain.
3. The bath may eventually be canceled, but it should be delayed first.
4. Delaying the bath accepts the client's present refusal to bathe; rest and pain reduction may make the client more amenable to hygienic care later in the day.

5-25 1. Donning a mask is not necessary for Standard Precautions and is not required for all Transmission-Based Precautions.
2. Wearing a gown is not part of Standard Precautions and is not required for all Transmission-Based Precautions.
3. Washing the hands before and after client care and whenever they are contaminated is the most important action for preventing the spread of microorganisms.
4. After visitors have been taught how to use Standard and Transmission-Based Precautions, they are permitted to visit clients with infections.

5-26 **1. Unconscious clients usually have dry mucous membranes of the oral cavity because they frequently breathe through the mouth, are not drinking fluids, and may be receiving oxygen; oral hygiene should be provided at least every 2 hours and more frequently as necessary.**
2. Every 4 hours is too long a period between sessions of oral care for an unconscious client; drying, sores, and lesions of the mucous membranes can occur.
3. Once per shift is too infrequent for providing oral care for an unconscious client.
4. Twice a day is too infrequent for providing oral care for an unconscious client.

5-27 1. Addressing a client by name meets the client's need for self-esteem.
2. Accepting an expression of feelings, including anger, meets the client's self-esteem needs. Limits may be set on feelings that escalate and place the client and/or others in danger.
3. This action meets the client's basic physiological need for adequate nutrients for body processes.
4. Knowing what will happen and why meets the client's security needs; also, this is a client's right. The unknown can be frightening.

5-28 1. The chart is a secondary source; it also contains primary health-care providers' prescriptions, which are dependent functions of the nurse.
2. The primary and most important source for obtaining information referring to a client is the client. The independent functions of the nurse include interventions that relate to human responses, which are identified by direct contact with the client.
3. A nurse is a secondary source; independent functions of the nurse can be performed independently of others.
4. A surgeon is a secondary source of information. The nurse is performing a dependent function when implementing a surgeon's prescription.

5-29 1. A confrontation may take away the client's current coping mechanisms; this may leave the client defenseless.
2. A client who is grieving is using defenses to cope with the crisis; these defenses should be supported.
3. Avoiding the client is a form of abandonment; the nurse should be present to provide support.
4. Setting limits may take away the client's coping mechanisms; this may leave the client defenseless.

5-30 1. Identifying a conclusion is not planning. Planning occurs after the assessment and analysis phases of the nursing process.
2. Assessing involves collecting data, which must be gathered before they can be analyzed and a conclusion made.
3. Data must be clustered and interpreted to identify human responses that indicate potential or actual health problems that can be treated by the nurse; statements that indicate actual or potential health problems treatable by the nurse require analysis and the making of a conclusion.

4. Implementation is putting the plan of care into action, which occurs after assessment, analysis, and planning.

5-31 **1. The elbow is a hinge joint. Flexion occurs when the elbow is bent to move the forearm toward the upper arm and shoulder.**

2. The elbow is a hinge joint. Extension occurs when the elbow is straightened so that the forearm is brought forward and downward, away from the upper arm and shoulder.
3. Supination occurs when the hand and forearm are rotated so that the palm is facing toward the ceiling while the elbow is flexed at a 90° angle.
4. Abduction occurs when the arm is raised laterally with the elbow straight to the side of the head with the palm facing outward.

6 The Nursing Process

Problem solving is a process that provides a framework for identifying solutions to complex problems. It is a step-by-step process that uses a systematic approach. One might say that problem solving is a "blueprint" that can be followed to identify and solve problems. The concept of problem solving is not used exclusively by nurses. It is used by other professionals to find solutions within the context of their job responsibilities. Nurses use the problem-solving process to identify human responses and to plan, implement, and evaluate nursing care. When scientific problem solving is used within the context of nursing, it is known as the *nursing process*, also called *clinical judgment*. The process of clinical judgment includes six steps, very much like the nursing process. Both processes are very similar and overlap with each other. See Chapter 8 for more information on the steps of clinical judgment.

The nursing process contains five steps:

1. Assessment
2. Analysis
3. Planning
4. Implementation
5. Evaluation

The nursing process incorporates critical thinking used by nurses to meet clients' needs, so items on nursing examinations are designed to test the use of this process. Test items are not written haphazardly. They are carefully designed to test your knowledge of a specific concept, skill, theory, or fact from the perspective of one of the five steps of the nursing process. When you read an item, being able to recognize its place within the nursing process should help you identify what the test item is asking. To do this, you must focus on the critical words within the item.

In this chapter, the five steps of the nursing process are explored. Sample items demonstrate item construction relating to each step of this process. Critical words associated with the steps of the nursing process are illustrated within the sample items. Try to identify critical words and variations of critical words within a sample item that indicate activities associated with the step of the nursing process presented in an item. Practice answering the questions. The better you understand the focus of an item, the better you will be at identifying what is being asked and the greater your chances of identifying the correct answer. For all sample items presented in this chapter, the correct answers and the rationales for all options appear at the end of the chapter.

ASSESSMENT

During assessment, data must be accurately collected, verified, and documented. Assessment activities identify the data about the client on which nurses base the subsequent steps of the nursing process. Assessment items are designed to test your knowledge of information, theories, principles, and skills related to appraising a client.

Assessment questions ask you to do the following:

- Obtain vital statistics
- Perform a physical assessment
- Collect specimens
- Identify clinical findings that are objective or subjective

- Identify client communications that are verbal or nonverbal
- Identify clinical findings that are expected (normal) or unexpected (abnormal)
- Use various data collection methods
- Identify sources of data
- Verify critical findings
- Identify commonalities and differences in response to illness
- Document information about assessments

Critical words and phrases that indicate a test item is focused on assessment include **inspect, identify, verify, observe, determine, notify, check, inform, question, verbal and nonverbal, signs and symptoms, stressors, adaptations, responses, clinical findings, clinical manifestations, sources, perceptions,** and **assess.** See whether you can identify variations of these critical words in the sample items in this chapter.

Most testing errors on assessment items occur because options are selected that:

- Collect insufficient data
- Have data that are inaccurately collected
- Use unscientific methods of data collection
- Rely on a secondary source rather than the primary source—the client
- Contain irrelevant data
- Fail to verify data
- Reflect bias or prejudice
- Fail to document data accurately

Collect Data

METHODS OF DATA COLLECTION

Collecting data is the first part of assessment. The nurse collects data through specific methods, such as performing a physical examination, interviewing the client and significant others, and reviewing records.

A **physical examination** includes the assessment techniques of inspection, palpation, auscultation, and percussion. Also, it includes obtaining vital signs and recognizing acceptable and unacceptable parameters of obtained values.

An **interview** collects data using a formal approach (e.g., obtaining a health history) or an informal approach (e.g., exploring feelings while providing other nursing care).

Review of records includes consideration of reports such as laboratory test results, diagnostic procedures, and assessments or consultations by other members of the health-care team.

SAMPLE ITEM 6-1

While making rounds, the nurse finds a client on the floor in the hall. Which should be the nurse's initial response?

1. Inspect the client for injury
2. Transfer the client back to bed
3. Move the client to the closest chair
4. Report the client's condition to the nurse manager

This item tests your ability to recognize that, in an emergency situation, the nurse must first assess (inspect) the condition of the client. This principle is basic to any emergency response by a nurse. Moving a client before an assessment may worsen an injury. This item demonstrates how a basic concept related to assessment can be tested.

SAMPLE ITEM 6-2

When getting a client out of bed, the nurse should:
1. put nonskid socks on the client's feet.
2. determine the strength of the client before the activity.
3. raise the side rail on the opposite side of the client's bed.
4. have the client sit on the side of the bed for a minute before standing.

This item tests your ability to recognize the concept that the nurse must assess a client before implementing care (option 2). The three distractors (options 1, 3, and 4) are all concerned with implementing care. This question also tests your ability to recognize a physical examination as a method of collecting data about the status of a client. If the nurse is already aware of the client's strength before the activity, it would not be necessary to determine the client's strength at this time (option 2). However, the stem does not indicate that the nurse is familiar with this client. As such, the test taker must answer the question as a general rule. A basic rule of client safety is to be aware of the client's abilities before implementing an activity.

SAMPLE ITEM 6-3

Which assessment by the nurse indicates that a client is having difficulty breathing?
1. 18 breaths per minute and inhaled through the mouth
2. 20 breaths per minute and shallow in character
3. 16 breaths per minute and deep in character
4. 28 breaths per minute and noisy

This item tests your ability to identify the option that reflects a respiratory rate and characteristic that are outside expected parameters. To answer this question successfully, you need to know the rate and characteristics of acceptable and unacceptable respirations.

SAMPLE ITEM 6-4

Which should a nurse always do when taking a rectal temperature?
1. Allow self-insertion of the thermometer
2. Position the client on the left side
3. Use an electronic thermometer
4. Lubricate the thermometer

Option 4 identifies what must be done (a critical element) to take a rectal temperature safely. The three distractors may or may not be done when obtaining a rectal temperature. Although this appears to be an implementation question because it involves an action, it is actually an assessment question because it is concerned with collecting information (i.e., rectal temperature).

SAMPLE ITEM 6-5

A nurse is assessing a client's ideal body weight. Which significant factor should be taken into consideration when performing this assessment?
1. Daily intake
2. Body height
3. Clothing size
4. Food preferences

This item tests the understanding that to calculate a client's ideal body weight the nurse must also know his or her height. The ideal body weight reflects the range of weight that is considered appropriate in relation to the client's height. The ideal body weight is the measurement against which the client's present weight is compared to determine if the client is underweight or obese. Although the question does not address these concepts, the nurse also must know the client's age and extent of bone structure.

SOURCES OF DATA

Data can be gathered by different methods as well as from different sources. Sources of data available to the nurse may be primary, secondary, or tertiary. There is only one **primary source**—the client. The client is the most valuable source of information because the data collected are the most current and specific to him or her.

A **secondary source** produces information from someone or something other than the client and is valuable for gathering supplementary information about a client. A family member is a secondary source who can contribute information about the client's likes and dislikes, ethnic and cultural background, changes in behavior, and level of function before and during the health problem. The client's medical record (chart) is another example of a secondary source. It is a legal document containing information on the client's physical, psychosocial, religious, and economic histories and documents the client's physical and emotional responses. Controversy surrounds whether diagnostic test results in a chart represent primary or secondary sources. Although the chart itself is a secondary source, diagnostic test results are direct objective measurements of the client's status and therefore are considered by some health-care professionals to be a primary source. The nurse must remember that the information in a chart is history and does not reflect the current status of the client because people are dynamic and constantly changing.

A **tertiary source** provides information from outside a client's frame of reference. Examples of tertiary sources include textbooks, the nurse's experience, and accepted commonalities among clients with similar physical and emotional responses. The nurse's or other health-care team members' responses to the client are tertiary sources of client data.

SAMPLE ITEM 6-6

From which source is the nurse seeking information when asking a client's wife specific questions about the client's health status before admission?

1. Primary source
2. Tertiary source
3. Subjective source
4. Secondary source

This item tests your ability to identify that a family member is a secondary source of information. Secondary sources provide information that is supplemental to the information collected from the client.

TYPES OF DATA

When a client is assessed, the data collected can be objective or subjective and verbal or nonverbal.

Objective data are measurable assessments. They are collected by nurses when they use sight, touch, smell, or hearing to acquire the information. Examples of objective data include an excoriated perineal area, diaphoresis, the ammonia odor of urine, crackles, and vital signs. **Subjective data** can be collected only when the client shares feelings, perceptions, thoughts, and sensations about a health problem or concern. Examples of subjective data include client statements about pain, shortness of breath, or feeling depressed.

SAMPLE ITEM 6-7

A nurse is performing a physical assessment of a newly admitted client. Which client statement communicates subjective data?
1. "I have sores between my toes."
2. "I dye my hair, but it is really gray."
3. "My joints hurt when I get up in the morning."
4. "My left leg drags on the floor when I am walking."

This item tests your ability to differentiate between subjective and objective data. The nurse should know the types of data collected for the purposes of future clustering and determining their significance. Any information that the client shares regarding feelings, thoughts, and concerns is subjective; the nurse cannot "see" the client's feelings or thoughts. Any information that the nurse verifies using the senses (e.g., vision, hearing, smell, and touch) or via some form of instrumentation (e.g., thermometer, pulse oximetry, laboratory data) is objective; it can be seen like an "object."

Communication can be verbal or nonverbal. **Verbal data** are collected via the spoken or written word. For example, statements made by a client to a nurse are verbal data. **Nonverbal data** are collected via transmission of a message without words. Crying, a fearful facial expression, a client's appearance, and gestures are all examples of nonverbal data.

SAMPLE ITEM 6-8

Which is an example of nonverbal communication?
1. Letter
2. Holding hands
3. Noise by the client
4. Telephone message

This item tests your ability to identify that holding hands is a form of nonverbal communication. Touch, gestures, posture, and facial expressions are examples of nonverbal communication. Nonverbal communication does not use words or sounds.

Verify Data

After data are collected, they must be verified. Information may be confirmed by collecting additional data, questioning prescriptions, obtaining judgments and/or conclusions from other team members when appropriate, and collecting data oneself rather than relying on technology. Verifying data ensures authenticity and accuracy. For example, when a vital statistic is outside the expected range, the nurse must substantiate the results first by collecting the data again and then by collecting additional data to supplement the original information.

SAMPLE ITEM 6-9

A nurse takes a client's blood pressure and records a diastolic pressure of 120 mm Hg. Which should the nurse do first?
1. Notify the primary health-care provider
2. Retake the blood pressure
3. Notify the nurse in charge
4. Take the other vital signs

This item tests your ability to identify that you must verify data when they are unexpectedly outside the acceptable range. Your first action should be to wait 2 minutes and then retake the blood pressure level. An error may have been made when taking the person's initial blood pressure reading.

Document Information About Assessments

The last component of assessment includes the nurse's ability to document information obtained from assessment activities. Sharing vital information about a client is essential to alert members of the health-care team about the client's current status. Communication methods vary (e.g., progress notes, verbal notification, flow sheets); however, they should all be accurate, concise, thorough, current, organized, and confidential.

SAMPLE ITEM 6-10

A client returns to the surgical unit from the postanesthesia care unit after abdominal surgery. In addition to other prescriptions, the surgeon prescribes IV fluids and measurement of intake and output (I&O). Two hours after surgery, the client voids 400 mL of amber urine. What should the nurse do with this information?

1. Report this information to the primary health-care provider
2. Record this amount on the client's intake and output flow sheet
3. Document this information on the client's vital signs flow sheet
4. Communicate this event verbally to the other members of the health-care team

This item tests your knowledge about the necessity of documenting a client's status and on which part of the client's clinical record the information should be placed.

ANALYSIS

Analysis, the second step of the nursing process, is the most difficult component. Analysis requires that data be validated and clustered and that their significance be determined. Analyzing data requires a strong foundation in scientific principles related to nursing theory, social sciences, and physical sciences. You need to know the commonalities and differences in clients' responses to various stresses. You must use reasoning to apply your knowledge and experience when answering analysis items. After the initial analysis of data, sometimes additional data should be collected and analyzed. Only after all the data have been analyzed should a conclusion or nursing diagnosis be made.

Analysis questions ask you to do the following:

- Validate the interrelationship of data
- Cluster data
- Identify clustered data as meaningful
- Interpret validated and clustered data
- Identify when additional data are needed to further validate clustered data
- Formulate conclusions/nursing diagnoses
- Communicate conclusions/nursing diagnoses to others

Critical words within a test item that indicate it is focused on analysis include **valid, organize, categorize, cluster, reexamine, pattern, formulate, nursing diagnosis, reflect, relate, problem, interpret, contribute, relevant, decision, significant, deduction, statement,** and **analysis.** See whether you can identify variations of these critical words in the sample items in this chapter.

Testing errors occur on analysis items when options are selected that:

- Omit data
- Cluster data prematurely
- Formulate a conclusion or make a nursing diagnosis before all significant data have been clustered
- Force a conclusion or nursing diagnosis to fit the signs and symptoms collected

Cluster Data

Clustering data means grouping related information together. Information is more meaningful when its relationship with other data is established. Clustering enables the nurse to organize data; eliminate that which is insignificant, irrelevant, or redundant; and reduce the data into manageable categories. First, data must be organized into general categories, such as physiological, sociocultural, psychological, and spiritual. Data can then be grouped into specific categories. For example, physiological data can be further grouped into categories such as nutrition, mobility, and elimination.

Data can be obvious and easy to cluster or obscure and difficult to cluster. Some data are clustered easily because the information collected is clearly related to only one system of the body. For example, hard stool, a feeling of rectal fullness, and straining on defecation all relate to intestinal elimination. These clinical manifestations are easy to group and lead to the interpretation that the client may be constipated. Other data are more difficult to cluster because the client's clinical manifestations may involve a variety of body systems. A weak, thready pulse; weight loss; hypotension; and dry mucous membranes can be grouped together. At first, this information may not appear to be related because the clinical findings cross several body systems. However, with a thorough analysis, the nurse should conclude that the data are interrelated and indicate that the client may be dehydrated. Established frameworks such as Marjory Gordon's functional health patterns (1994) and Abraham Maslow's hierarchy of needs (1970) (Fig. 6-1) provide structures for organizing and clustering data.

SAMPLE ITEM 6-11

A client had a brain attack (i.e., stroke, cerebrovascular accident) that resulted in paralysis of the right side. When clustering data, the nurse grouped these data: drooling of saliva and slurred speech. Which information is significant to include with these clustered data?

1. Receptive aphasia
2. Inability to ambulate
3. Difficulty swallowing
4. Incontinence of bowel movements

This item tests your ability to cluster clinical findings that indicate a client is at risk for aspiration. Oxygenation is a basic physiological need. A client who is drooling saliva and has slurred speech, right-sided paralysis, and difficulty swallowing is at serious risk for aspiration of material into the respiratory tract. Although the other options are all problems that must be addressed by the nurse, they are not data related to oxygenation and have no significance to this specific cluster.

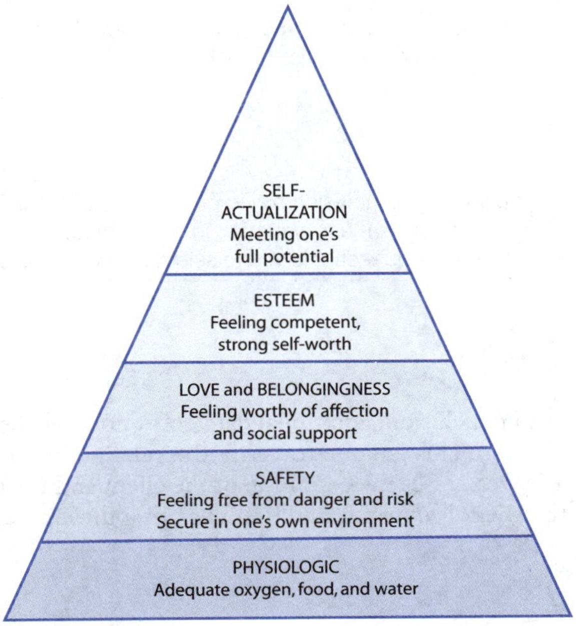

Figure 6–1. Maslow's Hierarchy of Human Needs

SAMPLE ITEM 6-12

Clients with which issue are at risk for developing a pressure ulcer?
1. Are immobilized
2. Have psychiatric diagnoses
3. Experience respiratory distress
4. Need close supervision for safety

This item tests your ability to identify the relationship between immobility and the formation of pressure ulcers. It tests your knowledge of the fact that prolonged pressure on a site interferes with cellular oxygenation, which causes cell death, resulting in a pressure ulcer.

Interpret Data

Interpretation of data is critical in the analysis step of the nursing process. It is associated with the nurse's ability to determine the significance of clustered data. *Significance* in this context refers to some consequence, importance, implication, or gravity connected to the cluster as it relates to the client's health problem. Finally, the interpretation of the significant clustered data should lead to a conclusion. Conclusions are the opinions, decisions, or inferences that result from the interpretation of data.

SAMPLE ITEM 6-13

A nurse is caring for a dying client who has a loss of appetite (anorexia), difficulty falling asleep (insomnia), and decreased interest in activities of daily living. Which feeling reflects these clinical findings?
1. Anger
2. Denial
3. Depression
4. Acceptance

This item tests your ability to come to a conclusion based on a cluster of data. The word *reflect* in the stem cues you to the fact that this is an analysis question. You need to draw from your knowledge of commonalities of human behavior and theories of grieving to arrive at the conclusion that the client probably is depressed.

SAMPLE ITEM 6-14

A client who is debilitated and unsteady when standing insists on walking to the bathroom without calling for assistance. This behavior best reflects a need to be:
1. alone.
2. accepted.
3. independent.
4. manipulative.

This item tests your ability to come to a conclusion based on a cluster of data. To answer this question, you must analyze and interpret the information in the stem and come to a conclusion. Your knowledge of human behavior should enable you to select the correct answer.

Collect Additional Data

After you arrive at an initial conclusion, additional data collection may be indicated to support the suspected conclusion. This is done to verify the relationship among the original data. The nurse continually reassesses the condition of the client and the presence of needs, while recognizing that the client is dynamic and ever changing throughout all phases of the nursing process.

SAMPLE ITEM 6-15

A nurse assesses that a postoperative client has a decreased blood pressure level and weak, thready pulse. The nurse concludes that the client may be hemorrhaging. For which additional signs of hemorrhage should the nurse assess the client?
1. Pain
2. Jaundice
3. Tachycardia
4. Hyperthermia

This item tests your understanding of the need for reassessment of the client to reinforce the proposed conclusion of hemorrhage. Hypotension, tachycardia, and a weak, thready pulse are related to a decreased blood volume, which is associated with postoperative hemorrhage.

Identify and Communicate Nursing Diagnoses

Converting a conclusion into a diagnostic statement changes it from a general statement of a problem into a specific statement—or a nursing diagnosis. A **nursing diagnosis** is a statement of a specific health problem that a nurse is legally permitted to treat. The diagnostic statement should include the problem and the factors that contributed to its development.

The contributing factors must be included because, although two clients may have the same problem, it may have been caused by different stresses. This concept is important because the nature of the contributing factors generally drives the choice of interventions that are planned. For example, two clients have impaired skin integrity. However, one client's skin problem is related to incontinence and edema, and the other client's skin problem is related to immobility and pressure. The interventions may be very different because the factors contributing to the problem are different. This is discussed in more detail in the section in this chapter titled "Planning."

Some nurses use the taxonomy of nursing diagnoses developed by NANDA International as a blueprint. This taxonomy provides standards for classifying nursing problems, standardizing language, facilitating communication, and focusing on an individualized approach to identifying and meeting a client's nursing needs. The following are examples of nursing diagnoses:

- Risk for impaired skin integrity, related to incontinence
- Feeding self-care deficit, related to bilateral arm casts
- Ineffective airway clearance, related to excessive secretions

Nurses must communicate nursing diagnoses to other nurses via a written plan of care. The plan should include the nursing diagnosis, expected outcomes, and planned interventions. The next section discusses outcomes and planned nursing interventions in more detail.

SAMPLE ITEM 6-16

A client who experienced a brain attack (i.e., stroke, cerebrovascular accident) has left-sided hemiparesis and is incontinent of urine. Which is an appropriately worded nursing diagnosis for this client?
1. The client has a need to maintain skin integrity.
2. The client had a stroke evidenced by hemiparesis and incontinence.
3. The client will be clean and dry and will receive range-of-motion exercises every 4 hours.
4. The client is at risk for impaired skin integrity related to left-sided hemiparesis and incontinence.

This item tests your ability to identify language used in the NANDA taxonomy. To answer this item correctly, you must be able to identify the differences among a client need, an expected outcome, a nursing intervention, and a properly stated nursing diagnosis associated with a cluster of data.

PLANNING

Planning is the third step of the nursing process. It involves identifying goals, projecting expected outcomes, setting priorities, identifying interventions, ensuring that the client's health-care needs will be appropriately met, modifying the plan of care as needed, and collaborating with other health-care team members. To plan care, you must have a strong foundation of scientific theory, understand the commonalities and differences in response to nursing interventions, and know theories related to establishing priority of needs.

You should use your knowledge and clinical experience when answering planning questions, which ask you to:

- Involve the client in the planning process
- Set goals
- Establish expected outcomes against which results of care can be compared for the purpose of evaluation
- Plan appropriate interventions based on their effects
- Establish priorities of nursing interventions
- Anticipate client needs
- Collaborate with others
- Coordinate planned care with health-care workers in other disciplines
- Recognize that plans must be flexible and modified on the basis of changing client needs

Critical words within a test item that indicate it is focused on planning include **achieve, desired, plan, effective, desired result, goal, priority, develop, formulate, establish, design, prevent, strategy, select, determine, anticipate, modify, collaborate, arrange, coordinate, expect,** and **outcome.** See whether you can identify variations of these critical words in the sample items in this chapter.

Testing errors occur during the planning phase when options are selected that:

- Do not include the client in setting goals and priorities
- Are inappropriate goals
- Misidentify priorities
- Reflect goals that are unrealistic
- Reflect goals that are not measurable
- Reflect planned interventions that are inappropriate or incomplete
- Fail to include family members and significant others when appropriate
- Fail to coordinate and collaborate with other health-care team members

Identify Goals

A **goal** is a broad, nonspecific statement concerning the desired result of nursing care. It is a general statement that directs nursing interventions and stimulates motivation. Goals can be long term or short term. A **long-term goal** is one that takes time to achieve (months or years). A **short-term goal** is one that can be achieved relatively quickly (usually within hours, days, or weeks). Goals should be:

- Client centered
- Specific (measurable)
- Realistic
- Achievable within a time frame

A short-term goal for a client who has a respiratory tract infection might state, "The client will independently use the incentive spirometer every hour for the next 4 hours." Or, "The client's sputum culture will be negative within 1 week." "The client" is the subject of the statement, and therefore the goal is client centered. "Sputum culture will be negative" is specific, realistic, and measurable. The phrase "within 1 week" establishes a time frame for the goal. A long-term goal for a client who has a respiratory tract infection might state, "The client will be free of infection within 1 month." "The client" is the subject of the statement, and therefore the goal is client centered. Being "free of infection" is specific, realistic, and measurable. The phrase "within 1 month" indicates the time frame in which the goal should be achieved.

Eventually, a goal can be further developed to become an expected outcome. An outcome provides a standard of measure to determine whether the goal has been reached. An expected outcome for the long-term goal listed above might be, "The client's sputum culture will be negative within 2 weeks." Outcomes are discussed in more detail next.

SAMPLE ITEM 6-17

A nurse is caring for a client with a new temporary colostomy. Which is a realistic short-term goal for this client?

1. The client will have regular bowel elimination.
2. The client's bowel will function within 2 days.
3. The client is at risk for impaired skin integrity.
4. The client's skin will remain intact around the stoma.

This item tests your ability to identify a short-term goal. To answer this question, you need to know commonalities related to caring for a client with a new temporary colostomy and be able to identify the differences among short- and long-term goals and a nursing diagnosis.

Project Expected Outcomes

Outcomes are any responses (positive or negative) to an intervention by an individual, family, or community. **Expected outcomes** are the predicted positive changes that should occur in response to the care given. Expected outcomes are derived from goal statements, but they are more specific because they describe behaviors to be demonstrated or data to be collected. Expected outcomes are the benchmarks against which the client's actual outcomes are compared to determine the effectiveness of the interventions provided.

Sometimes, nurses may state goals and outcomes together. For example, "The client will continuously maintain effective airway clearance as evidenced by expectoration of sputum, clear lung fields, and noiseless breathing." The first part of the statement is the goal, and what follows "as evidenced by" are the expected outcomes. The first part of the statement is general, and the second part is specific.

The Center for Nursing Classification and Clinical Effectiveness develops Nursing Outcome Classifications (NOCs) that use standardized nursing terminology for outcomes across clinical settings and nursing care specialties. The NOC system identifies outcomes, each of which includes a definition, a list of specific indicators that can be used to evaluate client status in relation to the outcome, a target outcome rating, and a measurement scale(s) to measure client status. With the evolving practice of nursing and the use of computers in the delivery of client care, this taxonomy of standardized outcome classifications has numerous advantages. The NOC system is research based, standardized, comprehensive, and flexible for clinical use when caring for individuals, families, or communities.

SAMPLE ITEM 6-18

A nurse is caring for a client experiencing insomnia. Which statement is an expected outcome?

1. "The client has a disturbed sleep pattern."
2. "The client can identify techniques to induce sleep."
3. "The client will have privacy when attempting to sleep."
4. "The client will report an optimal balance of sleep and activity."

This item tests your ability to identify a statement that reflects an expected outcome. To answer this question, you should know the commonalities of caring for a client with insomnia. You also need to understand the differences among a goal, an expected outcome, a nursing diagnosis, and a nursing intervention.

Set Priorities

Setting priorities is an important step in the planning process. After client needs and goals are identified, they must be ranked in order of importance. Maslow's hierarchy of needs (1970) is helpful in establishing priorities. Basic physiological needs are ranked first, with safety and security, belonging and love, self-esteem, and self-actualization following in rank order. It is important to understand, however, that at a given point in time, any one of Maslow's needs may take priority depending on the needs of the individual client. Obviously, if someone is choking on food, clearing the airway is the priority. However, there are times when the immediate need of the client is in the psychological dimension. The nurse must identify the client's perceptions and perspective when setting priorities because clients are at the center of the health-care team. When possible, the client should always be involved in setting priorities.

SAMPLE ITEM 6-19

A client has just returned from surgery with an IV solution infusing and does not have a gag reflex. Which planned intervention takes priority?

1. Observe the dressing for drainage.
2. Ensure adequacy of air exchange.
3. Check for an infiltration.
4. Monitor vital signs.

This item tests your ability to prioritize care. All of these planned interventions are important. However, oxygenation is essential to sustain life; therefore, maintaining a patent airway is the priority.

Identify Interventions

After priorities have been established, a plan for nursing action must be formulated. To plan appropriately, the nurse must rely on scientific information, clinical judgment, and knowledge about the client. By relying on this background, the nurse determines what nursing measures will be most effective in assisting the client to achieve a goal or outcome. Some nurses use the Nursing Interventions Classification (NIC) system, which is an evidence-based, standardized classification of nursing interventions for use in all settings and specialties. The NIC system defines a nursing intervention as "any treatment, based on clinical judgment and knowledge that a nurse performs to enhance client outcomes." Each intervention is composed of a label, a definition, and a set of activities that a nurse can perform to implement it. As a result of the evolving practice of nursing and the enhanced interdisciplinary nature of health-care delivery, this standardized system uses language that promotes communication among health-care professionals and provides for continuity of care. In addition, these interventions are coded so they can be used in documentation and reimbursement.

When using clinical judgment to identify an appropriate nursing intervention, a nurse must understand the rationale for that intervention. For example, when caring for a client with a pressure ulcer, the nurse reasons, "If I turn and reposition the client and rub around the area with lotion every 2 hours, then circulation will increase and healing will be promoted." When planning care, the nurse must know the scientific rationales for nursing interventions so the most appropriate interventions for the client-care situation are selected. It is not enough to just know how; you also must know why.

When making decisions, the nurse must consider the concepts of "cause and effect," "risk and probability," and "value of the consequence to the client." The action you plan is the "cause." The client's response is the "effect." The likelihood of either a positive or negative effect is the "probability." The probability of the client suffering harm from the action is the "risk." The value of the effect in relation to its probability of occurring influences the degree of risk one is willing to take to achieve the effect.

To facilitate this process of problem solving, an **information-processing model of decision making** should be used.

- First, identify all possible nursing actions (cause) that may help the client.
- Second, identify all possible positive and negative consequences (effect) associated with each action.
- Third, determine the odds (probability) that each consequence will occur. This includes determining the probability of a negative effect occurring (risk).
- Fourth, arrive at a judgment based on the value of each effect to the client.
- Fifth, choose the action that is "best" for the client. The "best" action is one that has the lowest risk and the highest probability of helping the client achieve the expected outcome (effect).

The concept of probability versus risk can be applied to buying a lottery ticket. If you buy one lottery ticket for $1, your chances of winning are small (low probability). If you do not win, your risk will be small because you will lose only $1 (low risk). On the other hand, if you spend your entire paycheck on lottery tickets, you will not dramatically increase your chances of winning (low probability). However, if you do not win, you will lose your whole paycheck and have no money to pay your bills (high risk). When making clinical decisions, you want to choose an action that has the highest probability of success with the lowest risk to the client.

Also, the appropriateness of clinical decisions depends on the quality of the data collected and the accuracy of the inferences made in the earlier steps of the nursing process. **Each step of the nursing process relies on the quality and accuracy of the preceding step.**

SAMPLE ITEM 6-20

Which is the most effective way that nurses can prevent the spread of microorganisms in a hospital?

1. Washing the hands
2. Implementing contact precautions
3. Using disposable equipment for procedures
4. Using linen hampers with foot-operated covers

This item tests your ability to identify that hand hygiene is the single most effective measure to prevent the spread of microorganisms. This question focuses on a specific action that can help protect all clients from the risk of infection.

SAMPLE ITEM 6-21

A client on bed rest needs a complete change of linen. Which should the nurse plan to do?

1. Make an occupied bed
2. Change the draw sheet and top sheet
3. Use a mechanical lift to raise the client
4. Transfer the client to a chair during the linen change

This item tests your ability to identify the needs of a client on bed rest and therefore to plan to make an occupied bed. The word *plan* used in the stem is an obvious clue that this is a planning question.

SAMPLE ITEM 6-22

The nurse should make an occupied bed for a client who is:

1. obese.
2. in a cast.
3. immobile.
4. on bed rest.

This item is similar to Sample Item 6-21; however, the content of the stem and the correct option are reversed. This item is more difficult to identify as a planning item because the word *plan* is not in the stem.

Ensure That Health-Care Needs Will Be Met Appropriately

The nurse is obligated to take an action that will ensure the provision of appropriate care. If adequate care cannot be administered because a nursing team member's expertise is unrelated to the client's needs, a nursing team member is inexperienced in caring for a client with a particular problem, or there is inadequate staffing, then a client may be placed at risk. This might require the nursing unit manager to rearrange the assignment, or it might require intervention by the assistant director of nursing. Once the nurse embarks on a "duty of care," he or she is obligated to provide a standard of care defined by the Nurse Practice Act in the state in which he or she works.

SAMPLE ITEM 6-23

The nursing unit manager arrives on duty and discovers that several staff members have just called in sick. Which is the appropriate response by the nursing unit manager?

1. Identify which clients need care and assign staff accordingly
2. Inform the assistant director of nursing and ask for additional staff
3. Explain to clients that when the unit is short-staffed, only essential care can be provided
4. Provide the best care possible, but refuse to accept responsibility for the standard of care delivered

This item tests your ability to identify your responsibility to ensure that clients' needs are met appropriately. Once the nursing unit manager perceives a risk to client safety, an action must be taken to ensure that appropriate care is provided.

Modify the Plan of Care as Needed

Planning generally takes place before care is given. However, client needs sometimes change while the nurse is in the process of implementing care, and a plan must be immediately modified. Modification of the plan of care also may take place after evaluation. The original plan may have been inadequate or inappropriate, or the client's condition may have improved. It is important to recognize that a plan of care is not set in stone but is modified in response to the changing needs of the client. A client's needs are dynamic, so the nursing plan also is dynamic. It must continually be changed to remain current by substituting new goals and planned interventions as indicated by the client's changing needs.

SAMPLE ITEM 6-24

A client is diaphoretic and is receiving oxygen by nasal cannula. During a bath, the client experiences dyspnea and reports feeling tired. Which should the nurse do?

1. Give a complete bath quickly
2. Continue with the bath as planned
3. Bathe only the body parts that need bathing
4. Arrange for several rest periods during the bath

This item tests your ability to identify the need to modify a plan of care based on new data.

Collaborate With Other Health-Care Team Members

Another component of planning comprises consultation and collaboration with other health-care team members to brainstorm, seek additional input, and delegate and coordinate the delivery of health services. The nurse is responsible for coordinating the members of the nursing team as well as the entire health-care team. The nurse manages the members of the nursing team by appropriately delegating and supervising nursing interventions. The plan also identifies and coordinates the services of other health-care professionals. The nurse is responsible for ensuring that services such as laboratory tests, radiological studies, and physical therapy are performed within the context of the client's physical and emotional abilities. For example, the nurse may arrange for a client to go to physical therapy in the morning before becoming tired or the nurse may consult with the dietitian to design a menu that incorporates a client's preferences. Effective planning contributes to the delivery of client care that has continuity and is client centered, coordinated, and individualized.

SAMPLE ITEM 6-25

A nurse is caring for a client with a large pressure ulcer that has not responded to common nursing interventions. With whom should the nurse consult first to best deal with this problem?
1. Surgeon
2. Physical therapist
3. Clinical nurse specialist
4. Primary health-care provider

This item tests your ability to identify that planning nursing care may require seeking the expertise of a nurse specialist. A clinical nurse specialist is educated and prepared to provide expert advice and lend problem-solving and educational skills to find solutions to difficult clinical nursing problems. Although the nurse consults with health-care team members of other disciplines for various reasons, the nurse should consult with a clinical nurse specialist or other resources in nursing first for assistance in solving nursing problems.

IMPLEMENTATION

Implementation is the step of the nursing process in which planned actions are initiated and completed. It includes tasks such as organizing and managing planned care; providing total or partial assistance with activities of daily living (ADLs); counseling and teaching the client and significant others; providing planned care; supervising and coordinating the delivery of care by the nursing staff; and recording and sharing data related to the care implemented.

To implement safe nursing care designed to achieve goals and expected outcomes, the nurse must understand and follow the implementation process. In addition, the nurse must have knowledge of scientific rationales for nursing procedures, the psychomotor skills to implement procedures safely, and the ability to use different strategies to implement care effectively. Implementation questions ask you to do the following:

- Identify steps in the implementation process
- Identify independent, dependent, and interdependent actions of the nurse
- Implement a procedure or treatment
- Respond to common or uncommon outcomes of an intervention
- Respond to life-threatening or adverse events
- Prepare a client for a procedure, treatment, or surgery
- Choose the approach that is most appropriate when implementing care
- Identify safe or unsafe practices
- Rationalize a step in a procedure
- Identify or apply concepts associated with teaching
- Identify or apply concepts associated with counseling
- Identify or apply principles associated with motivation
- Identify or apply techniques for therapeutic communication
- Identify when an intervention must be modified in response to a change in the client's condition
- Identify when additional assistance is required to provide safe care
- Identify the nurse's responsibility in supervising care delivered by those to whom interventions have been delegated
- Identify how and when to document or report care given as well as the client's response

Critical words within a test item that indicate it is focused on implementation include **dependent, independent, interdependent, change, assist, counsel, teach, give, supervise, perform, method, procedure, treatment, instruct, strategy, facilitate, provide, inform, refer, technique, motivate, delegate,** and **implement.** See whether you can identify variations of these words indicating implementation activities in the sample items.

Testing errors occur on implementation items when options are selected that:

- Implement actions outside the definition of nursing practice
- Fail to respond to an adverse or life-threatening situation
- Fail to modify interventions in response to the changing needs of the client
- Fail to identify when additional assistance is required for the delivery of safe care
- Reflect a lack of knowledge to implement interventions safely
- Do not accurately document the client's response to the care given
- Fail to supervise and evaluate the delivery of delegated interventions

Legal Parameters of Nursing Interventions

Implementation occurs when the nurse uses an intervention to help a client meet expected outcomes. Nursing interventions can be dependent, independent, or interdependent.

Dependent interventions are interventions that require a prescription by a primary health-care provider with a prescriptive license (e.g., physician, nurse practitioner, physician's assistant, dentist, or podiatrist). Administering a medication, providing IV fluids, and removing a nasogastric tube are examples of dependent interventions because they all require a legal prescription. When implementing a dependent intervention, the nurse does not blindly follow the prescription but determines whether it is appropriate. A nurse who does not question and carries out an inappropriate prescription is contributing to the initial error and will be held accountable.

Independent interventions (nurse-prescribed) are those actions that a nurse is legally permitted to implement with no direction or supervision from others. Independent interventions do not require a primary health-care provider's prescription. Tasks related to collecting data and determining their significance, providing assistance with ADLs, teaching regarding health, and counseling are in the realm of independent legal nursing practice. Encouraging coughing and deep breathing, encouraging expression of fears, teaching principles related to nutrition, tracking intake and output, and providing a bed bath are examples of independent nursing interventions.

Interdependent interventions (collaborative) are actions implemented in partnership with other appropriate professionals. An example of an interdependent intervention is implementing actions identified in standing protocols. These situations delineate the parameters within which the nurse is permitted to administer to the client. Standing protocols are commonly found in emergency and critical care areas. Another example of an interdependent intervention is an order from a primary health-care provider, such as "Out of bed as tolerated." When assisting this client to ambulate, the nurse must assess the client's response to the activity. Depending on the client's response, the nurse can decide to terminate the activity or to increase the time and/or distance to be ambulated.

SAMPLE ITEM 6-26

A primary nurse assigns a staff nurse to insert an indwelling urinary (Foley) catheter. Which is the first thing the staff nurse should do?

1. Check the primary health-care provider's prescription
2. Bring equipment to the client's bedside
3. Explain the procedure to the client
4. Wash the hands thoroughly

This question tests your ability to identify that the insertion of a urinary catheter is a dependent nursing intervention that requires a primary health-care provider's prescription.

Types of Nursing Interventions

Nursing actions associated with the implementation step of the nursing process include the following:

- **Assisting With Activities of Daily Living:** ADLs refer to activities associated with eating, dressing, hygiene, grooming, toileting, and movement/exercise. Situations associated with ADL assistance can be acute, chronic, temporary, permanent, or related to maintaining or restoring function. ADLs are an integral part of daily life; therefore, their implementation often is tested.
- **Teaching:** To teach effectively in the cognitive (learning new information), psychomotor (learning new skills), and affective (developing new attitudes, values, and beliefs) domains, the nurse must apply teaching/learning principles to motivate clients to learn and grow. Health teaching activities are incorporated throughout the health-illness continuum, in a variety of health-care delivery settings, and across the life span. For these reasons, teaching principles often are incorporated into client situations in test questions.
- **Responding to Life-Threatening Situations:** Responding to adverse or life-threatening situations requires the use of clinical judgment and decision making. Activities such as stopping the administration of an antibiotic in response to a client's allergic reaction, initiating cardiopulmonary resuscitation, implementing the abdominal thrust procedure (Heimlich maneuver), and administering emergency medication per protocol are examples of measures that may be implemented in life-threatening situations. Most of these interventions address basic physiological needs required for survival and therefore are frequently tested.
- **Implementing Preventive Actions:** Preventive actions are activities that help the client avoid a health problem. Administering immunizations, applying an allergy bracelet, employing medical and surgical asepsis, ensuring physical safety, and leading a group on weight reduction are examples of preventive measures. Today's society emphasizes health, wellness, and illness prevention, so these topics often are tested.
- **Performing Technical Skills:** The nurse must know how and when to implement a procedure and the expected outcomes of the procedure. Inserting a urinary catheter, providing an enteral feeding, administering medication, performing an enema, and preparing a client for a diagnostic test are examples of procedures implemented by the nurse. Steps, principles, rationales, and expected and potential adverse outcomes associated with procedures are concepts that often are tested in nursing questions.
- **Implementing Interpersonal Interventions:** Interpersonal activities conducted by the nurse help clients adapt to changes caused by loss, illness, disability, or stress. Emotional care is provided by activities such as promoting a supportive environment, motivating a client, providing privacy, and addressing spiritual needs. Counseling also is a component of interpersonal interventions. To counsel effectively, the nurse must apply therapeutic communication principles to explore clients' feelings and meet their emotional needs. Another aspect of interpersonal interventions is coordinating health-care activities. When the nurse collaborates with others to coordinate these activities, he or she functions as the client's advocate. People are complex human beings, and nursing care must address the mental, physical, emotional, spiritual, and legal/ethical realms. These realms are important, so associated nursing interventions often are tested in nursing questions.
- **Supervising and Evaluating the Effectiveness of Delegated Interventions:** Occasionally, a nurse who formulates a plan of care delegates all or part of its implementation to other members of the nursing team. Uncomplicated and basic interventions, particularly those associated with ADLs, are often delegated to a nursing assistant or licensed practical nurse. The nurse who delegates is responsible for the plan of care and is accountable for ensuring that the care is delivered according to standards of the profession. With changing roles in health-care delivery, the importance of the nurse as manager is increasing and therefore is tested.
- **Reporting and Recording:** After care has been given, it is recorded along with an assessment of the client's response to the care. Written communication establishes a permanent document of the care clients receive and their responses. In addition to

documentation, the nurse may verbally report to other health-care team members the care that was provided along with the client's responses. Also, verbal reports are given at the change of shifts, when responding to an emergency, or when transferring responsibility for a client to another nurse. Communication and documentation are essential to the provision of quality care, so they often are tested.

SAMPLE ITEM 6-27

A client has a prescription for a 2-gram sodium diet. Which should the nurse teach this client to limit in the diet?

1. Salt
2. Sugar
3. Liquids
4. Margarine

This item tests your ability to identify information that needs to be taught to a client. Teaching is performed by the nurse to assist a client in meeting a health need. Mainly, this question tests your ability to identify that salt is sodium and thus should be limited when a client is receiving a 2-gram sodium diet. The use of the word *limited* indicates that the stem of this question has negative polarity.

SAMPLE ITEM 6-28

A client vomits while in the supine position. Which should the nurse do?

1. Position the client's head between the knees
2. Raise the client to a low Fowler position
3. Transfer the client to the bathroom
4. Turn the client to the side

This item tests your ability to respond appropriately to an event. To answer this question, you must understand the importance of assisting the client in expectorating the vomitus to avoid aspiration. In addition, you need to know that a side-lying position is the best position to facilitate drainage of matter from the mouth. Questions that address a response to an event represent the implementation step of the nursing process.

SAMPLE ITEM 6-29

A client reports feeling nauseated. Which should the nurse do to provide support for this client?

1. Give mouth care every hour
2. Delay meals until the feeling passes
3. Position an emesis basin within easy reach
4. Explain that the feeling will lessen with time

Actions that anticipate an event are a type of implementation. The word *provide* in the stem is a clue that this is an implementation question. To answer this question correctly, you must understand that feeling nauseated is a precursor to vomiting and that providing an emesis basin will support a client who is nauseated.

SAMPLE ITEM 6-30

Which is the underlying rationale for a nurse changing a client's position every 2 hours?

1. Relieve pressure
2. Assess skin condition
3. Ensure that the skin is dry
4. Provide massage to bony prominences

This item tests your ability to identify the correct rationale for a nursing procedure. Relieving pressure is the rationale for regularly changing a client's position. To implement safe and effective care, nurses must have a strong understanding of the scientific rationales for nursing actions.

SAMPLE ITEM 6-31

A nurse is administering medications to a group of clients. Which is the safest way for the nurse to identify a client?
1. Ask the client his or her name
2. Check the identification bracelet
3. Double-check the medication administration record
4. Observe the response after stating the client's name

This item tests whether you can correctly identify a step in a procedure. Although more than one of the options may be implemented by the nurse, the question asks you to choose the best answer from all the options presented. In this set of options, checking the identification bracelet is the most reliable and safest method to verify a client's identity.

SAMPLE ITEM 6-32

Which should the nurse do to provide aseptically safe perineal care to all female clients?
1. Use a different part of the washcloth for each stroke
2. Employ a circular motion when applying soap
3. Apply deodorant spray to the perineal area
4. Sprinkle talcum powder on the perineum

This item tests your ability to identify a step in a procedure based on a specific scientific principle (asepsis). To answer this question correctly, you need to know that medical asepsis is promoted when the spread of microorganisms is limited. Using one area of the washcloth for each stroke when washing the perineum contributes to aseptically safe perineal care. Identifying a step in a procedure is an implementation question.

SAMPLE ITEM 6-33

A registered nurse (RN) delegates the insertion of an indwelling urinary catheter (Foley) to a licensed practical nurse (LPN). Which statement is accurate about the delegation of this procedure to the LPN?
1. The RN should have implemented the planned care and not have delegated it to the LPN.
2. The LPN will not be held accountable for the task because it was delegated by the RN.
3. The LPN should have respectfully refused to implement this task.
4. The RN will be held responsible for the delegated care.

This item tests your ability to understand that an RN who delegates care to another nursing staff member is responsible for supervising and evaluating the delivery of that care. This is an important component of implementation and is a concept that may be tested.

SAMPLE ITEM 6-34

A nurse signs a turning and positioning schedule form for a client. What does this documentation indicate?
1. The client received a back rub with lotion.
2. The client was turned at the time initialed.
3. The client received range-of-motion exercises.
4. The client was encouraged to turn to a different position.

This question tests your ability to understand the purpose of a turning and positioning flow sheet. Documenting the care given is a component of the step of implementation.

EVALUATION

Evaluation is the fifth and final step of the nursing process. Evaluation consists of four steps that must be implemented after care has been delivered to determine its effectiveness. The evaluation process includes identifying client responses to care (actual outcomes), comparing a client's actual outcomes with the expected outcomes, analyzing the factors that affected the outcomes for the purpose of drawing conclusions about the success or failure of specific nursing interventions, and modifying the plan when necessary.

Evaluation questions will ask you to do the following:

- Identify the steps in the evaluation process
- Identify whether an outcome has been met or not met
- Identify progress or lack of progress toward a goal and/or expected outcome
- Identify the need to modify the plan of care in response to a change in the client's status or when the plan is ineffective
- Understand that the process of evaluation is continuous
- Understand that the nursing process is dynamic and cyclical

Critical words within a test item that indicate it is focused on evaluation include **expected, met, desired, compared, succeeded, failed, achieved, modified, reassess, ineffective, effective, response,** and **evaluate.** See whether you can identify variations of these words indicating evaluation activities in the sample items.

Most testing errors occur on evaluation items when options are selected that:

- Do not thoroughly and accurately reassess the client after care has been implemented
- Fail to cluster new data appropriately
- Fail to determine the significance of new data
- Come to inappropriate or inaccurate conclusions when comparing actual outcomes with expected outcomes
- Fail to modify the plan of care in response to the changing needs of the client or in response to an ineffective plan

Identify Client Responses (Actual Outcomes)

The process of evaluation begins with a reassessment to collect new information. After nursing care has been implemented, the client is reassessed and new clusters of data are identified and their significance determined. In the nursing literature, the word *evaluation* is often used interchangeably with the word *assessment*, which causes confusion. It is important to remember that the collection of new information about a client (assessment) is only one component in the evaluation process. The nurse must first reassess to identify the client's responses (actual outcomes). Actual outcomes are the client's responses to nursing care.

SAMPLE ITEM 6-35

A client on a bland diet reports a reduced appetite. Which is an initial way for the nurse to determine whether the client's nutritional needs have been met?

1. Institute a 3-day food intake study.
2. Weigh the client at the end of the week.
3. Request a prescription for a dietary assessment.
4. Compare a current weight with the weight history.

This item tests your ability to identify a common way to evaluate one aspect of a client's nutritional status. In this situation, the results of nutritional care are determined by comparing a current weight assessment with a previous weight assessment to identify any gain or loss in the client's weight. After a change in status has been identified, a conclusion about the effectiveness of care can be determined from the data.

Compare Actual Outcomes With Expected Outcomes to Determine Goal Achievement

Expected outcomes and goals are the criteria established for future evaluation of nursing care. A comparison is made between the client's actual outcomes and the expected outcomes to determine the effectiveness of nursing interventions. When you reassess the client after care and compare these new data with the expected outcomes, it is possible to determine which expected outcomes have been achieved and which have not been achieved. The closer the client's actual outcomes are to the expected outcomes, the more positive the evaluation. When expected outcomes are achieved, the goal has been attained. Negative evaluations reflect situations in which the expected outcomes are not achieved. When expected outcomes are not achieved, the goal is not attained. Negative evaluations indicate that the nursing care was ineffective.

For example, the goal may be that "The client will be free of a wound infection when discharged 5 days after abdominal surgery"; the outcomes may be "as evidenced by the presence of a normal white blood cell count, approximation of wound edges with granulated tissue, and vital signs within expected limits." If the client's actual outcomes meet these expected outcomes, the goal has been achieved. If the client's actual outcomes indicate increased vital signs; an increased white blood cell count; and/or the presence of purulent exudate, erythema, or unapproximated wound edges at the incision site, the goal has not been achieved.

SAMPLE ITEM 6-36

A nurse teaches a client about the foods permitted on a 2-gram sodium diet. Which food selected by the client indicates an understanding of the teaching?

1. Celery
2. Fresh fruit
3. Vegetables
4. Luncheon meat

This item tests your ability to identify that of all the options presented, fruit has the least amount of sodium. In addition, the stem is worded in such a way that the nurse must evaluate the correctness of the client's response. The action described in the stem is an attempt to evaluate the client's understanding of the teaching provided.

Analyze Factors That Affect Actual Outcomes of Care

After the effectiveness of care has been determined, the nurse must come to some conclusions about the potential factors that contributed to the success or failure of the plan of care. If a plan of care has been ineffective, the nurse must examine what contributed to its failure. This requires the nurse to start at step 1 of the nursing process—assessment—and work through the entire process again to identify why the plan was ineffective. Questions the nurse must ask include "Was the original assessment accurate?" "If a conclusion was made, was it accurate?" "Was the goal realistic?" "Were the proposed outcomes measurable?" and "Were the planned interventions consistently implemented?"

SAMPLE ITEM 6-37

A client returns to the clinic after taking a 7-day course of antibiotic therapy and is still exhibiting signs of a urinary tract infection. The nurse's first action should be to:

1. make an appointment for the client to be seen by the primary health-care provider.
2. arrange for the primary health-care provider to prescribe a different antibiotic.
3. obtain another urine specimen for culture and sensitivity testing.
4. determine if the client took the medication as prescribed.

This item tests your ability to identify that the nurse must analyze the factors that influence outcomes of care. Options 1, 2, and 3 can be eliminated because these actions immediately move to an intervention before collecting more information. They may be unnecessary, depending on the information gleaned from the client. Option 4 is the correct answer because adherence with a medication administration schedule will influence the effectiveness of the medication.

Modify the Plan of Care

After it has been determined that a plan of care is ineffective, the plan must be modified. Changes in the plan of care are based on new client assessments, analysis of new data, goals, outcomes, and nursing strategies designed to address the changing needs of the client. The modified plan must then be implemented, and the whole evaluation process begins again. The process of evaluation is continuous.

SAMPLE ITEM 6-38

A recently admitted client was provided with a regular diet consisting of three traditional meals a day. After several days, it was identified that the client was eating only approximately 50% of the meals and was losing weight. What should the nurse do?

1. Assist the client until meals are completed
2. Schedule several between-meal supplements
3. Change the plan of care to provide five small meals daily
4. Secure an order to increase the number of calories provided

This item tests your ability to identify that the nursing plan of care must be changed when care is ineffective. The new actions must be within the legal definition of nursing and must address the specific needs of the client.

SUMMARY

The nursing process is one of the cornerstones of nursing practice. It provides a foundation for collecting data (Assessment), analyzing data (Analysis), planning nursing care (Planning), implementing nursing care (Implementation), and evaluating nursing care (Evaluation). The nursing process is a systematic approach that requires the use of critical thinking and problem solving to deal with complex client situations. The nursing process provides a blueprint for the delivery of nursing care, so nursing examinations contain test items that reflect the "thinking" and "doing" inherent throughout the process. When you can identify the step of the nursing process reflected in a test item, you should be better able to identify what is being asked. Understanding what is being asked in the stem of a test item will increase your ability to analyze the options presented in relation to the stem as well as your ability to select the correct answer.

Assessment

6-1 **1. Before a client is moved, an assessment must be made to determine whether any intervention is necessary to stabilize an injured body part; moving an injured person can exacerbate an injury.**
2. Transferring the client back to bed before other nursing interventions can exacerbate an injury.
3. Moving the injured client before other nursing interventions is unsafe because it can exacerbate an injury.
4. Reporting the incident should be done after the client is safe.

6-2 1. Although putting nonskid socks or shoes on the client's feet should be done, this action is premature at this time.
2. Nurses must always assess a client before a transfer to ensure that the client has the strength to stand and ambulate safely.
3. Although raising the side rail on the opposite side of the client's bed should be done, this action is premature at this time.
4. Although a client should sit on the side of the bed for a minute before getting out of bed to allow the circulatory system to adjust to the upright position, this action is premature at this time.

6-3 1. 18 breaths per minute is within the expected range for an adult. Breaths can be inhaled through the mouth or nose.
2. 20 breaths per minute is within the expected range for an adult. The depth is not significant as long as the respirations appear effortless.
3. 16 breaths per minute is within the expected range for an adult. The depth is not significant as long as the respirations appear effortless.
4. 28 breaths per minute is outside the expected range for an adult; expected respirations should be between 12 and 20 per minute, effortless, and noiseless. This client may be experiencing respiratory distress.

6-4 1. A nurse may permit an alert and capable client to insert a rectal thermometer; however, if the client has physical or cognitive deficits, this may not be possible. When a client self-inserts an electronic thermometer, the handle of the probe must be decontaminated after use.
2. When a rectal temperature is taken, the client can be safely positioned on either the right or the left side.
3. The use of an electronic thermometer is not always practical. Electronic thermometers usually are not used in isolation because of the inconvenience of decontaminating equipment after use.
4. Lubricating a rectal thermometer is always done to facilitate entry into the rectum; a lubricant reduces resistance when the thermometer is inserted through the anal sphincters.

6-5 1. Daily intake reflects the amount of food/fluid the client is ingesting; this information does not contribute to the calculation of ideal body weight.
2. To calculate ideal body weight, the nurse must know the client's height, age, and extent of bone structure.
3. Clothing size is determined by weight and by inches reflecting circumference of the chest and waist; this information does not contribute to the calculation of ideal body weight.
4. Determining food preferences supports the client's right to make choices about care; this information does not contribute to the calculation of ideal body weight.

6-6 1. The primary source is the client, not the wife.
2. A tertiary source provides information outside the client's frame of reference.
3. The wife is not a subjective source. As used here, *subjective* refers to a type of data; subjective data are collected when the client shares feelings, perceptions, sensations, and thoughts.
4. Family members are secondary sources. Secondary sources provide supplemental information about a client.

6-7 1. The nurse can examine between the client's toes and visually verify the presence of sores. The sores can be visually verified, so this information is objective.
2. Hair color can be visually verified and therefore is considered objective information.
3. The experience of pain is subjective information because it can be verified only by the client.

4. An altered gait can be visually verified and therefore is considered objective information.

6-8 1. A letter is considered verbal communication; words are written.
2. Holding hands is nonverbal communication; a message is transmitted without using words.
3. Sounds may or may not communicate meaning; however, a sound that communicates meaning is considered verbal communication.
4. A telephone message is verbal communication; words generally are spoken in a telephone message.

6-9 1. Notifying the primary health-care provider may eventually be necessary, but it is not the priority.
2. The reading should be verified by retaking the blood pressure level because the nurse may have made a mistake when taking the original blood pressure reading.
3. Notifying the nurse in charge may be done after the blood pressure reading has been verified and all the vital signs have been taken.
4. Other vital signs are obtained after the initial blood pressure reading has been taken a second time; once one vital sign has been identified as outside the expected range, all vital signs should be assessed.

6-10 1. The primary health-care provider does not need to be notified at this time. The primary health-care provider should be notified if a client does not void within 6 to 8 hours after surgery.
2. When a primary health-care provider writes a prescription for I&O, every fluid that goes into the client (e.g., oral fluids, IV fluids, nasogastric instillations) is considered intake and every fluid that comes out of the client (e.g., urine, vomitus, wound drainage) is considered output. The amount of urinary output must be documented in the client's clinical record.
3. The vital signs (e.g., temperature, pulse, respirations, blood pressure, and sometimes bowel movements) are recorded on the vital signs flow sheet.
4. Although this may be done, it does not provide a written record. Written documentation is necessary for a permanent record and to communicate the information to appropriate health-care team members who are not working on the surgical unit.

Analysis

6-11 1. Receptive aphasia is not associated with the data cluster presented in the stem. Receptive aphasia is an inability to understand either spoken or written language.
2. An inability to ambulate is not associated with the data cluster identified in the stem; this is associated with the inability to bear weight on the right leg because of hemiplegia.
3. Difficulty swallowing can increase the risk for aspiration; it is associated with the data identified in the stem (paralysis of the right side, drooling, slurred speech), and together they present a significant cluster of information.
4. Incontinence of stool is not associated with the data cluster identified in the stem; this is associated with hygiene needs and supports the fact that the client is at risk for impaired skin integrity, not aspiration.

6-12 **1. Clients who are immobilized are subject to increased pressure over bony prominences with a subsequent decrease in circulation to the tissues.**
2. A psychiatric diagnosis is unrelated to the development of pressure ulcers.
3. Respiratory distress is unrelated to the development of pressure ulcers.
4. A need for close supervision for safety is unrelated to the development of pressure ulcers.

6-13 1. Acting-out behaviors commonly reflect anger.
2. Refusing to believe or accept a situation is reflective of denial.
3. Clinical manifestations commonly associated with depression include avoiding contact with others, withdrawal, loss of appetite (anorexia), and difficulty falling asleep (insomnia).
4. Acceptance is related to the final step of grieving; a client reconciles and accepts the situation and is at peace.

6-14 1. The client is not trying to be left alone. Avoiding others reflects this need.
2. A client who wants to be accepted usually will follow directions.
3. The client is attempting to perform self-care to demonstrate the ability to be self-sufficient and independent.
4. Manipulation is associated with intrigue, scheming, and conniving. This client's behavior is clear and direct.

6-15 1. Pain generally is not associated with hemorrhage.
2. Jaundice is associated with a problem with the liver or biliary system.
3. Tachycardia, an increased heart rate, is a compensatory mechanism to increase oxygen to all body cells and is associated with hemorrhage.
4. Hyperthermia, increased body temperature, is unrelated to hemorrhage.

6-16 1. This statement identifies a need, not a nursing diagnosis.
2. This statement is an incorrectly worded nursing diagnosis; a stroke is not something a nurse can diagnose or treat.
3. This statement is a combination of an expected outcome and an intervention, not a nursing diagnosis.
4. This statement is an appropriately worded nursing diagnosis that uses NANDA terminology; it contains a health problem appropriate for nursing interventions.

Planning

6-17 1. This is a long-term goal, not a short-term goal. Also, the statement does not contain a time frame.
2. This is correct wording for a goal, but it is unrealistic; it takes 3 to 5 days for a new colostomy to function.
3. This is a problem statement, the first part of a nursing diagnosis.
4. This is a short-term goal; it is client centered and specific, and the word *remain* reflects the time frame.

6-18 1. This is the problem statement of a nursing diagnosis, not an expected outcome.
2. This statement is an expected outcome. It is specific knowledge the client should demonstrate that may help attain the ultimate goal of relief from insomnia.
3. This statement is a planned nursing intervention, not an expected outcome.
4. This statement is not an expected outcome. This statement is an incomplete goal; it does not have a time frame.

6-19 1. Observing the dressing for drainage is important, but it is not the priority.
2. Providing for a client's oxygenation is essential to maintain life and is always the priority.
3. Checking for infiltration is important, but it is not the priority.
4. Monitoring vital signs is important, but it is not the priority.

6-20 **1. Washing the hands with soap and water mechanically removes microorganisms from the skin; hand hygiene is the most effective way to prevent cross contamination.**
2. Usually contact precautions are necessary only when the client has a virulent microorganism.
3. Although use of disposable equipment can help prevent cross contamination, it is not the most effective action presented.
4. Although foot-operated linen hampers contain and limit the spread of microorganisms, they are not the most effective action to prevent cross contamination.

6-21 **1. An occupied bed is made for a client on complete bed rest; this client is not permitted out of bed.**
2. All the linens should be changed regularly and whenever necessary.
3. An occupied bed can be made without a mechanical lift just by turning the client.
4. A client on bed rest is not allowed out of bed for any reason unless directed by a primary health-care provider's prescription.

6-22 1. An obese client can be transferred out of bed while the linen is changed.
2. A client in a cast can be transferred out of bed while the linen is changed.
3. An immobile client can be transferred out of bed while the linen is changed.
4. Clients on bed rest must remain in bed when the linens are changed; this is called "making an occupied bed."

6-23 1. All clients must have their needs met.
2. The nursing unit manager has an obligation to ensure that all clients' needs are appropriately met; this is the only option that addresses this concept.

3. Providing only essential care does not ensure that appropriate care is provided; this action will increase anxiety and cause clients to doubt the quality of care being provided.
4. Once assuming a course of duty, the nurse is responsible for the care that is delivered.

6-24 1. Giving care as quickly as possible will increase the demand on the client's cardiopulmonary system. This increases activity, which in turn increases oxygen needs; rushing may cause the client to decompensate.
2. The client's dyspnea cannot be ignored. Continuing with the bath as planned will further jeopardize the client's status.
3. This does not address the client's physical needs. The client needs a full bath because of the diaphoresis.
4. Providing rest periods conserves energy; this reduces the strain of activity by decreasing the demand for oxygen, which in turn decreases the rate and labor of respirations.

6-25 1. When a client does not respond to common nursing interventions for a large pressure ulcer, resources other than a surgeon are more appropriate and available for consultation.
2. The physical therapist is a specialist in assisting a client to achieve or maintain physical mobility and is not an expert in providing nursing care.
3. The clinical nurse specialist is educated and prepared to provide expert assistance when other members of the health-care team seek solutions to difficult clinical nursing problems.
4. A primary health-care provider is responsible for the client's medical care and is not an expert in providing nursing care.

Implementation

6-26 **1. Inserting an indwelling urinary catheter is a dependent nursing intervention that requires a prescription. The nurse must verify the prescription before it can be implemented.**
2. Bringing equipment to the client's bedside is premature.
3. There are other things the nurse must do first.
4. Washing the hands is not the first step in this procedure.

6-27 **1. Salt used to season meals contains sodium; sodium must be limited when a client is receiving a 2-gram sodium diet.**
2. Sugar is limited when a client is receiving a reduced-calorie or diabetic diet, not a 2-gram sodium diet.
3. Fluids are limited when a client has fluid restrictions, not when receiving a 2-gram sodium diet; however, the client must be alert to avoid fluids that are high in sodium, such as diet sodas.
4. Margarine should be limited when a client is receiving a low-fat diet, not a 2-gram sodium diet.

6-28 1. Positioning the head between the knees may exacerbate vomiting because the pressure of the abdomen against the chest and the force of gravity promote the flow of gastric content toward the mouth.
2. The low Fowler position should be avoided because it will allow vomitus to collect in the posterior oropharynx and increase the risk of aspiration.
3. Vomiting takes energy and can cause the client to become weak during the transfer.
4. Turning the client to the side drains the mouth via gravity and reduces the risk of aspiration.

6-29 1. Oral hygiene is sufficient every 8 hours and whenever necessary.
2. Delaying meals is inappropriate; nausea may be a long-standing problem.
3. An emesis basin provides physical and emotional comfort; the emesis basin collects vomitus rather than soiling the bed linens and reduces the client's concern regarding soiling.
4. This action provides false reassurance; the nurse cannot predict when nausea will subside.

6-30 **1. Changing a client's position relieves pressure from body weight and permits circulation to return to the area; prolonged pressure can cause cell death from lack of oxygen and nutrients needed to sustain cellular metabolism.**
2. Although skin condition should be assessed, it is not the primary reason for changing a client's position every 2 hours.
3. The nurse should ensure the skin is clean and dry, but this is not the primary

reason for changing a client's position every 2 hours.
4. Massage should be performed around, not on, bony prominences.

6-31 1. Asking a client his or her name is unsafe; the client may be cognitively impaired.
2. Checking the identification band is the safest method to identify a client; it is the most reliable method because each client on admission receives an identification bracelet with his or her name and identification number.
3. Checking the medication administration record will not verify the name of the person.
4. Calling the client's name and observing the response are unsafe interventions because the client may be cognitively impaired.

6-32 **1. When washing a client, using different parts of the washcloth with each stroke provides a clean surface for each stroke; it avoids contaminating the meatus with soiled portions of the cloth.**
2. Using a circular motion is unsafe because it may bring soiled matter into contact with the urinary meatus.
3. Applying deodorant spray to the perineal area can be irritating to some clients and can contribute to impaired skin integrity; also it does not remove bacteria.
4. Talcum powder is contraindicated because its application may aerosolize toxins that can be inhaled, contributing to lung disease. Also, talcum powder has been identified as a contributing factor to ovarian cancer.

6-33 1. An RN can delegate tasks to other qualified nursing staff members as long as the delegated tasks are within the scope of practice of the staff member, the staff member is supervised, and the delivery of care is evaluated.
2. An LPN always is held responsible for care provided to clients and always works under the direction of an RN.
3. It is inappropriate to refuse to implement delegated tasks as long as the tasks are within the legal scope of LPN practice and the LPN can safely implement them. This procedure is within the scope of practice of an LPN.
4. This is an accurate statement; the delegating RN is responsible for supervising and evaluating the delivery of delegated tasks.

6-34 1. Although a back rub with lotion should be implemented when a client is turned and positioned, it is not the purpose of a turning and positioning schedule form.
2. This indicates that turning and positioning were implemented as planned.
3. Although the client should receive range-of-motion exercises, this is not the purpose of a turning and positioning schedule form.
4. A client must actually be turned and positioned before the nurse signs the turning and positioning flow sheet; although a client may be encouraged to turn, it does not mean that the client was actually turned.

Evaluation

6-35 1. A food intake diary for 3 days might be done later if initial reassessments are inadequate.
2. It is unnecessary to wait until the end of the week; the client's nutritional status can be assessed immediately.
3. It is not necessary to request a dietary assessment. The client's nutritional status can be done easily and immediately by the nurse.
4. Measuring a client's weight and comparing the result with a previous weight is a quick and easy way to determine the person's nutritional status.

6-36 1. Celery has more sodium than the nutrient in the correct option.
2. Fruit has the least amount of sodium compared with the other options.
3. Vegetables have more sodium than the nutrient in the correct option.
4. Luncheon meat is high in sodium because of the ingredients used to process it.

6-37 1. Making an appointment for the client with the primary health-care provider is inappropriate before collecting additional data on the present plan of care.
2. Arranging for the primary health-care provider to prescribe a different antibiotic is inappropriate before collecting additional data on the present plan of care; this may be necessary later.

3. Obtaining another urine sample for a culture and sensitivity test is inappropriate before collecting additional data on the present plan of care.
4. **Determining adherence to the antibiotic regimen is the priority. To maintain adequate blood levels of the drug, antibiotics must be taken routinely and consistently for the full course of treatment.**

6-38 1. Clients must not be forced to eat; the portions may be too large for a client with anorexia to ingest.
2. Adding between-meal supplements is a dependent intervention and requires a primary health-care provider's order.
3. **Arranging for five small meals daily is an interdependent nursing intervention. The primary health-care provider ordered a regular diet, and the nurse is providing this diet over five meals a day rather than the traditional three meals a day. Small, frequent feedings spread the meals throughout the day and provide a volume that is not as overwhelming as a full meal.**
4. The problem is not the number of calories provided on the tray but the amount of food the client is able to ingest at any one time.

7 Test-Taking Techniques

Performing well on nursing questions requires both roots and wings. The information in the previous chapters provided you with roots by giving you information about formulating a positive mental attitude, using critical thinking, employing time-management strategies, exploring a variety of study skills, and developing an understanding of the multiple-choice question and the nursing process. In this chapter, an attempt is made to provide you with the wings necessary to "fly through" multiple-choice questions. Flying through multiple-choice questions has nothing to do with speed; it relates to being test wise and able to navigate through complex information with ease.

Nursing tests involve complex information that has depth and breadth. In addition to having its own body of knowledge, nursing draws from a variety of disciplines, such as sociology, psychology, and anatomy and physiology. To perform well on a nursing examination, you must understand and integrate the subject matter. Nothing can replace effective study habits or knowledge about the subject being tested. However, being test wise can maximize the application of the information you possess. Being test wise entails specific techniques related to individual question analysis and general techniques related to conquering the challenge of an examination. One rationale for learning how to use these techniques is to acquire skills that increase your command over the testing situation. If you are in control, you will maintain a positive attitude, which will affect your performance in a positive manner. When you have knowledge and are test wise, you should fly through a test by gliding and soaring, rather than by flapping and fluttering.

GENERAL TEST-TAKING TECHNIQUES

A general test-taking technique is a strategy that is used to conquer the challenge of an examination. To be in command of the situation, you must manage your internal and external domains. The test taker who approaches a test with physical, mental, and emotional authority is in a position to regulate the testing situation, rather than to be dominated by it.

Follow Your Regular Routine the Night Before a Test

Follow your usual routine the night before a test. This is not the time to make changes that may disrupt your balance. If you do not normally eat pepperoni pizza, exercise, or study until 2 a.m., do not start now. Go to bed at your usual time. Avoid the temptation to have an all-night cram session. Studies have demonstrated that sleep deprivation decreases reaction times and cognitive skills. An adequate night's sleep is necessary to produce a rested mind and body, which provide the physical and emotional energy required to maximize performance on an examination.

Do Not Drive to the Test With a Friend

Car-pooling to a test can add stress if your friend finishes the test before you do. You don't want to feel pressure to finish so your friend doesn't need to wait. In addition, don't make dinner or travel plans for after you take the test, since this deadline could also put pressure on yourself to finish sooner.

Arrive Early for the Examination

Plan your schedule so that you arrive at the testing site 15 to 30 minutes early. Arrange extra time for unexpected events associated with traveling. There may be a traffic jam, a road may have a detour, the car may not start, the train may be late, the bus may break down, or you may have to park in the farthest lot from the testing site. If the location of the testing site or classroom is unfamiliar to you, it is wise to take a practice run at the same time of day as the scheduled test and locate the room. On the day of the examination, this should help you avoid getting lost or being late.

By arriving early, you have an opportunity to visit the restroom, survey the environment, and collect your thoughts. Anxiety is associated with an autonomic nervous system response, so you may have urgency, frequency, or increased intestinal peristalsis. Visit the restroom before the test to avoid using testing time to meet physical needs. The test may or may not be administered in the room in which the content is taught. Arriving early allows you to become more comfortable in the testing environment. If seats are not assigned, decide where you want to sit. Students have preferences such as sitting by a window, being in the back of the room, or surrounding themselves with friends. Selecting your own seat allows you to manipulate one aspect of your environment. In addition, this time before the test provides you with an opportunity to collect your thoughts. You may want to review content on a flash card, perform relaxation exercises, or reinforce your positive mental attitude.

Avoid comparing notes with other students. They may have inaccurate information or be anxious. Remember, anxiety is contagious. If you are the type who is affected by the anxiety of other people, avoid these people until after the test.

Bring the Appropriate Tools

To perform a task, you need adequate tools. A pen may be required to complete the identifying information on a form or answer sheet. If you are taking a paper-and-pencil test that uses a computer answer form, a pencil is necessary to record your answers. Use No. 2 pencils because they have soft lead that facilitates computer scoring of the answer sheet. Bring at least two pens and two or more pencils. Backup equipment is advisable because ink can run out and points can break. Have at least one eraser. You may decide to change an answer or need to erase extraneous marks that you make on the question book or answer sheet. When a clock is not available in the room or on the computer, a watch also is a necessary tool if permitted. Depending on your individual needs, other tools may include eyeglasses or a hearing aid. If you are taking the test using a computer, students often are not permitted to bring anything into the testing environment. All electronic devices, including watches and calculators, must be left outside the room. A clock and calculator may be accessed on the computer when desired. Assemble all your equipment the night before the test, and be sure to take them with you to the testing site.

Understand All the Directions for the Test Before Starting

It is essential to understand the instructions before beginning the test. On some tests, you are responsible for independently reading the instructions, whereas on others the proctor verbally announces the instructions. However, more often than not, you will have a written copy of the instructions while the proctor reads them aloud. In this instance, do not read ahead of the proctor. The proctor may elaborate on the written instructions, and you do not want to miss any additional directions. If you do not understand a particular part of the instructions, immediately request that the proctor explain it again. You must completely understand the instructions before beginning the examination.

Some examinations, such as the NCLEX-RN®, provide a tutorial or practice test so test takers can become acquainted with the computer-administered examination and the various question formats used. Computerized practice tests are available from proprietary companies on the Internet. A tutorial or practice test can provide a unique experience that will familiarize you with an examination on the computer and reduce the anxiety that tends to accompany the unknown.

Manage the Allotted Time to Your Advantage

All tests have a time limit. Some tests have severe time restrictions in which most test takers do not complete all the questions. These are known as "speed tests." Other tests have a generous time frame during which the majority of test takers have ample time to answer every question. These are known as "power tests." Most nursing examinations, which are designed to identify how much information the test taker knows about nursing care, are power tests. Regardless of the type of test, you must use your time well.

To manage your time on an examination, you must determine how much time you have to answer each item while leaving some time for review at the end of the testing period if permitted. To figure out how much time you should allot for each item, divide the total time you have for the test by the number of items on the test. For example, if you have 90 minutes to take a test that has 50 items, divide 90 by 50. This allots 1 minute and 48 seconds for each item. If you allot 1.5 minutes per item, you will leave 15 minutes for a final review. Be aware of the time as you progress through a test. For example, if you determine that you have approximately 1.5 minutes for each question, by the time you have completed 10 items, 15 minutes should have passed. Pace yourself so that you do not spend more than 1.5 minutes on an item if possible. If you answer an item in less than 1.5 minutes, you can use the extra time for another item that may take slightly longer than 1.5 minutes or add this time to the end for review.

The allocation of time for test completion depends on the complexity of the content, the difficulty of the reading level, and the number of options presented in the items. Read each item slowly and carefully, including all the options presented. It may be necessary to read the question twice. If you process items too quickly, you may overlook important words, become careless, or arrive at impulsive conclusions. If you find that you are spending too much time, you may want to immediately eliminate obvious distractors and not try to make them fit. Then work with only the remaining viable options. In addition, you want to avoid getting bogged down on a difficult question because you can lose valuable time, become flustered, and lose focus and concentration when upset. Clearly mark the question so that you can return to it later if permitted. Move on; this puts you back in control! Some computerized tests do not allow you to review past items. In this situation, a question must be answered before the next question is presented. Answer the question to the best of your ability, and then move on.

Work at your own pace. Do not be influenced by the actions of other test takers. If other test takers complete the examination early, ignore them and do not become concerned. Just because they finished early does not indicate they will score well on the test. They may be imprudent speed demons. A cautious and discriminating approach is to your advantage. Be your own person, and remember that time can be your friend rather than your enemy.

For tests taken on a computer, time allocation varies. The NCLEX-RN® examination allots a total time of 6 hours, and the NCLEX-PN® examination allots a total time of 5 hours. The allotted time includes a tutorial, all optional breaks taken, and the time the test taker uses to answer test items. The length of the NCLEX-RN® examination varies from 75 to 265 questions depending on the test taker's ability. It is recommended that test takers spend no more than 1 to 2 minutes per question to maintain a pace of 1.5 minutes per question. This pace is recommended to ensure adequate time if the test taker requires the maximum number of questions. Most test takers finish the test with plenty of time to spare (https://www.ncsbn.org/ngn-resources.htm).

Concentrate on the Simple Before the Complex

If possible, answer the easy questions before the difficult questions. This is not an option with the NCLEX® examination, but might be an option in your nursing program. This technique uses the basic teaching/learning principle of moving from the simple to the complex. By doing this, you can maximize your use of time and maintain a positive mental attitude.

Begin answering questions. When you are confronted with a difficult item, have already used your allotted time to answer it, and still do not know the answer, then skip over this item and move on to the next one. Make a notation on scrap paper, next to the item in the question booklet, next to the number of the skipped item on the answer sheet, or in the appropriate location on a computer-administered examination so that you can return to this item later in the test if permitted. When you reach the end of the test, return to the items that you saved for the end. You should have time to spend on these items, and you may have accessed information from other items that can assist you in answering these questions. Concentrating on the simple before the complex permits you to answer the maximum number of items in the time allocated for the examination.

The strategy to skip a complex question and return to it later in the test may not be applicable on computer-administered tests, such as NCLEX® examinations. You may be required to enter an answer before the next item will appear on the screen.

Avoid Reading Into the Question

A nursing question has two parts. The first part is known as the *stem*. The stem is the statement that asks a question. The second part contains the possible responses, which are called *options*. The stem of a question also has two parts. One part presents information about a clinical event, topic, concept, or theory. The other part asks you to respond in some way. The response part asks you to choose the option that answers the question on the basis of the information presented in the stem. The information presented in the stem needs to be separated in your mind from the response part of the stem. In some questions, the information and response parts of the question are very clear. Other questions are presented in a manner that makes it less clear which is the information part and which is the response part.

The questions that follow illustrate the difference between the information and the response parts of the stem. In each example, the information part of the stem is **boldfaced** and the response part is *italicized.*

While walking, a client becomes weak, and the client's knees begin to buckle. *What should the nurse do?*

Which is an example of **a client goal?**

What should the nurse do first **before administering medication for pain?**

Questions generally are designed to test common principles and concepts. Therefore, it is important that you avoid overanalyzing the facts in the question. In an attempt to achieve this goal, consider the following suggestions:

When reading the stem:

- Identify the important words.
- Do not add information from your own mind and/or experience.
- Do not make assumptions (read between the lines) about the information presented in the stem.

When reading the options:

- Read all the options before choosing the correct answer.
- Refer back only to the words that you identified as being important in the stem.
- Do not add information to an option.
- Relate an option only to what is being asked in the response part of the stem.
- Focus on commonalities, principles, and concepts associated with the level of learning that is being tested.
- Do not focus only on your experiences, which may be too narrow for a point of reference.
- Recognize that although an option may contain correct information, it may or may not have anything to do with the information and response parts of the stem.

When reading options, it is important that you read all of them before selecting the correct answer. This may sound like a ridiculous suggestion; however, we found that students often selected options 1, 2, or 3 over option 4. We tested this theory by placing the correct answer as option 1 on one test and then placing it as option 4 on a different examination.

When the correct answer was 4 instead of 1, fewer students selected the correct option. When students answered incorrectly on items for which the correct answer was option 4, we asked if they had examined the final option; some students admitted that they had not read all the options.

Don't try to see a pattern in the correct option order. In other words, if the correct answers have been option 2 in two questions in a row, don't assume that option 2 will not be the correct answer in the third question, as well. Just focus on each question as an individual unit.

Most students find it helpful to separate the information part of a question from the response part of the question. By incorporating this suggestion, you should be better able to identify what information is in the stem and what you are being asked to do. As a result, your chances of answering the question correctly, without reading into the question, should increase.

Make Educated Guesses

An educated guess is the selection of an option using partial knowledge, without knowing for certain that it is the correct answer. When you have reduced the final selection to two options, usually it is to your advantage to reassess these options in the context of the knowledge you do possess and make an educated guess. Of the two options, consider "What does not make sense about this option?" as you decide between the options, to help in making your final selection. Making a wild guess by flipping a coin or choosing your favorite number should be limited to tests that do not have a penalty for guessing.

Some examinations assign credit when you answer a question correctly and do not assign credit when you answer a question incorrectly. The directions for these examinations may state that only correct answers will receive credit, that you should answer every question, that you should not leave any blanks, or that there are no penalties for guessing. In these tests, it is to your advantage to answer every question. First, select answers based on knowledge. If you are unsure of the correct answer, reduce the number of options using test-taking techniques and then make an educated guess. If you have absolutely no idea what the answer is, then make a wild guess because you will not be penalized for a wrong answer.

Other tests assign credit when you answer a question correctly and subtract credit when you answer a question incorrectly. The instructions for these examinations may inform you not to guess or may state that credit will be subtracted for incorrect answers or that there is a penalty for guessing. In these tests, a statistical manipulation is performed to mathematically limit the advantage of guessing. When taking these tests, it is still to your advantage to make an educated guess when, through knowledge, you can reduce your final selection to two options. However, wild guessing is not to your advantage because your chance of selecting the correct answer is only 25% when there are four options.

Maintain a Positive Mental Attitude

It is important that you foster a positive mental attitude and a sense of relaxation. A little apprehension can be motivating, but too much can interfere with your attention, concentration, and problem-solving ability. To enhance relaxation and a positive mental attitude, use the positive techniques you have practiced and that work for you. For example, enhance relaxation by employing diaphragmatic breathing for several deep breaths, rotating your shoulders, or flexing and extending your head. Foster a positive mental attitude by telling yourself, "I am prepared to do this well!" or "I know I have studied hard, and I will be successful!"

Check Your Answers and Answer Sheet

It is important to record your answers accurately, particularly when using a computer scoring sheet. Paper-and-pencil computer-scored tests usually use separate answer sheets on which numbers or letters represent the corresponding responses to each item in the test. You do not want to lose points because you placed your answer in the wrong row. You should verify the number of the question with the number on the answer sheet at least two times when recording your answer. You should conscientiously do this every time you record an answer.

At the end of the examination, again review your answer sheet for accuracy. Make sure that every mark is within the lines, is heavy and full, and is in the appropriate space. Erase any extraneous marks on the answer sheet. Additional pencil marks, inadequately erased answers, and marks outside the lines will confuse the computer and alter your score. Also, make sure that you have answered every question, especially on tests that do not penalize you for guessing. An effective and thorough review should leave you with a feeling of control and a sense of closure at the end of the examination.

When you take an examination on a computer, you may be required to answer a question before moving on to the next question. On other computer examinations, you may be permitted to skip a question and answer it later or answer a question and go back and change your answer. Whenever you submit your final choice on a computer examination, double-check your selected response before hitting the key that finalizes your answer.

SPECIFIC TEST-TAKING TECHNIQUES

A specific test-taking technique is a strategy in which skill and forethought are used to analyze a test item before an answer is selected. A technique is not a gimmick but a method of examining a question with consideration and thoughtfulness to help you select the correct answer. When an item has four options, the chance of selecting the correct answer is one out of four, or 25%. When you eliminate one distractor, the chance of selecting the correct answer is one out of three, or 33.3%. If you are able to eliminate two distractors, the chance of selecting the correct answer is one out of two, or 50%. Each time you successfully eliminate a distractor, you dramatically increase your chances of correctly answering the question.

Before you attempt to answer a question, break it into its components. First, read the stem. What is it actually asking? It may be helpful to paraphrase the stem to focus on its content. Then, try to answer the question in your own words before looking at the options. Often, one of the options will be similar to your answer. Then examine the other options and try to identify the correct answer.

If you know, understand, and can apply the information being tested, you often can identify the correct answer. However, do not be tempted to select an option too quickly, without careful thought. An option may contain accurate information, but it may not be correct because it does not answer the question asked in the stem. Be careful! Each option deserves equal consideration.

Use test-taking techniques for every question in conjunction with your knowledge base. When you select an answer based on your knowledge, have confidence in your answer. However, the use of test-taking techniques becomes more important when you are unsure of the answer because each distractor that you are able to eliminate increases your chances of selecting the correct answer. Most nursing students are able to reduce the number of plausible answers to two. Use everything in your arsenal to conquer the multiple-choice question test: effective studying, a positive mental attitude, and last but not least, test-taking techniques.

The correct answers for the sample items in this chapter and the rationales for all the options are presented at the end of the chapter.

Identify the Word in the Stem That Indicates Negative Polarity

On a nursing examination, read each question stem slowly and carefully. Look for key words that indicate negative polarity such as **not, except, never, avoid, violate,** and **least.** Some words that indicate negative polarity are not as obvious as others, such as **unacceptable, contraindicated, unrelated,** and **irrelevant.** The stem of a question containing a word that indicates negative polarity is asking a question that is concerned with what is false. A negatively worded stem asks you to identify an exception, detect an error, or recognize nursing interventions that are unacceptable or contraindicated. If you read a stem and several of the options appear correct, reread the stem because you may have missed a key negative word. These words are sometimes brought to your attention by an underline (<u>not</u>), italic font (*except*), boldface font (**never**), or capital letters (VIOLATE). Many nursing examinations avoid questions with negative polarity. However, examples of these items are included for your information.

SAMPLE ITEM 7-1

Which action violates medical asepsis when the nurse makes an occupied bed?

1. Returning unused linen to a linen closet
2. Wearing gloves when changing the linen
3. Tucking clean linen against the frame of the bed
4. Using the old top sheet for the new bottom sheet

The key term in this stem is *violates.* The stem is asking you to identify the option that does not follow correct medical aseptic technique. If you miss the word *violates* and look for the answer that indicated correct medical aseptic technique, there will be more than one correct answer. When this happens, reread the stem for a word with negative polarity. To answer this item correctly, you have to be particularly careful because the word *violates* is not emphasized for your attention.

SAMPLE ITEM 7-2

A client is receiving a low-sodium diet. Which food should the nurse teach the client to avoid because it is high in sodium?

1. Stewed fruit
2. Luncheon meats
3. Whole-grain cereal
4. Green, leafy vegetables

The key word in this stem is *avoid;* it is brought to your attention because it is italicized. The stem is asking you to select the food that a client receiving a low-sodium diet should not eat. If you miss the word *avoid* and look for foods that are permitted on a low-sodium diet, there will be more than one correct answer. When there appears to be more than one correct answer, reread the stem for a key negative word that you may have missed.

SAMPLE ITEM 7-3

When rubbing a client's back, the nurse should never:

1. apply pressure over vertebrae.
2. use continuous strokes.
3. wipe off excess lotion.
4. knead the skin.

The key word in this stem is *never.* The stem is asking you to identify which option is not an acceptable practice associated with a back rub. If you miss the word *never* and look for what the nurse should do for a back rub, there will be more than one correct answer. This should alert you to the fact that you missed a key negative word.

Identify the Word in the Stem That Sets a Priority

Read the stem carefully while looking for key words such as **first, initially, best, priority, safest, highest, support,** and **most.** These words modify what is being asked. This type of question requires you to put a value on each option and then place them in rank order. If the question asks what the nurse should do first, what the initial action by the nurse should be, or what the best response is, then rank the options in order of importance from 1 to 4, with the most desirable option as number 1 and the least desirable option as number 4. The correct answer is the option that you ranked number 1. If you are having difficulty ranking the options, eliminate the option that you believe is most wrong among all the options. Next, eliminate the option you believe is most wrong among the remaining three options. At this point, you are down to two options, and if only one option is correct, your chance of selecting the correct answer is 50%. When key words such as *most important* are used, frequently two or more of the options are appropriate nursing care for the situation. However, only one of the options is the *most* important. When all the options appear logical for the situation, reread the stem to identify a key word that asks you to place a priority on the options. These words occasionally are emphasized by an underline, *italic font,* **boldface font,** or CAPITAL LETTERS.

Answering a test question that asks you to establish a priority requires you to make a decision using clinical judgment. You must use perceptual, inferential, and/or diagnostic judgment to arrive at the correct answer according to the data in the question and options. To do this, you must draw on your knowledge of theory, concepts, principles, and nursing standards of practice. The student who has a strong foundation of knowledge and who is a critical thinker is best equipped to arrive at the correct answer. For additional information about making clinical decisions and types of clinical judgments, refer to Chapter 2, "Critical Thinking," in the section "Clinical Judgments," and Chapter 8, in the section "Clinical Judgment Question Formats Reflective of Next Generation NCLEX." A strategy to help you answer priority questions is to refer to basic guiding theories that are part of the foundation of nursing. Maslow's hierarchy of needs, the nursing process, Kübler-Ross's theory of death and dying, man as a unified being, the theory that the client is the center of the health-care team, teaching/learning theory, emotional support and communication theory, and the ABCs (Airway, Breathing, Circulation) of prioritizing physical care, to name a few, present clear parameters of practice that are the foundation of nursing practice. Choosing which theory or principle to draw on when answering a test question comes with practice. You first have to identify "what is happening" and "what should I do." You then have to identify which theory or principle applies best in the scenario presented in the question in light of the options presented.

You should keep these theories in mind when answering test questions, while recognizing the following concepts:

- Physiological needs generally need to be met first, before higher-level needs.
- Disbelief and denial are generally a person's first responses to news of a loss or anticipated loss.
- Meeting the needs of the client comes first over other tasks.
- Client readiness to learn must be assessed first, before designing a teaching program.
- A client's emotional status must be assessed as part of the first step in the nursing process.
- Nurses need to use interviewing techniques to communicate effectively in a nonthreatening way with clients.
- The nurse must deliver care in a nonjudgmental manner.
- Maintaining a client's airway is always a priority.
- The client's safety is always a priority.
- A thorough assessment must be completed before other steps in the nursing process.

Practice the questions in Chapter 11 that ask you to set a priority, and study the rationales for the right and wrong answers. Priority questions are identified by the statement "Identify key words in the stem that set a priority," which appears in the TEST-TAKING TIP after the question. This will help you build a body of knowledge based on what the nurse should do first in different clinical situations presented in practice questions.

SAMPLE ITEM 7-4

Which should the nurse do first before administering an enema?
1. Collect the appropriate equipment
2. Inform the client about the procedure
3. Ensure the client's bathroom is empty
4. Verify the prescription for the procedure

The key word in this stem is *first.* Each of these options includes a step that is part of the procedure for administering an enema. You must decide which option is the *first* step among the four options presented. Before you can teach a client, collect equipment, or actually administer the enema, you need to know the type of enema prescribed. The type of enema will influence the other steps of the procedure. If option 4 were different, such as "Use medical asepsis to dispose of contaminated articles," the correct answer among these four options would be option 2. You can choose the first step of a procedure only from among the options presented.

SAMPLE ITEM 7-5

An older adult client has significant short-term memory loss and does not remember the primary nurse from day to day. The client asks the nurse, "Who are you?" Which is the most appropriate response by the nurse?
1. "You know me. I take care of you every day."
2. Say nothing, because it probably will upset the client.
3. State your name and say, "I am the nurse caring for you."
4. Place a sign with your name on it on the wall across from the client's bed.

The words *most appropriate* in the stem set a priority. You are asked to select the most suitable response from among the four options presented. You may dislike all of the statements. You may even think of a response that you personally prefer to the presented options. YOU CANNOT REWRITE THE QUESTION. You must select your answer from the options presented in the item. The words *most appropriate* are not highlighted in this item; therefore, you must be diligent when reading the stem.

SAMPLE ITEM 7-6

A nurse is caring for a client who just had a long leg cast applied for a compound fracture of the femur. Which is the **most** important nursing intervention when caring for this client?
1. Turn and position every 4 hours
2. Take pulses proximal to the casted area
3. Cover rough edges of the cast with tape
4. Inspect the cast for signs of drainage or bleeding

The word *most* in the stem sets a priority. Use the ABCs (Airway, Breathing, and Circulation) to identify the *most* important option. No options are associated with airway or breathing. However, options 2 and 4 are associated with circulation. If you identify that assessing a distal, not proximal, pulse is important, then you can eliminate option 2. You have arrived at the correct answer.

Identify Key Words in the Stem That Direct Attention to Content

Generally, the stem of an item is short and contains only the information needed to make it clear and specific. Therefore, the use of a word or phrase in the stem has significance. A key word or phrase provides information that leads you to the correct answer. Sometimes a key word or phrase modifies another word or phrase in the stem. A key word or phrase takes a broad concept and focuses the reader's attention on a more specific aspect of the concept (see Sample Item 7-7). Other times, a word or phrase in the stem is significant because it is similar to or a paraphrase of a word or phrase in the correct answer (see Sample Item 7-8).

Occasionally, a word or phrase in the stem is identical to a word or phrase in the correct answer and is called a **clang association** (see Sample Item 7-9). Every word in the stem is important, but some words are more significant than others. The identification of key words and the analysis of the significance of these words in relation to the stem and the options require critical thinking.

SAMPLE ITEM 7-7

Which should the nurse do to meet a client's basic physiological needs according to Maslow's hierarchy of needs?

1. Maintain the client's body in functional alignment
2. Pull the curtain when the client is on a bedpan
3. Respond to a call light immediately
4. Raise both side rails on the bed

An important word in the stem is *physiological*. It is an intentional use of a word to specifically limit consideration to one aspect of Maslow's theory.

SAMPLE ITEM 7-8

Which should the nurse do to help meet a client's self-esteem needs?

1. Encourage the client to perform self-care when able
2. Ask family members to visit the client more often
3. Anticipate needs before the client requests help
4. Give the client a complete bath

An important term in the stem is *self-esteem*. The term *self-esteem* is similar to the term *self-care*. Thoughtfully examine option 1. An option that incorporates words that are similar to words in the stem is often the correct answer. In addition, the term *self-esteem* in the stem intentionally focuses on one aspect of Maslow's theory. This question exemplifies the use of two clues in the stem when answering a question.

SAMPLE ITEM 7-9

Which should the nurse do to meet a client's basic physical needs?

1. Pull the curtain when providing care
2. Answer the call bell immediately
3. Administer physical hygiene
4. Obtain vital signs

An important word in the stem is *physical*. It is a clue that should provide a hint that option 3 is the correct *answer*. The use of the word physical in both the stem and the correct option is called a *clang association*. It is the repetitious use of a word. Examine option 3 because when a clang association occurs, it is often the correct answer.

Identify the Central Person in the Question

Test questions usually require the nurse to respond to the needs of a client. When a stem is limited to just the client and the nurse, the client usually is the central person in the question. However, some questions focus on the needs of others, such as a child, parent, spouse, or roommate. To select the correct option, you have to identify the central (significant) person in the stem. The significant person is the person who is to receive the care. The inclusion of others may set the stage for the question or test your ability to discriminate. Mention of these people also may distract you from who is actually the significant person in the stem. Therefore, to answer the question accurately, you must determine WHO is the central person in the question.

SAMPLE ITEM 7-10

A nurse will be going on vacation. Which is the **best** response by the nurse to involve the client in the excitement?

1. "Tell me about some of your favorite past vacations."
2. "Do you want to hear about the plans for my trip?"
3. "I'll bring the brochures for you to see."
4. "What do you think about vacations?"

There are two people in this stem, the client and the nurse. There are two clues in the stem. The first clue is "involve the client." To involve the client, the client must be active. Therefore, options 2 and 3 can be eliminated because they focus on the nurse, who is not the central person in the question. The second clue is the word best. The word best is asking you to set a priority. More than one option may include appropriate nursing care, but only one is the "best" action. Options 1 and 4 include appropriate nursing care. However, option 1 requires a more detailed response than option 4. Reminiscing involves more than just giving an opinion.

SAMPLE ITEM 7-11

A client who has experienced the surgical removal of a breast (mastectomy) says to the nurse, "My husband can't look at my incision and hasn't suggested having sex since my surgery." Which should be the initial action of the nurse?

1. Arrange to speak with the husband about his concerns
2. Plan to teach the husband that the wife needs his support
3. Explore the client's feelings about her husband's behavior
4. Make an appointment with Reach for Recovery for the client

There are three people in this stem: the client, the husband, and the nurse. There are two clues in the stem. The first clue is the quoted statement by the client about her husband's behavior. The second clue is the word *initial*. The word *initial* is asking you to set a priority. The situation may require one or more of these responses, but only one of them should be done first. The client's statement reflects the client's concern. Addressing the client's concern should come first. The client is the central person in this question, not the husband. Options 1 and 2 focus on the husband, who is not the central person in this question, and can be eliminated. In option 4, the nurse is using a referral to evade the issues involved and avoid professional responsibility.

SAMPLE ITEM 7-12

A client is friendly and appears happy. However, when the client's daughter visits, the client cries and reports the presence of pain. The daughter's eyes are filled with tears, and she is visibly upset when she leaves her mother's room. Which should the nurse do?

1. Explore the situation with the daughter
2. Encourage the client to be more positive
3. Tell the daughter that the client usually does not cry
4. Observe the interaction between them without intervening at this time

There are three people in this situation: the client, the daughter, and the nurse. The question expects the nurse to follow one course of action when the daughter becomes upset. The phrase "she is visibly upset" shifts the focus of the question to the daughter. Options 1 and 3 focus on the daughter. By eliminating two options (options 2 and 4), you have increased your chances of getting this question correct to 50%.

Identify Client-Centered Options

Nursing is a profession that provides both physical and emotional care to clients. Therefore, the nurse's concern usually is focused on the client. Items that test your ability to be client-centered tend to explore the client's feelings, identify the client's preferences, empower the client, afford the client choices, or in some other way put the emphasis on the client. The client is the center of the health-care team and, therefore, generally is the priority.

SAMPLE ITEM 7-13

When a client who recently had an above-the-knee amputation is assisted with a transfer into a chair, the client starts to cry and says, "I am useless with only one leg." Which is a therapeutic response by the nurse?

1. "Losing a leg can be very difficult."
2. "You still have the use of one good leg."
3. "A prosthesis will make a big difference."
4. "You'll feel better when you can use crutches."

Option 1 is client-centered. It focuses on the client's feelings by using the interviewing technique of reflection. Option 2 denies the client's feelings, and options 3 and 4 provide false reassurance. When a client's feelings are ignored or minimized, the nurse is not being client-centered. To be client-centered, the nurse should concentrate on the client's feelings or concerns.

SAMPLE ITEM 7-14

A client who is oriented states, "I always forget the questions I want to ask when my doctor visits me." Which is the nurse's **best** response?

1. Offer to stay when the doctor visits
2. Remind the client of the doctor's next visit
3. Give the client materials to write questions to ask the doctor
4. Suggest that a family member be available to question the doctor

Option 3 is client-centered. It focuses on the client's ability, fosters independence, and empowers the client. Option 2 does not address the client's concern, and options 1 and 4 promote dependence, which can lower self-esteem. Avoiding client concerns and promoting dependence are not client-centered actions. To be client-centered, the nurse should encourage self-care.

SAMPLE ITEM 7-15

Which should the nurse do first when combing a female client's hair?

1. Use tap water to moisten the hair
2. Apply a hair conditioner before combing
3. Comb the client's hair using long strokes
4. Ask the client how she prefers to wear her hair

Option 4 is client-centered. It allows choices and supports the person as an individual. Options 1, 2, and 3 do not take client preferences into consideration. A procedure that is begun before determining client preferences is not client-centered. The Patient Care Partnership (formerly the Patient's Bill of Rights) mandates that the client has a right to considerate and respectful care and to receive information before the start of any procedure and/or treatment.

SAMPLE ITEM 7-16

A client enjoys television programs about animals. After one of these programs, the client cries and sadly talks about a beloved cat that died. Which should be the nurse's initial response?

1. Tell the client a story about a cat
2. Hang a picture of a cat in the client's room
3. Ask the client to share more about the cat she loved
4. Obtain a book about cats for the client from the library

Option 3 is client-centered. It encourages the client to communicate further. Options 1, 2, and 4 may eventually be done because they take into consideration the client's interest in cats. However, they should not be the initial action because they do not focus on the client's feelings at this time. The nurse is being client-centered when encouraging additional communication and expression of feelings and concerns from the client.

Identify Specific Determiners in Options

A specific determiner is a word or statement that conveys a thought or concept that has no exceptions. Words such as **just, always, never, all, every, none,** and **only** are absolute and easy to identify. They place limits on a statement that generally is considered correct. Statements that use all-inclusive terms frequently represent broad generalizations that are false. *Frequently, options that contain a specific determiner are incorrect and can be eliminated.* However, some absolutes, such as "All clients should be treated with respect," are correct. Nevertheless, there are few absolutes in this world, so options that contain specific determiners should be examined carefully. Be discriminating.

SAMPLE ITEM 7-17

A nurse is giving a client a bed bath. How can the nurse best improve the client's circulation during the bath?

1. Use firm strokes
2. Utilize only hot water
3. Keep the client covered
4. Apply soap to the washcloth

In option 2, the word *only* is a specific determiner. It allows for no exceptions. Hot water can burn the skin and also is contraindicated for clients with sensitive skin, such as children, older adults, and people with dermatological problems. Option 2 allows for no exceptions, so it can be eliminated as a viable option.

SAMPLE ITEM 7-18

Which action protects nurses from microorganisms when providing perineal care for clients?

1. Washing the hands before giving care
2. Disposing of contaminated water in the toilet
3. Wearing clean gloves when providing perineal care
4. Encouraging clients to provide all of their own care

In option 4, the word *all* is a specific determiner. It is a word that obviously includes everything. Expecting clients to provide all of their own care is unreasonable, is unrealistic, and may be unsafe. Option 4 can be eliminated. This increases your chances of choosing the correct answer because you have to choose from among three options rather than four.

SAMPLE ITEM 7-19

A client states that the elastic straps of the oxygen face mask feel too tight. How should the nurse respond?

1. Explain the face mask must always stay firmly in place
2. Replace the face mask with a nasal cannula
3. Pad the straps with gauze
4. Adjust the straps

In option 1, the word *always* is a specific determiner. It is an absolute term that places limits on a statement. This option can be eliminated. By deleting option 1, the chances of selecting the correct answer become 33.3% rather than 25%.

Identify Opposites in Options

Sometimes an item contains two options that are the opposite of each other. They can be single words that reflect extremes on a continuum, or they can be statements that convey converse messages. When opposites appear in the options, they must be given serious consideration. One of them may be the correct answer, or they both can be eliminated from consideration. *When options are opposites, more often than not, but not always, one of them is the correct answer.* When one of the opposites is the correct answer, you are being asked to differentiate between two responses that incorporate extremes of a concept or principle. When an opposite is a distractor, it is attempting to divert your attention from the correct answer. If you correctly evaluate opposite options, you can increase your chances of selecting the correct answer because you have reduced the plausible options to two or three. However, the test-taking technique, *Identify Opposites in Options*, usually cannot be applied to options that reflect numerical values (e.g., heart rates, blood pressure levels, respiratory rates, laboratory values). The sample items that follow provide various examples of how opposites appear in options.

SAMPLE ITEM 7-20

Which of the following descriptions reflects the progress of growth and development in all older adults?

1. Slips backward
2. Moves forward
3. Becomes slower
4. Remains stagnant

Options 1 and 2 are opposites. They should be considered carefully in relation to each other and then in relation to the other options. These options are the reverse sides of a concept, movement in relation to growth and development. Options 3 and 4, although true for some individuals, are not true statements about all older adults as indicated in the stem. You now must select between options 1 and 2. Option 2 is the correct answer. By focusing on options 1 and 2 and then progressively examining and deleting options 3 and 4, you have systematically scrutinized this item.

SAMPLE ITEM 7-21

Antiembolism stockings are ordered for a client. When should the nurse apply the antiembolism stockings?

1. While the client is still in bed
2. Once the client reports having leg pain
3. When the client's feet become edematous
4. After the client gets out of bed in the morning

Options 1 and 4 are opposites. Examine these options first. They are contrary to each other in relation to before or after an event, getting out of bed. Now assess options 2 and 3. These options expect the nurse to apply antiembolism stockings after a problem exists. The purpose of these stockings is to foster venous return, thereby preventing dependent edema. Options 2 and 3 can be omitted from further consideration. The final selection is between options 1 and 4. You have increased your chances of correctly answering the question from 25% to 50%. Lower extremity edema can occur when the legs and feet are dependent; as a result, antiembolism stockings should be applied before, not after, the client gets out of bed. You have arrived at the correct answer, option 1, using a methodical approach.

SAMPLE ITEM 7-22

A school nurse is teaching a health class about nutrition. Which is the primary reason that protein foods are used by the body and should be included in the discussion?
1. Energy
2. Growth
3. Excretion
4. Catabolism

Options 2 and 4 are obscure opposites. Protein intake is related to the construction phase of metabolism, contributing to repair and growth of the body (anabolism). Anabolism is the opposite of catabolism. Catabolism (think of the word "cut") is related to the destructive phase of metabolism, when complex substances are reduced to simpler substances, releasing energy. Examine options 2 and 4 carefully because, more often than not, an option that is an opposite is the correct answer.

Identify Equally Plausible or Unique Options

Sometimes items contain two or more options that are similar. It is difficult to choose between two similar options. One option is no better or worse than the other option in relation to the statement presented in the stem. When analyzing options, use the "If → Then" technique. Ask yourself, "If I perform this intervention in the option, then what will be the outcome?" In equally plausible options, the outcomes also are frequently the same or similar. *Usually, equally plausible options are distractors and can be eliminated from consideration.* You have now improved your chances of selecting the correct answer to 50%.

If you find three equally plausible options on initial examination, the fourth option probably is different from the others and appears unique. Children's activity books present a game based on this concept. Four pictures are presented, and the child is asked to pick the one that is different. "Which one of these is not like the others? Which one of these is not the same?" For example, the picture may contain three types of fruit and one vegetable, and the child is asked to identify which one is different. The correct answer to a test item can sometimes be identified by using this concept of similarities and differences.

SAMPLE ITEM 7-23

Which should the nurse do to effectively help meet a client's basic safety and security needs?
1. Serve adequate food
2. Provide sufficient fluid
3. Place the call bell near the client
4. Store the client's valuables in the bedside table

Options 1 and 2 are similar because they both provide nutrients. They are equally plausible when compared with each other and particularly when assessed in relation to the concepts of safety and security; neither relates to meeting a client's safety and security needs. These options are distractors and can be eliminated from consideration. By having to choose between only options 3 and 4, you have raised your chances of correctly answering the question to 50%.

SAMPLE ITEM 7-24

How can the nurse promote circulation when providing a back rub?
1. Place the client in the prone position
2. Use moisturizing cream
3. Apply Keri Lotion
4. Knead the skin

Options 2 and 3 use substances when performing the back rub. Ask yourself, "If I use moisturizing cream, then what is the outcome?" Ask yourself, "If I use Keri Lotion, then what is the outcome?" In both instances the outcome is that the skin will become less dry and more supple. Because the outcomes are similar, the options are equally plausible. Equally plausible options usually are distractors; therefore, you can delete these options. Now evaluate the remaining options. One of them is the correct answer.

SAMPLE ITEM 7-25

Nurses understand that passive range-of-motion exercises are performed to:
1. increase endurance.
2. prevent loss of mobility.
3. strengthen muscle tone.
4. maximize muscle atrophy.

Options 1, 3, and 4 all include words (*increase, strengthen,* and *maximize*) that address improvement of something (endurance, muscle tone, and atrophy). They are alike. Option 2 is different. It prevents something from happening, loss of mobility. Option 2 is unique compared with the presentation of the other options, and it should be given careful consideration. Even if you do not know the definition of "atrophy" and do not understand that the loss of muscle mass should not be maximized, you can still use the test-taking technique of identifying similar and unique options. "Which one of these is not like the others? Which one of these is not the same?"

SAMPLE ITEM 7-26

Which should the nurse plan to do immediately before performing any client procedure?
1. Shut the door
2. Wash the hands
3. Close the curtain
4. Drape the client

Options 1, 3, and 4 are similar in that they all somehow enclose the client. Ask yourself about the outcome of each intervention (If → Then). Options 1, 3, and 4 all provide for client privacy. They are all plausible interventions when providing client care. It is difficult to choose the most correct answer from among these three options. Option 2 is different. It relates to microbiological safety rather than emotional safety (privacy). This option is unique compared with the other options, so it should be thoroughly examined in relation to the stem because it is likely the correct answer.

Identify the Global Option

A global option is more comprehensive and general than the other options. Although unspoken, the global option may include under its mantle a specific concept identified in one or more of the other options. Identifying global options is similar to identifying unique options. The global option usually is a broad general statement, whereas the three distractors generally are specific. You must pick out the option that is different. "Which one of these is not like the others? Which one of these is not the same?"

SAMPLE ITEM 7-27

Which is the most effective way for the nurse to prevent the spread of infection in a nursing home?
1. Administer antibiotics to sick clients
2. Limit the spread of microorganisms
3. Isolate clients who are sick
4. Keep all unit doors closed

Options 1, 3, and 4 are all incorrect as indicated in the rationales. However, if you did not know that they were incorrect and you just examined the four options, you should have noticed that options 1, 3, and 4 all identify specific actions, whereas option 2 is broad and general and is different from the other options. Also, note that option 4 contains the word *all*, which is a specific determiner.

SAMPLE ITEM 7-28

Which is the **most** important principle of body mechanics when the nurse is repositioning a client?
1. Elevating the arms on pillows
2. Maintaining functional alignment
3. Preventing external rotation of the hips
4. Placing a small pillow under the lumbar curvature

Options 1, 3, and 4 are something the nurse might do to support a client in a specific position. However, option 2 is comprehensive and broad and identifies something the nurse should do when positioning all clients regardless of the specific position.

Identify Duplicate Facts Among Options

Sometimes items are designed so that each option contains two or more pieces of information. Usually, identical or similar pieces of information appear in at least two of the four options. If you identify a piece of information as incorrect, you can eliminate all the options that contain this piece of information. By deleting distractors, you increase your chances of selecting the correct answer.

SAMPLE ITEM 7-29

The nurse is making the occupied bed of a client who has a vest restraint. To promote client safety, the nurse should:
1. untie the vest restraint and lower both side rails.
2. keep the vest restraint tied and lower both side rails.
3. untie the vest restraint and lower the rail on the working side of the bed.
4. keep the vest restraint tied and lower the rail on the working side of the bed.

This item is testing two concepts: whether a vest restraint should be tied or untied when providing direct care and whether one or both side rails should be lowered when providing direct care. If you know only that the side rail should be lowered just on the side on which you are working, you can eliminate options 1 and 2. If you know only that a vest restraint can be untied when the nurse is at the bedside providing direct care, you can eliminate options 2 and 4. In either case, you can eliminate two options as distractors, and you have increased your chances of selecting the correct answer from 25% to 50%.

SAMPLE ITEM 7-30

A 2-gram sodium diet is prescribed for a client. Which group of nutrients is **most** appropriate for this diet?

1. Fruit, vegetables, and bread
2. Hot dogs, mustard, and pickles
3. Hamburger, onions, and ketchup
4. Luncheon meats, rolls, and vegetables

This item is testing your knowledge about the sodium content of foods. If you know that hot dogs and luncheon meats are both processed foods that are high in sodium, you can eliminate options 2 and 4. If you understand that ketchup and mustard are both condiments that are high in sodium, you can delete options 2 and 3. By knowing either piece of information you can reduce the final selection to two options. The similarities between these options would be clearer if the parts were identical, but the technique of identifying duplicate facts in options can still be used.

SAMPLE ITEM 7-31

A nurse is monitoring a client who is at risk for hemorrhage. For which clinical manifestations should the nurse assess the client?

1. Warm, dry skin; hypotension; bounding pulse
2. Hypertension; bounding pulse; cold, clammy skin
3. Weak, thready pulse; hypertension; warm, dry skin
4. Hypotension; cold, clammy skin; weak, thready pulse

This item is testing your knowledge about client responses associated with hemorrhage. Three client responses are presented: the condition of the skin, the blood pressure, and the characteristic of the pulse. If you know that hypotension is associated with hemorrhage, you can eliminate options 2 and 3. If you know that cold, clammy skin is related to hemorrhage, you can delete options 1 and 3. If you know that a weak, thready pulse is associated with hemorrhage, you can eliminate options 1 and 2. If you know only one or two of the pieces of information presented, you can maximize your chance of correctly answering this type of item. Options that have two or three parts work to your advantage if you use the technique of identifying duplicate facts in options.

Identify Options That Deny Clients' Feelings, Concerns, or Needs

Nurses are human and caring and primarily want their clients to get well; thus, they often assume the role of champion, protector, or savior. However, by inappropriately adopting these roles, nurses often diminish clients' concerns, provide false reassurance, and/or cut off further client communication. To be a client advocate, the nurse cannot always be a Pollyanna. Pollyanna, the heroine of stories by Eleanor Hodgman Porter, was a person of irrepressible optimism who found good in everything. Sometimes nurses must focus on the negative rather than the positive, acknowledge that everything may not have a desired outcome, and concentrate on clients' feelings as a priority. Options that imply everything will be all right deny the client's feelings, change the subject raised by the client, encourage the client to be cheerful, or transfer nursing responsibility to other members of the health-care team usually are distractors and can be eliminated from consideration.

SAMPLE ITEM 7-32

The day before surgery for a hysterectomy, a client says to the nurse, "I am worried that I might die tomorrow." Which response by the nurse is therapeutic?

1. "It is really routine surgery."
2. "The thought of dying can be frightening."
3. "You need to tell your surgeon about this."
4. "Most people who have this surgery survive."

Options 1 and 4 minimize the client's concern because these messages imply that there is nothing to worry about; the surgery is routine, and most clients survive. In option 3, the nurse avoids the opportunity to encourage further discussion of the client's feelings and surrenders this responsibility to the surgeon. After collecting more information, the nurse should inform the surgeon of the client's concern about death. Options 1, 3, and 4 deny the client's feelings and can be eliminated because they are distractors. Option 2 is the correct answer because it encourages the client to focus on the expressed feelings about death.

SAMPLE ITEM 7-33

After surgery, a client reports mild incisional pain while performing deep breathing and coughing exercises. Which is the nurse's **best** response?

1. "Each day it will hurt less and less."
2. "This is an expected response after surgery."
3. "With a pillow, apply pressure against the incision."
4. "I will get the pain medication that was prescribed."

Option 1 is a Pollyanna-like response that may provide false reassurance. The nurse does not know that the pain will get less and less for this client. Option 1 can be deleted from consideration. Although option 2 is a true statement, it cuts off communication because it diminishes the client's concern and does not explore a solution for minimizing the pain. Option 2 can be eliminated as a distractor. You now must choose between options 3 and 4. The stem indicates that the client has pain when coughing; the pain is not continuous. Option 4 can be deleted because it is inappropriate to administer an analgesic at this time. Mild pain should subside after the activity is completed. The correct answer is option 3 because it recognizes the mild pain and offers an intervention to help relieve the temporary discomfort. Each time you eliminate an option that denies a client's feelings, you increase your chances of selecting the correct answer.

SAMPLE ITEM 7-34

An older woman with a right-sided hemiplegia and tears in her eyes sadly states, "I used to brush my hair 100 strokes a day, and now I have to rely on others to do it." Which should be the initial response by the nurse?

1. "It's hard not being able to do things for yourself."
2. "Let me brush your hair, and then I'll help you with breakfast."
3. "With physical therapy you will be able to brush your own hair someday."
4. "That's true, but there are lots of other things you are capable of doing for yourself."

Option 3 is a Pollyanna-like response because it implies that everything will be all right eventually. Option 2 changes the subject and cuts off communication. Option 4 initially accepts the client's statement but then attempts to refocus the client on the positive. In one way or another, options 2, 3, and 4 deny the client's feelings, concerns, and/or needs. The correct answer is option 1 because it is an open-ended statement that focuses on the client's feelings.

Use Multiple Test-Taking Techniques

You have just been introduced to a variety of test-taking techniques. As you practice applying each of these techniques to test items, you will become more test wise. As you become better at applying test-taking techniques, you can further maximize success in choosing the correct option if you use more than one test-taking technique within an item.

SAMPLE ITEM 7-35

A client's plan of care indicates that active range-of-motion (AROM) exercises of the right leg are to be done every 4 hours while the client is awake. Which should the nurse do?

1. Explain that all clients do AROM exercises by themselves
2. Take the client to physical therapy for the AROM exercises
3. Move the client's leg through AROM exercises as prescribed
4. Demonstrate for the client how to implement AROM exercises

Option 1 includes the specific determiner *all* and should be carefully evaluated. Some clients are able to perform AROM exercises themselves, and others require assistance. Since there are exceptions to the statement in option 1, as some clients cannot totally perform AROM exercises independently, option 1 can be deleted from consideration using the technique *Identify Specific Determiners in Options.* Option 2 transfers the responsibility for care that the nurse is educated and licensed to provide. This option can be eliminated from consideration by using the technique *Identify Options That Deny Client Feelings, Concerns, or Needs.* By using two test-taking techniques, you have eliminated options 1 and 2, reduced the number of options to two, and increased your chances of selecting the correct answer to 50%.

SAMPLE ITEM 7-36

Which client responses are unexpected in relation to the general adaptation syndrome?

1. Dilated pupils and bradycardia
2. Mental alertness and tachycardia
3. Increased blood glucose level and tachycardia
4. Decreased blood glucose level and bradycardia

By carefully reading the stem, you should identify that *unexpected* is a significant word in this item. You have just used the test-taking technique *Identify the Word in the Stem That Indicates Negative Polarity.* If you know that tachycardia is associated with the general adaptation syndrome, you can eliminate options 2 and 3. This reasoning uses the test-taking technique *Identify Duplicate Facts Among Options.* If you identify that options 3 and 4 are opposites, you should give these options particular consideration. By seriously considering these options, you are using the test-taking technique *Identify Opposites in Options.* A variety of test-taking techniques can be applied to analyze and answer this item.

SAMPLE ITEM 7-37

Which client need is being met when the nurse administers a back rub to reduce the physical discomfort of a backache?

1. Safety
2. Security
3. Self-esteem
4. Physiological

By thoughtfully reading the stem, you should identify that the important words are "reduce the physical discomfort of a backache." When reviewing the options, you should recognize that the word *physiological* in option 4 is closely related to the word *physical* in the stem. Option 4 should be given serious consideration. This reasoning uses the test-taking technique *Identify Key Words in the Stem That Direct Attention to Content.* Also, the use of physical in the stem and physiological in option 4 is a clang association. Options 1 and 2 present the words *safety* and *security.* They are comparable, and choosing between them is difficult. They are distractors. This reasoning uses the test-taking technique *Identify Equally Plausible Options.* Options 1, 2, and 3 all begin with the letter "S," whereas option 4 begins with the letter "P." Option 4 is different from the others and should be considered carefully because it may be the correct answer. You have just used the test-taking technique *Identify the Unique Option.* The use of multiple test-taking techniques when considering an item can facilitate the deletion of distractors and the selection of the correct answer.

SUMMARY

Nursing examinations involve extensive complex information that crosses clinical disciplines and the life span. As a result, they may challenge your ability to remain calm and in control. General test-taking techniques will help you manage your internal and external environments and maximize your approach to the testing situation. In addition, it is impossible for you to experience every clinical situation that may be included on an examination. Therefore, you must use critical thinking to integrate the knowledge you do possess and employ specific test-taking techniques to help you analyze a test item and determine which options are distractors and which option is the correct answer. A nursing examination is a challenging experience. General and specific test-taking techniques can help you conquer this challenge.

ANSWERS AND RATIONALES FOR SAMPLE ITEMS IN CHAPTER 7

7-1 **1. Linens cannot be returned to a linen storage area once they have been removed because they are exposed to microorganisms in the hallways and/or client rooms.**
2. Used linens may be contaminated with body secretions; wearing gloves is part of standard precautions.
3. Tucking clean linen against the frame of the bed is an acceptable practice; the entire bed is washed with a disinfectant between clients.
4. Reusing a top sheet for the bottom sheet is an acceptable practice if the sheet is not wet or soiled.

7-2 1. Stewed fruit is low in sodium.
2. Luncheon meats generally are processed with large amounts of sodium.
3. Whole-grain cereal is low in sodium.
4. Green, leafy vegetables are low in sodium.

7-3 **1. Applying pressure over the vertebrae should be avoided because it can cause unnecessary pressure over bony prominences; back rub strokes should massage muscle groups, not vertebrae.**
2. Using continuous, firm strokes is soothing and relieves muscle tension; this action is based on the gate-control theory of pain relief.
3. Excess lotion left on the skin can be an irritant and should be removed.
4. Kneading the skin increases circulation and should be part of a back rub unless contraindicated.

7-4 1. Collecting equipment is not done first because each type of enema requires different equipment.
2. Informing the client about the procedure is not done first because the nurse's explanation depends on the type of enema being administered.
3. Arranging for an empty bathroom should be done after the equipment and client are prepared and ready.
4. The prescription should be verified first. It is essential that the specific type of enema prescribed be given; enemas have different solutions, volumes, and purposes.

7-5 1. This statement is a demeaning response and does not answer the client's question.
2. Not responding may upset the client more; the client has a right to know who is providing care.
3. This statement answers the question, which meets the client's right to know; also, it is a respectful response.
4. Although this eventually may be done, it does not answer the client's question. Also, a cognitively impaired older adult may not comprehend the symbols used in writing or may not have acceptable vision to see the sign.

7-6 1. The client should be turned and positioned every 2 hours to help minimize venous stasis, which may contribute to deep vein thrombosis, as well as to relieve pressure, which can contribute to skin breakdown.
2. Distal, not proximal, pulses should be taken to ensure that the client's circulation is not compromised by the pressure of the cast.
3. Although it is important to cover rough edges of the cast with tape, this intervention is not the priority.
4. Bleeding may occur with a compound fracture. Drawing a ring around the drainage on the cast and adding the date, time, and nurse's initials helps to establish the degree of bleeding or discharge over time.

7-7 **1. Maintaining functional alignment supports a basic physiological need; this reduces physical strain and potential injury to joints, muscles, ligaments, and tendons and can prevent the formation of contractures.**
2. Pulling the curtain supports the client's need for self-esteem; it provides privacy.
3. Responding to the call light immediately supports the client's need for security and safety; clients should know that help is available immediately when needed.
4. Raising both side rails on the bed supports the client's need for safety and security; bed rails prevent a client from falling out of bed.

7-8 **1. Self-care encourages a client's independence, which increases self-esteem.**
2. Family member visits generally meet the client's need for love and belonging, not self-esteem.
3. When a person is dependent on another, such dependency often lowers self-esteem. Clients should be encouraged to voice requests and make decisions associated with the delivery of their daily health care.

4. Providing a complete bath promotes dependency; the client should be as independent as possible.

7-9 1. Pulling a curtain when providing care supports the client's self-esteem needs.
2. Answering a call bell immediately meets the client's safety needs.
3. Administering hygiene meets the client's basic physiological need to be clean.
4. Vital signs are not a physiological need of the client. They are an assessment done by the nurse to determine the client's needs.

7-10 1. This response directly involves the client and invites reliving a past vacation.
2. This response focuses on the nurse rather than the client.
3. This response focuses on the nurse's vacation rather than focusing on the client.
4. This question by the nurse asks for an opinion, which can be answered with a short response.

7-11 1. Speaking with the husband might be done later. It is not the initial action.
2. Eventually, the husband also will need support; however, the client's needs should be met first.
3. The fact that the client raised these issues about her husband indicates that she is concerned about his behavior. Her feelings need to be explored and her self-esteem supported.
4. Making an appointment with Reach to Recovery is not the initial intervention. This may be done eventually, after the client's initial needs have been met.

7-12 1. Exploring the situation gives the daughter an opportunity to express her feelings regarding her mother's behavior. All behavior has meaning, and talking about the situation may provide insight. Eventually, the situation should be explored with the client and the daughter together.
2. Encouraging the client to be more positive denies the client's feelings and ignores the daughter's feelings; both cut off communication.
3. This information may further upset the daughter and may precipitate feelings such as guilt or anger.
4. The nurse has a responsibility to intervene.

7-13 1. This statement focuses on the client's feelings by using the interviewing technique of reflection.
2. This statement denies the client's feelings.
3. This statement is an assumption and offers false reassurance.
4. The nurse cannot predict that the client will feel better. This response offers false reassurance.

7-14 1. Although this eventually may be done, it does not promote independence; also, if the questions are personal, it may violate the client's privacy.
2. Reminding the client of the primary health-care provider's next visit does not address the client's concern; the client forgets the questions to be asked, not the time of the primary health-care provider's next visit.
3. Providing a paper and pen to write down questions promotes independence, self-esteem, and privacy.
4. This may foster feelings of dependence and may violate the client's privacy if the questions to be asked are personal.

7-15 1. Moistening the hair may be done after obtaining the client's permission.
2. Applying a hair conditioner may be done if desired by the client. The procedure should be explained and the client's consent obtained before beginning a procedure.
3. Initially, short strokes, beginning at the ends and progressively moving toward the roots as tangles are removed, should be used to comb/brush the hair.
4. Seeking preferences promotes individualized care by allowing personal choices.

7-16 1. This intervention is not client-centered. This intervention focuses on the nurse's perspective, not the client's perspective.
2. Although this may eventually be done if desired by the client, it is not the primary intervention.
3. This intervention is client-centered. Asking the client to share more encourages the expression of feelings.
4. The nurse may eventually do this if the client expresses an interest in reading a book about cats.

7-17 **1. Pressure and friction produce local heat, which dilates blood vessels, improving circulation.**
2. Hot water can damage delicate tissue and should be avoided; bath water should be between 110°F and 115°F.
3. Keeping the client covered prevents chilling; it does not promote circulation.
4. Soap lowers the surface tension of water, which promotes cleaning.

7-18 1. Hand hygiene before care protects the client from the nurse.
2. If not wearing personal protective equipment, the nurse is still exposed to body secretions when discarding contaminated water.
3. Gloves are a barrier against body secretions and are used with standard precautions.
4. Expecting clients to provide all of their own care is unreasonable and inappropriate; some clients require assistance with meeting their needs.

7-19 1. Straps and a mask that are firm against the skin can cause tissue trauma.
2. Changing the method of oxygen delivery requires a primary health-care provider's order.
3. Padding the straps with gauze without adjusting the straps will make the mask tighter against the face.
4. Loosening the elastic straps will reduce the pressure of the mask against the face; the elastic straps can be adjusted for comfort while keeping the edges of the mask gently against the skin.

7-20 1. Aging is progressive and does not move backward.
2. Aging, from conception to death, advances and moves onward.
3. Although this may be true for some older adults, it is not true for all.
4. Although this may be true for some older adults, it should not be generalized to the entire population of older adults.

7-21 **1. Dependent edema is minimal while the feet are elevated; antiembolism stockings should be applied before the legs are moved to a dependent position.**
2. The purpose of antiembolism stockings is to promote venous return, not reduce pain.
3. This will cause tissue trauma because of the presence of fluid in the interstitial compartment; antiembolism stockings are applied to prevent, not treat, dependent edema.
4. In clients with peripheral vascular disease or congestive heart failure, fluid will accumulate in a dependent extremity. When there is fluid in the interstitial compartment, the application of antiembolism stockings will cause tissue trauma.

7-22 1. Carbohydrates, not proteins, are the main fuel source for energy. Athletes competing in endurance events often adhere to a diet that increases carbohydrates to 70% of their diet for the 3 days before a race (carbohydrate loading) to maximize muscle glycogen storage.
2. Anabolism, the process by which the body's cells synthesize protoplasm for growth and repair, requires amino acids, which are the essential components of proteins.
3. Although adequate amounts of food from all the food groups are necessary for maintaining healthy, functioning systems within the body, effective kidney function and an adequate fluid balance are necessary for excretion. The increased load of nitrogenous wastes associated with excessive protein intake burdens the kidneys, rather than facilitating excretion.
4. Protein is ingested to prevent, not promote, catabolism. Catabolism occurs when complex substances break down into simpler substances, releasing energy.

7-23 1. Serving adequate food meets basic physiological needs, not safety and security needs.
2. Providing sufficient fluid meets basic physiological needs, not safety and security needs.
3. Being able to summon help when needed provides a sense of security and physical safety for the client.
4. The bedside table is not a secure place to store valuables.

7-24 1. Placing the client in the prone position exposes the entire area to permit a thorough back rub; it does not promote circulation.

2. Moisturizing creams hold moisture within the skin, making it supple; they do not promote circulation.
3. Keri Lotion is a moisturizing lotion that helps make skin supple. Keri Lotion does not promote circulation.
4. **Kneading causes friction and pressure against the skin, which promotes localized heat and precipitates vessel dilation, improving circulation.**

7-25 1. Active range-of-motion (AROM), not passive range-of-motion (PROM), exercises can increase endurance.
2. **PROM exercises prevent shortening of muscles, ligaments, and tendons, which causes joints to become fixed in one position, limiting mobility.**
3. AROM, not PROM, exercises can strengthen muscle tone.
4. Maximizing muscle atrophy will never be a client goal. Atrophy is the loss of muscle mass due to lack of muscle contraction. AROM exercises will minimize, not maximize, muscle atrophy.

7-26 1. Shutting the door provides privacy and prevents drafts, but it may contaminate the nurse's hands.
2. **Between clients and before and after providing care, the nurse must wash the hands to remove dirt and microorganisms; otherwise, equipment and the client will be affected by cross contamination. Medical asepsis is a priority. Hand washing also is known as *hand hygiene*.**
3. The curtain should be closed before washing the hands; curtains are considered contaminated.
4. Draping the client provides privacy and prevents chilling; however, if the nurse's hands are not clean, they will contaminate the linen and the client.

7-27 1. Antibiotics are administered to treat clients with infections, not all sick clients.
2. **This is a broad statement that incorporates many different actions that may prevent the spread of microorganisms.**
3. Isolating a client is not necessary unless a communicable disease is diagnosed; implementing standard precautions is sufficient.
4. Keeping all unit doors closed is unnecessary; this action is not part of standard precautions. Closing the door is part of airborne precautions.

7-28 1. This is not required for all positions. The arms are supported when a client is placed in a lateral or a semi-prone position.
2. **Functional alignment refers to maintaining the body in an anatomical position that supports physical functioning; minimizes strain and stress on muscles, tendons, ligaments, and joints; and prevents contractures.**
3. This is not required for all positions. External rotation of the hips is prevented when a client is in the supine (dorsal recumbent) position.
4. This is not required for all positions. A pillow is placed under the lumbar curvature when a client is in the low Fowler or supine (dorsal recumbent) position.

7-29 1. Although the vest restraint can be untied while the nurse is at the bedside, lowering the rail on the side opposite to which the nurse is working may result in the client falling out of bed.
2. Both actions may injure the client. The client may partially fall out of bed on the side opposite the nurse. A restrained client may sustain an injury when moved.
3. **Untying a vest restraint permits free movement, which limits stress on the client's musculoskeletal system. Lowering the side rail on the working side of the bed allows the nurse to provide direct care. Keeping the side rail raised on the opposite side to which the nurse is working prevents the client from falling out of bed.**
4. Although the side rail on the working side of the bed can be lowered, a restrained client may sustain an injury when moved.

7-30 1. **These foods—fruits, vegetables, and bread—contain the least amount of sodium compared with the foods listed in the other options.**
2. Hot dogs, mustard, and pickles all contain high levels of sodium and should be avoided.
3. Ketchup is high in sodium and should be avoided.

4. Luncheon meats are processed foods that contain a high level of sodium and should be avoided.

7-31 1. During hemorrhage, the client's skin will be cold and clammy, not warm and dry, and the pulse will be weak and thready, not bounding. Hypotension is associated with hemorrhage because of hypovolemia.
2. As a result of the reduced blood volume associated with hemorrhage, the client's blood pressure will decrease, not increase, and the pulse will be weak and thready, not bounding. Cold, clammy skin is associated with hemorrhage because of peripheral vasoconstriction.
3. A weak, thready pulse is associated with hemorrhage because of hypovolemia. When hemorrhage occurs, the client's blood pressure will decrease, not increase, and the skin will be cold and clammy, not warm and dry.
4. As a result of the decreased blood volume associated with hemorrhage, the client's blood pressure will be reduced and the pulse will be weak and thready; because of the autonomic nervous system response and the constriction of peripheral blood vessels, the client's skin will be cold and clammy.

7-32 1. This statement denies the client's feelings about death and cuts off further communication.
2. This statement uses reflective technique because it focuses on the underlying feeling expressed in the client's statement.
3. This statement abdicates the responsibility of the nurse (to explore the client's feelings) to the surgeon; it cuts off communication and does not meet the client's immediate need to discuss fears of death; eventually, the surgeon should be notified of the client's feelings.
4. This statement minimizes the client's concern about dying; it cuts off communication.

7-33 1. Although this is true for most clients, it may not be true for this client. This is a Pollyanna-like response that may provide false reassurance.
2. Although this is a true statement, it cuts off communication and does not present an intervention to help limit the client's discomfort.
3. This response recognizes the mild pain and offers the client an intervention to help limit the temporary discomfort.
4. This response is inappropriate at this time. If more than mild pain is expected, analgesics should be administered before pain-inducing activities, not after.

7-34 **1. This response identifies the client's concern and offers an opportunity to discuss the topic further.**
2. This response offers a solution before allowing the client to discuss concerns, thereby cutting off communication.
3. This is a Pollyanna-like response that provides false reassurance; the client may never be able to brush her own hair.
4. This response is premature. After the client's present feelings are explored, then pointing out the client's abilities is appropriate.

7-35 1. Some clients are not capable of performing AROM exercises, depending on the strength of the affected and unaffected extremities and their physical, mental, and/or emotional status.
2. Taking the client to physical therapy every 4 hours is unrealistic and transfers the nurse's responsibility to another member of the health-care team.
3. AROM exercises should be performed by the client. PROM exercises should be performed by a nurse.
4. Assisting clients with mobility issues is within the scope of nursing practice. A demonstration by the nurse and a return demonstration by the client will ensure that the client knows how to perform AROM.

7-36 1. Tachycardia, not bradycardia, is associated with general adaptation syndrome; dilated pupils are expected.
2. Both mental alertness and tachycardia are expected autonomic nervous system responses during the alarm stage of general adaptation syndrome. These are part of the "fight-or-flight" mechanism.
3. Both increased blood glucose level and tachycardia are expected autonomic nervous system responses that occur during the alarm stage of the general adaptation syndrome. These are part of the "fight-or-flight" mechanism.

4. During the alarm stage of general adaptation syndrome, both the blood glucose level and heart rate of the client increase, not decrease.

7-37 1. Safety and security needs, the second level of needs according to Maslow, are met when the client is protected from harm.

2. Security needs are related to safety needs, the second level of needs according to Maslow. A client will feel protected and safe when safety and security needs are met.

3. Self-esteem needs, a third-level need, are met when the client is treated with dignity and respect.

4. Being free from pain or discomfort is a basic physiological need; a back rub improves local circulation, reduces muscle tension, and limits pain.

8 Testing Formats Other Than Multiple-Choice Questions

Teachers make many decisions that influence students. Some are instructional decisions, such as, "What strategies should be used to teach certain content?" Some decisions are curricular. These include, "What information should be included in a unit of instruction?" The decisions teachers make that produce the most anxiety in the most students are those involving measurement and evaluation of the student. "What does the student know? What can the student do?" To make these decisions, teachers use tests to appraise progress toward curricular goals, assess mastery of a skill, and evaluate knowledge of what was learned in a course. Three factors are involved in making measurement and evaluation decisions.

1. **What knowledge or ability is to be measured?** Generally, that which is most important or relevant is measured. Examples include the expected range of vital signs in an adult, the principles of client teaching, the legal and ethical implications of health-care delivery, and client safety. You can usually identify what is most significant by the emphasis placed on the material. Content in a textbook that is highlighted, boldfaced, capitalized, or repeated several times is usually important. Information that appears in the textbook and is incorporated into the teacher's classroom instruction is also significant. Concepts that are introduced in the classroom setting and then applied in a classroom laboratory or clinical setting are critical concepts. By paying attention to these factors, you can often predict the content that will be on a test and therefore use your study time more efficiently.
2. **How can the identified knowledge or ability be measured?** A set of operations must be devised to isolate and display the knowledge or ability that is to be measured. Examples include multiple-choice questions, true-false questions, completion items, matching columns, extended essay questions, and the performance of a procedure. In addition, the teacher may include clinical judgment questions in a format designed by National Council of State Boards of Nursing (NCSBN), which develops the National Council Licensure Examination (NCLEX®). This can help you to not only become familiar with the steps in the NCSBN model as you prepare for the licensing test, but more important, it will imbed the steps in your ongoing professional judgment. Clinical judgment questions will be part of the NCLEX® test, beginning in 2023, and are discussed in more detail later in this chapter. For more information, refer to the NCSBN Web site (https://www.ncsbn.org/ngn-resources.htm).

   To feel in control when taking tests, you should be familiar with the various testing formats. Dealing with a particular test format is a skill, and to develop a skill you must practice. Student workbooks that accompany required textbooks, questions at the end of chapters, and books devoted to testing usually contain numerous questions. Practice answering these questions. Experience promotes learning, and practice makes perfect!
3. **How can the results of the devised operations be measured or expressed in quantitative terms?** In other words, the unit of measure that indicates a passing grade or an acceptable performance must be identified by the instructor. Examples of acceptable results include a grade within 10% of the average grade in the class, a grade of 80%, or the correct performance of previously identified steps (critical elements) of a procedure. When taking tests, you should be aware of the criteria for scoring them. You should ask the following questions: What is the passing grade? How many points are allocated to each question? Can partial credit be received for an answer? Is there a

penalty for guessing? What critical steps must be performed for each skill in order to pass the test? Answers to these and other questions can help you make decisions, such as how much time to devote to certain questions or whether to make an educated guess at an answer.

In previous chapters, the multiple-choice question was discussed in detail. In this chapter, testing formats other than multiple-choice questions are presented. Test questions can be classified as structured-response questions, restricted-response questions, extended essay questions, or performance appraisals. In addition, alternate question formats that measure clinical judgment and are reflective of the NCLEX® examinations are discussed in this chapter.

A **structured-response question** requires you to select the correct answer from among available alternatives. Multiple-choice, multiple-response, true-false, and matching items are examples of structured-response questions.

A **restricted-response question** requires you to write a short answer. The response is expected to be a word, phrase, sentence, or product of a mathematical calculation. Short-answer, completion, and fill-in-the-blank items are examples of restricted-response questions.

An **extended essay question** requires you to generate the answer to a question or problem via a free-response format.

A **performance appraisal** presents a structured situation and requires you to demonstrate part or all of a skill.

The answers and rationales for all the sample items in this chapter are presented at the end of the chapter. Test-taking tips do not always apply to alternate question format items. When applicable, test-taking tips are presented and discussed.

STRUCTURED-RESPONSE QUESTIONS

A structured-response item is one that asks a question and requires you to select an answer from among the options presented. These items include multiple-choice, multiple-response, true-false, and matching questions. These formats usually are efficient, dependable, and objective. As multiple-choice questions are discussed in Chapter 5, only multiple-response, true-false, clinical judgment, and matching questions are presented here.

Multiple-Response Questions

A multiple-response question is a variation of a regular multiple-choice question. A regular multiple-choice question asks a question and then provides three or four potential answers. The test taker must select the one correct answer from among the presented potential answers. A *multiple-response* question is similar in that it presents a question and potential answers. However, it varies in that it requires the test taker to identify more than one correct answer from among numerous potential answers (usually five or six).

TEST-TAKING TIP: See Multiple-Response Items Under Alternate Question Formats Reflective of NCLEX® on page 140 for Test-Taking Tips.

SAMPLE ITEM 8-1

The nurse identifies the extent of tissue damage when assessing a stage III pressure ulcer. **Select all that apply.**

1. _______ Undermining of adjoining tissue
2. _______ Damage to subcutaneous tissue
3. _______ Limited partial-thickness loss
4. _______ Extension through the fascia
5. _______ Damage to muscle

SAMPLE ITEM 8-2

A nurse is caring for a client who has primary pulmonary tuberculosis and is receiving airborne precautions. Which action must be implemented by the nurse to meet the criteria of airborne precautions? **Select all that apply.**

1. _______ Donning a gown when entering the room
2. _______ Putting on gloves when delivering a food tray
3. _______ Placing a mask on the client during transport
4. _______ Admitting the client to a private room that has negative air pressure
5. _______ Wearing a respiratory device when entering the room (N95 respirator)
6. _______ Keeping the door to the room closed except when entering or leaving

SAMPLE ITEM 8-3

The nurse is assessing a newborn with a cephalohematoma who was born 48 hours ago at 36 weeks gestation due to the mother's severe preeclampsia. The newborn's face and chest appear to be slightly orange. The mother reports that she plans on exclusive breastfeeding, but the baby is not breastfeeding very well. She attributes this to her 24-hour labor and inexperience as a first-time mother. The nurse identifies four predisposing factors for neonatal jaundice in this newborn. **Select four.**

1. Gestational age
2. Maternal preeclampsia
3. Length of labor
4. Cephalohematoma
5. Maternal primiparity
6. Newborn fluid intake

True-False Questions

In a true-false question, a statement is presented and only two options are given from which to select an answer. True-false questions frequently are used to test knowledge of facts because the response must be absolutely true or false. It can be a demanding format because no frame of reference is provided. The question usually is constructed out of context, and the truth or falsity of the statement can be difficult to evaluate. However, true-false questions can work to your benefit because you have a 50% chance of getting the answer right. If you do not know the answer and there is no penalty for guessing, make an educated guess. Never leave an answer blank if there is no penalty for guessing. Follow the instructions for selecting the correct answer; for example, you may be told to circle your answer or to place an X on a line next to your answer.

SAMPLE ITEM 8-4

When providing a bed bath, the nurse understands that soap helps in cleaning because it decreases the surface tension of water. Place an X on the line that indicates your answer.

True _______ False _______

SAMPLE ITEM 8-5

A nurse should assume a broad stance when transferring a client from the bed to a wheelchair. Circle your answer.

True False

SAMPLE ITEM 8-6

The nurse should teach a client experiencing insomnia that exercising just before going to bed promotes sleep. Place an X on the line that indicates your answer.

True _______ False _______

SAMPLE ITEM 8-7

When obtaining a client's vital signs, the nurse understands that pulse pressure is the difference between the apical and radial pulse rates. Circle your answer.

True False

Variations of true-false items have been developed to simplify and clarify what is being asked. These questions may also obtain more information about what you know and limit guessing. Test items that **highlight a word or phrase in the question** (by CAPITALIZING it or by using **bold type,** *italic font*, or <u>underlining</u>) is a simple variation that helps to reduce ambiguity for the test taker. You can also use this technique when answering true-false questions in which certain words are not highlighted. Underline key words, as well as terms that modify key words, to focus your attention on the most important part of the statement.

SAMPLE ITEM 8-8

Palpation is the examination of the body using the sense of **touch.** Place an X on the line that indicates your answer.

True _______ False _______

SAMPLE ITEM 8-9

The process in which solid, particulate matter in a fluid moves from an area of increased concentration to an area of decreased concentration is known as <u>osmosis</u>. Circle your answer.

True False

The grouping of short true-false items under a common question, another variation of the true-false question, attempts to arrange affiliated information together. It is an effective approach to assess knowledge about related categories, classifications, or characteristics. Each statement that is being evaluated must be considered in relation to the original question. This variation reduces the amount of reading and provides a greater frame of reference for evaluating each statement. This type of question also increases specificity and clarity.

SAMPLE ITEM 8-10

Indicate if the following choices are true or false in relation to the introductory statement. Place an X on the lines that indicate your answers.

Surgical asepsis is maintained when the nurse:

1. removes the drape from a sterile package by touching the outer 1 inch with ungloved hands.

   True _______ False _______
2. dons the first sterile glove by touching just the inside of the glove.

   True _______ False _______
3. keeps hands below the elbows during a surgical hand scrub.

   True _______ False _______
4. holds a sterile object below waist level.

   True _______ False _______

SAMPLE ITEM 8-11

Signify whether or not each procedure employs the principle of positive pressure. Circle your answers.

1. Mechanical ventilation

   True False
2. Continuous bladder irrigation

   True False
3. Chest tubes (chest drainage system)

   True False
4. Instillation of fluid into a nasogastric tube with a piston syringe

   True False

Requiring the test taker to correct false statements is another variation of the true-false question. With this type of item, you are instructed to rewrite the question whenever you determine that the statement is false. This approach guarantees that you understand the information underlying a false statement. It also decreases guessing because you will receive credit only if you are able to revise the question to make it a correct statement. This variation is sometimes combined with the true-false variation that highlights a word or phrase in the original question.

SAMPLE ITEM 8-12

Mark your answer with an X in the space provided. If you identify the statement as false, revise the statement so that it is accurate.

The expected range of the heart rate for an adult is 70 to 110 beats per minute.

True _______ False _______

Correction ____

SAMPLE ITEM 8-13

Indicate with an X if the statement is true or false. Correct the underlined words if the statement is false.

The central task of <u>young adulthood</u> is *identity* versus *role confusion* according to Erikson's developmental theory.

True _______ False _______

Correction ____

True-false items can be asked in relation to specific stimulus material included with the question. This variation of the true-false question provides a frame of reference for the specific questions being asked within the item. Examples of stimulus material include a graph, map, chart, table, or picture. Memorization of information generally is not sufficient for answering these types of questions because they test more than the recall or regurgitation of facts. These questions test comprehension, interpretation, application, and reasoning, which are higher levels of cognitive ability.

SAMPLE ITEM 8-14

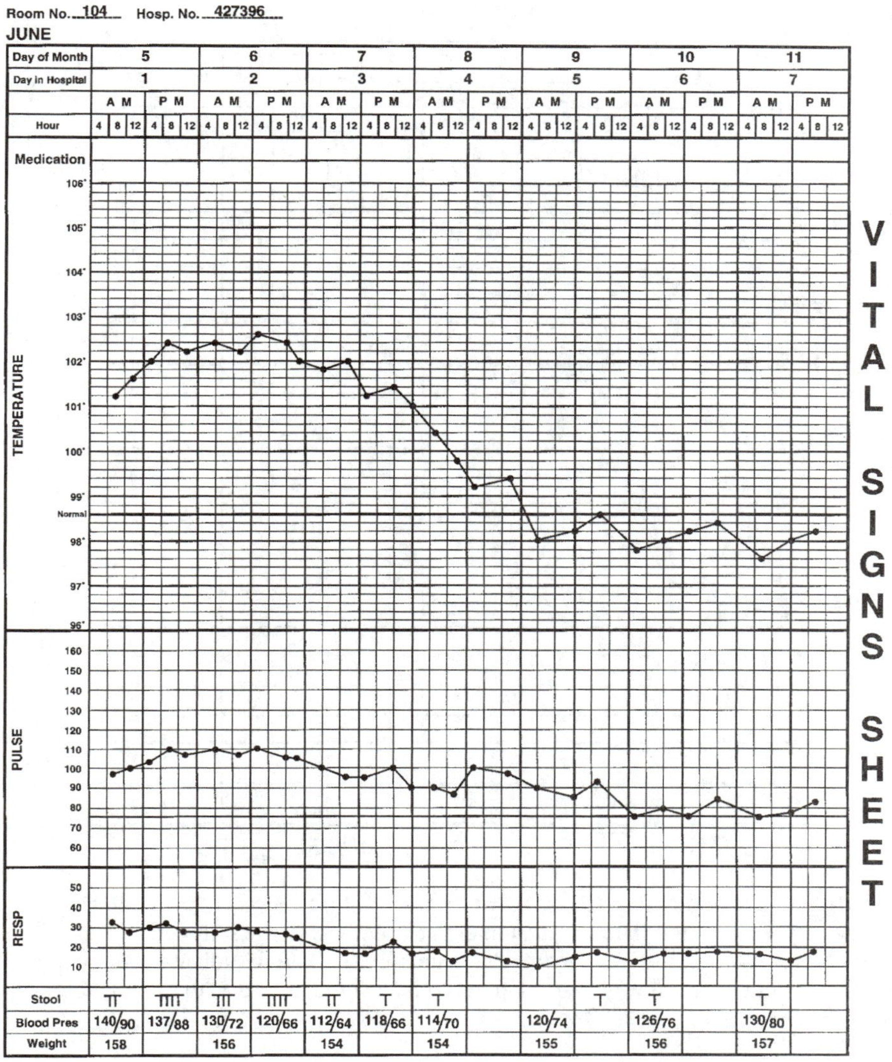

The vital signs sheet reflects an adult client's 7-day hospitalization. Determine whether each statement is true or false in relation to the information plotted on the vital signs sheet. Circle your answers.

1. On June 7 at 10 p.m., the client's temperature was 101.2°F.

   True False

2. During the last 3 days of the client's hospitalization, the client's temperature reflected a normal circadian rhythm.

   True False

3. During the first 4 days of the client's hospitalization, the client's blood pressure was consistent with a developing deficient fluid volume.

   True False

4. During hospitalization, the client's pulse rate ranged from 76 to 110 beats per minute.

   True False

5. The client's baseline pulse rate on admission to the hospital was within expected limits.

   True False

6. When the client's temperature increased during the acute phase of the illness, the client's respirations decreased.

   True False

SAMPLE ITEM 8-15

DAILY INTAKE AND OUTPUT RECORD

DATE JUNE 5

INTAKE								OUTPUT			
I.V. FLUIDS							ORAL	URINE	EMESIS	N.G. TUBE	HEMOVAC
Time	Bottle	Amount	Solution	Medication and Dosage	* ABS.	∓ LIB					
8	1	1000	NS	20 mEq KCl	↓			650			
8:30							360				
10:00							120				
11:30							240	150			
12:00									160		
1:40									90		60
2:15								250			
3:00					525	475					45
7-3 TOTAL		8-HR TOTAL			525	475	720	1050	250		105
3-11 TOTAL		8-HR TOTAL									
11-7 TOTAL		8-HR TOTAL									
24 HOUR TOTAL											

INTAKE GRAND TOTAL ______ OUTPUT GRAND TOTAL ______

* ABS. = amount absorbed ∓ LIB = Left in bag

A client's daily intake and output (I&O) record for the 7 a.m. to 3 p.m. shift is illustrated above. Identify whether the following statements correctly or incorrectly reflect the information presented in the I&O record. Place an X on the line to indicate your answer.

1. If the intravenous solution was infused at an equal volume per hour, the hourly rate was 75 mL per hour.

   True _______ False _______

2. If the client had 4 ounces of orange juice with breakfast at 8:30 a.m., the client also drank another 10 ounces of fluid with breakfast.

   True _______ False _______

3. The client's intake and output were equal at the completion of the 7 a.m. to 3 p.m. shift.

   True _______ False _______

4. The additive to the client's intravenous solution was 20 mg of vitamin K.

   True _______ False _______

Matching Questions

A matching question begins by establishing a frame of reference for the question. It explains the topic of the question and the basis on which matches should be made. The item then divides into a double-column format. It presents a statement in Column I and then requires you to select a related statement from a list of possible options in Column II. (See Sample Item 8-16.) Usually the question assesses information about related categories, classifications, or characteristics. Sometimes the items in the two columns are equal in number, and sometimes Column I has fewer statements than Column II. When the columns are equal in length, the format can work either for you or against you. If the columns have seven items each and you know six of the answers, you will automatically get the last answer correct.

On the other hand, if you make an incorrect choice, you will automatically get at least two answers wrong. These problems are minimized if the response column (Column II) has more options than the question column (Column I). The matching question is a relatively superficial testing format that lends itself to factual information that usually is memorized. Some sample items present statements in Column II and then require you to select a related statement from a list of possible options in Column I. (See Sample Item 8-17.)

TEST-TAKING TIPS:

- **Read the directions for matching questions carefully because they specify the basis for the matching. In addition, they tell you where to place the correct answer and the number of times an option can be selected.**
- **Cover Column II and for each item in Column I attempt to recall the memorized information without being cued by the content in Column II. Hopefully, the information you memorized will appear as an option in Column II. By doing this, you may become less confused or distracted by the list of options.**
- **Match items you are absolutely certain are correct matches. This leaves a reduced list on which to focus. Now consider the remaining options, moving from the simple to the complex as determined by your frame of reference.**
- **Make an educated decision if you do not know an answer.**

SAMPLE ITEM 8-16

Column I contains terminology used to describe types of breathing exhibited by clients. Match each term to its correct description in Column II. Place the number you select from Column II on the line at the left of the term in Column I. Use each number only once.

Column I	Column II
_______a. Bradypnea	1. Respirations that are increased in depth and rate
_______b. Apnea	2. Difficulty breathing
_______c. Hyperpnea	3. Respiratory rate less than 10 breaths per minute
_______d. Tachypnea	4. Absence of breathing
_______e. Eupnea	5. Respiratory rate greater than 20 breaths per minute
_______f. Dyspnea	6. Normal breathing
	7. Shallow breathing interrupted by irregular periods of apnea

SAMPLE ITEM 8-17

Column I lists types of exercises. Match a type of exercise with its **most** therapeutic value or outcome. In the space provided, indicate the number from Column I that matches the letter in Column II. Options from Column I can be used more than once.

Column I—Exercises	Column II—Outcomes
1. Passive range of motion	a. Promotes urinary continence (__________)
2. Aerobic	b. Improves strength of pelvic floor muscles (__________)
3. Isometric	c. Promotes pulmonary functioning (__________)
4. Kegel	d. Improves cardiovascular conditioning (__________)
	e. Increases muscle mass, tone, and strength of an extremity in a cast (__________)
	f. Maintains joint mobility (__________)

RESTRICTED-RESPONSE QUESTIONS

Restricted-response questions are also known as free-response questions. Completion and short-answer questions are examples of restricted-response questions. These test items pose a question for which you are expected to furnish the answer. The response can be a word, phrase, sentence, or product of a mathematical calculation. These types of questions usually have an uncomplicated, direct format; thus, they are most effective for assessing the understanding of simple concepts, the definition of terms, the knowledge of facts, or the ability to solve mathematical problems.

Completion Questions

A completion question generally is a short statement with one or more blanks. You are required to furnish the word, words, or phrase that accurately completes the sentence. In a completion question, the key word or words are the ones that are omitted. This forces you to focus on the important information reflected in the question rather than on trivia. This type of question does not permit flexibility or creativity in your response. The question anticipates a particular word or phrase that will produce an accurate statement.

SAMPLE ITEM 8-18

The condition of flexion and fixation of a joint is called a ____________.

SAMPLE ITEM 8-19

Postural drainage uses gravity to drain secretions from the ____________.

SAMPLE ITEM 8-20

The expected respiratory rate for an adult is ____________ to ____________ breaths per minute.

The inclusion of two possible answers to fill in the blank is a simple variation of a completion question. This format resembles an alternate-response question because you are asked a question and two choices are presented from which to pick an answer. This type of question gives you an advantage because the words presented are clues. These words nudge your memory and the recall of information necessary to answer the question. When faced with a question that has only two possible options, the chance of selecting the correct answer is 50%.

SAMPLE ITEM 8-21

When describing "radiating pain," the nurse is referring to its (intensity/location).

SAMPLE ITEM 8-22

The feeling that a person needs to void immediately is called (frequency/urgency).

Short-Answer Questions

A short-answer question is a free-response item because it asks a question, and you are expected to compose an answer. It provides some flexibility and creativity because the response does not have to complete a sentence or fill in a blank. You usually can use anywhere from one word to several sentences to answer the question. A short-answer question that requires only a word or a phrase as a response is similar to a completion question, but the original question is a complete sentence rather than an incomplete sentence. A short-answer question that requires several sentences to answer the question goes beyond the standards or criteria of a completion question, but it still focuses on knowledge of facts, terminology, simple concepts, or the ability to perform mathematical computations.

Short-answer and completion questions can be used interchangeably to address the same content. For example, compare Sample Items 8-18 through 8-20 with Sample Items 8-23 through 8-25, respectively.

TEST-TAKING TIP: Write as much relevant information as the format permits in the hope that what you include answers the question and contains the specific information expected. The more relevant information you include in the response, the better you can demonstrate comprehension of the information being tested.

SAMPLE ITEM 8-23

What is the definition of the word *contracture?*

Answer: ______________________________

SAMPLE ITEM 8-24

What is the purpose of postural drainage?

Answer: ______________________________

SAMPLE ITEM 8-25

What is the normal range of respirations per minute in an adult?

Answer: ______________________________

SAMPLE ITEM 8-26

An intravenous solution of 1000 mL of D_5W to be administered at 100 mL/hr is ordered for a client. The drop factor of the intravenous administration set is 15 drops/mL. How many drops per minute should the client receive? Show all work.

Answer: __________ drops/min

EXTENDED ESSAY QUESTIONS

An extended essay question is a free-response question because the answer is drafted by you in reply to a question. It requires higher cognitive skills than just recall and comprehension. You must be able to write in order to answer an extended essay question. Essay questions require you to select, arrange, organize, integrate, synthesize, and compare or contrast information. You must be able to use language constructively, be creative when solving problems, and use critical thinking to manipulate complicated information. The extended essay is most suitable for evaluating mastery of complex material.

Instructors measure your knowledge by evaluating an end product such as a written assignment or an essay question on an examination. They generally examine your writing from the viewpoint of **writing for evaluation.** To answer an essay question, you must be able to put your thoughts on paper in a logical manner using correct spelling, grammar, and punctuation. There is no easy way to develop effective writing skills without practice. Seek assistance from your professor or other resources available in your school if you need assistance with developing your writing abilities. Most learning institutions today have writing centers staffed by specialized faculty to assist you with writing activities. To maximize your success in formulating written assignments, you must view writing from the perspectives of **learning to write** and **writing to learn.**

Learning to Write

When learning to write, you are not looking at an end product that will be evaluated by the instructor but rather focusing on the process of writing. Writing requires a basic understanding of the English language. For example, you need to have an adequate vocabulary, understand the rules of grammar and punctuation, and be able to spell. When learning to write, you also must focus on the organizational and analytical skills that help you to assess, advise, teach, argue a point of view, and challenge new and old theories. Critical thinking is an essential skill needed to process the information that is to be written. For client care papers, formatting one's response with the six steps of the clinical judgment format discussed below will demonstrate critical thinking and the clinical judgment process. Techniques that promote learning to write include brainstorming, setting priorities, and editing and revising previously written material.

Brainstorming is a method of exploring a topic by spontaneously listing thoughts or ideas. Making lists of words or phrases that relate to a topic allows you to explore the topic and your perspectives on it. For example, when we asked a group of nursing students to make a list of everything and anything relevant to client progress notes, interesting insights developed. Some students were content oriented and listed things such as vital signs, nursing care provided, and clients' responses to care. Other students were process oriented and stated that notes should be objective, specific, and comprehensive. Brainstorming helps you not only to learn to write but also to explore topics through writing. If you take the time to examine what you have written, it also may tell you a lot about yourself.

Setting priorities is an analytical skill that requires you to compare and contrast information and identify that which is most important or significant. Use a systematic method or theoretical base to make priority setting easier. Maslow's hierarchy of needs is an excellent framework because it also helps to organize information. Data can be clustered in each of the five levels or categories of needs. These needs are ranked according to how critical they are to survival. The physiological needs are the most basic and carry the highest priority; safety and security, love and belonging, self-esteem, and self-actualization follow. You can practice setting priorities daily just by ranking your activities for the day in order of importance.

Analyzing, editing, and revising previously written material are other ways to learn to write. Consider writing directly on a computer. Initially, don't edit your thoughts for grammar, punctuation, or spelling, just put them down for later review. On a computer, it is easy to move around words, phrases, and sentences as you edit and revise your writing. Seeing your words in print helps to separate you from your own handwriting and makes it easier to examine the content of your writing. When you have the luxury of time, it is always to your advantage to write an assignment one day and then several days later review this first draft. Your analytical skills may improve; you may have acquired new information since you first wrote the material; or your perspective may be different or clearer. Also, you probably will be more open to constructive criticism when it comes from within. Analyzing, editing, and revising your own written work are excellent ways to improve your writing abilities.

The hardest thing to overcome when engaging in learning-to-write activities is the feeling that, because you may not have completed a project, you have not learned. Remember, learning takes place in the learner and is a lifelong process.

Writing to Learn

When writing to learn, you are focusing on what you will eventually understand or remember, not on the process of writing. You learn content by the very act of writing because at least two cognitive domains are being integrated: cognitive (thinking) and psychomotor (writing). You learn the course content you are writing about and discover what you know, what you need to know, and what you think about certain topics. When you are writing to learn, you are writing for yourself, and what you learn is the end product. Techniques that can promote writing to learn include writing lists, writing journals, posing and answering questions, and note taking.

Writing a list can be a simple or complex task. Simple lists include repetitiously writing a phrase or fact in an effort to reinforce learning. This requires a low-level thinking process that involves the recall of information—for example, writing common equivalents (30 mL = 1 ounce). A complex list might require the writer to discriminate between the commonalities and differences of content material. This requires higher levels of the thinking process and includes comprehension, application, and analysis. An example is making a list of nursing interventions that use the concept of gravity (intravenous infusion, urinary catheter, elevation of an extremity to promote venous return). To compile this list, you must comprehend a concept and be able to identify the commonalities among the applications of this concept.

Writing a journal focuses on the use of words, the expression of ideas and feelings, and the documentation of activities; no consideration should be given to format, grammar, or punctuation. For 5 to 10 minutes each day, write a diary. It will improve your thinking and learning as well as document where you have been, where you are, and where you are going. Capture the things you are currently most worried about knowing or doing while learning to be a nurse. When you review these entries weeks or months later, you can easily see how you have grown as a student, when many of these things are no longer worrisome.

Posing and answering questions can improve understanding of the content you are learning along with your critical thinking and clinical judgment skills. Many textbooks have a companion study guide or workbook. Answering questions from these books and answering questions that you make up for yourself are excellent ways to reinforce understanding of the information. Putting your thoughts into concrete words and using the psychomotor skill of writing help you to learn. Pretend you are explaining concepts or conditions to a client, and answer the questions out loud, even if nobody is listening.

Note taking can be a simple or complex task. A simple note-taking strategy is the rewriting of class notes. When you rewrite notes, you revise information so that it is more organized and clear. A complex note-taking strategy is to add relevant information from the textbook to your class notes. You can even add your own thoughts and reactions to your notes.

TEST-TAKING TIPS:

- **Learn to write.**
- **Write to learn.**
- **Follow a three-part format when answering an extended essay question.**
  - ***Write an introduction.* An introduction should, in a general way, indicate what will be discussed. It introduces the topic and serves as a preface for what will follow. In a client care situation, the introduction might begin with, "Postpartum hemorrhage (PPH) is a common and potentially life-threatening condition." Consider giving statistics and risks for the condition to support your statement. Then, "This paper will examine the most common symptoms of PPH, including appropriate assessments and nursing care."**
  - ***Write the central part of the answer.* The central part of the answer should explore all the information that is being presented to answer the question. Organize this part of the answer by writing a topical outline. This blueprint promotes an orderly flow of information, prevents departure from your script, and ensures that significant material is included. You have already given the reader an idea of the outline in the last sentence of your opening paragraph above. Continue by using the six steps of clinical judgment (discussed in detail later in this chapter). Each of the questions in bold can be used as a subheading for each individual section, following the correct format.**
    1. When caring for a client with these symptoms, or with this condition, **What matters most?** (What are the symptoms of concern?)
    2. **What could it mean?** (Is it a fluid balance, respiratory, metabolic, or other concern?)
    3. **Where do I start?** (What is the most urgent symptom that requires intervention?)

4. **What can I do?** (Based on the setting, what is a list of things I can do?)
5. **What will I do?** (Of all of these options, which one is the most urgent to save a life?)
6. **How will I know if it helped?** (What will I see to note improvement?)

- ***Write a summary.* The summary should recap what was discussed and should come to several conclusions. It serves as a finale and brings closure to your answer. Your final sentence might be something like, "Although postpartum hemorrhage is a serious condition, the prudent nurse can prevent morbidities and mortalities by knowing the client's risk factors, anticipating the condition, and completing prudent assessments and treatments appropriately."**

SAMPLE ITEM 8-27

Compare and contrast critical thinking and clinical judgment and include at least three characteristics of each.

PERFORMANCE APPRAISAL

Nursing care is an art and a science. Nurses must not only comprehend information but also be able to perform skills safely. Therefore, testing the ability to identify and accurately implement steps in a procedure is essential in evaluating the achievement of skills. It is impossible physically to demonstrate an entire psychomotor skill on paper-and-pencil or computer-administered examinations. However, skills can be tested in a variety of ways. Questions that require you to identify a step in a procedure can be asked in the typical multiple-choice format. An example is "A nurse must make an unoccupied bed. Which is the first step of the procedure for making the bed?" This question requires you to select one correct answer out of four presented options. (See Sample Item 4-2 in Chapter 4.) Questions that require you to select related steps in a procedure also can be presented in the multiple-response format. An example is "Which action must be implemented by the nurse to meet the criteria of airborne precautions?" This question requires you to select one or more options to answer the question. (See Sample Item 8-2.)

Questions that ask you to demonstrate knowledge about a skill in relation to a realistic image, such as an illustration or a photograph, require you to respond in some way. An example is "Place an X over the area where the nurse should insert the needle of the syringe when utilizing the *vastus lateralis* muscle." This question directs the test taker to implement just one step of a procedure in relation to a visual cue. (See Sample Item 8-31.) Another question format that can test knowledge about the steps of a procedure is the drag-and-drop/ordered-response question. To evaluate your knowledge about a skill, a drag-and-drop question asks you to place the options presented in the question into the order in which they should be performed: for example, "A nurse discovers a fire in the dayroom where a client is watching television. Rank the following actions from 1 to 5 in the order in which they should be performed in accordance with the RACE acronym associated with fire safety." (See Sample Item 8-32.)

Performance appraisals also can be performed by implementing a procedure on a simulator manikin. This type of performance appraisal evaluates your ability to complete all the steps of a psychomotor skill. (See "The Computer As a Simulator" and "The Computer As an Evaluator" in Chapter 9). Obtaining a blood pressure reading, changing a sterile dressing, administering a tube feeding, performing tracheal suctioning, and obtaining a client's temperature are examples of psychomotor skills. When evaluating these skills, the criteria (critical elements) for passing should be identified before you attempt the procedure.

A **critical element** is any step that must be performed accurately to receive a passing score. Critical elements may be general or may list very specific criteria. For example, general critical elements for obtaining a temperature reading may include maintaining medical asepsis, providing for physical safety, and ensuring privacy. These are less specific because there are numerous ways to meet each of these critical elements. Specific critical elements may include use of a probe cover on the thermometer before placement in the client's mouth, holding the thermometer while it is in place, or pulling the curtain around the client before obtaining a rectal temperature.

TEST-TAKING TIPS:

- **Use clinical techniques/skills textbooks when practicing procedures and preparing for performance appraisals. A clinical checklist of step-by-step critical elements can be used by another student to assess your performance of a psychomotor skill in a laboratory setting. This supports reciprocal study relationships.**
- **Practice psychomotor skills using a simulator manikin. Practicing a skill on a manikin and talking to the manikin provides a nonthreatening hands-on experience. It also provides an opportunity to simulate a testing situation and helps with desensitization, which may give you a feeling of control. Some environments with a simulator manikin have the ability to videotape your performance. This allows you to review your performance and identify whether the steps were performed correctly.**

TEST-TAKING TIPS FOR ALTERNATE QUESTION FORMATS REFLECTIVE OF NCLEX®

Before April 2003, all of the questions on NCLEX® examinations were presented in the typical single-answer, multiple-choice format. This type of question requires you to select one correct answer from four presented options. In April 2003, the NCSBN incorporated item formats other than the typical multiple-choice question. These questions are called *alternate item formats*. **Alternate item formats** use computer technology to assess knowledge by requiring you to identify multiple answers, perform a calculation, prioritize information, or respond to a question in relation to a graphic image, picture, audio recording, video, or exhibit. The NCSBN believes that test takers can demonstrate their entry-level nursing competence in ways that are different from and more readily and authentically evaluated than the typical multiple-choice format.

In this section of the book, "Test-Taking Tips for Alternate Question Formats Reflective of NCLEX®," the focus is on the original fill-in-the-blank items, hot spot items, multiple-response items, graphic and illustration items, drag-and-drop/ordered-response items, and exhibit items. The sample questions that follow illustrate these alternate question formats. The next section, "Clinical Judgment Question Formats Reflective of Next Generation NCLEX," will give examples of Next Generation (NGN)® formats.

Fill-in-the-Blank Items

A fill-in-the-blank item requires you to perform a mathematical computation and type in your answer. You are directed to include a whole number or told the number of decimal places that should be used. Only numbers and decimal points can be entered. If the test is taken on a computer, you usually can access an online calculator to assist you with your computation.

TEST-TAKING TIPS:

- **Memorize important formulas when studying for a test.**
- **When beginning a test, immediately write several important formulas or equivalent conversions on provided scrap paper or an erasable note board.**

OR

- **When confronted with a calculation question, visualize the formula required to answer the question and write it down before answering the question.**
- **Insert the information presented in the scenario into the formula and perform the computation using a calculator. DO NOT PERFORM MATHEMATICAL CALCULATIONS IN YOUR HEAD.**

- **Read the question carefully to identify the unit of measure required and determine whether the answer should be a whole number or should have one or more decimal places.**
- **Review your answer to ensure that it is in the unit of measure requested in the question. Some questions provide the unit of measure in the area in which the answer is to be inserted.**
- **Ensure that the numerical answer is presented accurately:**
  - **If the answer is less than a whole number, place a 0 before the decimal point (e.g., 0.25). Some computer programs automatically insert the 0.**
  - **If instructed to use one or two decimal places, ensure that only one or two numbers follow the decimal point (e.g., 0.2, 0.25).**
  - **If the question asks that the answer be a whole number and the mathematical calculation results in an answer that is not a whole number, you must round up or down to the next whole number. To round up a tenth of a number, it has to end in .5 to .9. For example, 21.75 should be rounded up to 22. To round down a whole number, it has to end in .1 to .4. For example, 21.3 should be rounded down to 21.**
  - **Ensure that the answer is realistic.**

SAMPLE ITEM 8-28

A primary health-care provider orders 1500 mL to be administered IV every 24 hours. At what hourly rate should the nurse set the infusion pump? **Record your answer using a whole number.**

Answer: _________ mL/hr

SAMPLE ITEM 8-29

A primary health-care provider prescribes 500 mg of an antibiotic to be administered IVPB every 6 hours. One gram of the medication is supplied in a vial that states "Add 2.5 mL of sterile water to yield 3 mL of solution." How much solution should the nurse administer? Record your answer using one decimal place.

Answer: _________ mL

Hot Spot Items

A hot spot item asks a question in relation to a presented illustration. When the test is taken on a computer, you need to place the cursor on the area you want to select and left-click on the mouse.

TEST-TAKING TIPS:

- **Read the question twice to ensure that you understand what it is asking. Briefly look at the visual cue (e.g., illustration, photograph).**
- **Visualize the anatomy and consider its associated physiology in relation to the question being asked.**
- **In your mind, identify the location of your answer. Then examine the visual cue provided in the question and insert your answer.**

SAMPLE ITEM 8-30

A client is on complete bed rest in the semi-Fowler position because of excessive fluid volume and difficulty breathing. Place an X over the area of the body that is at the **highest** risk for dependent edema.

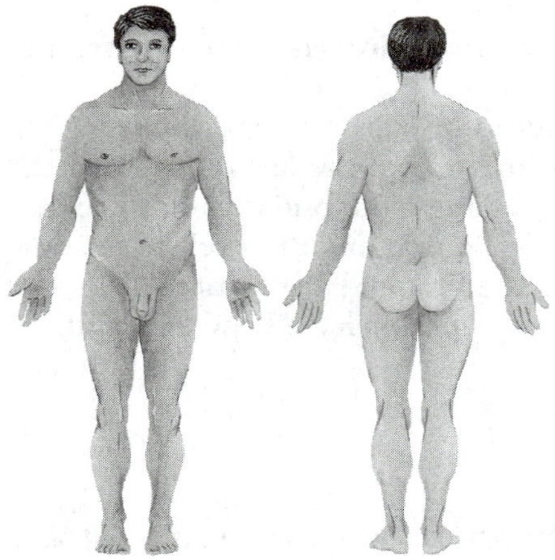

SAMPLE ITEM 8-31

The nurse must administer an intramuscular injection. Place an X over the area where the nurse should insert the needle of the syringe when utilizing the *vastus lateralis* muscle.

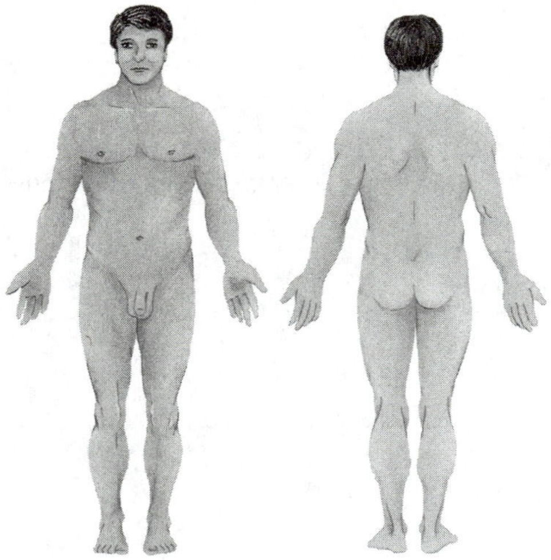

Drag-and-Drop/Ordered-Response Items

A drag-and-drop item presents a situation followed by a list of statements. You are asked to place them in order of priority. For example, it may be steps in a procedure or actions that need to be placed in order of importance. When a test is taken on a computer, each option must be highlighted and dragged with your mouse and then dropped in a designated area in rank order. When included on a written test, you may be asked to write the numbers of the options in the rank order that you identify.

TEST-TAKING TIPS:

- **Explore priorities related to nursing care when studying (e.g., washing your hands before a procedure, maintaining a patent airway, and assessing a client before planning or implementing care). Also, explore a variety of actions that may**

be performed last (e.g., leaving a bed in the lowest position, washing your hands after removing gloves, documenting all care provided, and positioning a call bell near the client before leaving the room).

- **Use theories or scientific processes to help prioritize options, for example, the ABCs (Airway, Breathing, and Circulation), Maslow's hierarchy of needs, and the steps of the nursing process.**
- **If the question is about a procedure, visualize yourself performing the procedure and then analyze the options.**
- **Place all options in order of priority or importance by beginning with your first selected option and progressing to the last one among the options presented. If you have difficulty progressing from one through five or six options, select the option you believe should be first and then select the one you think should be last. Alternate selecting the first and last options from the remaining options until one option is left or all the options have been selected.**

SAMPLE ITEM 8-32

A nurse discovers a fire in the dayroom where a client is watching television. Rank the following actions from 1 to 5 in the order in which they should be performed in accordance with the RACE acronym associated with fire safety.

1. Pull the fire alarm.
2. Shut the doors on the unit.
3. Move all clients off the unit.
4. Take the client out of the dayroom.
5. Move clients in adjacent rooms to an area down the hall.

Answer: __________

SAMPLE ITEM 8-33

Place the following protective devices in order from the **least** restrictive to the **most** restrictive.

1. Waist belt
2. Safety vest
3. Finger control mitt
4. Wheelchair lap hugger
5. Four-point leather cuffs

Answer: __________

Multiple-Response Items

A multiple-response item requires you to identify one or more correct options from among a list of presented options. It is similar to a multiple-choice question except that it has more than four options and there are one or more correct options. All the correct options must be identified to receive credit for the question.

TEST-TAKING TIPS:

- **Use test-taking techniques that apply to traditional multiple-choice questions, such as identifying specific determiners in options, identifying opposites in options, and identifying options that deny client feelings, concerns, or needs.**
- **Identify each option you know is a correct answer. Then identify each option you know is an incorrect answer. Finally, examine any remaining options and make an educated guess as to whether they are correct or incorrect.**
- For each selected option, ask yourself, "Where does this *not* make sense?"

OR

- **Identify one option you know is a correct answer. Then identify one option you know is an incorrect answer. Continue to alternate the identification of correct and incorrect options until all options have been determined to be correct or incorrect or you cannot classify any remaining options as correct or incorrect. Then examine these final options and make an educated determination as to whether they are correct or incorrect.**

SAMPLE ITEM 8-34

A nurse determines that a client has a deficient fluid volume. Which assessment **supports** this conclusion? **Select all that apply.**

1. _________ Tenting of skin
2. _________ Decreased pulse
3. _________ Sudden weight loss
4. _________ Increased blood pressure
5. _________ Longitudinal furrows in the tongue

SAMPLE ITEM 8-35

A nurse manager of a medical/surgical unit is making the assignments for the day for the nursing members of the health-care team. Which activity can be delegated to a nursing assistant? **Select all that apply.**

1. _________ Massaging the back of a client who is on complete bed rest
2. _________ Transferring a client from the bed to a chair by using a mechanical lift
3. _________ Changing the linen of a client with a continuous passive motion machine
4. _________ Teaching a client who is receiving an opioid how to prevent constipation
5. _________ Replacing a client's wound dressing that is saturated with a bloody discharge
6. _________ Obtaining vital signs of a client who is returning from the postanesthesia care unit

Exhibit Items

An exhibit item presents a situation and asks a question. It provides information that can be accessed via a variety of tabs. Each tab must be reviewed to collect information within that tab. When the test is taken on a computer, you must click on one tab to collect the information within that tab before moving to the next tab. When an exhibit item is included on a written test, you probably will be able to view the information within all the tabs at the same time. You must identify significant information within each tab and integrate the important details from all of the tabs. From this analysis, you can make inferences, deductions, and/or conclusions that eliminate options and support the correct answer.

TEST-TAKING TIPS:

- **Read the stem of the question carefully to determine what the question is asking. Identify important words that focus your attention on significant information in the tabs that follow.**
- **Read all the information presented in the tabs of the exhibit item. This may include laboratory results, vital signs, prescriptions for medications, primary health-care provider orders, client assessment, client statements, or progress notes. Identify significant data, such as abnormal laboratory values, vital signs that are outside expected values, medications that may have drug-to-drug interactions, inappropriate prescriptions or orders, and client concerns.**
- **Reread the stem of the question and compare and contrast the information in the stem with the information in the tabs.**
- **Compare and contrast your conclusions about significant information in the stem and the tabs with the information in each option.**

- **Ensure that the option you select has a relationship with the main topic of the question in the stem and with the information presented in one or more tabs.**

SAMPLE ITEM 8-36

A 90-year-old man is admitted to the hospital with a diagnosis of change in mental status. A family member states that the client has not eaten much for the last week and seemed very confused this morning. The nurse completes a physical assessment and reviews the client's clinical record. The nurse determines that the client is exhibiting:

1. dehydration.
2. hypervolemia.
3. urinary tract infection.
4. increased blood glucose level.

Laboratory Results

Sodium: 155 mEq/L
White blood cells (WBCs): 8000 cells/mcL
Hematocrit (Hct): 60%
Fasting blood sugar (FBS): 94 mg/dL

Vital Signs at 2:00 p.m.

Temperature: 100°F
Pulse: 88 beats/min, regular
Respirations: 24 breaths/min

Progress Note

Client is oriented to place and person but is easily distracted, is unable to follow directions, and voided a small amount of clear amber urine; the tongue has furrows, and there is tenting of the skin.

SAMPLE ITEM 8-37

A client comes to the emergency department with concerns about extreme fatigue and prolonged episodes of menstruation. The primary health-care provider performs a battery of tests. The nurse reviews the client's clinical record and identifies that the client has an oxygen problem. Which impaired physiological mechanism has precipitated the client's oxygen problem?

1. Osmosis
2. Diffusion
3. Transport
4. Ventilation

Laboratory Results

Red blood cells (RBCs): 2.9 cells/mcL
White blood cells (WBCs): 7000 cells/mcL
Hemoglobin (Hb): 8.5 g/dL
Hematocrit (Hct): 34%

Radiology Report

Chest radiograph: normal findings; all bones aligned and symmetrical; normal positioned soft tissues, mediastinum, lungs, pleura, heart, and aortic arc.

Vital Signs Sheet

Temperature: 98.8°F (oral)
Pulse: 92 beats/min, regular rhythm
Respirations: 24 breaths/min, regular rhythm, unlabored

Graphic Items

A graphic item presents a question with several options as potential answers. Each option contains a graphic image rather than textual material. You must analyze the images and select the correct answer from the presented options. In a graphic item, the illustrations appear in the options.

TEST-TAKING TIPS:

- **Within your textbook or other resources, graphic materials such as illustrations often are presented to support written content. Concentrate on these images and commit them to memory when studying because they reinforce the content you are learning. Examples include illustrations of range-of-motion exercises, the chain of infection, or a person with Parkinson's disease. Remember that "a picture is worth a thousand words."**
- **When confronted with a question with graphic material, recall similar visual images you have studied, and draw on your knowledge related to those visual images to answer the question.**

SAMPLE ITEM 8-38

Which of the following procedures requires the use of medical aseptic technique?

1. 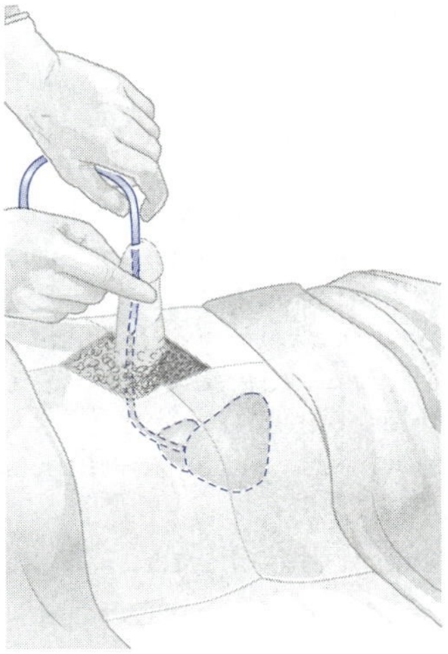

2. 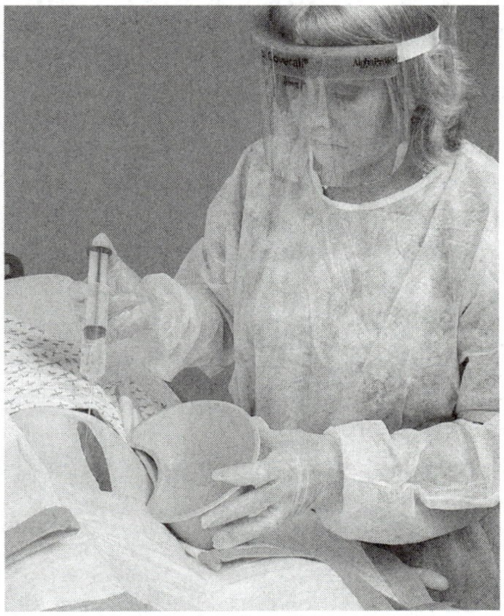

3. 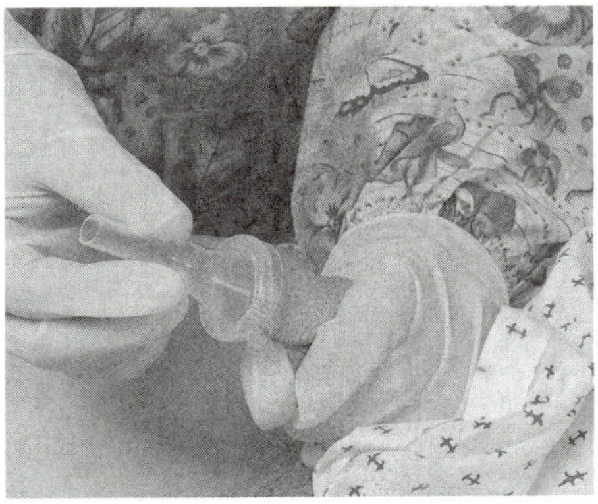

4. 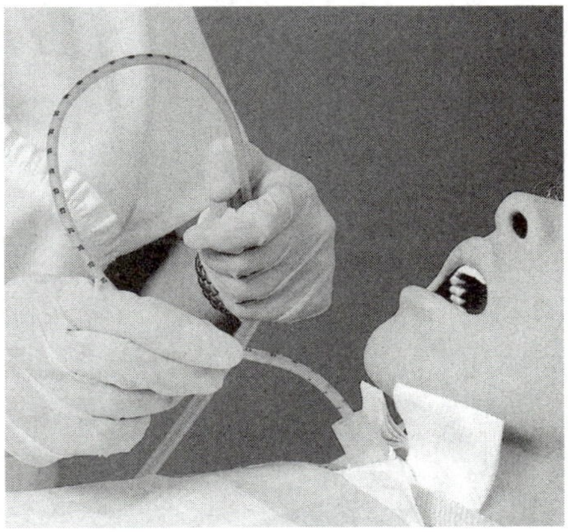

SAMPLE ITEM 8-39

Which syringe should a nurse use when administering 1 mL of a medication via the Z-track technique?

1. 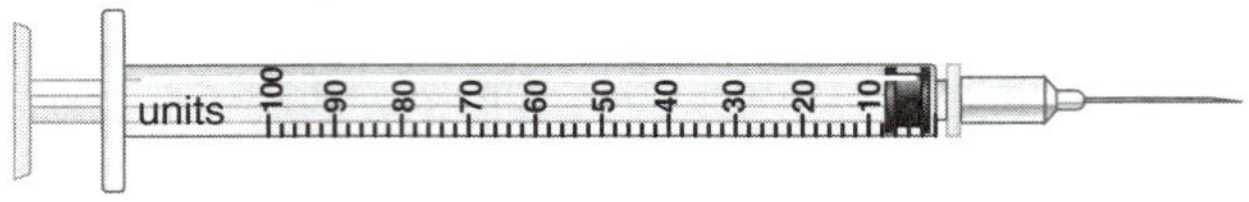

2. 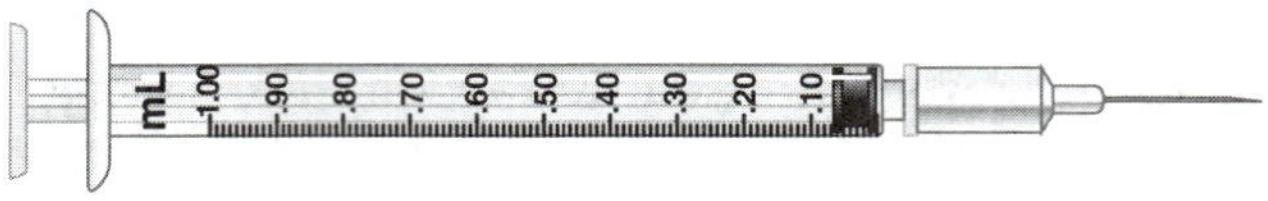

3. 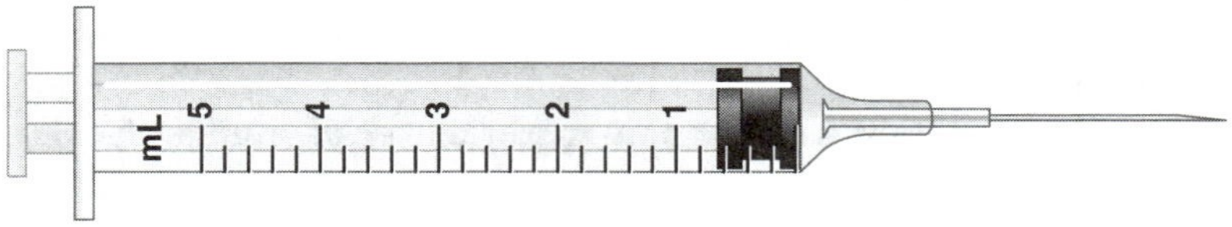

4. 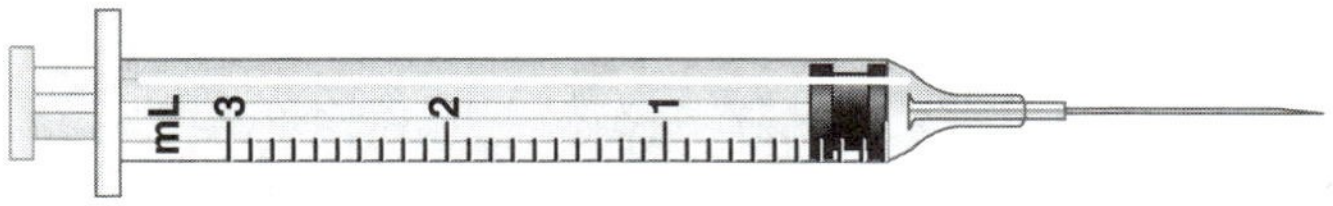

Multimedia in Multiple-Choice and Alternate Question Format Items

Multimedia uses more than one means of expression or communication. Usual word-based (textual) material is combined with content presented in the form of an illustration (e.g., chart, table, image, graphic, photograph), an audio clip, or a video. An illustration item is a variation of a graphic item. It presents a question accompanied by a chart, table, or visual image. You must analyze the options in relation to the illustration before selecting the option you believe is the correct answer. Illustrations can appear in a variety of formats, such as multiple-choice items (see Sample Item 8-40), drag-and-drop/ordered-response items (see Sample Item 8-41), multiple-response items (see Sample Item 8-42), and fill-in-the-blank items (see Sample Item 8-43); however, the illustration will always be part of the stem of the question.

TEST-TAKING TIPS: See Test-Taking Tips under Graphic Items in this chapter.

SAMPLE ITEM 8-40

A nurse is caring for a client who demonstrated a fluctuating temperature over a 24-hour period. At what hour did the client demonstrate a temperature of 100.4°F?

1. 5th hour
2. 14th hour
3. 18th hour
4. 21st hour

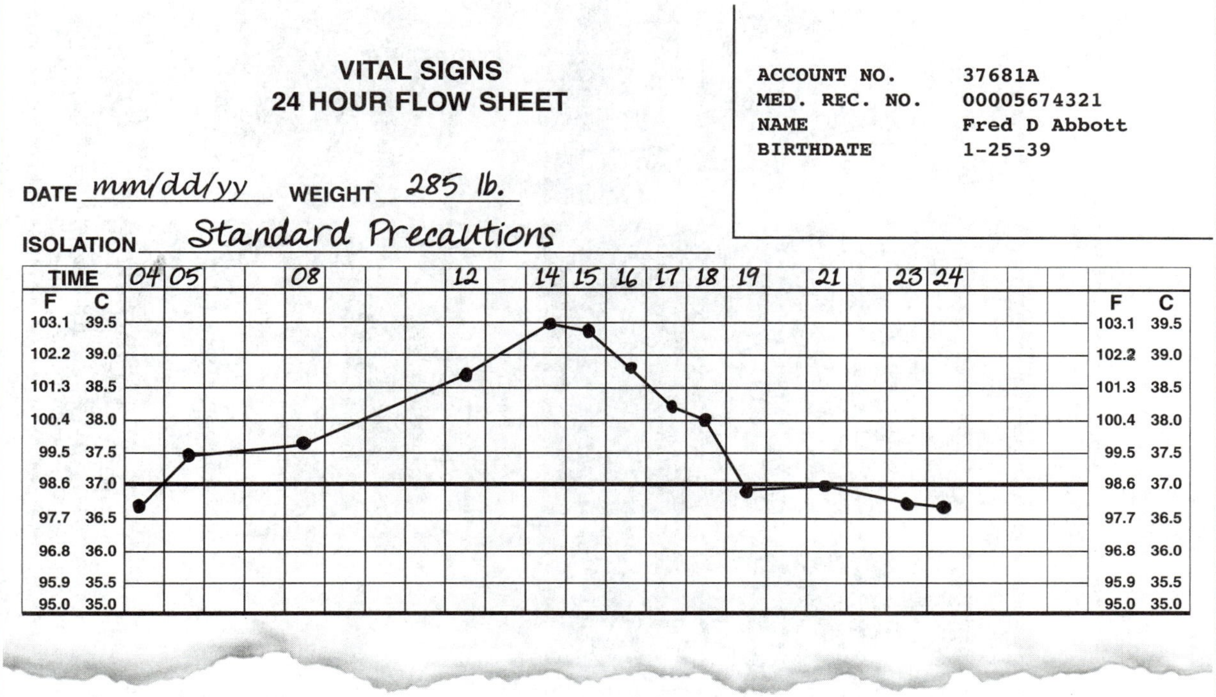

SAMPLE ITEM 8-41

A nurse is caring for a client who has an order for intravenous fluids. Place the following photographs in the order in which the actions should be implemented when initiating a peripheral intravenous infusion.

1.
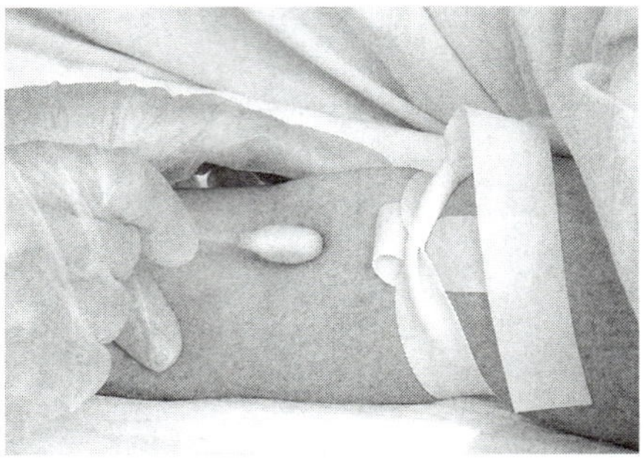

2.
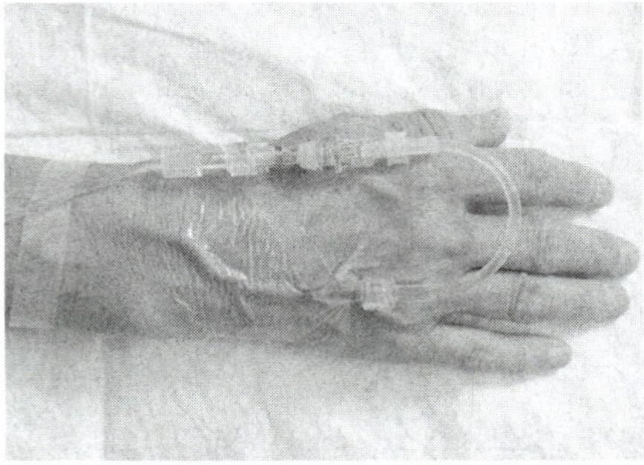

3.
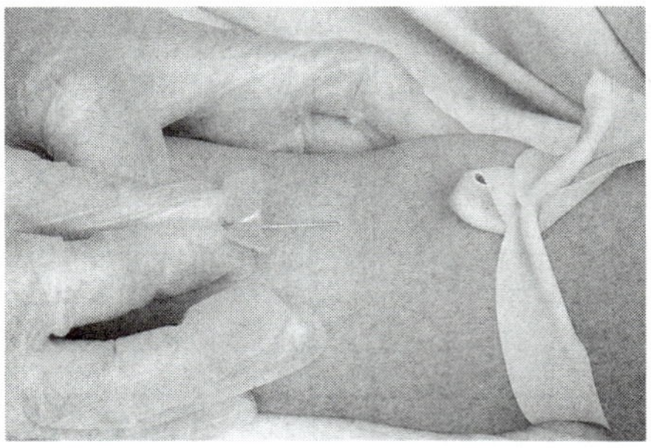

4.
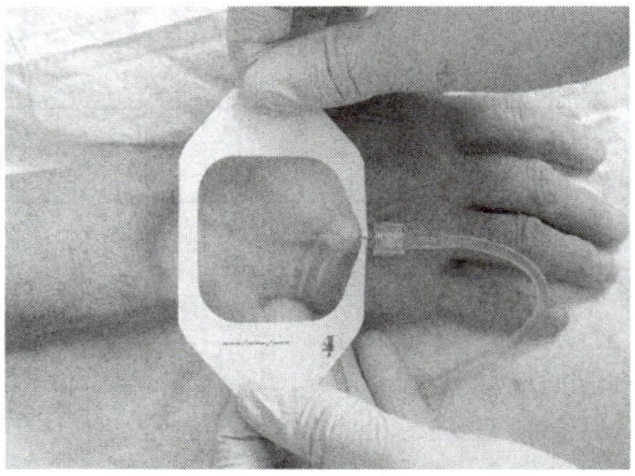

5.
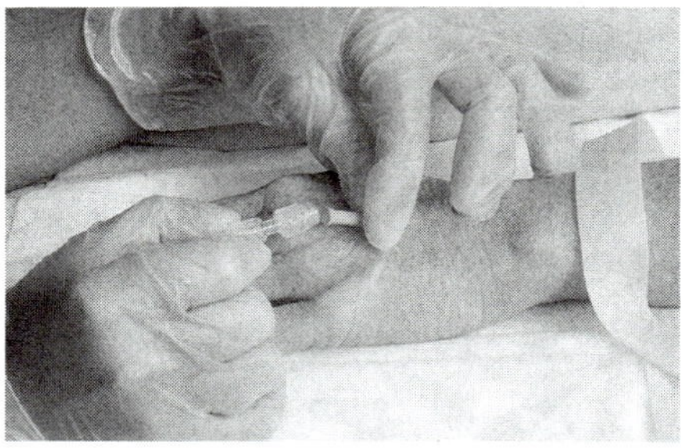

Answer: __________

SAMPLE ITEM 8-42

Identify the position used by the nurse that reflects correct body mechanics to help prevent stress and strain on back muscles. **Select all that apply.**

1. _____ 2. _____ 3. _____ 4. _____ 5. _____

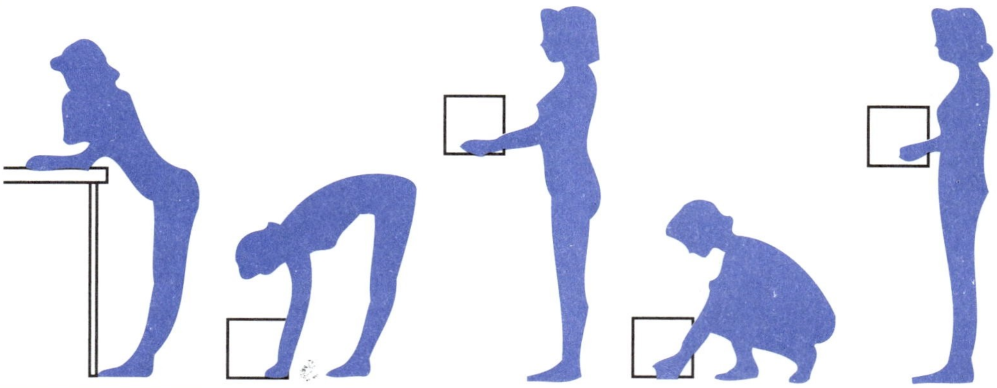

SAMPLE ITEM 8-43

Refer to the I&O flow sheet for a client admitted at 8 a.m. What was the client's total fluid intake for the 7 hours between 8 a.m. and 3 p.m.? **Record your answer using a whole number.**

DAILY INTAKE AND OUTPUT RECORD

DATE JUNE 5

INTAKE								OUTPUT			
I.V. FLUIDS							ORAL	URINE	EMESIS	N.G. TUBE	HEMOVAC
Time	Bottle	Amount	Solution	Medication and Dosage	* ABS.	∓ LIB					
8	1	1000	NS	20 mEq KCl	↓			650			
8:30							360				
10:00							120				
11:30							240	150			
12:00									160		
1:40									90		60
2:15								250			
3:00					525	475					45
7-3 TOTAL		8-HR TOTAL			525	475	720	1050	250		105
3-11 TOTAL		8-HR TOTAL									
11-7 TOTAL		8-HR TOTAL									
24 HOUR TOTAL											

INTAKE GRAND TOTAL ____ OUTPUT GRAND TOTAL ____

* ABS. = amount absorbed ∓ LIB = Left in bag

Answer: ______ mL

CLINICAL JUDGMENT QUESTION FORMATS REFLECTIVE OF NEXT GENERATION NCLEX

The NCSBN has developed and rigorously tested a Clinical Judgment Measurement Model (NCJMM®) to measure clinical judgment. In 2023 the NCLEX examination will include question items that have been shown to measure the clinical judgment skills of newly graduated nurses (https://www.ncsbn.org/ngn-resources.htm). These item types will be given in addition to the traditional multiple-choice format currently in use.

The case study format presents a case study with all six steps of the NCJMM® format presented in a series of six questions. Responses to each of the six questions reveal the test taker's multiple clinical decisions along the steps of the NCJMM®. These six steps are as follows:

1. Recognize cues—what matters most?
2. Analyze cues—what could it mean?
3. Prioritize hypotheses—where do I start?
4. Generate solutions—what can I do?
5. Take action—what will I do?
6. Evaluate outcomes—did it help?

Step 5 is where the end result of the nurse's clinical judgment becomes evident, when the nurse takes action. An example of this case study item type is given in Sample Items 8-44 through 8-49. The six steps of the NCJMM® will not be identified as such in the

NCLEX examination, but are built into each item. It is important to note that the six steps do not replace the nursing process, but follow the same process very closely.

Some of the NGN item types are similar to traditional multiple choice, but the test taker is required to prioritize a limited number of answers, when several valid options for nursing care may be given. Generally, the best option is the one most closely related to client survival.

The seven new item types, as noted in *Fundamentals Success*, 6th edition (Nugent & Vitale, 2022, p. 6), are briefly explained here. The item names are not important for you to remember. Many of the formats might be familiar to you already, in one form or another.

1. **Cloze.** For this item type, the test taker will select words from a drop-down list of up to six options. Generally, the most serious condition affecting the client's life is the best answer. The questions might read as follows:
   - "The nurse is initiating the plan of care. The nurse should first address the client's (select one from the list) followed by the client's (select one from the list). (See Sample Item 8-46.)
   - This item type might also be a knowledge check. A case study might be given, followed by a question like this: "Based on the case study, the nurse should recognize that the labor contractions may (select one from the list) and the fetal heart rate may (select one from the list) upon rupture of membranes." Because this question is about spontaneous rupture of membranes, you will have a choice such as "become stronger" for the contractions, and the choice of "decrease suddenly" for the fetal heart rate. This will demonstrate that you know to anticipate the effects of ruptured membranes.
2. **Enhanced hot spot.** This is very similar to using a highlighter. The test taker clicks on selected information to highlight his or her response. Here are two examples:
   - The question may provide a case study and progress notes. The instructions could be: "Click to highlight the findings that would indicate the client is not progressing as expected" and the test taker will highlight the appropriate findings, whether it is lab results, assessments in the nurse's progress notes, client comments, and so on. Once clicked, the information is highlighted in yellow.
   - The question may provide a case study, and then a page from the *Physician's Desk Reference* (PDF) to ask about medication administration. "Which drug reference information supports your decision to withhold the medication? Highlight the text that supports your decision." The test taker will highlight conditions given in the case study that are contraindications to administering the medication.
3. **Extended drag and drop.** A box with two columns is given, following a case study. The test taker will be asked to "Drag each (given) potential issue that the client is at risk for, to the box on the right."
4. **Extended multiple choice.** This format will be familiar. The question that follows a case study may be, "The nurse is preparing the client for a pacemaker implant. Which of the following actions should the nurse take? **Check all that apply.**" (See Sample Item 8-48.)
5. **Matrix.** This item type requires the test taker to prioritize care and other clinical decision making. As an example, a table with four columns may be given. In response to a case study, the first column may have a provider's order on each line. To the right will be two or three columns with labels such as "anticipated, nonessential, or contraindicated," or some other Likert-type labels. In this example, the test taker must click in the appropriate column beside each provider's order to indicate whether it is anticipated, nonessential, or contraindicated. (See Sample Item 8-47.)
6. **Bowtie.** This is one of two so-called *stand-alone* item types. More than one of the six steps in the NCJMM® are addressed in one question. (See *NGN News*, Fall 2021, at https://www.ncsbn.org/ngn-resources.htm for more information.) The bowtie item type presents as five boxes that appear similar to a bowtie shape. After reading the given clinical scenario, the test taker will begin by dragging the *most likely condition* a client is experiencing to the middle box of the bowtie. Next, one answer is dragged to each of the boxes on the left that correspond with the *actions* the nurse should take to address

that condition. Finally, the test taker drags the two *priority parameters to monitor* into the boxes on the right. (See Sample Items 8-50–8-52.)

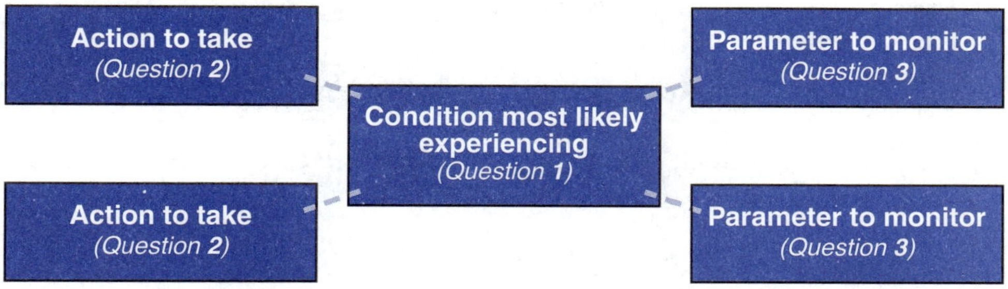

7. **Trend.** This is the second stand-alone item type. This item type presents one or more of the NCJMM® components in one question. The test taker will assess a client's trend of symptoms, lab results, for example, and determine such things as a worsening or improving condition.

Case Study Item Type Examples

The nurse is assuming care of a 26-year-old client with an obstetrical history of G1 P1001 who delivered 45 minutes ago. Her prenatal course was uncomplicated. The client was induced with oxytocin at 41 weeks gestation. Her labor lasted 20 hours and pain relief was provided per epidural. Vital signs during labor were T 99°F (37.2°C), P 88, R 18, BP 116/80.

She pushed for 3 hours before the provider placed low forceps in response to a nonreassuring fetal heart rate. A baby weighing 9 lb 12 oz (4422 grams) was delivered in the occiput posterior position and is currently stable in the father's arms. The provider was called away for another delivery immediately after the birth and did not inspect the placenta at that time.

Her quantitative blood loss at the time of delivery was 450 mL. An oxytocin infusion of 20 units in 1000 mL lactated Ringer's solution is running at 100 mL/hour by pump. The previous nurse has changed the client's peri pad two times over the past 20 minutes. Each time, the pad was soaked with bright red blood and dark red blood. The client's fundus is reported as firm at the umbilicus and deviated to the right. Her current pulse rate is 110 and her BP is 100/70. The client's epidural catheter is still in place. She states she feels "shaky."

SAMPLE ITEM 8-44: Recognize Cues

Which of the following require immediate follow-up? **Select two.**

1. Fundal tone
2. Cumulative blood loss
3. Current lochia amount
4. Fundal position
5. Client's report of shakiness

SAMPLE ITEM 8-45: Analyze Cues

Client Findings	(a) Retained Placental Tissue	(b) Obstetric Laceration	(c) Bladder Fullness
1. Soaking pad every 10 min			
2. Fundal deviation			
3. Fundal tone			
4. Bright red blood			

SAMPLE ITEM 8-46: Prioritize Hypotheses

The nurse should first address the client's **(select one):**
1. Fundal tone
2. Bladder
3. Bleeding
4. Blood sugar
Followed by the client's **(select one):**
a) Fundal tone
b) Bladder
c) Bleeding
d) Blood sugar

SAMPLE ITEM 8-47: Generate Solutions

Potential Order	(a) Anticipated	(b) Nonessential
1. Prepare client for surgery		
2. Insert large-bore venous access device (VAD)		
3. Run additional intravenous fluids		
4. Administer additional uterotonics		
5. Type and cross 2 units, PRBCs		
6. Perineal shave prep		
7. NPO		

The client was catheterized for 400 mL urine. Her fundus remains firm at the umbilicus and is no longer deviated to the right. The nurse notes continued bright red blood trickling from the vagina. The client has saturated another pad within 10 minutes. Blood pressure is now 96/80, pulse 115. Oxygen saturation is 96% on room air. The provider was notified to come STAT and has examined the client at the bedside. The client has been diagnosed with a long cervical laceration. The client's cumulative blood loss is now 900 mL. The provider and nurse are discussing the treatment plan for the client. For each potential order, select whether it is anticipated or nonessential.

SAMPLE ITEM 8-48: Take Action

The placenta was saved for the provider, who examined it and determined that it was delivered intact. The provider has asked the nurse to prepare the client for a surgical repair of the cervical laceration as soon as possible. Which of the following actions should the nurse take? **Select all that apply.**

1. Inform the client about surgery risks and benefits
2. Obtain client's signature on surgical permit
3. Complete perineal shave prep
4. Confirm patency of venous access devices (VADs)
5. Perform medication reconciliation
6. Preoperative and postoperative teaching

SAMPLE ITEM 8-49: Evaluate Outcomes

The client is now 24 hours postoperative, following a forceps delivery of a macrosomic baby, followed by a cervical laceration repair. Her epidural was still functional and was used for surgical anesthesia. She has not received a blood transfusion. Identify the nursing documentation entries below that indicate the client is not progressing as expected. **Select all that apply.**

1. Client complains of perineal tenderness.
2. Unsteady with ambulation, requiring assistance.
3. Temperature 101°F (38.3°C), BP 100/70, and pulse 95.
4. States cramping is relieved with ibuprofen.
5. Complains of discomfort at epidural insertion site.

Note: The nurse's documentation is given in this example by numbered sentences. In the NCLEX® examination, the nurse's notes will be in paragraph format. The test taker will be asked to click on the findings within the paragraph to highlight the correct responses.

Stand-Alone Item Type Examples, Bowtie

The same information in this case study (above) could be presented in bowtie format:

SAMPLE ITEM 8-50

The nurse is assuming care of a 26-year-old client with an obstetrical history of G1 P1001 who delivered 45 minutes ago. Her prenatal course was uncomplicated. The client was induced with oxytocin at 41 weeks gestation. Her labor lasted 20 hours and pain relief was provided per epidural. Vital signs during labor were T 99°F (37.2°C), P 88, R 18, BP 116/80.

She pushed for 3 hours before the provider placed low forceps in response to a nonreassuring fetal heart rate. A baby weighing 9 lb 12 oz (4422 grams) was delivered in the occiput posterior position and is currently stable in the father's arms. The provider was called away for another delivery immediately after the birth and did not inspect the placenta at that time.

Her quantitative blood loss at the time of delivery was 450 mL. An oxytocin infusion of 20 units in 1000 mL lactated ringer's solution is running at 100 mL/hour by pump. The previous nurse has changed the client's peri pad two times over the past 20 minutes. Each time, the pad was soaked with bright red blood and lochia. The client's fundus is reported as firm at the umbilicus and deviated to the right. Her current pulse rate is 110 and her BP is 100/70. The client's epidural catheter is still in place. She states she feels "shaky."

Select a complication which the client is likely experiencing.

1. Hypoglycemia
2. Infection
3. Postpartum hemorrhage

SAMPLE ITEM 8-51

Which of the following actions should the nurse take to address that condition? **Select two.**

1. Increase the oxytocin infusion rate
2. Perform fundal massage
3. Offer the client orange juice
4. Empty client's bladder
5. Notify provider for STAT bedside consultation

SAMPLE ITEM 8-52

Specify two parameters the nurse should monitor to reduce the risks of the identified complication.
1. Vital signs
2. Blood sugar
3. Urinary output
4. Bleeding

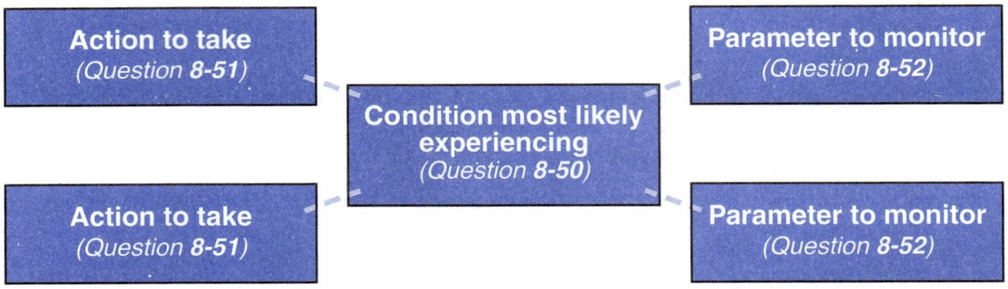

SUMMARY

To promote success when challenged by an examination with a variety of testing formats, it is wise to be familiar with the various formats. Structured-response, restricted-response, extended essay, and performance-appraisal formats are commonly used in schools of nursing in addition to the alternate item formats found on the NCLEX®, such as fill-in-the-blank, multiple-response, hot spot, drag-and-drop/ordered-response, graphic and illustration, and exhibit items. Multimedia such as charts, tables, and graphics can be used in multiple-choice questions and all types of alternate item formats. These questions have some commonalities, but each is unique. Understanding the commonalities and differences in these formats and using a variety of test-taking techniques facilitate a feeling of control, which contributes to a positive mental attitude.

8-1 Answer: 1 and 2.

1. **Undermining of adjoining tissue can occur with a stage III pressure ulcer. Undermining is a wider area of tissue damage that extends under and beyond the opening of a wound (under the surface of adjoining tissue). With undermining, the wound is more extensive than what is visible from the surface.**
2. **A stage III pressure ulcer involves full-thickness skin loss (through the dermis and epidermis), with damage or necrosis extending to the subcutaneous tissue.**
3. A stage III pressure ulcer is not limited to partial-thickness loss. A wound with just a partial-thickness loss (e.g., blister, abrasion, shallow crater) is associated with a stage II pressure ulcer.
4. A stage III pressure ulcer does not involve damage through the fascia. A stage IV pressure ulcer involves damage to muscle, bone, or supporting tissue (e.g., a tendon or capsule of a joint). Undermining and sinus tracts (tunneling) are relatively common with a stage IV pressure ulcer.
5. A stage III pressure ulcer does not involve muscle damage. A stage IV pressure ulcer involves damage to muscle, bone, or supporting tissue (e.g., a tendon or capsule of a joint). Undermining and sinus tracts (tunneling) are relatively common with a stage IV pressure ulcer.

8-2 Answer: 3, 4, 5, and 6.

1. Donning a gown when entering a room where airborne transmission–based precautions are required is unnecessary unless there is a likelihood of splashing of blood, body fluids, body secretions, or excretions.
2. Putting on gloves when delivering a food tray where airborne transmission–based precautions are required is unnecessary unless there is a likelihood of splashing of blood, body fluids, body secretions, or excretions.
3. **A client requiring airborne transmission–based precautions must wear a surgical mask when being transported outside the room; this protects others from the client's respiratory microorganisms.**
4. **A client requiring airborne transmission–based precautions must be cared for in a monitored negative air pressure room that maintains 6 to 12 air changes per hour. A negative air pressure room prevents room air from flowing through the door to the hallway; it expels room air to the outside environment, unless a high-efficiency particulate air (HEPA) filtration system is used.**
5. **An N95 respirator mask must be worn when entering a room where airborne transmission–based precautions are required. An N95 respirator mask protects the wearer from the transfer of oral and nasopharyngeal organisms from the client. N95 respirators demonstrate a filtration efficiency of the most penetrating particle size (0.1 to 0.3 micrometers) at 99.5% to 99.75%.**
6. **The door to a room with monitored negative air pressure must be kept closed at all times except when entering or exiting the room. This prevents air in the room from flowing through the door to the hallway and expels the room air to the outside environment, unless a high-efficiency particulate air (HEPA) filtration system is used.**

8-3 Answer: 1, 2, 4, 6

1. **Infants born between 34 and 37 weeks gestation ("late preterm") are at higher risk for neonatal jaundice due to immaturity of the liver (Lee & Barfield, 2021). In addition, they have fewer bowel movements because their intake is low. As a result, the level of bilirubin builds up, creating a yellow tinge to their skin. Bilirubin is made of the yellow pigment in bile. Jaundice is caused by too much bilirubin in the blood.**
2. **Maternal preeclampsia is a risk factor for neonatal jaundice (Boskabadi et al., 2020).**
3. A long labor by itself is not a risk factor for neonatal jaundice.
4. **A cephalohematoma is the result of blood vessels rupturing under the baby's scalp. A long labor can contribute to this condition; however, most babies born after a long labor do not develop a cephalohematoma. As the**

baby's body reabsorbs the broken blood cells, bilirubin levels rise and circulate throughout the baby's body.

5. Maternal primiparity by itself is not a risk factor for neonatal jaundice.
6. **The mother's report of "poor breast-feeding" could be a clue that the newborn has inadequate fluid intake. Without adequate intake, the new-born has fewer or smaller bowel move-ments. The excretion of bilirubin in the stool is reduced and the bilirubin can be reabsorbed back into the cir-culation (Academy of Breastfeeding, 2017).**

8-4 TRUE
Soap decreases the surface tension of water. Surface tension is the tendency of a liquid to minimize the area of its surface by contract-ing. Decreasing the surface tension increases the ability of water to wet another surface.

8-5 TRUE
A broad stance widens the nurse's base of support, which promotes stability.

8-6 FALSE
Exercise is a stimulating activity that should be avoided before bedtime. Ade-quate exercise during the day promotes sleep later in the day.

8-7 FALSE
Pulse pressure is the difference between the systolic and diastolic blood pressures. Pulse deficit is the difference between the apical and radial pulse rates.

8-8 TRUE
Palpation is a technique in which the examiner applies the fingers or hands to the body to assess the texture, size, con-sistency, and location of body parts.

8-9 FALSE
The process in which solid particulate matter in a fluid moves from an area of increased concentration to an area of decreased concentration is known as *diffusion.* The process in which a pure solvent, such as water, moves through a semipermeable membrane from an area that has a decreased solute concentration to one that has an increased solute concentration is known as *osmosis.*

8-10 1. TRUE
The outer border of a drape is consid-ered contaminated. After sterile gloves are donned, the nurse can touch only inside this border to maintain sterility of the field.

2. TRUE
The nurse understands that the hands are not sterile and avoids contaminating the sterile glove by touching only the inside of the glove. The second sterile glove is donned by touching just the outside of the glove with the hand that is already covered by the first sterile glove.

3. FALSE
During a surgical hand scrub, the hands are held above the elbows; this allows water to flow downward by gravity without contaminating the nurse's hands. Hand hygiene associated with medical asepsis requires the hands to be held below the elbows.

4. FALSE
Sterile objects held below the waist are not within the nurse's direct visual field and inadvertently may become contaminated.

8-11 1. TRUE
Mechanical ventilation uses positive pressure to push air and/or oxygen into the lungs during the inspiratory phase of the respiratory cycle. Positive pressure is pressure greater than that of the atmosphere.

2. FALSE
A continuous bladder irrigation uses the principle of gravity to instill fluid into the bladder as well as to promote the flow of fluid out of the bladder through the triple-lumen indwelling urinary catheter. Gravity is the force that draws all masses in the earth's sphere toward the center of the earth.

3. FALSE
Chest tubes (chest drainage systems) exert negative pressure to remove air and fluids from the pleural space. Negative pressure is pressure less than that of the atmosphere, and it is the opposite of positive pressure.

4. TRUE
Positive pressure is exerted when the plunger of a piston syringe is pushed toward its cone tip.

8-12 FALSE
This statement can be revised in the fol-lowing way: The expected range of the heart rate for an adult is *60 to 100* beats per minute.

8-13 FALSE
To revise this question as directed, the words *young adulthood* must be changed to *adolescence*. You will not receive credit for this question if you changed *identity versus role confusion* to *intimacy versus isolation*. Although this statement is accurate, the instructions for revising the statement have not been followed.

8-14 1. FALSE
The client's temperature was 101.4°F. Each line above 101 is 0.2 of a degree.

2. TRUE
Body temperature varies throughout the day, with the lowest temperature in the early morning and the highest temperature between 8 p.m. and midnight. A circadian rhythm (diurnal variation) is a pattern based on a 24-hour cycle.

3. TRUE
With deficient fluid volume, the volume in the intravascular compartment decreases (hypovolemia), resulting in decreased blood pressure (hypotension).

4. TRUE
This client's pulse rate ranged from 76 (on June 10 and 11) to 110 (on June 5 and 6) beats per minute.

5. TRUE
A pulse rate of 98 beats per minute is within the expected range of 60 to 100 beats per minute.

6. FALSE
During the acute phase of the illness, the client's temperature, pulse, and respirations were all increased.

8-15 1. TRUE
The intravenous solution was hung at 8 a.m. and infused 525 mL over the next 7 hours. The total volume (525 mL) divided by the number of hours (7) equals 75 mL/hr.

2. FALSE
If each ounce is equal to 30 mL, 4 ounces is equal to 120 mL. When you subtract 120 mL from the total volume of fluid taken at 8:30 a.m. (360 mL), the amount of additional fluid consumed was 240 mL. When you divide 240 mL by 30 mL, it equals 8 ounces, not 10 ounces.

3. FALSE
The intake was 525 + 720 = 1245 mL. The output was 1050 + 250 + 105 = 1405 mL. The output exceeded the intake by 160 mL.

4. FALSE
The additive to the client's intravenous solution was 20 mEq of potassium chloride.

8-16 a. 3
Bradypnea is abnormally slow breathing with a regular rhythm (respiratory rate less than 10 breaths/min).

b. 4
Apnea is the temporary cessation of breathing (absence of breathing).

c. 1
Hyperpnea is deep, rapid, labored respirations, usually associated with strenuous exercise.

d. 5
Tachypnea is abnormally rapid breathing with a regular rhythm (respirations that are increased in depth and rate).

e. 6
Eupnea is breathing that is expected at a rate of 12 to 20 breaths per minute and depth with a tidal volume of approximately 500 mL (normal breathing).

f. 2
Dyspnea is characterized by an increased effort and use of accessory muscles (difficulty breathing).
The phrase *Shallow breathing interrupted by irregular periods of apnea* is an extra option included in Column II that does not have a matching term in Column I.

8-17 a. 4
Kegel exercises consist of repetitive contractions of the muscles of the pelvic floor. These muscles facilitate voluntary control of urination.

b. 4
Kegel exercises, which are performed by voluntarily starting and stopping the urinary stream, tone the perineal muscles of the pelvic floor.

c. 2
Aerobic exercises involve activity that demands that oxygen be taken into the body at a rate greater than that usually required by the body, promoting respiratory functioning.

d. 2
Aerobic exercises involve sustained muscle movements that increase blood flow, heart rate, and metabolic demand for oxygen over time, which promotes cardiovascular functioning.

e. 3
Isometric exercises cause a change in muscle tension but no change in muscle length; no muscle or joint movement occurs.

f. 1
Passive range-of-motion exercises occur when another person moves each of the client's joints through their full range of movement, maximally stretching all muscle groups within each plane over each joint.

8-18 ***Contracture* is the only acceptable answer to this question.**
Contractures are permanent flexion deformities of joints caused by disuse, atrophy, and shortening of muscles.

8-19 ***Respiratory passages* or *lung* are both acceptable answers to this question.**
With postural drainage, the client is placed in various positions to promote the movement of secretions from smaller to larger pulmonary airways, where they can be removed by coughing or suctioning.

8-20 **The correct answer for this question is *12* to *20*.**

8-21 **The correct answer is *location*.**
Radiating pain is a description that relates to where the pain is experienced in the body. It includes the initial site of the pain and its extension to other parts of the body. Intensity refers to the perceived severity of the pain; intensity is commonly measured on a scale of 0 (no pain) to 10 (severe pain).

8-22 **The correct answer is *urgency*.**
Urgency is the feeling that the person must void immediately whether or not there is much urine in the bladder. It is precipitated by psychological stress and/or irritation of the vesical trigone and/or urethra. Frequency is the increased incidence of voiding.

8-23 **Acceptable answers include permanent flexion and fixation of a joint or an abnormal shortening of a muscle that results in limited range of motion of a joint and eventually ankylosis.**
Compare this item with Sample Item 8-17.

8-24 **Acceptable answers include mobilize respiratory secretions; loosen pulmonary secretions to facilitate their expectoration; or promote a clear airway by draining respiratory secretions toward the oral cavity.**
Compare this item with Sample Item 8-18.

8-25 **Acceptable answers include just stating the numbers 12 to 20.**
A more complex answer might be stated as follows: The expected (normal) number of breaths per minute for an adult ranges from 12 to 20 with an average of 16. Compare this item with Sample Item 8-19.

8-26 **Answer: 25 drops/min.**

$$\frac{\textbf{Volume to be infused}}{\textbf{Number of hours}} \times \frac{\textbf{drop factor}}{\textbf{60 minutes}}$$

$$\frac{100 \times 15}{1 \times 60}$$

$$\frac{1500}{60} = 25 \text{ drops/min}$$

8-27 **To answer this question, use the three-part format:**
INTRODUCTION: The introduction functions as a preface, preamble, or prologue for the information that follows.

Although there are many detailed definitions of the practice of nursing, in the simplest terms nursing consists of helping people meet their needs. To do this, nurses must employ cognitive skills such as critical thinking and clinical judgment. The commonalities and differences of critical thinking and clinical judgment will be discussed.

CENTRAL PART: The central part of the answer presents and explores the information necessary to answer the question. Make a topical outline of the facts to be included, and then write a narrative that incorporates and elaborates on the information in the outline.

Definition of critical thinking
Definition of clinical judgment
Commonalities of critical thinking and clinical judgment
  Strong knowledge base
  Attitude of inquiry and intellectual humility

Purposeful process
Use of reasoning
Distinguishing features of critical thinking
Is proactive
Uses thinking processes to clarify and improve understanding
Is open-ended
Distinguishing features of clinical judgment
Is reactive
Uses the mental operation of critical thinking to explore possibilities
Starts with a problem and ends with an enlightened conclusion

SUMMARY: The summary should briefly recap or review the general theme of the discussion and come to one or more conclusions. It serves to close the response to the essay question.

The nurse of today and especially of the future must be able to integrate critical thinking and clinical judgment to maximize human potential. Although they have a common foundation, each mode of thinking is unique. Nurses should blend them into a repertoire of cognitive strategies.

ALTERNATE QUESTION FORMATS REFLECTIVE OF NCLEX®

Fill-in-the-Blank Items

8-28 **Answer: 63 mL/hr**
The question directed you to use a whole number for your answer. 1500 ÷ 24 = 62.5 mL. When a portion of a milliliter is .5 or greater, round up to the next full number.

8-29 **Answer: 1.5 mL**
The question directed you to use one decimal place in your answer. One gram is equal to 1000 mg. Solve the problem using ratio and proportion.

$$\frac{\text{Desired}}{\text{Have}} \quad \frac{500\text{ mg}}{1000\text{ mg}} = \frac{x\text{ mL}}{3\text{ mL}}$$

$$1000x = 1500$$
$$x = 1500 \div 1000$$
$$x = 1.5\text{ mL}$$

Hot Spot Items

8-30 **For this client, the sacral area (shaded) is at the highest risk for dependent edema. Excess fluid volume increases capillary pressures that cause fluid to move from the intravascular compartment into the interstitial tissue. Fluid flows by gravity, so edema is observed in dependent tissues. A client who has difficulty breathing is generally positioned in a semi- or high-Fowler position. In the Fowler position, the sacrum is the most dependent area and therefore is at highest risk for interstitial edema.**

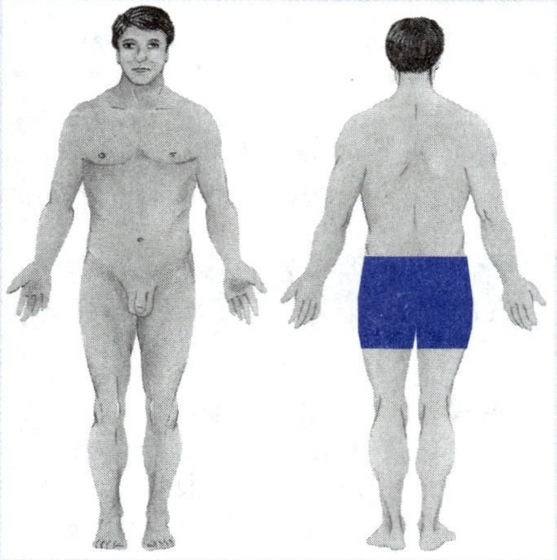

8-31 **The *vastus lateralis* site (shaded) is located in the middle third and anterior lateral aspect of the thigh, one handbreadth above the knee (from the lateral femoral condyle) and one handbreadth below the greater trochanter.**

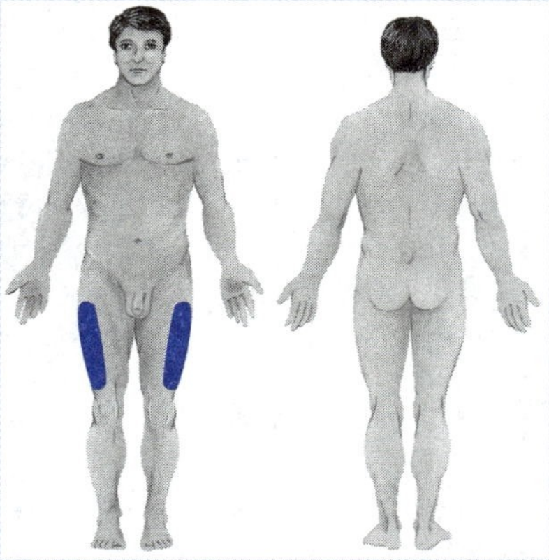

Drag-and-Drop/Ordered-Response Items

8-32 Answer: 4, 1, 2, 5, and 3.

4. *Take the client out of the dayroom*—Remove: The priority is to remove the client, who is in the immediate vicinity of the fire and is at risk for injury.
1. *Pull the fire alarm*—Activate: Once the client is protected from harm, the fire alarm can be activated.
2. *Shut the doors on the unit*—Contain: After the client is protected from harm and the alarm is sounded, actions can be implemented to contain the fire such as closing doors.
5. *Move clients in adjacent rooms to an area down the hall*—Evacuate: This is necessary only after the previous three steps have been implemented and if it is determined that clients are at risk.
3. *Move all clients off the unit*—Evacuate: This is necessary if the fire escalates and the clients are at risk.

8-33 Answer: 4, 3, 1, 2, and 5.

4. A wheelchair lap hugger can be removed by the client and is the least restrictive of the options presented. It supports upper body alignment and posture. Also, it is used to remind the client to call for help before attempting to rise. Upon rising, a wheelchair lap hugger self-releases and therefore is not considered a restraint.
3. A finger control mitt allows free range of motion of the fingers within the mitt, but it limits the ability to grasp objects. Also, it allows range of motion of the wrist(s) and shoulder(s). A finger control mitt is not considered a restraint because it is not tied to an immovable object, such as the frame of a bed. A finger control mitt becomes a restraint when it is tied to an immovable object. At this point, it becomes as restrictive as a wrist restraint.
1. A waist belt is tied to each side of a bed frame but is designed to permit the client to move all four extremities and to fully turn from side to side for comfort.
2. A safety vest allows a bedbound client to move all four extremities and turn slightly from side to side. A safety vest is tied to an immovable object, such as a bed frame.
5. Of the options listed, four-point limb leather cuffs are the most restrictive restraint. All four extremities are restrained and cannot be moved through range of motion. They are tied to an immovable object, such as the frame of a bed.

Multiple-Response Items

8-34
1. Tenting of the skin occurs because of the decrease in interstitial and intracellular fluid.
2. The pulse increases, not decreases, to compensate for hypovolemia.
3. One liter of fluid weighs 2.2 pounds. The client will lose weight as fluid is excreted.
4. The blood pressure decreases because of the decreased, not increased, intravascular fluid volume.
5. Interstitial and intracellular fluid shifts to the intravascular compartment to maintain cardiovascular function. As a result, the tongue becomes furrowed and dry.

8-35
1. Providing a back rub is considered an activity of daily living, which is within the scope of practice of a nursing assistant.
2. Assisting clients with activities of daily living, which include transferring clients from the bed to a chair, is within the scope of practice of a nursing assistant.
3. Assisting clients with activities of daily living, which include maintaining clean linen for a client with a continuous passive motion machine, is within the scope of practice of a nursing assistant.
4. Client teaching is an independent role of a nurse, not a nursing assistant. For appropriate nursing interventions, teaching requires knowledge of anatomy, physiology, pharmacology, teaching/learning principles, and rationales.
5. Caring for surgical dressings, which requires the use of sterile technique,

is not within the scope of practice of a nursing assistant. In addition, a nurse, not a nursing assistant, is educationally prepared to assess a wound and to determine whether a client is hemorrhaging.

6. Although nursing assistants can take routine vital signs of clients who are physiologically stable, immediate postoperative clients and clients who are physiologically unstable should have their vital signs assessed by a nurse.

Exhibit Items

8-36

Laboratory Results

Sodium: 155 mEq/L
White blood cells (WBCs): 8000 mcL
Hematocrit (Hct): 60%
Fasting blood sugar (FBS): 94 mg/dL

Vital Signs at 2:00 p.m.

Temperature: 100°F
Pulse: 88 beats/min, regular
Respirations: 24 breaths/min

Progress Note

Client is oriented to place and person but is easily distracted, is unable to follow directions, **and** voided a small amount of clear amber urine; the tongue has furrows, and there is tenting of the skin.

ANSWER AND RATIONALES

1. The physical assessment and laboratory results indicate that the client is dehydrated. Oliguria, furrows of the tongue, tenting of the skin, and increased vital signs are all signs of dehydration. The serum sodium level that is higher than the expected range of 135 to 145 mEq/L and the Hct that is higher than the expected range of 40% to 54% indicate hemoconcentration associated with dehydration.
2. With hypervolemia, the client's Hct will be decreased, indicating hemodilution.
3. With a urinary tract infection, there is not just an increase in temperature; the WBC count also will be increased, and the urine will be cloudy.
4. The physical assessment data do not support the inference that the client has hyperglycemia. The FBS is within the expected limits of 70 to 100 mg/dL, and there is an absence of polyuria, polyphagia, polydipsia, fatigue, weakness, and vision changes.

8-37

Laboratory Tests

Red blood cells (RBCs): 2.9 cells/mcL
White blood cells (WBCs): 7000 cells/mcL
Hemoglobin (Hb): 8.5 g/dL
Hematocrit (Hct): 34%

Radiology Report

Chest radiograph: normal findings; all bones aligned and symmetrical; normal positioned soft tissues, mediastinum, lungs, pleura, heart, and aortic arc.

Vital Signs Sheet

Temperature: 98.8°F (oral)
Pulse: 92 beats/min, regular rhythm
Respirations: 24 breaths/min, regular rhythm, unlabored

ANSWER AND RATIONALES

1. Osmosis is unrelated to this client situation. Osmosis is related to fluid balance. It is the movement of water through a semipermeable membrane from an area of decreased concentration of constituents to an area of increased concentration of constituents.
2. The client's respiratory status—an unlabored respiratory rate of 24 breaths/min with a regular rhythm—does not reflect a problem with diffusion. The slight increase in respiratory rate is a compensatory response to the decreased number of red blood cells that carry oxygen to all body cells. The chest radiograph rules out primary lung disease and indicates that problems with diffusion do not exist.
3. The client has a problem with oxygen transport because of an inadequate number of red blood cells; the hemoglobin component of red blood cells carries oxygen to body cells. When the client's laboratory results are compared with the expected values below, the results indicate that the client's RBCs, Hb, and Hct are all decreased, reflecting a reduced ability to transport oxygen on the hemoglobin molecule of the red blood cells. The expected ranges for these laboratory tests for women are as follows:
   RBCs: 3.6 to 5.0 cells/mcL
   WBCs: 5000 to 7000 cells/mcL
   Hb: 12.0 to 16.0 g/dL
   Hct: 36% to 48%
4. Although increased pulse rate and respirations may indicate a problem with ventilation, the fact that the respirations are unlabored and the chest radiograph results are within expected limits shows there is not a problem with ventilation.

Graphic Items

8-38
1. The insertion of a catheter into a sterile body cavity (urinary bladder) requires the use of surgical, not medical, asepsis.
2. Irrigation of a wound requires the use of surgical, not medical, asepsis.
3. **Application of a condom catheter requires the use of medical asepsis. A sheath is placed over the penis to collect urine after it passes through the urinary meatus. A body cavity is not entered.**
4. Insertion of a catheter into a body cavity (trachea and bronchi) requires the use of surgical, not medical, asepsis.

8-39
1. This syringe is an insulin syringe. The length of the needle of an insulin syringe is designed to enter subcutaneous tissue. The needle is too short to enter a muscle.
2. This syringe is a tuberculin syringe. The length of the needle of a tuberculin syringe is designed for intradermal injections. The needle is too short to enter a muscle.
3. This syringe is a standard 5-mL syringe. Although the needle is 1.5 inches long and can enter a muscle, the volume of the syringe is beyond the volume necessary to administer the prescribed 1 mL of medication.
4. **This syringe is a standard 3-mL syringe. The needle is 1.5 inches long and can enter a muscle. It can hold the prescribed volume of 1 mL of medication.**

Multimedia in Multiple-Choice and Alternate Question Formats

8-40
1. At the 5th hour, the client's temperature was 99.5°F.
2. At the 14th hour, the client's temperature was 103.1°F.
3. **This is the correct answer. At the 18th hour, the client's temperature was 100.4°F.**
4. At the 21st hour, the client's temperature was 98.6°F.

8-41 **Answer: 1, 3, 5, 4, and 2.**

1. Of the options presented, this photograph depicts the first step when initiating a peripheral IV infusion. Applying a tourniquet helps to "fill-dilate" the veins to allow for easier location of an infusion site. An antiseptic scrub at the insertion site removes microorganisms and minimizes the risk of them entering the vascular site during venipuncture.

3. Of the options presented, this photograph depicts the second step when initiating a peripheral IV infusion. The needle is inserted by piercing the skin directly over the vein.

5. Of the options presented, this photograph depicts the third step when initiating a peripheral IV infusion. The IV administration set (tubing) is connected to the IV catheter.

4. Of the options presented, this photograph depicts the fourth step when initiating a peripheral IV infusion. The insertion site and the hub of the catheter are covered with a transparent dressing (preferred over a gauze dressing because the site can be assessed). The transparent dressing should be gently pinched around the catheter hub and smoothed over the skin to ensure adherence. The transparent dressing should not cover the junction of the needle hub with the administration tubing. This ensures that the junction is accessible when tubing has to be changed.

2. Of the options presented, this photograph depicts the fifth step when initiating a peripheral IV infusion. The tubing is secured with tape to prevent tension on the insertion site.

8-42
1. ___ Bending over without bending the knees places undue stress and strain on the lower back muscles and should be avoided. This illustration demonstrates correct body mechanics.

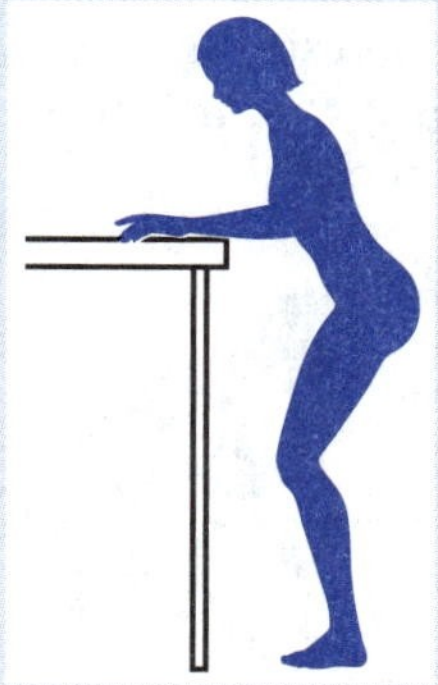

2. ___ Lifting an object without bending the knees and standing close to the object should be avoided. It requires upper body muscles to lift the object, causing undue stress and strain on upper body structures. In addition, the center of gravity is outside the base of support. This illustration demonstrates correct body mechanics.

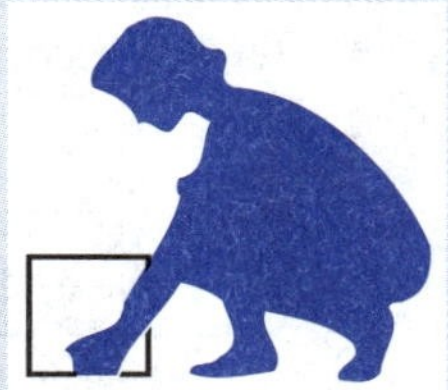

3. ___ Holding objects in front of and away from the body places the center of gravity outside the base of support, which places undue stress and strain on muscles of the upper body and should be avoided. In addition, balance is less stable when the line of gravity falls outside the base of support. This illustration demonstrates correct body mechanics.

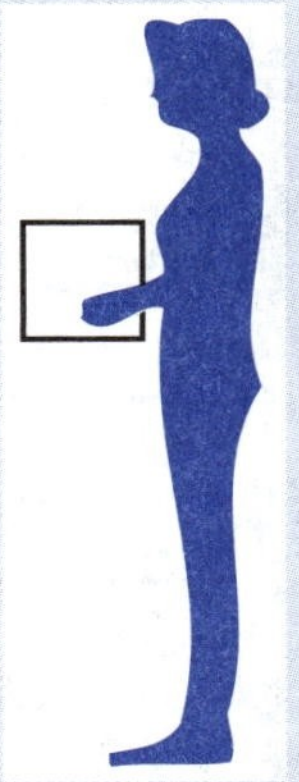

4. X Standing close to an object to be lifted, flexing the knees and hips, and then straightening the knees and hips cause the large muscles of the legs to bear most of the burden. Doing so places less stress and strain on the muscles of the back. This illustration demonstrates correct body mechanics.

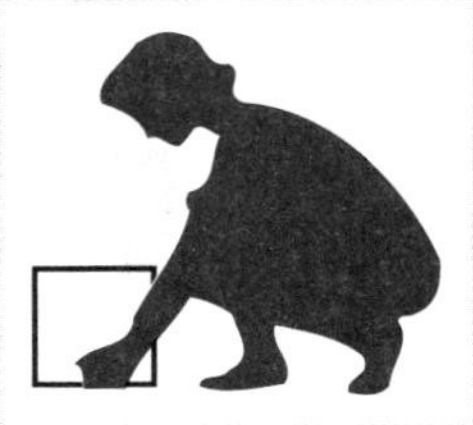

5. X Holding objects close to the body places the line of gravity closer to the base of support, facilitating balance and reducing stress and strain on the muscles of the back. This illustration demonstrates correct body mechanics.

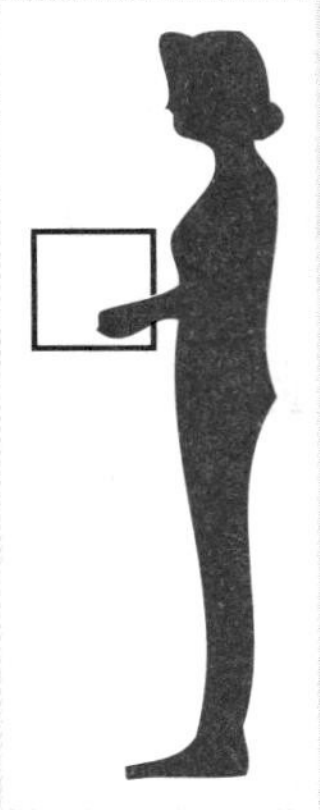

8-43 Answer: 1245 mL.
To arrive at the total intake for the 7 hours between 8 a.m. and 3 p.m., the nurse has to add the 525 mL of IV fluid absorbed (indicated in the box at the bottom of the "Abs" column in the row labeled "7-3 total") and the 720 mL of oral intake (indicated in the box at the bottom of the "ORAL" column in the row labeled "7-3 total"): 525 mL of IV fluids plus 720 mL of oral intake equals 1245 mL of total fluid intake for the 7 hours between 8 a.m. and 3 p.m.

DAILY INTAKE AND OUTPUT RECORD

DATE JUNE 5

INTAKE								OUTPUT			
I.V. FLUIDS							ORAL	URINE	EMESIS	N.G TUBE	HEMOVAC
Time	Bottle	Amount	Solution	Medication and Dosage	* ABS.	∓ LIB					
8	1	1000	NS	20 mEq KCl				650			
8:30							360				
10:00							120				
11:30							240	150			
12:00									160		
1:40									90		60
2:15								250			
3:00					525	475					45
7-3 TOTAL		8-HR TOTAL			525	475	720	1050	250		105
3-11 TOTAL		8-HR TOTAL									
11-7 TOTAL		8-HR TOTAL									
24 HOUR TOTAL											

INTAKE GRAND TOTAL [ ]   OUTPUT GRAND TOTAL [ ]

* ABS. = amount absorbed   ∓ LIB = Left in bag

8-44 **Answers 3 and 4**
Which of the following require immediate follow-up? **Select two.**

1. Note that the test taker is not asked to select responses in any particular order at this point. This question is asking, "What is unexpected?" Since the fundus has remained firm, it is not a cue of something that needs urgent intervention.
2. The cumulative blood loss is important to follow up on, but is not one of the **two** most important cues. The client must be stabilized first.
3. **The cue of saturating a pad every 10 minutes for the past 20 minutes indicates something is not right. If this rate of bleeding continues, it could threaten the client's safety.**
4. **The fundal position at the umbilicus is an expected finding. However, a fundus that is deviated to the right is not expected. A deviated fundus generally indicates a full bladder that can prevent the uterus from contracting adequately. This can lead to increased bleeding or hemorrhage, threatening the client's safety.**
5. The client's report of shakiness is a normal finding this soon after a birth.

8-45 **Answers: 1(a)(b)(c), 2(c), 3(b), 4(b)**
For each client finding below, click to specify if the finding is consistent with the complication of Retained placental tissue, Obstetric laceration, or Bladder fullness. Each finding may support more than one condition. Each column must have at least one selection.

Client Findings	(a) Retained Placental Tissue	(b) Obstetric Laceration	(c) Bladder Fullness
1. Soaking pad every 10 min	X	X	X
2. Fundal deviation			X
3. Fundal tone		X	
4. Bright red blood		X	

1(a) **Retained placental tissue can prevent the uterus from contracting appropriately and the client can experience continued bleeding in spite of what feels like a firm fundus. If the provider had had time to inspect the placenta before being called away and found it intact, this would not be one of the considerations.**

1(b) **A firm fundus in spite of heavy bleeding suggests a source other than the uterus. The nurse must ask, "Where does this not make sense?" For this client, the delivery of a macrosomic baby in the posterior position with the use of forceps suggests an obstetric laceration is possible. This could be a cervical or vaginal wall laceration.**

1(c) **A full bladder can contribute to heavy bleeding by preventing the uterus from contracting efficiently, even though it may feel firm. Because of the epidural, the client is unable to sense how full her bladder has become, making it vital for the nurse to anticipate when the bladder is full.**

2(c) **A fundus that is deviated to the right suggests the bladder is full. None of the other options apply.**

3(b) **As noted in option 1(b), vaginal bleeding in spite of a firm fundus suggests the bleeding is from a cause other than fundal atony.**

4(b) **Persistent, *bright red* bleeding suggests an acute obstetric laceration. This is different from the characteristics of lochia, which is dark red and often will contain small clots. Lochia consists of blood, tissue, and mucus from inside the uterus, giving it the darker coloration.**

8-46 **Answers: 2 and c**
Unlike Sample Item 8-44, this question asks for nursing assessments *in order*.
The nurse should first address the client's **(select one):**

1. The fundus has remained firm, so this is not a priority assessment at this time. Something else is going on.
2. **Because a full bladder can contribute to excess blood loss, and a deviated fundus suggests a full bladder, this is the most obvious intervention the nurse should complete first.**

3. The amount of bleeding and its persistence is important to assess, but is not the first assessment to make.
4. The client's blood sugar does not need to be checked. This is a distractor. For this client, shakiness is not a threat to her life.

Followed by the client's **(select one)**:

a. As noted above, fundal checks are important. This might be the third assessment the nurse completes after the bleeding, just to confirm that it remains firm.
b. Bladder emptying should be the first thing the nurse addresses.
c. **Bleeding amounts after bladder emptying will confirm whether or not the uterus was impacted by a full bladder. This information will give further clues to the source of the bleeding.**
d. As noted above, the blood sugar is a distractor.

8-47 Answers: 1(a), 2(a), 3(a), 4(b), 5(a), 6(b), 7(a)

Potential Order	(a) Anticipated	(b) Nonessential
1. Prepare client for surgery	X	
2. Insert large-bore venous access device (VAD)	X	
3. Run additional intravenous fluids	X	
4. Administer additional uterotonics		X
5. Type and cross 2 units, PRBCs	X	
6. Perineal shave prep		X
7. NPO	X	

1(a) The nurse can anticipate that the client will need a surgical repair for the cervical laceration.

2(a) The nurse can anticipate an order for an additional VAD because of the cumulative blood loss and anticipated, ongoing blood loss that will continue until the repair is completed. The client's dropping blood pressure and rising pulse suggest that inserting a large-bore needle for blood transfusions and other hemodynamic resuscitation fluids, if needed, is a prudent decision.

3(a) The nurse can anticipate that additional intravenous fluids are necessary, given the dropping blood pressure and rising pulse rate.

4(b) Because the client's fundus has remained firm throughout the immediate postpartum phase, additional uterotonics are not essential. The excess bleeding is related to bleeding from a nonuterine site. Once the repair is completed, the client's bright red bleeding should be absent, although normal amounts of lochia will still be expected.

5(a) The nurse can anticipate an order to type and crossmatch at least 2 units of packed red blood cells (PRBCs) in case they are needed to stabilize the client's hemodynamic status during or after surgery. Note this is not an order for blood; it is an order to have the laboratory type and crossmatch blood for use when/if needed.

6(b) A perineal shave prep is not essential for an obstetric laceration repair, whether it is on the cervix or along the vaginal vault.

7(a) The nurse should anticipate giving the client nothing by mouth (NPO) once surgery seems inevitable, and certainly once the decision for surgery has been made. Although the procedure will likely be completed with epidural anesthesia while the client is awake, it is considered prudent to keep the client NPO until the procedure has been completed.

8-48 Answers: 2, 4, 5, & 6

1. It is the responsibility of the provider, not the nurse, to inform the client about surgery risks and benefits.
2. **After the client has discussed the procedure with the provider, the nurse may obtain the client's signature on the surgical permit.**
3. A perineal shave prep is not necessary for a cervical laceration repair.
4. **The nurse must confirm patency of the VADs, especially the one that was inserted at the start of the labor and may have become bent or infiltrated during the labor and birth.**

5. **The nurse must perform a medication reconciliation before moving the client to surgery.**
6. **The nurse must perform brief preoperative and postoperative teaching as the client's condition and urgency of the procedure allow. The test taker must answer the question with best practices in mind and not read anything into the stem such as a possible lack of time.**

8-49 Answers: 2 and 3

1. Perineal tenderness is expected after a forceps delivery. The nurse will make a careful assessment, but tenderness alone does not indicate abnormal progression of client condition.
2. **The client's unsteadiness is unexpected at this point. It could indicate symptomatic anemia or nerve issues related to the epidural.**
3. **The client's temperature is elevated. Her blood pressure is lower than before her hemorrhage, and her pulse is fairly rapid. This indicates that the client is not progressing as expected. These are new cues that direct the nurse to a new round of the six steps of clinical judgment to determine possible hypotheses related to these findings.**
4. Relief of cramping with ibuprofen is a positive report.
5. Discomfort at the epidural insertion site is not uncommon. The nurse will make a careful assessment to identify possible infection or bruising at the insertion site and notify the anesthesia provider if indicated, but tenderness alone does not indicate abnormal progression of client condition.

8-50 Answer: 3

1. The client is not experiencing hypoglycemia. The case study does not indicate she has diabetes. The test taker must not assume that the macrosomic infant is a "clue." Her shakiness is a distractor.
2. The client is ultimately at risk of infection, but there are no symptoms suggestive of infection at this time as given in the case study. Of the three response options, number three is the most likely condition.
3. **The client is experiencing a postpartum hemorrhage. Traditionally, a blood loss amount greater than 500 mL for a vaginal delivery was defined as a postpartum hemorrhage (PPH). In 2017, the American College of Obstetricians and Gynecologists revised that definition to define PPH as an amount of 1000 mL or more, in addition to symptoms of hypovolemia in the first 24 hours after the birth (Wormer et al., 2022). With this client's history of 450 mL blood loss at the birth and multiple saturated pads, she has no doubt lost nearly 1000 mL of blood already. This is why careful weighing of the pads by the nurse for quantitative blood loss tracking is essential for every delivery.**

   The client's risk factors for PPH as given in the case study include the oxytocin induction, fetal macrosomia (weight of more than 4000 grams), forceps use, and cervical laceration. The test taker will drag the answer "Postpartum hemorrhage" to the center box labeled "Condition most likely experiencing," as indicated in the diagram below.

8-51 Answers: 4, 5

1. The important cue in the case study is that the fundus is firm. As such, the oxytocin infusion does not need to be increased. As noted, the combination of firm fundus with continued bleeding suggests that the source of the hemorrhage is not from the uterus, but from some other cause. The client's risk factors suggest that an obstetric laceration could be the source of the bleeding.
2. The client's fundus is firm, so it does not need massage. In fact, continuous fundal massage can lead to uterine atony and more bleeding.
3. The client's shakiness is a distractor. Her shakiness is most likely a normal reaction that follows childbirth as a result of adrenaline and other hormones. She should be given nothing by mouth from this point on, in case she needs surgical intervention by the provider.
4. **The client's fundus was deviated to the right. This suggests that the bladder is full. Although the client's fundus is currently firm, a full bladder can reduce the ability of the fundus to *remain* firm, so the client's bladder should be emptied in order**

to maintain fundal tone. In addition, if she needs a surgical repair, the bladder should be empty to provide unimpeded visualization of the cervix for the provider. The test taker will drag the answer "Empty client's bladder" into one of the boxes on the left labeled "Action to take."

5. **A provider's examination is warranted STAT. Because the nurse cannot diagnose an obstetric laceration, a provider's examination is necessary. With the client's persistent blood loss and vital sign changes, the provider should be paged for a STAT bedside consultation. The test taker will drag the response, "Notify provider for STAT bedside consultation" to one of the boxes on the left, labeled "Action to take."**

8-52 Answers: 1, 4

1. **Vital signs must continue to be monitored to confirm the success of the interventions and/or to guide the addition of additional interventions to reduce morbidity and mortality. The test taker will drag the response "Vital signs" to the first box on the right.**
2. The blood sugar does not need to be monitored.
3. Once the bladder has been emptied, frequent assessment of urinary output is not a necessary assessment.
4. **The bleeding must continue to be monitored closely to provide the health-care team with information about appropriate interventions. The test taker will drag the response "Bleeding" to the second box on the right. The test taker will note that unlike knowledge assessment questions, this question does not include all the parameters to monitor, since it is not a teaching method in this case. For example, ongoing fundal checks are also important parameters to assess, but they are not included in the options for this question.**

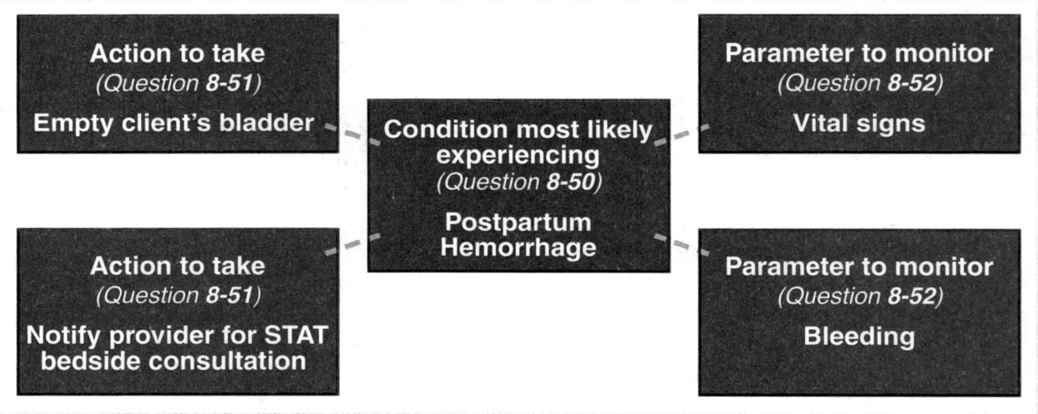

9 Computer Applications in Education and Evaluation

We are members of an informational society in which information is created, stored, retrieved, manipulated, and communicated. Exploding knowledge and technology, emerging health-care reform initiatives, and the intensified and diversified role of the nurse all add to the complexity of functioning within this informational society. To process information effectively and economically, computers are essential. They have become a reality in every aspect of our world and are used in private homes, educational settings, industry, and health-care facilities. To prepare for a career in nursing, you must have the basic skills to use computers in a comfortable manner and be a willing learner to keep pace with rapidly advancing computer technology. Although computers are used in the practice of nursing, this chapter focuses on the use of computers only in relation to education and evaluation.

Computing across the curriculum is not new in the educational setting. Educators immediately identified the potential of interactive participation to facilitate learning. Programmed-instruction textbooks were the predecessors of computer programs. These textbooks presented information within blocked narrative material. Each grouping of material was called a *frame*. Each frame required a response from the learner before moving on to the next narrative frame. These textbooks required active involvement by the learner. Computers make this programmed approach more interactive by increasing the potential, richness, and variety of frame styles, which has improved the effectiveness of the lesson. Computers also use graphics, color, and sound to facilitate learning in a way that programmed-instruction textbooks were unable to do because of the limitations of the written format.

Students generally enjoy using the computer to facilitate learning because programs hold their attention, provide immediate feedback, and never become impatient. Also, they are accessible, challenging, and fun. Computer-based instruction is not designed to replace the more traditional forms of teaching in most settings, but to augment them. Computers allow you to review difficult material at your own rate, increase critical thinking, experience simulated clinical situations, and assess your knowledge and judgment. The greatest advantage of computer-based instruction is that you become an active participant, not just a passive spectator.

To be an active participant, you should have a simple understanding of a few essential keyboard keys. Most programs are "user-friendly" and include on-screen instructions, help menus, and/or tutorials. Generally, students do not have difficulty manipulating the keyboard or mouse. However, some students have "computer anxiety." Only exposure to computers in a secure and positive learning environment can lessen computer anxiety and promote computer literacy.

The computer can enhance student learning by accessing professional resources, managing information, teaching, simulating clinical situations, and evaluating knowledge. Examples of how computers can be used in education and evaluation follow.

THE COMPUTER AS A RESOURCE TOOL

The computer is a resource tool that can be used to obtain information for academic assignments. A computerized literature search that uses national databases or networks can provide rapid access to current literature in nursing and its related fields. A modem (a device that allows transmission of data between computers over a telephone or cable line) connects you to the information retrieval system, and specific protocols may be required to gain entry to a database. These searches can be conducted in most libraries with the assistance of the research librarian. However, cost may be a factor because lines must be maintained to transmit and receive information. Most systems also have online connect charges for accessing the database as well as for the length of time the database is being used, and a fee may be charged for online or off-line printing. However, many college and hospital libraries pay this fee and students may access the information at no cost. Online printing provides an immediate hard copy of the desired information, whereas off-line printing provides a hard copy that is sent by mail at a later date. If the library does not have a subscription to a specific journal the student is interested in, the student can pay a fee to obtain the information. Sometimes, however, the fees incurred are beyond the financial means of the average student. It is prudent to find other sources, instead. Literature searches on the computer save time and energy. Therefore, you must decide whether these activities are cost-effective for you by measuring the time saved against the money spent.

THE COMPUTER AS AN INFORMATION MANAGER

The computer has revolutionized the way in which information is managed, not only outside the home but also inside the home. Many people now compose written material immediately on the computer. This is possible because you no longer need to have strong keyboard skills or expend extensive time and energy to learn how to use software programs. Today, user-friendly software programs have on-screen commands and effective help menus. Touch, a stylus, or a mouse also facilitate computer use. The personal computer can be used for word processing, spreadsheets, data processing, creating graphs of data, and so on. You can now manipulate data, words, and images to complete your academic assignments with ease.

THE COMPUTER AS AN INSTRUCTOR

Computer-assisted instruction (CAI) is an excellent addition to the repertoire of strategies available to educators and nursing students to facilitate the learning process. In CAI, information is communicated from the computer to the learner without direct interaction with the teacher. These instructional delivery systems can present principles and theory, enhance comprehension, promote creative problem solving, and provide immediate feedback to enrich independent learning.

Some computer programs display information in a textual format that requires limited interaction between you and the computer. These programs really function as an automated textbook. Other tutorial approaches present new information in small steps or frames and then require you to respond to demonstrate your comprehension of the material just delivered. Such programs function as an automated programmed-instruction textbook. These types of programs generally use a linear format that proceeds from the beginning of the program to the end of the program without deviation. They present information in a straight line, with one beginning and one end, and every student is exposed to the same information. Although valuable, these programs do not recognize the learner as an individual with specific needs, interests, and abilities.

Interactive videodisc instruction (IVD, IVI), a sophisticated form of CAI, uses computer technology to enrich the clinical situation presented. Programs that use a branching format allow you to select a path that focuses on information relevant to your ability and interest, as well as encourage the highest degree of interaction between you and the computer. Studies have demonstrated that there is a highly significant degree of student satisfaction with IVD instruction and that a positive mental attitude is significant to the learning process because of its influence on student motivation, learning rate, and retention and application of information.

THE COMPUTER AS A TOOL FOR DISTANCE EDUCATION

Computers and the technology that affects their use are revolutionizing existing parameters about what is a teaching/learning environment. The age of the Internet has enabled a shift from the typical classroom setting to distance learning/education via the Internet/World Wide Web.

Distance education, also known as *distributed learning*, *e-learning*, *online learning*, and *virtual classroom*, has created communities of learning that maximize communication between and among students and faculty. Many colleges and universities offer distance education courses to meet the needs of students who have part-time or full-time jobs, family responsibilities, or study-time constraints or who are geographically isolated. Originally, distance education involved print materials; instruction via audio or video cassettes; and communication via telephone, voice mail, and faxing. Today, technological advances, including fixed computer media (e.g., CD-ROM), room-based video conferencing (e.g., interactive television), desktop video conferencing, and the World Wide Web (e.g., Internet-based programming), provide multimedia methods of instruction that many students find more challenging and interesting than the traditional text-based materials. These new methods of delivery promote learning in the cognitive (thinking), affective (feeling), and psychomotor (skills) domains inherent in nursing practice, which is an intellectually challenging and social, behavioral, and practice-oriented profession. During the COVID-19 pandemic, the use of computer simulation to replace some of the in-patient clinical experiences for nursing students became more widely used and approved, out of necessity, by state boards of nursing. Understanding that simulations do not provide real-time multitasking required of nurses, many hospitals provided longer orientation times for newly graduated nurses in their first year of employment.

Distance education has both advantages and disadvantages and requires a special type of learner.

Advantages of distance education include the following:

- Accessibility to education for those who are geographically isolated
- Opportunities for learning within a flexible time frame
- Individualized pace of learning
- Active participation
- Self-motivation
- Development of computer literacy

Disadvantages of distance education include the following:

- Lack of face-to-face communication
- Sense of isolation
- Difficulty with course content in the affective (feelings) and psychomotor (skills) learning domains
- Inability to adjust to innovative teaching/evaluation strategies
- Pressure to master the technology

Students who participate successfully in distance education are:

- Risk takers
- Assertive
- Self-directed
- Responsible

The computer as a tool for distance education has unlimited potential and has already revolutionized higher education. Distance education, particularly in the nursing curriculum, is gaining momentum and acceptance. Important questions still exist regarding student financial aid, confidentiality, source of finances for infrastructure, availability of qualified nursing faculty, transferability of credit, delivery of academic support services, appropriate/effective clinical experiences, and valid and reliable methods of evaluation. These concerns have legal and ethical implications that must be addressed for distance education to continue to be a viable alternative for students who want to become nurses. Only the future will tell whether computers in relation to distance education will increase the number of graduate nurses and help reverse the nursing shortage.

THE COMPUTER AS A SIMULATOR

The role of the nursing educator is to assist you in moving beyond the mere memorization of facts to the application of information in clinical situations. To do this, you must use critical thinking to integrate information into a meaningful frame of reference. Computer simulations are designed to enhance your ability to use critical thinking and safely make sound clinical judgments in a fabricated situation. These simulation programs provide a supportive environment in which to practice procedures, because they usually produce less anxiety than caring for a client in a clinical setting. Also, a student can learn from mistakes without compromising the safety of a client. Although computer simulation has long been used in aeronautics and flight training, it is in its adolescence in simulating experiences within the health-care professions.

Nursing simulations may present a client database that requires you to input, sort, and retrieve data. Simulations may focus on the application of information processing skills, which assist you in selecting appropriate sources of data, classifying data, clustering and sequencing data, and even evaluating data. Simulations may focus on components of critical thinking. A program addressing critical thinking may require you to identify relationships, recognize commonalities and differences, and use deductive and inductive reasoning to support inferences. Simulations also may be designed to improve decision making by requiring you to identify the nature of a problem, choose a course of action from multiple options, establish priorities, and evaluate the outcome of the final decision.

These simulations are maximized by the use of simulator manikins that can be programmed to reflect human responses. Manikins have been used in nursing education since 1911, when a simple manikin called *Mrs. Chase* was introduced. Mrs. Chase manikins are still used today to practice basic fundamental nursing skills. In 1960, Resusci Anne (simulator) was developed to teach, practice, and evaluate the performance of cardiopulmonary resuscitation (CPR). Numerous forms now available include adult, child, and infant manikins. Resuscitation manikins are more advanced than the Mrs. Chase manikin but are not as advanced as high-fidelity integrated manikins. SimMan computerized manikins were not routinely used in nursing education until approximately 2009. At that time, they became more affordable, and the National Council of State Boards of Nursing issued a position paper that advocated the inclusion of innovative teaching strategies in nursing education. The computer within the manikin was preprogrammed and/or faculty could program the manikin to produce human responses, such as palpable pulses; normal and abnormal heart, lung, and bowel sounds; the chest rising and falling; blinking eyes; changing pupillary accommodation; and speaking. Preprogrammed scenarios were available that allowed students to practice simulated experiences in preparation for clinical experiences or evaluations on the simulator.

The original simulation manikins were obsolete within several years and were replaced by more sophisticated simulation manikins that can present complex clinical situations that are difficult to present in a classroom setting or events that a student may not have had the opportunity to experience in the clinical setting. Curricula cannot guarantee that every student will have an opportunity to experience each and every situation that may be important to learning. However, computer simulations help to fill this void.

THE COMPUTER AS AN EVALUATOR

Evaluation (test-taking) programs are designed to measure your knowledge, skills, and abilities in relation to the practice of nursing. They can be self-administered or administered by a person in authority. Programs devised to be self-administered generally contain both a learning mode and a self-evaluation mode.

In the learning mode, you are presented with a question and are asked to select the correct answer. After you select an option, the program provides immediate feedback regarding the correctness of the choice. Rationales for the correct and wrong answers may be provided, depending on how the program is designed. The learning mode that provides rationales for all the choices has the potential to promote new learning or reinforce previous learning. These types of programs are a form of CAI.

The evaluation mode enables you to conduct an assessment of your test-taking abilities regarding a specific body of knowledge addressed in the program. The evaluation mode also allows you to experience a testing situation. Some programs provide rationales for all the options at the completion of the program. Other, more detailed programs allow you to design self-tests according to specific parameters (e.g., number of questions, clinical specialty, and parameters reflective of the NCLEX® test plan, nursing process, client need, and cognitive level). Also, programs may supply an individualized analysis of your performance after you take a test. This analysis may include information on the questions you got wrong with rationales, the content areas that you need to study further, your performance in relation to that of other nursing students, or predictions for passing future examinations. Self-administered evaluation programs are particularly successful because they focus on competency and provide immediate feedback.

An evaluation program conducted by a person in authority may be administered to assess your ability to pass a course of study or to demonstrate your competency for certification or licensure. These programs use computer technology and replace paper-and-pencil tests. Some programs use question and answer testing formats, and others use simulator manikins. Computer programs that present questions that require the test taker to select an answer are used to evaluate the competency of a nursing student. Some programs may use a format in which you and every other test taker are confronted with the exact same questions. Other programs may use **computerized-adaptive testing** (CAT), a unique format in which your examination is assembled interactively as you answer each question. This is the format used in the NCLEX® licensing examination. In a typical CAT format, all the questions in the test bank have a calculated level of difficulty. You are presented with a question. If you answer the question correctly, you are presented with a slightly more difficult question. If you answer that question incorrectly, you are presented with a slightly easier question. This process is repeated for each question until a pass-or-fail decision is determined statistically by the computer. Passing depends on your demonstration of knowledge, skills, and abilities in relation to a standard of acceptable performance. The advantages of the CAT format are that it individualizes each test, provides for self-paced testing, and produces greater measurement precision. In addition, test takers who answer a high number of the more difficult questions correctly are presented with fewer questions, reducing the amount of time needed to complete the test. The disadvantages of the CAT format are that you cannot review the entire test before starting, you cannot skip difficult questions and return to them at a later time, and you cannot go back and change an answer once it has been selected and entered. However, the questions presented in the new, Next Generation NCLEX® (NGN) format will allow for partial credit scoring when several responses are required (see the Summer 2021 Issue of *Next Generation NCLEX News* for more information at https://www.ncsbn.org/ngn-resources.htm).

Simulator manikins often are used by faculty to evaluate a nursing student's ability to perform specific skills, assess a client, and/or use clinical judgment in a simulated scenario. Evaluations using a simulator manikin can be a stressful experience. Therefore, students should take every opportunity to use these simulator manikins to advance their knowledge, "clinical experience," and ability to think critically when making clinical judgments.

In 1994 the NCLEX-RN® and the NCLEX-PN®, the licensure examinations for registered nurses and practical nurses, respectively, changed from standard paper-and-pencil tests to examinations using CAT. Although no previous computer experience is necessary to take a test using CAT, it is always better to be familiar with the particular testing format used. Many commercial products that use the CAT format are available on the Internet. Practice can only improve your performance on future CAT examinations.

SUMMARY

Computers are causing major changes in the traditional ways health-care education and evaluation are provided. In our information-savvy society, some certainties exist: We are on information overload; the manipulation of information has become more sophisticated than ever before; and computers will be used more extensively in nursing education, evaluation, and practice in the future. You must become computer literate and be willing to learn about new computer technology as it emerges. The most important implication of computer applications in learning, practice, and evaluation is that you can use the computer and simulator manikins to increase the efficiency of your work and study, thereby leaving more time to interact with instructors, peers, and clients.

Analyze Your Test Performance

10

Students work hard at studying course content and learning and using test-taking strategies. However, they seldom progress to the important step of analyzing their test performance to determine their knowledge and information-processing strengths and needs. When reviewing a wrong answer, usually you are able to identify when you did not know the principles being tested. However, without a performance analysis, you may not identify any trends in your knowledge gaps because you are lacking the "big picture." In addition, errors occur more often because of inept information processing than because of lack of knowledge. When reviewing an examination, you might say, "What a silly mistake. I knew that content." This suggests that you probably made an information-processing error. Unless you identify your knowledge gaps and information-processing errors and take corrective action, you probably will continue to make the same mistakes over and over.

Students frequently do not review their test performance because they believe it is time-consuming, or they feel traumatized by their bad score and want to forget about it, or they review their test performance in a haphazard, rather than a systematic, manner. A methodical analysis of your test performance is well worth the time and effort. It does take time because you have to stop and think critically about each item you answered incorrectly. However, ***you must spend time to save time.*** When you focus your study, you will study "better," not longer or harder. Also, an analysis of your test performance should identify your information-processing errors. When you are aware of these errors, you can correct them, which should improve your test-taking abilities and ultimately your test grades.

You may find it threatening to analyze your test performance because it requires you to admit that you may be doing something wrong or that you are unprepared in some manner. This kind of negative thinking will not promote your success. Finding fault is not the focus of a performance review. We all make mistakes. If we were perfect, we would not be human. The important point is that you must learn from your mistakes in order to improve. This will be true in your future professional environment, as well. If you are having difficulty with controlling negative thoughts, review Chapter 1, "Empowerment." Your goal is to improve your test performance. Identifying your knowledge deficits and information-processing errors should provide a focus for corrective action. This places you in a position of control, which is essential if you are to be successful.

In this chapter, two tools are presented to analyze questions that you answered incorrectly. The first tool, **Information-Processing Analysis,** focuses on the "process" of test taking. This tool has two parts: Processing Errors and Personal Performance Trends. It discloses processing errors in relation to the stem of a question and the options in a question. It also addresses trends in your personal performance in relation to time management, concentration, empowerment, decisiveness/indecisiveness, and clusters of errors. It includes a section for you to make notes about your reactions or questions that you may want to explore with your instructor. The second tool, **Knowledge Analysis,** focuses on the "content" aspect of a test. It may identify clusters of errors in specific knowledge categories as well as errors in the steps of the nursing process.

This chapter also contains corrective action guides that address each tool. These guides discuss how to correct your identified errors in the "Analysis" tools and direct you to sections in the text that will help you avoid these errors in the future.

INFORMATION-PROCESSING ANALYSIS TOOL

The Information-Processing Analysis Tool has two parts: Processing Errors and Personal Performance Trends. Processing Errors focus on mistakes in scrutinizing a question when selecting a final answer. Personal Performance Trends focus on the personal tendencies that affect your test performance.

Information-Processing Analysis Tool

Processing Errors	Question Number	Total
STEM		
Missed word indicating negative polarity		
Missed word that set a priority		
Missed key words that direct attention to content		
Misinterpreted information presented		
Missed the central point/theme		
Missed the central person		
Read into the question		
Missed the step in the nursing process (NP)		
Incompletely analyzed the stem; read it too quickly		
Did not understand what the question was asking		
Did not know or did not remember the content associated with the question		
OPTIONS		
Answered quickly without reading all the options		
Failed to respond to negative polarity in the stem		
Misidentified the priority		
Misinterpreted information		
Read into the option		
Did not know or did not remember the content		
Knew content but inaccurately applied concepts and principles		
Knew the right answer but recorded it inaccurately		

Personal Performance Trends	Comments
1. I finished the examination with time to review. YES { } NO { }	
2. I was able to focus with little distraction. YES { } NO { }	
3. I felt calm and in control. YES { } NO { }	
4. When I changed answers, I got more questions right rather than wrong. YES { } NO { }	
5. Identify error clusters: a. First third of examination { } b. Middle third of examination { } c. Last third of examination { } d. "Runs" of errors { } e. No clusters identified { }	

Complete the Processing Errors portion of the Information-Processing Analysis Tool in the following way:

- Review a question you got wrong, and determine which processing error caused you to answer the question incorrectly.
- Place the number of the question in the first box to the right of the identified processing error on the tool.
- If you cannot decide between two processing errors or more than one error was involved, put the number of the question next to more than one processing error.
- When another question you got wrong has the same processing error, place the number of the subsequent question in the box to the right of the number of the previous question.
- Insert the number of every question you got wrong on the examination into the Processing Errors portion of the Information-Processing Tool.
- Tally the total number of answers you got wrong for each processing error in the last column on the right. Students often notice a clustering of errors in one area or another.

You can individualize this tool to reflect your specific processing error. For example, if you find that you frequently got questions wrong because you "Read into the question," you can subdivide this area into "Added information from my own mind" and/or "Made assumptions."

Complete the Personal Performance Trends portion of the Information-Processing Analysis Tool in the following way:

- Answer questions 1, 2, 3, and 4. Identify your answer as either YES or NO by placing a mark in the brackets accompanying each question.
- Divide the number of questions in the test by 3 to determine how many questions are in the first, middle, and last thirds of the test.
- Count the number of questions you got wrong in the first third of the examination and enter that number in the brackets next to 5.a. Do the same for 5.b. and 5.c.
- Look at the questions you got wrong, and identify whether two or more occurred in a row or whether three or more occurred in close proximity. Enter the number of "runs" you identify in the brackets next to 5.d.
- If no error clusters are identified, place a mark in the brackets next to 5.e.
- In the Comments column of the Personal Performance Trends portion of this tool, add your own analysis regarding your performance in relation to these questions.

CORRECTIVE ACTION GUIDE FOR THE INFORMATION-PROCESSING ANALYSIS TOOL

The Corrective Action Guide for the Information-Processing Analysis Tool has two parts: one that addresses Processing Errors and another that addresses Personal Performance Trends. Both of these mirror what is in the Information-Processing Analysis Tool. Before you can use the Corrective Action Guide, you have to first assess your performance on an examination and insert the questions you answered incorrectly and answer the questions in the Personal Performance section of the Information-Processing Analysis Tool. Now you can investigate how to improve your examination performance.

Corrective Action Guide for Processing Errors in the Information-Processing Analysis Tool

The Corrective Action Guide for Processing Errors has three columns:

- Column 1 lists Processing Errors, which are identical to the Processing Errors in column 1 of the Information-Processing Analysis Tool.
- Column 2 refers you to the chapters and sections in this textbook that address information related to the Processing Errors listed in column 1.
- Column 3 indicates the pages where you can find the information listed in column 2.

This portion of the guide directs you to information that you can review to correct your information-processing problems. For example, if you have multiple "Xs" in the row related to "Missed word that set a priority," you should review the information in the section titled "Identify the Word in the Stem That Sets a Priority," which is included in Chapter 7, "Test-Taking Techniques." Review the sections in the book included in column 2 for every processing error that you identify that relates to your performance.

The Processing Errors section of the guide directs you to information that you can review to enhance your scrutiny of the stem of a question and explore the options presented to arrive at the correct answer.

Corrective Action Guide for Processing Errors in the Information-Processing Analysis Tool

Processing Errors	Review the Following Sections	Page Number
STEM		
Missed word that indicates negative polarity	**Chapter 7** Test-Taking Techniques (Identify the Word in the Stem That Indicates Negative Polarity)	100
Missed word that set a priority	**Chapter 7** Test-Taking Techniques (Identify the Word in the Stem That Sets a Priority)	102
Missed key words that direct attention to content	**Chapter 7** Test-Taking Techniques (Identify Key Words in the Stem That Direct Attention to Content)	103
Misinterpreted information presented	**Chapter 2** Critical Thinking (Practice Critical Thinking and Apply Critical Thinking to Multiple-Choice Questions)	15 15
	Chapter 8 Testing Formats Other Than Multiple-Choice Questions (Clinical Judgment Question Formats Reflective of Next Generation NCLEX)	147
Missed the central point/theme	**Chapter 2** Critical Thinking (Practice Critical Thinking and Apply Critical Thinking to Multiple-Choice Questions)	15 15
Missed the central person	**Chapter 7** Test-Taking Techniques (Identify the Central Person in the Question)	104
Read into the question	**Chapter 7** Test-Taking Techniques (Avoid Reading Into the Question)	98
	Chapter 2 Critical Thinking (Avoid Reading Into the Question)	16
Missed the step in the nursing process (NP)	**Chapter 6** The Nursing Process (Focus on the step of the nursing process that you misidentified in the knowledge analysis tool)	72
Incompletely analyzed the stem; read it too quickly	**Chapter 7** Test-Taking Techniques (Avoid Reading Into the Question and Identify Key Words in the Stem That Direct Attention to Content)	98 103
	Chapter 2 Critical Thinking (Apply Critical Thinking to Multiple-Choice Questions)	15

Corrective Action Guide for Processing Errors in the Information-Processing Analysis Tool—cont'd

Processing Errors	Review the Following Sections	Page Number
Did not understand what the question was asking	**Chapter 7** Test-Taking Techniques (Identify Key Words in the Stem That Direct Attention to Content and Avoid Reading Into the Question)	103 98
	Chapter 2 Critical Thinking (Practice Critical Thinking and Apply Critical Thinking to Multiple-Choice Questions)	13 15
	Chapter 8 Testing Formats Other Than Multiple-Choice Questions (Clinical Judgment Question Formats Reflective of Next Generation NCLEX)	147
	Chapter 11 Practice Questions With Answers and Rationales (Study answers and rationales for practice questions related to content in the questions you got wrong)	187
Did not know or did not remember the content associated with the question	**Chapter 4** Study Techniques (Specific Study Techniques Related to Cognitive Levels of Nursing Questions)	41
	Chapter 8 Testing Formats Other Than Multiple-Choice Questions (Clinical Judgment Question Formats Reflective of Next Generation NCLEX)	147
	Chapter 11 Practice Questions With Answers and Rationales (Study answers and rationales of practice questions)	187
OPTIONS		
Answered quickly without reading all the options	**Chapter 7** Test-Taking Techniques (Avoid Reading Into the Question)	98
Failed to respond to negative polarity in the stem	**Chapter 7** Test-Taking Techniques (Identify the Word in the Stem That Indicates Negative Polarity)	100
Misidentified the priority	**Chapter 7** Test-Taking Techniques (Identify the Word in the Stem That Sets a Priority)	102
	Chapter 11 Practice Questions With Answers and Rationales (Study answers and rationales for practice questions related to content in the questions you got wrong)	187
Misinterpreted information	**Chapter 2** Critical Thinking (Practice Critical Thinking and Apply Critical Thinking to Multiple-Choice Questions)	13 15
	Chapter 8 Testing Formats Other Than Multiple-Choice Questions (Clinical Judgment Question Formats Reflective of Next Generation NCLEX)	147
Read into the options	**Chapter 7** Test-Taking Techniques (Avoid Reading Into the Question)	98
	Chapter 2 Critical Thinking (Avoid Reading Into the Question)	16

Continued

Corrective Action Guide for Processing Errors in the Information-Processing Analysis Tool—cont'd

Processing Errors	Review the Following Sections	Page Number
Did not know or did not remember the content	**Chapter 4** Study Techniques (Specific Study Techniques Related to Cognitive Levels of Nursing Questions)	41
	Chapter 8 Testing Formats Other Than Multiple-Choice Questions (Clinical Judgment Question Formats Reflective of Next Generation NCLEX)	147
	Chapter 11 Practice Questions With Answers and Rationales (Study answers and rationales for practice questions related to content in the questions you got wrong)	187
Knew content but inaccurately applied concepts and principles	**Chapter 2** Critical Thinking (Apply Critical Thinking to Multiple-Choice Questions)	15
	Chapter 8 Testing Formats Other Than Multiple-Choice Questions (Clinical Judgment Question Formats Reflective of Next Generation NCLEX)	147
	Chapter 11 Practice Questions With Answers and Rationales (Study answers and rationales for practice questions related to content in the questions you got wrong)	187

Personal Performance Trends	Comments
1. I finished the examination with time to review. YES { } NO { }	
2. I was able to focus with little distraction. YES { } NO { }	
3. I felt calm and in control. YES { } NO { }	
4. When I changed answers, I got more questions right rather than wrong. YES { } NO { }	
5. Identify error clusters: a. First third of examination { } b. Middle third of examination { } c. Last third of examination { } d. "Runs" of errors { } e. No clusters identified { }	

Corrective Action Guide for Personal Performance Trends in the Information-Processing Analysis Tool

The Correct Action Guide for Personal Performance Trends provides a global perspective of your functioning throughout the examination rather than your performance on specific test items. After you have completed the Personal Performance Trends portion of the Information-Processing Analysis Tool, investigate your results with the corrective actions suggested here.

This section of the guide includes issues such as the following:

- Time management. (I finished the examination with time to review.)
- Concentration. (I was able to focus with little distraction.)

- Empowerment. (I felt calm and in control.)
- Decisiveness/indecisiveness. (When I changed answers, I got the questions right rather than wrong.)
- Error clusters. (I had no error clusters; I had error clusters in the first, middle, or last third of an examination or "runs" of error clusters.)

This portion of the guide focuses on issues that can promote or hinder your performance on an examination. Each Personal Performance Trend statement is accompanied by the following:

- Comments that specifically relate to the trend being discussed
- Questions you must ask yourself if you answered NO to statements 1 through 4 or if you identified error clusters in statement 5
- A **REVIEW** that refers you to content in the book that explores information related to the Personal Performance Trend being discussed

1. I finished the examination with time to review.

If your answer was YES, you have managed your time well. If your answer was NO, you are not managing your time effectively, and you need to identify why you are taking too long to proceed through the examination. You must answer the following questions:

- Am I taking too much time to answer each question?
- Am I getting bogged down and spending too much time on a few difficult questions that prevent me from finishing or reviewing the examination?
- (Other) Identify your own questions.

REVIEW

Chapter 7, "Test-Taking Techniques," "Manage the Allotted Time to Your Advantage," page 97.

Chapter 7, "Test-Taking Techniques," "Concentrate on the Simple Before the Complex," page 97.

2. I was able to focus with little distraction.

If your answer was YES, you have sufficient concentration and the ability to block out distractions. If your answer was NO, you must answer the following questions:

- Am I fatigued before and/or during examinations?
- Do distractions in the environment cause me to lose focus?
- Am I physically uncomfortable during examinations?
- (Other) Identify your own questions.

REVIEW

Chapter 1, "Empowerment," "Establish Control Before and During the Test," page 6.

3. I felt calm and in control.

If your answer was YES, you have anxiety under control and were able to focus on the examination rather than having to cope with anxious responses. If your answer was NO, you must answer the following questions:

- Do I experience uncomfortable, fearful responses during examinations?
- Do I experience internal mental stressors (negative self-talk) that block my confidence?
- Do I get flustered when confronted with a question that I am unable to answer?
- (Other) Identify your own questions.

REVIEW

Chapter 1, "Empowerment," "Develop a Positive Mental Attitude," page 6.

Chapter 7, "Test-Taking Techniques," "Maintain a Positive Mental Attitude," page 99.

4. When I changed answers, I got more right rather than wrong.

Some examinations, especially those taken on a computer, do not permit a review of previously answered questions. However, others allocate time for a short review at the end of the examination. During review of your answers at the end of an examination, you may be tempted to change your original answer to another option that you now believe is the correct answer. It is important for you to know whether you are changing correct answers to wrong answers or wrong answers to correct answers when reviewing questions. If you answered YES to the question "When I changed answers, I got more questions right rather than wrong," you are able to change answers on the basis of careful review of the stem and options. If you answered NO to the question, you must ask yourself the following questions:

- What causes me to change my answers?
- Do I lack confidence when I answer a question?
- Why do I keep changing answers when I know I always change correct answers to wrong answers?
- (Other) Identify your own questions.

Analyze whether changing answers works to your advantage. Every time you review an examination, evaluate your accuracy in changing answers. Keep score of how many answers you changed from wrong to right and how many you changed from right to wrong.

If the number of items you changed from wrong to right is greater than the number of items you changed from right to wrong, it is probably to your advantage to change answers you ultimately believe you answered incorrectly. Subsequent questions may have contained content that was helpful in answering a previous question, you may have accessed information you did not remember originally, or you may be better able to assess the question with more objectivity at the end of the examination, when you personally feel less pressure to finish.

If the number of items you changed from right to wrong is greater than the number of items you changed from wrong to right, you should avoid changing your answers unless you are absolutely positive that your second choice is the correct answer. As the end of an examination approaches, some people tend to experience more anxiety, not less, which interferes with perception and the processing of information. If you tend to change answers to the wrong options, leave your "eraser" home or sit on your hands so that you do not change the answers!

When considering changing an answer to a previously answered question, use test-taking techniques to increase your ability to focus on what the question is asking and eliminate distractors. A careful review may dissect the question into its component parts, thereby revealing a key word or clue that assists you in reconsidering your previous answer.

REVIEW

Chapter 7, "Test-Taking Techniques," page 95.

Chapter 8, "Testing Formats Other Than Multiple-Choice Questions," page 123.

Chapter 11, "Practice Questions With Answers and Rationales" (Most questions contain test-taking tips), page 187.

5. Identify error clusters.

The purpose of identifying error clusters is to determine whether anxiety or fatigue is affecting your performance. If you identify a group of errors at the beginning, middle, or end of an examination or you identify "runs" of incorrect answers (two or more incorrect answers in a row or three or more in close proximity), you need to analyze what is happening. You must ask yourself the following questions:

- Do I get anxious before or during an examination?
- Do I get tired?
- Do I get flustered when confronted with a difficult question?
- Do I lose my ability to concentrate?
- (Other) Identify your own questions.

REVIEW

Errors that occur in the first third of an examination: If your errors occur in the beginning of an examination, you may want to use techniques that allow you to control the testing environment or use anxiety reduction techniques just before the examination begins to feel more in control and therefore less anxious.

Chapter 1, "Empowerment," "Establish Control Before and During the Test," page 6.

Chapter 1, "Empowerment," "Develop a Positive Mental Attitude," page 1.

Errors that occur in the middle third of an examination or in clusters throughout an examination: If you find that errors occur in the middle third of the examination or runs of error clusters occur after every 20 or 30 questions, you may need to reduce tension and anxiety. We counseled a graduate nurse who did not pass the National Council Licensure Examination for Registered Nurses (NCLEX-RN®) after two attempts. When assessing her performance on a practice examination, we identified that every 30 minutes she made four or five errors in a row. We encouraged her to take a break every 25 minutes until she completed the examination. On her next attempt, she passed the NCLEX-RN®. A break every 25 minutes was the key change in her approach to the NCLEX-RN®. In the classroom setting, this may be impossible; therefore, you should engage in a relaxation technique that works for you for 2 or 3 minutes. In addition, you can visualize a person who supports you emotionally standing beside you and giving you encouragement during the examination or use positive self-talk by saying, "I can do this" or "I studied hard for this examination."

Remember, relaxation techniques must be practiced to be effective and should be conducted in a simulated testing situation before a real testing situation. Understand that if you implement relaxation techniques during a test, you must adjust the time you allot for each question and for your review.

REVIEW

Chapter 1, "Empowerment," "Challenge Negative Thoughts," page 2.

Chapter 1, "Empowerment," "Use Diaphragmatic Breathing," page 2.

Chapter 1, "Empowerment," "Perform Muscle Relaxation," page 4.

Chapter 1, "Empowerment," "Use Imagery," page 5.

Errors that occur in the last third of an examination: If you find that the majority of your errors occur during the last third of an examination, you may need to increase your test-taking stamina by practicing for longer periods of time. Stamina also can be increased by practicing test taking in a simulated testing environment.

REVIEW

Chapter 1, "Empowerment," "Exercise Regularly," page 6.

Chapter 4, "Study Techniques," "Simulate a Testing Environment," page 38.

Chapter 4, "Study Techniques," "Practice Test Taking," page 48.

KNOWLEDGE ANALYSIS TOOL

The Knowledge Analysis Tool has two parts: Knowledge Categories and Nursing Process. Knowledge categories include the range of basic information that is the foundation of nursing practice. The Nursing Process section of the tool includes the steps of the nursing process: assessment, analysis, planning, implementation, and evaluation. The nursing process provides a systematic approach to the delivery of nursing care.

Knowledge Analysis Tool

Knowledge Categories	Question Number	Total
Legal/ethical issues		
Health-care delivery systems		
Basic human needs		
Growth and development		
Communication		
Diversity, spirituality/religion		
Emotional needs		
Physical assessment		
Physical safety		
Mobility		
Hygiene		
Pain and comfort		
Rest and sleep		
Nutrition		
Fluid and electrolytes		
Urinary elimination		
Bowel elimination		
Oxygen		
Microbiological safety		
Administration of medications		
Pharmacology		
Perioperative		
Community setting		
Pathophysiology		
Anatomy and physiology		
Computations		
NURSING PROCESS		
Assessment		
Analysis		
Planning		
Implementation		
Evaluation		
CLINICAL JUDGMENT PROCESS		
Recognize cues		
Analyze cues		
Prioritize hypotheses		
Generate solutions		
Take action		
Evaluate outcomes		

Complete the Knowledge Categories portion of the Knowledge Analysis Tool in the following way:

- Review a question you got wrong, and determine which knowledge category best represents the content being tested in the question.
- Place the number of the question in the first box to the right of the identified knowledge category on the tool.
- If you cannot decide between two knowledge categories, put the number of the question next to more than one knowledge category.
- When another question you got wrong has the same knowledge category, place the number of the subsequent question in the box to the right of the previous question.
- Insert the number of every question you got wrong on the test into the Knowledge Categories portion of the Knowledge Analysis Tool.
- Tally the total number of answers you got wrong for each knowledge category in the last column on the right. Students often notice a clustering of errors in one or more categories.

If you find that you got many questions wrong in one of the categories, you may identify subdivisions to the category. For example, if you got many questions wrong in the area of perioperative nursing, which includes the time frame before, during, and after surgery, you could subdivide this area into "Preoperative," "Intraoperative," and "Postoperative."

Complete the Nursing Process portion of the Knowledge Analysis Tool in the following way:

- Review a question you got wrong, and determine which step of the nursing process best represents the content being tested in the question. Identify just one step of the nursing process for each question you got wrong.
- Place the number of the question in the first box to the right of the step in the nursing process you identified.
- When another question you got wrong reflects the same step of the nursing process, place the number of the subsequent question in the box to the right of the previous question.
- Insert the number of every question you got wrong on the examination into the Nursing Process portion of the Knowledge Analysis Tool.
- Tally the total number of answers you got wrong for each step of the nursing process in the last column on the right. Students often will notice a clustering of errors in one or two steps of the nursing process.

Complete the Clinical Judgment portion of the Knowledge Analysis Tool in the same way as you did for the Nursing Process portion:

- Review a question you got wrong, and identify which step of the clinical judgment process is being tested in the question.
- Place the number of the question in the first box to the right of the step in the clinical judgment process you identified.
- When another question you got wrong reflects the same step of the clinical judgment process, place the number of the subsequent question in the box to the right of the previous question.
- Insert the number of every question you got wrong on the examination into the Clinical Judgment Process portion of the Knowledge Analysis Tool.
- Tally the total number of answers you got wrong for each step of the clinical judgment process in the last column on the right. Students often will notice a clustering of errors in one or two steps of the clinical judgment process.
- For each condition you study, ask yourself the questions associated with the steps in the clinical judgment process:
    1. Recognize cues—which symptoms or complaints reported to me by my client matter the most and require more investigation?
    2. Analyze cues—in light of what I know, what is the most likely explanation for these symptoms?
    3. Prioritize hypotheses—what is the first assessment I should do? What is the next most important assessment?

4. Generate solutions—what actions can I take, and what can I anticipate the provider will order?
5. Take action—having identified the actions I can take, which ones will I do now? Which actions would not be helpful, or can be delayed?
6. Evaluate outcomes—did it help?

CORRECTIVE ACTION GUIDE FOR THE KNOWLEDGE ANALYSIS TOOL

This guide has two parts: Knowledge Categories and Nursing Process. Knowledge Categories include the broad areas of information that form the basics of nursing practice. Evaluating your performance using this section of the tool will help identify your gaps in knowledge. The Nursing Process portion of the tool reflects the steps of the nursing process: assessment, analysis, planning, implementation, and evaluation. Exploring your performance using this section of the tool will help identify your difficulties in performing critical thinking and problem-solving behaviors within the practice of nursing. Remember, the nursing process is a systematic approach that uses critical thinking to provide nursing care.

Corrective Action Guide for Knowledge Categories in the Knowledge Analysis Tool

First, complete the Knowledge Categories portion of the Knowledge Analysis Tool. Then, identify the knowledge categories that have question numbers indicating incorrect answers. The more wrong answers within a category, the less knowledge you have of the content within the category. The more categories in which you have wrong answers, the broader your lack of nursing knowledge. The related nursing content for each wrong answer should be explored. However, when time is limited, focus on those knowledge areas with the most wrong answers.

Studying is essential to learning, which is a complex activity. Most people study before a test. However, it is essential to also study *after* a test. By studying with the intention of improving your approach and asking focused questions as you learn, your chances of success are improved. When you identify a practice question that you answered incorrectly, reread your class notes and textbook regarding that topic. Discuss it with your instructor if you still do not understand the content. When you have a thorough understanding of the content being tested, you will be better able to identify the correct answer. In addition, you will have more confidence in the option you selected and be less likely to change your answer later during an examination.

One of the best ways to achieve a higher grade on an examination is to be overprepared. Compare and contrast class notes with information within your textbook. Study in a small group with your peers to obtain different perspectives on material in a specific knowledge category or when analyzing an examination item. Practice the questions in Chapter 11, and review the rationales for the correct and incorrect answers. Understanding complex concepts usually requires a variety of study approaches and repetition.

REVIEW

Chapter 4, "Study Techniques," "General Study Techniques," page 37.

Chapter 4, "Study Techniques," "Specific Study Techniques Related to Cognitive Levels of Nursing Questions," page 41.

Chapter 1, "Empowerment," "Overprepare for a Test," page 5.

Chapter 11, "Practice Questions With Answers and Rationales," page 187.

Corrective Action Guide for the Nursing Process in the Knowledge Analysis Tool

First, complete the Nursing Process portion of the Knowledge Analysis Tool. Then, identify the steps of the nursing process that have question numbers indicating answers that are incorrect. The more wrong answers within a particular step of the nursing process, the more significant your difficulties will be in answering questions that require the typical thinking behaviors associated with that step. For example, assessment questions may require you to collect or analyze data, whereas planning questions may require you to set goals or identify priorities.

Read the stem and each option carefully when taking a simulated practice examination. Determine which step of the nursing process is reflected by the question before even attempting to answer it. When you are able to identify the question's placement within the nursing process, it will provide a more in-depth review of the stem and options. It should facilitate your identification of what the test item is asking.

REVIEW

Chapter 2, "Critical Thinking," page 9.
Chapter 6, "The Nursing Process," page 67.

SUMMARY

You should use these test analysis tools to assess your test performance on a practice examination. You should then use these tools when reviewing every examination you take in class. Do not be shy about asking your instructor for help with your analysis. Nursing instructors who are student centered will help you with this analysis during class or office hours because instructors have a vested interest in your success. Analysis of your test performance is essential if you are to identify your own individual learning needs. After your learning needs have been identified using the presented tools, the Corrective Action Guides should direct you to information that can improve your abilities. ***Engaging in activities that analyze your test performance is time well spent!***

11 Practice Questions With Answers and Rationales

WORLD OF THE CLIENT AND NURSE

This section includes factors that influence the role of the nurse and the delivery of health care. Questions address ethics, legal aspects of nursing practice, the nursing process, responsibilities associated with the management of nursing practice (including delegation to and supervision of members of the nursing team), clients' rights, the difference between dependent and independent roles of the nurse, standards of nursing practice, and agencies that provide structure for the delivery of health care.

QUESTIONS

1. The client tells the nurse, "I can't find my mobile phone and I know I had it before my procedure." The nurse provides client-centered care by stating:
   1. "It is here somewhere. I will ask the staff."
   2. "I am sure you will find it. You are just foggy from your procedure."
   3. "I understand your concern about your phone. I will help you find it."
   4. "I did not see you with it before your procedure. You must have misplaced it."

   TEST-TAKING TIP: Identify the word in the stem that sets a priority. Identify the clang association. Identify the client-centered option that focuses on. Identify the option that denies the client's feelings, concerns, or needs.

2. During annual training at a health-care facility, all registered nurses are required to read and sign an agreement to abide by the state nurse practice act. The nurse understands that state nurse practice acts define what aspects of nursing? **Select all that apply.**
   1. Passing standards for NCLEX
   2. Defining criteria for safe nursing practice
   3. Investigating complaints of substandard care
   4. Standards of competence at initial licensure
   5. Standards of competence for licensure renewal

   TEST-TAKING TIP: Think about standards of care and minimum requirements to practice.

3. The nurse observes a client going into another client's room without permission, which upsets the other client. Which should the nurse do **first** when responding to the wandering client?
   1. Help the client to the correct room
   2. Place the client in restraints temporarily
   3. Determine the motivation for the client's behavior
   4. Share the observation about the client with the health-care team

   TEST-TAKING TIP: Identify the word in the stem that sets a priority. Identify the central person in the question. Identify client-centered options.

4. The nurse is caring for a client with type 2 diabetes mellitus who has developed neuropathy. The nurse places a consultation for wound care, educates the client on the use of foot creams, and speaks with case management about home health at discharge. The nurse is using which parts of the nursing process? **Select all that apply.**
   1. Assessment
   2. Diagnosis
   3. Planning
   4. Implementing
   5. Evaluating

5. The nonresponsive client in the intensive care unit needs a central line placed immediately. Rather than wait for the family to consent, the charge nurse directs the vascular access nurse to place the line now. Which is the most appropriate action by the vascular access nurse?
   1. Place the central line now
   2. Notify the Chief Nursing Officer
   3. Wait until informed consent is given
   4. Notify the provider who placed the order

   TEST-TAKING TIP: Identify opposites in options.

6. A client is legally determined to have died. The nurse should begin postmortem care:
   1. as soon as death is pronounced.
   2. after significant others have left.
   3. once the nursing supervisor is informed.
   4. only after the primary health-care provider is notified.

   TEST-TAKING TIP: Identify the option with a specific determiner. Identify the unique option.

7. The nurse is caring for a client who is 17 years of age and is scheduled to have surgery to amputate the right leg. The nurse attempts to obtain a signed, valid informed consent form for surgery. What question by the nurse reflects the element of disclosure?
   1. "Did the surgeon explain the risks, benefits, costs, and alternatives to you?"
   2. "Are you signing this consent voluntarily without pressure from others?"
   3. "Are you legally emancipated from your parents, married, or a parent?"
   4. "Can you repeat in your own words the details about the procedure?"

   TEST-TAKING TIP: Identify the word in the stem that directs attention to content.

8. The nurse has just arrived for their shift and is preparing to receive a hand-off report on four clients. Which should the nurse do first?
   1. Review each client's electronic medical record
   2. Review each client's medications due during the shift
   3. Perform the required controlled drug count with the nurse going off shift
   4. Visit each client's room with the outgoing nurse for report and to review client status

   TEST-TAKING TIP: Identify the word in the stem that sets a priority. Identify the key word in the stem that directs attention to content.

9. The nurse breaks a client's dentures because of carelessness. Which specific legal term applies to this action?
   1. Battery
   2. Assault
   3. Negligence
   4. Malpractice

10. The nurse is caring for a client who is often argumentative and demanding. Which is an appropriate nursing intervention when planning care for this client?
    1. Bring another nurse as a witness.
    2. Involve the client in decision making.
    3. Accept the behavior as probably a lifelong pattern.
    4. Explain that the staff would appreciate the client's cooperation.

    TEST-TAKING TIP: Identify key words in the stem that direct attention to content. Identify opposites in options. Identify the client-centered option. Identify the option that denies the client's feelings, concerns, or needs.

11. The provider ordered the new nurse caring for a 5-year-old client with a closed leg fracture to begin the sedation protocol for a closed reduction procedure while the provider cared for another client. Doing this would be against facility protocol. How should the nurse proceed?
    1. Find another provider to start the sedation protocol
    2. Follow the provider's orders and begin the sedation protocol
    3. Ask another nurse to assist in beginning the sedation protocol
    4. Wait to initiate the sedation protocol until the provider is in the room

12. A client with dementia needs assistance with hygiene, grooming, eating, and toileting. Which agency can meet this client's needs after discharge from the hospital?
    1. Nursing home
    2. Psychiatric institution
    3. Outpatient care facility
    4. Adult day-care program

    TEST-TAKING TIP: Identify key words in the stem that direct attention to content.

13. The nurse observes a multiple-vehicle collision in which several people are seriously injured and stops to offer assistance. Which legal principle is in operation in this situation?
    1. A legal trust that accompanies a nursing license applies to this situation.
    2. The nurse can be held legally responsible for care provided.
    3. Immunity is afforded because a contract does not exist.
    4. Immunity is provided by the Good Samaritan Law.

    TEST-TAKING TIP: Identify clang associations. Identify opposites in options. Identify equally plausible options.

14. The nurse left the client unattended in the shower. The client fell, obtained a head injury, and died 2 days later. Which intentional tort can the nurse be sued for?
    1. Assault
    2. Battery
    3. Slander
    4. Negligence

15. The nurse obtains a signed, valid informed consent form from a client who is to have an invasive procedure. Which does the nurse's signature on the informed consent form indicate?
    1. The surgeon described the procedure and its potential risks.
    2. The client knows and understands expected outcomes.
    3. The client actually signed the consent form.
    4. The surgeon is protected from being sued.

    TEST-TAKING TIP: Identify the clang association. Identify equally plausible options.

16. The nurse witnesses another nurse treating a client in an abusive manner. Which should the nurse do **first?**
   1. Tell the charge nurse and write a report
   2. Become a role model for the other nurse
   3. Discuss the incident with the other nurse
   4. Move the client away from the abusive nurse

   TEST-TAKING TIP: Identify the word in the stem that sets a priority. Identify the central person in the question. Identify the unique option. Identify the client-centered option.

17. The charge nurse notices the new graduate nurse attempting to transfer an unsteady client to a chair without using a gait belt. After helping to safely transfer the client, the charge nurse discusses the potential implications with the nurse to: **Select all that apply.**
   1. Mentor to provide safe, quality care.
   2. Establish an environment that maintains respect.
   3. Minimize risk that the client will take legal action.
   4. Maintain accountability for delegated nursing care.
   5. Remind the nurse that they are new and must do as the charge nurse dictates.

18. When obtaining a health history, the nurse identifies that a client has gained 10 pounds in the past week. Which step of the nursing process is performed when the nurse documents this information in the client's clinical record?
   1. Analysis
   2. Planning
   3. Evaluation
   4. Assessment

19. The nurse assigns a nursing assistant to a client who transfers to a chair with a mechanical lift. It has been a long time since the nursing assistant used a lift. To ensure the safety of the client, the nurse should:
   1. request that another nursing assistant assist with the client's care.
   2. ask the nursing assistant to demonstrate how to use the lift.
   3. explain to the nursing assistant how to use the lift.
   4. assign the client to another nursing assistant.

   TEST-TAKING TIP: Identify equally plausible options. Identify clang associations.

20. A male client has dementia. He is verbally and physically abusive and paranoid. Which should the nurse always do when providing care? **Select all that apply.**
   1. _____ Explore his preferences about the care to be given
   2. _____ Compliment him on how nice he looks
   3. _____ Administer nursing care at a slow pace
   4. _____ Explain what care is to be done
   5. _____ Tell him what he wants to hear

   TEST-TAKING TIP: Identify the word in the stem that sets a priority. Identify the key words in the stem that direct attention to content.

21. A client says, "I don't like anyone to go into my closet or drawers." Which should the nurse do when returning hygiene equipment to the client's bedside cabinet? **Select all that apply.**
   1. _____ Store the materials on the overbed table
   2. _____ Allow the client to put the equipment away
   3. _____ Provide reassurance that personal things will not be taken
   4. _____ Explain the hazard of not putting equipment away as it is being done
   5. _____ Request permission to return equipment to the client's bedside cabinet

   TEST-TAKING TIP: Identify the clang association. Identify client-centered options. Identify options that deny client feelings, concerns, or needs.

22. The primary nurse who is responsible for a group of clients is delegating responsibilities to the other members of the nursing team. Which task should the nurse include when formulating an assignment for the nursing assistant? **Select all that apply.**
1. _____ Monitoring clients' tube feedings
2. _____ Ambulating clients outside their rooms
3. _____ Regulating clients' intravenous solutions
4. _____ Assessing clients' skin for pressure ulcers
5. _____ Supervising clients when they are taking medications

TEST-TAKING TIP: Identify key words in the stem that direct attention to content.

23. The nurse is caring for a brain-dead client whose family wants to keep the client on life support indefinitely, creating an ethical dilemma between the family and the health-care facility. Using the nursing process as a guide to ethical decision making, place the steps presented in the order that the nurse should consider.
1. State the dilemma and clarify that the issue is ethical in nature
2. Evaluate the decisions and actions to identify what was learned from the process
3. Implement decisions and actions that have acceptable consequences
4. Identify and explore options with the consequences of each for each stakeholder
5. Gather and analyze data to interpret the situation

Answer: _____________

24. Which situation is an example of an intentional tort? **Select all that apply.**
1. _____ Forgetting to administer a STAT medication
2. _____ Performing a procedure without informed consent
3. _____ Carelessly administering a medication to the wrong client
4. _____ Threatening to withhold pain medication if a client does not behave
5. _____ Applying a restraint without a prescription when a client is at risk for self-harm

TEST-TAKING TIP: Identify key words in the stem that direct attention to content.

25. Which action by a nurse violates client confidentiality and privacy? **Select all that apply.**
1. _____ Interviewing a client in the presence of others
2. _____ Writing client statements in the progress notes
3. _____ Disclosing client information to family members
4. _____ Presenting the client's problems at a team conference
5. _____ Sharing data about a client at the change of shift report
6. _____ Performing a procedure for a client without pulling the curtain around the bed

TEST-TAKING TIP: Identify the word in the stem that indicates negative polarity. Identify key words in the stem that direct attention to content.

26. Nurses must respect the expectations and responsibilities of clients and inform them of the Patient Care Partnership (formerly Patient Bill of Rights). Which client expectation is included in the Patient Care Partnership? **Select all that apply.**
1. _____ Having a safe environment
2. _____ Requesting to know the identity of caregivers
3. _____ Being involved in decision making concerning care
4. _____ Receiving accurate information about a diagnosis
5. _____ Refusing a treatment prescribed by the primary health-care provider

27. The nurse's client is angry that another nurse on the unit shared the client's diagnosis with a visitor. The nurse is completing an Unusual Occurrence Report because of the breach in client confidentiality. Review the Unusual Occurrence Report and select the most appropriate "Occurrence Category" and the most appropriate "Contributing Factors" by placing a check in the boxes in the report that relate to this event.

Unusual Occurrence Report

Date of Event: __________ **Time of Event:** __________ **Department:** ____________________

Client Last Name:	**First Name:**	**MI:**
Client #:	**Attending Physician:**	
Visitor Last Name:	**First Name:**	**Phone #:**
Employee Name:	**Dept:**	
Physician Name:	**Specialty:**	

Occurrence Category (Check most appropriate)		
☐ Agency nurse-related	☐ AMA	☐ Delay in treatment
☐ Diet-related	☐ HIPAA compliance	☐ Loss of personal property
☐ Medication-related	☐ Narcotics-related	☐ Order not executed
☐ Client injury	☐ Peer-review related	☐ Restraint-related
☐ Staff injury	☐ Supplies/Equipment	☐ Visitor injury
☐ Other (please explain):		

Description of Occurrence:
A client overheard a nurse sharing information about the client's diagnosis and treatment to a visitor in the hall. The client reported this event to the nurse in charge and stated, "I am very upset".

Contributing Factors (Check all that apply)	
☐ Individual:	☐ System:
Knowledge, skills, and/or experience: ☐ Unclear ☐ Incomplete	Policies/procedures not in place: ☐ Unclear ☐ Outdated
☐ Non-adherence to standard of care or practice	Environmental: ☐ Staffing ☐ Client acuity ☐ Congestion
☐ Documentation incomplete or inadequate	Communications and work flow: ☐ Intradepartmental ☐ Interdepartmental
	☐ Equipment failure
Other (please explain):	

Submitted by:	**Dept:**	**Date:**

TEST-TAKING TIP: Identify the word in the stem that sets a priority.

28. The registered nurse is the leader of a team consisting of one licensed practical nurse and two nursing assistants. Which assignment should the registered nurse delegate to the licensed practical nurse? **Select all that apply.**
1. _____ Administer an enema to a client who is having surgery in the morning
2. _____ Give a medication via the direct IV push technique
3. _____ Perform a venipuncture to obtain a blood specimen
4. _____ Change a dressing on a pressure ulcer
5. _____ Collect clinical data about clients

TEST-TAKING TIP: Identify the words in the stem that direct attention to content.

29. Which activity is a dependent function of the nurse? **Select all that apply.**
1. _____ Ambulating a client down the hall
2. _____ Documenting perioperative nursing care
3. _____ Changing a sterile dressing that is soiled
4. _____ Providing oxygen for sudden shortness of breath
5. _____ Assisting with selection of choices on the menu

TEST-TAKING TIP: Identify the key word in the stem that directs attention to content.

30. A health-care facility may release patient health-care information (PHI) for purposes other than treatment, payment, and routine health care without the client's authorization if releasing the information is determined to be for the good of the general population. Which situations below allow for this type of release? **Select all that apply.**
1. A celebrity is being treated in the facility after a car accident
2. The medical record is needed for the investigation of a crime
3. A virus outbreak occurs among students at a local high school
4. Information is needed to identify victims of a tornado outbreak
5. The adult child of a schizophrenic client wants to help care for their parent

31. The nurse is formulating a nursing assistant assignment. Which activity should the nurse delegate to the nursing assistant? **Select all that apply.**
1. _____ Reporting unusual clinical manifestations to the nurse
2. _____ Ensuring that clients swallow their medication
3. _____ Orienting a new employee to the unit
4. _____ Teaching clients personal hygiene
5. _____ Distributing meal trays to clients
6. _____ Obtaining routine vital signs

TEST-TAKING TIP: Identify key words in the stem that direct attention to content.

32. An older adult female client who suffered a cerebrovascular accident (CVA) is constantly using her call light and yelling for help from the nursing staff. To provide the client with safe quality care, the nurse uses the nursing process to determine the client's presenting problem. Place the steps below in the correct order that the nurse uses to deliver the client's care according to the nursing process.
1. Assist the client to achieve the desired outcomes, promote wellness, and aid in coping with altered function
2. Collect data to determine the client's strengths and needs and their ability to manage their own care
3. Measure the extent to which the client has achieved outcomes and modify the plan of care as needed
4. Identify client outcomes to develop an individualized plan of care, establish priorities, and communicate the plan of care to the client
5. Develop a list of nursing diagnoses and problems that nursing interventions can resolve or prevent

Answer: __________

TEST-TAKING TIP: Identify key words in the stem that direct attention to content.

33. A nurse who is a member of a quality improvement committee reviews a chart detailing trends in four problem categories identified in Incident Reports over a 4-month period. Corrective action plans were implemented to address each problem category. The nurse analyzes the chart documenting trends for these categories over the successive months of March, April, and May. Which problem category should cause the **most** concern?
1. Falls
2. Medication errors
3. Violations of confidentiality
4. Failures to maintain standards of practice

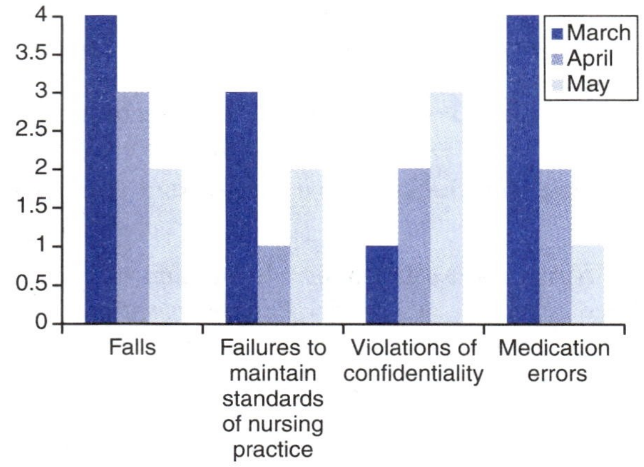

TEST-TAKING TIP: Identify the word in the stem that sets a priority.

34. During client assessments, the nurse gathers subjective and objective data to determine the client's problems and needs. Identify the examples of subjective data a nurse collects. **Select all that apply.**
1. ____ The client complains of tingling in their fingers and toes.
2. ____ The client states their pain is a 5 on a scale of 1 to 10.
3. ____ The client vomits three times within an hour.
4. ____ The client's ankles and feet are swollen.
5. ____ The client is crying with a rapid pulse.
6. ____ The client says they are nauseous.

TEST-TAKING TIP: Identify key words in the stem that direct attention to content.

35. Which action or inaction by a nurse is an example of an unintentional tort? **Select all that apply.**
1. _____ Failure to stop at an automobile collision to render first aid
2. _____ Failure to recognize a cluster of data that indicate a safety problem causing injury to a client
3. _____ Failure to identify the signs and symptoms of hyperglycemia causing a life-threatening situation
4. _____ Fracturing a client's rib while implementing cardiopulmonary resuscitation that followed appropriate standards of care
5. _____ Refusal to be transferred to a unit for which the nurse does not feel adequately prepared to provide an acceptable level of care

TEST-TAKING TIP: Identify key words in the stem that direct attention to content.

36. The registered nurse is the leader of a team consisting of two nursing assistants. Which assignment should the registered nurse keep rather than assign to one of the nursing assistants? **Select all that apply.**
1. _____ Evaluating a client's response to the administration of an analgesic
2. _____ Emptying the collection bag of a urinary retention catheter
3. _____ Obtaining a specimen of exudate from a draining wound
4. _____ Taking vital signs of clients who are unstable
5. _____ Teaching clients range-of-motion exercises

TEST-TAKING TIP: Identify the key words in the stem that direct attention to content.

37. An older adult is to be discharged from the hospital after being treated with IV antibiotics for pneumonia. A nursing case manager is assessing the client's physical, emotional, and socioeconomic needs. The nurse reviews the primary health-care provider's summary and interviews the client and the client's son. Which setting should the nurse explore with the client and son because it is the **most** appropriate setting for the client when discharged from the hospital?
1. Independent living facility
2. Assisted-living facility
3. Day-care program
4. Nursing home

CLIENT INFORMATION

Primary Health-Care Provider's Summary

The client is an 86-year-old woman who has emphysema and arthritis of the hands and knees. She is capable of performing activities of daily living but should use a wheelchair when going long distances. Her vital signs are within acceptable limits for an individual her age. She should continue medical supervision every 3 months.

Interview of Client

Client looking forward to discharge. She stated, "I like my privacy. I prefer to take care of myself." Client indicated difficulty getting to the store now that she no longer drives. She also stated, "I am a little lonely living by myself, and I am so sick of making the same old meals all the time."

Interview of Client's Son

Client's son works full-time and has an active social life on the weekends. He stated, "I would like her to live with me, but it really is impossible. I am never home." The son indicated that his mother has ample financial resources for whatever she decides to do.

TEST-TAKING TIP: Identify the word in the stem that sets a priority.

38. An emergency department nurse is caring for a client with a history of chronic pulmonary disease who presents with shortness of breath, a dry oral cavity, and furrows of the tongue. In addition, the client is using accessory muscles to breathe. Which action can be implemented independently by the nurse? **Select all that apply.**
1. _____ Taking the vital signs
2. _____ Encouraging fluid intake
3. _____ Monitoring oxygen saturation
4. _____ Placing the client in the high Fowler position
5. _____ Assessing the lungs for adventitious breath sounds

TEST-TAKING TIP: Identify key words in the stem that direct attention to content.

39. Which is an example of a goal identified by a nurse and client when planning care? **Select all that apply.**
   1. _____ "The client will state pain relief within 30 minutes after receiving an analgesic."
   2. _____ "The client should receive small, frequent feedings at least 5 times a day."
   3. _____ "The client needs assistance with meals."
   4. _____ "The client is at risk for weight loss."
   5. _____ "The client will gain 5 pounds."

40. The nurse is planning to delegate client care to a nursing assistant. Which is an appropriate activity for a nursing assistant? **Select all that apply.**
   1. _____ Evaluating vital signs
   2. _____ Making occupied beds
   3. _____ Monitoring tube feedings
   4. _____ Helping clients to eat a meal
   5. _____ Providing clients with physical hygiene
   6. _____ Assisting postoperative clients with their first ambulation

   TEST-TAKING TIP: Identify key words in the stem that direct attention to content.

1. **TEST-TAKING TIP:** ***Client-centered*** **is the key term to help identify the correct answer. Options 1, 2, and 4 deny the client's feelings, concerns, or needs. Option 3 is client-centered.**
   1. This response dismisses the client's feelings and concern and is not keeping the client at the center of the caregiving.
   2. This response is not therapeutic and does not establish a relationship of mutual respect. It does not promote the dignity of the client.
   3. **This is the correct response because both the client and the nurse share in the solution. This is therapeutic and client-centered because the nurse is demonstrating respect for the client.**
   4. This response dismisses the client's feelings and concerns. It is not client-centered care and dismisses the client's concerns.

2. **TEST-TAKING TIP: The nurse practice act in each state is the state-specific licensing and regulatory body that establishes standards of care and safe nursing practice.**
   1. **Nurse practice acts define the minimum criteria for safe nursing practice in each state.**
   2. **State boards of nursing, in their nurse practice acts, define the procedures to investigate and handle any disciplinary actions for nursing practice violations.**
   3. **State nurse practice acts define the minimum required competencies to be licensed in the state and issue licenses to qualified candidates.**
   4. **State nurse practice acts define the standards for safe nursing practice and care and decide the scope of practice for nurses within the jurisdiction. This includes minimum competencies for licensure renewal.**
   5. Passing standards for the National Council Licensure Examination for Nurses (NCLEX) are established by the National Council for State Boards of Nursing, not individual state nurse practice acts.

3. **TEST-TAKING TIP: The word** ***first*** **in the stem sets a priority. The client in the room is the client who was violated and is the central person in the question. Options 1 and 2 are client-centered because both actions protect the client in the room who was violated. Options 2 and 3 focus on the wandering client, not on the client who was violated. Restraints are inappropriate unless less-restrictive measures are tried first to control the wandering client's behavior; thus option 2 can be eliminated.**
   1. **Clients have a right to privacy and security for themselves and their belongings; helping the client to the correct room protects the other violated client.**
   2. Restraining clients for any reason other than their own physical safety or the safety of others is illegal; it is false imprisonment.
   3. This is not the priority. The nurse can explore the motivation for the behavior later.
   4. Sharing the observation with the health-care team does not address the immediate need. After the behavior has been addressed, it can be communicated.

4. **TEST-TAKING TIP: Think about each step in the Nursing Process and identify the priorities for each step.**
   1. **Assessment is the systematic and continuous collection of client data. The nurse has already assessed the client and is planning for future care.**
   2. **Diagnosis begins after the nurse has collected client data. In the diagnosis phase, the nurse analyzes and interprets data collected during the assessment phase. The nurse has already established nursing diagnoses and is planning outcomes based off of these diagnoses.**
   3. **In the planning phase, the nurse identifies care priorities, identifies client outcomes, and selects evidence-based interventions to create a plan of care. Placing the wound consultation identifies wound care as a priority. Consulting with case management plans for care after discharge.**
   4. **During implementation, the plan of care is carried out. Implementation helps the client achieve health outcomes, promotes and restores health, and facilitates client coping with alterations in health and functioning. The nurse educates the client on appropriate wound care creams as part of the implementation phase.**
   5. **During evaluation, the nurse and the client determine how well the client has achieved the outcomes identified in the**

plan of care. Factors that contribute to the client's ability to achieve the expected outcomes are reviewed and, if necessary, the plan of care is modified. The client is not in the evaluation phase.

5. **TEST-TAKING TIP: Options 1 and 3 are opposites.**
   1. Nurses have a legal responsibility to ensure consent is obtained before a procedure and may be held legally accountable for any deviation from their scope of practice. The nurse should not place the central line without consent.
   2. The nurse should notify administration only if the nurse in charge continues to insist that the task be performed, though an incident report should be submitted for follow-up.
   3. **Nurses must have informed consent with documentation before any treatment or intervention requiring consent is carried out.**
   4. This is not the most appropriate answer and does not resolve the situation between the nurse and charge nurse.

6. **TEST-TAKING TIP: Option 4 contains the word *only*, which is a specific determiner. In options 1, 3, and 4, the final word in the statements ends in "-ed." Option 2 is unique.**
   1. Postmortem care at this time is premature.
   2. **This allows the family members time to make a last visit before the body is prepared for transfer to a mortuary.**
   3. Postmortem care at this time is premature.
   4. Postmortem care does not have to be delayed until the primary health-care provider is notified.

7. **TEST-TAKING TIP: The word *disclosure* in the stem directs attention to content.**
   1. **This statement reflects the element of *disclosure*. It is the responsibility of the primary health-care provider to provide this information as well as answer all questions asked by the client.**
   2. This statement reflects the element of *voluntariness*. The client must willingly give consent.
   3. This statement reflects the element of *competence*. The client must be capable of understanding the information to make an informed decision. The person must be alert, have intact cognition, and be 18 years of age or, if younger, must be legally emancipated, a parent, or married.
   4. This statement reflects the element of *comprehension*. The client must be able to describe details about the procedure including risks, benefits, costs, and alternatives demonstrating understanding.

8. **TEST-TAKING TIP: The word *first* in the stem sets a priority. The word *arrived* is the key word in the stem that directs attention to content. It establishes a time frame.**
   1. **Before the nurse can prioritize care, the nurse must first know about each client's status during the bedside shift report. Once the nurse has received a full report on all clients for the day, the medical record can be reviewed to prioritize care.**
   2. **Part of prioritizing care will be medication administration. This is decided after the nurse has received a report and evaluated each client's status for safety and immediate needs.**
   3. **Controlled drugs can be counted at any time within the required timeline during a shift.**
   4. **Before care can be planned and implemented, the nurse must know the condition and immediate needs of clients. This information is given by the nurse who previously provided care for the clients during the bedside shift report.**

9.
   1. *Battery* is the purposeful, angry, or negligent touching of a client without consent.
   2. *Assault* is an act intended to provoke fear in a client.
   3. ***Negligence* occurs when actions do not meet appropriate standards and result in injury to a client or to the client's belongings; negligence can occur with acts of omission or commission.**
   4. *Malpractice* is misconduct performed in professional practice that results in harm to a client.

10. **TEST-TAKING TIP: The words *argumentative* and *demanding* are key words in the stem that direct attention to content. Options 2 and 4 are opposites. Option 2 offers the client choices, and option 4 implies that the client must comply with directives from staff members. Option 2 is client-centered. Option 4 denies the client's feelings, concerns, or needs.**
    1. This is a defensive response. All behaviors have meaning; the nurse should initially identify the reason for the behavior.

2. **The client is the center of the health-care team and has a right to be involved in decisions concerning care; this individualizes care and promotes self-esteem, which often prevents argumentative and demanding behavior.**
3. This is an assumption. The client's behavior may not be a lifelong pattern. Many people cope with anxiety by exhibiting this behavior. This behavior may be an attempt to gain control in a situation in which an individual feels out of control, and it should be addressed.
4. This response is judgmental and takes away the client's coping mechanism. The nurse should cooperate with the client to help meet individual needs.

11. **TEST-TAKING TIP: Think client safety and nursing accountability.**
1. This is not the correct option. The nurse should wait for the client's provider before beginning the sedation protocol.
2. This action undermines client safety and goes against facility protocol. Beginning the sedation protocol without the provider would not be within the nurse's scope of practice. If the client was harmed, there would be grounds for negligence.
3. This is not the correct option as not having the provider in the room is against facility protocol. Having another nurse assist places both nurses at risk for negligence.
4. **This is the correct answer. The nurse should identify the potential liabilities with starting the sedation protocol without the provider. The legal responsibility and accountability for nursing actions rest with the nurse. To avoid legal conflicts, nurses must practice within their scope of practice and confidence. Client safety must always be the priority, even if it means challenging other members of the health-care team protocol. Having another nurse assist places both nurses at risk for negligence.**

12. **TEST-TAKING TIP: The words *needs assistance with hygiene, grooming, eating, and toileting* are key words in the stem that direct attention to content because they indicate the significant level of assistance needed.**
1. **This client needs long-term nursing care as well as 24-hour supervision.**
2. A psychiatric institution is inappropriate for this client. Clients with dementia need supportive care for the rest of their lives. Today, psychiatric settings generally provide acute-care services for clients with a mental illness.
3. Outpatient care facilities usually provide acute-care services, not long-term nursing care or 24-hour supervision.
4. Many day-care programs function 5 days a week from 8 a.m. to 6 p.m. to assist working family members. No data given indicate the support of family members to meet the client's needs or the ability of the client to provide self-care when not at the day-care program.

13. **TEST-TAKING TIP: The words *legal* in the stem and in option 1 and *legally* in option 2 are clang associations. Option 2 is opposite of both options 3 and 4. Options 3 and 4 are equally plausible because they both provide immunity.**
1. Assistance at the scene of an accident is an ethical, not a legal, duty.
2. **Nurses are responsible for their own actions, and the care provided must be what any reasonably prudent nurse would provide under similar circumstances.**
3. A contract does not have to exist for a nurse to commit negligence.
4. The Good Samaritan Law does not provide legal immunity; the nurse can still be held accountable for gross departure from acceptable standards of practice or willful wrongdoing.

14. **TEST-TAKING TIP: Torts may be intentional or unintentional. Torts are subject to legal action in a civil court, usually settled with money.**
1. Assault is an attempt or threat to unjustifiably touch another person.
2. Battery is an assault that includes willful, forcible, or negligent touching of another's body or anything attached to the body. Pushing a patient into a chair is an example of battery.
3. Slander is defamation of character by spoken words.
4. **Negligence is the failure to do something a reasonably prudent nurse would do under similar circumstances or the commission of an act that a reasonably prudent nurse would not commit under similar circumstances.**

15. **TEST-TAKING TIP: The term *consent form* in the stem and option 3 is a clang association. Options 1 and 2 are equally plausible.**

1. The nurse's signature does not document that the surgeon described the procedure and its risks.
2. The nurse's signature does not document that the client was properly informed about expected outcomes. The client's signature documents that the client gives consent for the procedure.
3. **The nurse only witnesses the client's signature and examines the document for the correct date.**
4. The nurse's signature on an informed consent form does not protect the surgeon from being sued. Reasonably prudent practice protects the surgeon from being sued.

16. **TEST-TAKING TIP: The word *first* in the stem sets a priority. The client is the central person in the question, not the abusive nurse. Option 4 is unique because it is the only option that addresses the needs of the client. Option 4 is client-centered.**

1. Telling the charge nurse about the behavior and writing a report should be done later; another action is the priority.
2. Nurses should always be a role model for other nurses and exhibit professional, kind, and caring behaviors. Abusing a client is never accepted and the nurse should model professional behaviors, but this is not the priority.
3. This may be done later; it is not the priority at this time.
4. **Nurses must always be client advocates. The client is the priority at this time; after the client is protected and safe, the actions of the abusive nurse must be addressed.**

17. **TEST-TAKING TIP: Remember that care should always be safe, effective, and client-centered.**

1. **This is a correct option. It is crucial for nurses to understand the ethical dimensions of professional practice and potential legal pitfalls. The charge nurse can mentor the new nurse to support them in their development of critical thinking and nursing skills with the goal of providing high-quality, client-centered care.**
2. **This is a correct option. By speaking to the new nurse after transferring the patient, the charge nurse is maintaining the dignity of the new nurse while allowing for reflection and learning to prevent this from happening in the future.**
3. This is not a correct option. Discussing the potential implications is for the nurse to understand the ethical dimensions of their practice to provide client-centered, high-quality nursing care and to serve as an advocate for their client—not to lessen the chances a client may take legal action.
4. **This is a correct option. The experienced nurse transferred responsibility to the new nurse but is still accountable for the outcome. Appropriate delegation can result in safe and effective client care.**
5. This is not a correct option. The charge nurse is there to mentor and teach the new graduate nurse. This is an autocratic type of leadership and does not include the new nurse in decision making.

18.
1. Analysis involves interpretation of data, collection of additional data, and determining the significance of collected data. Analysis does not include documenting collected data.
2. Planning involves setting goals, establishing priorities, identifying expected outcomes, identifying interventions designed to achieve goals and outcomes, ensuring that a client's health-care needs are met appropriately, modifying the plan as necessary, and collaborating with other health-care team members to ensure that care is coordinated. Planning does not include documenting collected data.
3. Evaluation involves identifying a client's response to care, comparing a client's actual responses with the expected outcomes, analyzing factors that affected the actual outcomes for the purpose of drawing conclusions about the success or failure of specific nursing activities, and modifying a plan of care when necessary. Evaluation does not include documenting collected data.
4. **Communicating important assessment data to other health-care team members is a component of the assessment phase of the nursing process.**

19. **TEST-TAKING TIP: Options 1 and 4 are equally plausible. The words *used a lift* in the stem and *use the lift* in options 2 and 3 are clang associations.**

1. Another nursing assistant should not be held accountable for the care assigned

to another staff member. The nurse is directly responsible for ensuring that delegated care is safely delivered to clients.

2. **Demonstration is the safest way to assess whether the nursing assistant has the knowledge and skill to transfer a client safely using a mechanical lift.**
3. This teaching method does not take into consideration the need for the nursing assistant to practice the psychomotor skills associated with this task. Explaining is not sufficient.
4. This does not address the nursing assistant's need to know how to move a client safely with a mechanical lift.

20. **TEST-TAKING TIP: The word *always* in the stem sets a priority. *Abusive and paranoid* are the key words in the stem that direct attention to content.**
    1. **This intervention includes the client in the decision making and focuses on the client's preferences. Including a client who is paranoid in the decision-making process provides the client with a sense of control of the situation.**
    2. This may not be true; trust is based on honesty.
    3. **A slow pace allows the client time to comprehend what is being done. Rushing may increase the client's anxiety, which can intensify paranoia and abusive behavior.**
    4. **This explanation supports the client's right to know what care is being given and why. Explanations should be given before touching a client who is paranoid or abusive.**
    5. Telling a client what he wants to hear is patronizing; when clients feel they are being humored, trust deteriorates.

21. **TEST-TAKING TIP: The word *equipment* in the stem and in options 2, 4, and 5 is a clang association. Options 2 and 5 give the client control and therefore are client-centered options. Options 3 and 4 deny client feelings, concerns, or needs.**
    1. This intervention is unsafe. Equipment should be stored appropriately to protect it from pathogens in the environment.
    2. **This supports the client's right to control his or her personal space.**
    3. Unfortunately, this statement could be false reassurance. Items can be misplaced or thrown away because they are broken or considered by another to be insignificant.
    4. Logic generally does not reduce a client's concern; the client needs to feel in control, and this action does not support this need.
    5. **Requesting permission to enter the client's bedside cabinet allows the client to control the situation. The client can give or not give the nurse permission to return the equipment to the bedside cabinet.**

22. **TEST-TAKING TIP: The words *nursing assistant* are key words in the stem that direct attention to content.**
    1. Monitoring clients' tube feedings is the legal responsibility of the nurse, not the nursing assistant.
    2. **Nursing assistants are responsible for meeting clients' basic activities of daily living under the supervision of the nurse.**
    3. Regulating clients' IV solutions is the legal responsibility of the nurse, not the nursing assistant.
    4. Assessment of clients is within the scope of practice of the nurse, not the nursing assistant.
    5. Assisting clients with taking medication is the legal responsibility of the nurse, not the nursing assistant.

23. **Answer: Following the nursing process of assessment, diagnosis, planning, implementing, and evaluation, the correct steps are 5, 1, 4, 3, 2.**

    Refer to the Ethical Decision-Making Algorithm indicated below, which highlights the steps in the question as they appear in the algorithm.

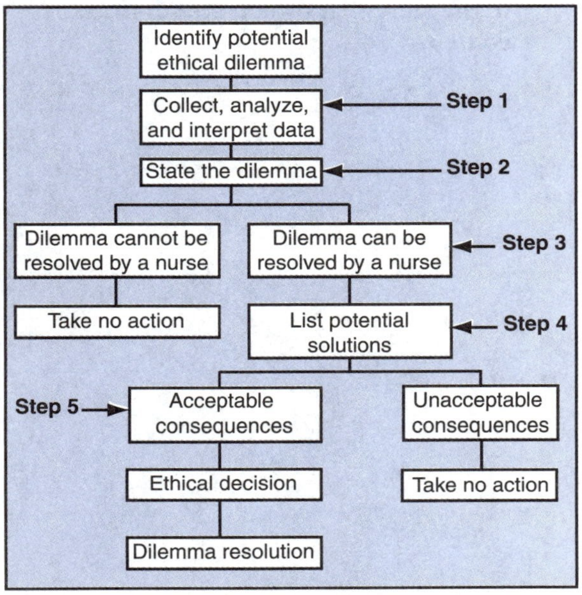

24. **TEST-TAKING TIP: The words *intentional tort* are key words in the stem that direct attention to content.**
   1. This is an unintentional tort. The nurse did not intentionally forget to administer the STAT medication.
   2. **This action is an intentional tort. Intentionally touching a client's body or clothing or anything held by or attached to a client in an angry, willful, negligent, or violent manner without consent or providing treatment without informed consent is battery.**
   3. This is an unintentional tort. The medication was carelessly, not intentionally, administered to the wrong client.
   4. **This action is an intentional tort. Intentionally threatening to harm or touch a client in an insulting, unjustifiable, or offensive manner is assault.**
   5. This action is not an intentional tort. This is appropriate nursing care. A nurse may apply a restraint without a prescription from a primary health-care provider in an emergency when a client is at risk of hurting self or others. The nurse is obligated to seek a prescription from a primary health-care provider as soon as possible.

25. **TEST-TAKING TIP: The word *violate* in the stem indicates negative polarity. The question is actually asking "Which actions do NOT support a client's right to confidentiality and privacy?" The words *confidentiality* and *privacy* are key words in the stem that direct attention to content.**
   1. **Interviewing a client in the presence of others violates confidentiality; others may overhear information that should be kept confidential.**
   2. Documenting statements in the client's medical record is an acceptable practice.
   3. **The nurse legally is not permitted to divulge client information to anyone without the client's consent.**
   4. A team conference enables professionals to share important information about clients and is an acceptable practice.
   5. Sharing information at a change of shift report notifies nursing team members of the client's changing status and is an appropriate practice.
   6. **Performing a procedure without pulling a curtain or closing the door allows others to view the procedure, which violates the client's right to privacy.**

26.
   1. **An agency must have policies and procedures that ensure client safety. Safety of clients is a priority and includes freedom from abuse and neglect.**
   2. **Clients have a right to know the names of caregivers and their roles.**
   3. **The client is the center of the health-care team and should be involved in all health-care decisions.**
   4. **Clients have a right to accurate information about their diagnosis, treatment, and prognosis in terms they can understand.**
   5. **Clients have a right to refuse care against medical advice; the primary health-care provider must explain to the client the risks involved in lack of treatment.**

27. **TEST-TAKING TIP:** The word *most* in the stem sets a priority. For the "Occurrence Category," *HIPAA compliance* is the correct choice. For "Contributing Factors," *Nonadherence to standard of practice* is the correct choice. The nurse disclosed confidential information by inappropriately discussing the client's diagnosis with a third party, which the client construed as an invasion of privacy. This disclosure could subject the nurse to legal liability. Most health-care facilities require health-care workers to have HIPAA training and sign confidentiality agreements. The nurse's breach of duty, the invasion of privacy, caused emotional harm to the client and is considered malpractice.

Unusual Occurrence Report

Date of Event: ___________ **Time of Event:** ___________ **Department:** ___________________

Client Last Name:	**First Name:**	**MI:**
Client #:	**Attending Physician:**	
Visitor Last Name:	**First Name:**	**Phone #:**
Employee Name:	**Dept:**	
Physician Name:	**Specialty:**	

Occurrence Category (Check most appropriate)

☐ Agency nurse-related	☐ AMA	☐ Delay in treatment
☐ Diet-related	☐ HIPAA compliance	☐ Loss of personal property
☐ Medication-related	☐ Narcotics-related	☐ Order not executed
☐ Client injury	☐ Peer-review related	☐ Restraint-related
☐ Staff injury	☐ Supplies/Equipment	☐ Visitor injury
☐ Other (please explain):		

Description of Occurrence:

A client overheard a nurse sharing information about the client's diagnosis and treatment to a visitor in the hall. The client reported this event to the nurse in charge and stated, "I am very upset".

Contributing Factors (Check all that apply)

☐ Individual:	☐ System:
Knowledge, skills, and/or experience: ☐ Unclear ☐ Incomplete	Policies/procedures not in place: ☐ Unclear ☐ Outdated
☑ Non-adherence to standard of care or practice	Environmental: ☐ Staffing ☐ Client acuity ☐ Congestion
☐ Documentation incomplete or inadequate	Communications and work flow: ☐ Intradepartmental ☐ Interdepartmental
	☐ Equipment failure
Other (please explain):	

Submitted by:	**Dept:**	**Date:**

28. **TEST-TAKING TIP: The words *licensed practical nurse* in the stem direct attention to content.**

1. **Licensed practical nurses can administer enemas. This procedure is within their scope of practice.**
2. Licensed practical nurses cannot administer medication via the direct IV push technique. Also, they cannot administer IV antineoplastic medications or the initial bag of an IV solution. These situations have a risk of untoward client effects that a licensed practical nurse is not prepared to address.
3. **Licensed practical nurses can perform a venipuncture to obtain a blood specimen. Licensed practical nurses learn anatomy and physiology, sterile technique, and how to perform simple nursing procedures.**
4. **Licensed practical nurses can change dressings on wounds. Licensed practical nurse educational programs include the principles of sterile technique and uncomplicated sterile nursing procedures. The clinical data obtained during a dressing change must be reported to a registered nurse for evaluation and intervention if necessary.**
5. **Licensed practical nurses can assess clients to collect clinical data, but they cannot interpret the information or determine which clinical action is required.**

29. **TEST-TAKING TIP: The word *dependent* is the key word in the stem that directs attention to content.**

1. **Ambulation of a client requires a primary health-care provider's prescription. Client activity (e.g., bed rest, out of bed to chair, out of bed) is a dependent function of a nurse.**
2. Documenting nursing care is an independent function of the nurse and does not require a primary health-care provider's prescription.
3. **Dependent activities of the nurse are activities that require a primary health-care provider's prescription; changing a sterile dressing requires a primary health-care provider's prescription.**
4. In an emergency, a nurse may administer oxygen to a client experiencing acute shortness of breath until a primary health-care provider's prescription is obtained.
5. Selecting among choices of foods offered within a diet is an interdependent function; however, the type of diet is a dependent function.

30. **TEST-TAKING TIP: All written or spoken information about clients is considered confidential, including diagnosis, treatments, and past medical information. To release the client's health information for purposes other than treatment, payment, and routine health care, the client must sign an authorization. This authorization rule has three exceptions in which authorization is not required to release client information: public health activities, law enforcement and judicial proceedings, and issues concerning deceased persons.**

1. A celebrity is being treated in the facility after a car accident
2. **The medical record is needed for the investigation of a crime**
3. **A virus outbreak occurs among students at a local high school**
4. **Information is needed to identify victims of a tornado outbreak**
5. The adult child of a schizophrenic client wants to help care for their parent

31. **TEST-TAKING TIP: The words *nursing assistant* are key words in the stem that direct attention to content.**

1. **The nursing assistant is trained to identify major abnormal or unexpected signs and symptoms and to notify the nurse when they have changed from the client's baseline; the nurse then completes a professional assessment of the client's condition.**
2. It is illegal for the nursing assistant to administer drugs, even if done under the supervision of the nurse.
3. A nursing assistant should not be responsible for the supervision or orientation of other employees.
4. The nursing assistant is not prepared for this responsibility. Teaching requires a strong scientific knowledge base and an ability to use scientific teaching/learning principles when planning and implementing an educational plan.
5. **Nursing assistants are permitted to distribute meal trays to clients. They just have to verify the client's name against the name on the menu on the tray.**
6. **Obtaining routine vital signs is within the scope of practice of nursing assistants. Nurses should obtain the vital**

signs of clients who are unstable, clients who are going to or returning from a procedure, and clients who are being admitted or discharged from a unit or facility.

32. **TEST-TAKING TIP: The words *nursing process* are key words in the stem that direct attention to content.**

Answer: 2, 5, 4, 1, 3

2. **Assessment, the first step of the nursing process, involves collecting, verifying, and documenting client information/data; this includes vital signs and physical assessments.**
5. **Diagnosis, the second step of the nursing process, involves clustering and analyzing data and arriving at conclusions about the significance of the data.**
4. **Planning, the third step of the nursing process, involves setting goals, objectives, and expected outcomes. In addition, priorities of care are identified and interventions are planned to meet the goals, objectives, and expected outcomes.**
1. **Implementation, the fourth step of the nursing process, involves the actual delivery of nursing care. It includes activities such as executing the proposed plan of care, performing dependent and independent interventions, reacting to life-threatening/adverse responses, and communicating with or teaching clients.**
3. **Evaluation, the fifth step of the nursing process, involves identifying client responses to care, comparing actual client outcomes with expected outcomes, determining factors that affected outcomes, and modifying the plan of care if necessary.**

33. **TEST-TAKING TIP: The word *most* in the stem sets a priority.**

1. The *Falls* category demonstrates a downward trend in the number of events, indicating improvement. This indicates a positive trend and is not a cause for concern.
2. The *Medication errors* category demonstrates a downward trend in the number of events, indicating improvement. This indicates a positive trend and is not a cause for concern.
3. **The *Violations of confidentiality* category results should cause the most concern. The chart indicates that the number of events increased rather than decreased each month in spite of the implementation of a corrective action plan.**
4. The *Failures to maintain standards of nursing practice* category initially demonstrates improvement in April; however, it indicates an increase in events in May compared with April. Although this is a concern, it is not as alarming as the progressively negative trend demonstrated in another problem category.

34. **TEST-TAKING TIP: Identify the key word in the stem that directs attention to the content.**

1. **The client complains of tingling in their fingers and toes. This is subjective data because it is what the client says about themselves. The nurse cannot physically observe or assess tingling through measurement, inspection, palpation, percussion, or auscultation.**
2. **The client states their pain is a 5 on a scale of 1 to 10. This is subjective data because the client is relaying their pain through a self-assessment to the nurse but their actual pain cannot be validated on a pain scale.**
3. The client vomits three times within an hour. This is objective data. The nurse can physically observe the client vomiting.
4. The client's ankles and feet are swollen. This is objective data. The nurse can physically observe through inspection and palpation of the client's ankles and feet.
5. The client is crying with a rapid pulse. This is objective data. The nurse can observe the client crying and measure the client's pulse rate.
6. **The client says they are nauseous. This is subjective data because it is what the client says about themselves. Nausea cannot be assessed.**

35. **TEST-TAKING TIP: The words *unintentional tort* are key words in the stem that direct attention to content.**

1. A nurse is not obligated to stop at the scene of an accident to render first aid.
2. **This is an example of an unintentional tort. The nurse's lack of action failed to meet standards of care established by a job description, agency policy or procedures, the state's nurse practice act, or standards established by professional organizations, which caused the client to experience an injury.**

3. **This is an example of an unintentional tort. The nurse's lack of action failed to meet standards of care established by a job description, agency policy or procedures, the state's nurse practice act, or standards established by professional organizations, which caused the client to experience a life-threatening event.**
4. Although an unintentional injury occurred, there are no grounds for a tort because appropriate standards of care were followed.
5. This is not an unintentional tort. A client is not involved. This is associated with management. State nurse practice acts protect a nurse from suspension, termination, disciplinary action, and/or discrimination when refusing to do or not do something because he or she believes it is inappropriate and could be harmful.

36. **TEST-TAKING TIP: The words *registered nurse* are the key words in the stem that direct attention to content.**
1. **Evaluating client responses to medications is the responsibility of a licensed nurse. Nursing assistants do not have the educational background related to the expected and nontherapeutic effects of medications.**
2. Nursing assistants are taught to follow medical aseptic principles when performing basic skills, such as emptying the collection bag of a urinary retention catheter.
3. **Obtaining a specimen of exudate from a draining wound involves the use of sterile technique. The use of sterile technique is beyond the scope of practice of a nursing assistant.**
4. **Nurses must take the vital signs of unstable clients because of the multitude of factors that can affect vital signs. Nursing assistants are capable of taking the vital signs of clients who are stable. Obtained vital signs are then reported to the registered nurse, who evaluates the values obtained by the nursing assistant.**
5. **Teaching clients range-of-motion exercises is within the scope of practice of nurses because it requires knowledge of anatomy and physiology and teaching principles.**

37. **TEST-TAKING TIP: The word *most* in the stem sets a priority.**
1. **Each client in an independent living facility has a separate apartment. It can be as small as one room with a kitchenette, sitting area, and sleeping area or as large as a one-, two-, or three-room apartment. These facilities usually provide two or three meals a day and social activities. This client has difficulty getting to the store, is bored with meal preparation, is lonely, and has ample financial resources. An independent living facility can best meet the client's needs after discharge from the hospital.**
2. An assisted-living facility is unnecessary for this client at this time. This client is capable of performing her own activities of daily living (e.g., bathing, toileting, and dressing), and she prefers privacy. This type of facility may be appropriate in the future if her emphysema or arthritis is progressively debilitating.
3. Most day-care programs function only 5 days a week and may require clients to supply their own transportation to and from the program. Also, many day-care programs are designed for cognitively impaired individuals. No data indicate that this client is cognitively impaired.
4. This client does not require the services of a nursing home. The client is able to perform activities of daily living and has no health problems that require either skilled nursing care or custodial nursing care.

38. **TEST-TAKING TIP: The words *implemented independently* are key words in the stem that direct attention to content.**
1. **Taking the vital signs provides important information about the overall status of the client and is an independent function of a nurse.**
2. The intake of fluid and food requires a prescription by the primary health-care provider and is a dependent function of the nurse.
3. **Pulse oximetry is a noninvasive procedure that measures the oxygen saturation level in the blood. It is commonly used to assess the oxygen status of a client, the effect of medications on the respiratory system, and a client's tolerance to a change in activity level. Pulse oximetry does not require a prescription by a primary health-care provider and is within the scope of independent nursing practice.**
4. **The high Fowler position facilitates respirations by using gravity to lower abdominal organs away from the**

diaphragm, thereby improving expansion of the thoracic cavity on inspiration. The greater expansion of the thoracic cavity facilitates gas exchange, promoting oxygenation of body cells. Positioning clients appropriately is an independent function of the nurse and does not require a prescription by a primary health-care provider.

5. **Assessing a client's lung sounds is an independent function of the nurse. Identifying various breath sounds, such as rales, rhonchi, stridor, or wheezing, can assist the primary health-care provider in planning medical intervention. In addition, nurses can evaluate the outcomes of interventions such as position changes; encouragement of coughing; increased fluid intake; and nebulizer treatments and other medications, such as bronchodilators, on the basis of improvement or lack of improvement in breath sounds.**

39.
1. **This goal statement is specific and measurable and contains a time frame. "Thirty minutes after the administration of an analgesic" is the time frame.**
2. This statement identifies an intervention in response to an identified problem, not a goal.
3. This statement identifies a client need, not a goal.
4. This statement is an inference about the client's status, not a goal.
5. This statement is incomplete because it does not have a time frame.

40. **TEST-TAKING TIP: The words *nursing assistant* are key words in the stem that direct attention to content.**

1. Evaluating vital signs requires professional nursing judgment. The nurse, not the nursing assistant, is educationally prepared to determine the significance of vital sign measurements.
2. **Making occupied and unoccupied beds is within the role of nursing assistants. Nursing assistants are taught to perform this activity safely.**
3. It is not legal for a nursing assistant to monitor tube feedings; this action is within the legal practice of a licensed nurse.
4. **Helping clients to eat a meal is within the scope of practice of a nursing assistant. Nursing assistants often help clients with activities of daily living.**
5. **Nursing assistants are trained to provide basic hygiene measures under the direction of a nurse.**
6. Nurses should ambulate postoperative clients for the first time after surgery; nurses have the knowledge to analyze a client's response to ambulation postoperatively. Nursing assistants can ambulate clients who have simple, noncomplex needs.

COMMON THEORIES RELATED TO MEETING CLIENTS' BASIC HUMAN NEEDS

This section includes questions related to the work of theorists such as Kübler-Ross, Maslow, Selye, Dunn, Engel, Kohlberg, and Erikson. It also includes questions related to principles of teaching, growth and development, and stress and adaptation and the definition of health.

QUESTIONS

1. A 78-year-old male client who fell and fractured his hip while shoveling snow states, "Leave me alone. I do not need help and can take care of myself like I have been doing for years." According to Erikson's Theory of Psychosocial Development, how should the nurse proceed?

1. Plan interventions to help the client contribute to society.
2. Plan interventions to foster a sense of fulfillment and purpose.
3. Plan interventions to initiate new learning so the client can care for himself.
4. Plan interventions for the client to establish his identity and sense of direction.

TEST-TAKING TIP: Identify key words in the stem that direct attention to content.

2. A nurse is teaching a client with diabetes mellitus how to self-monitor blood glucose levels. What is the **most** important factor when predicting the success of a teaching program regarding the learning of this skill?

1. Interest of the learner
2. Extent of family support
3. Amount of reinforcement
4. Level of learner's cognitive ability

TEST-TAKING TIP: Identify the word in the stem that sets a priority. Identify clang associations.

3. The emergency department nurse is using development theories while precepting a new nurse about caring for clients of all ages and stages of development. Which statements reflect key points of developmental theories? **Select all that apply.**

1. Health status influences growth and development.
2. People are only sometimes orderly and predictable.
3. There are no definitive stages of developmental theory.
4. The progress and behaviors of a person within each developmental stage are unique.
5. Heredity and the emotional and physical environment influence growth and development.

TEST-TAKING TIP: Identify equally plausible options.

4. A 22-year-old client is undergoing intensive physical and occupational therapy after an automobile accident. The client needs assistance dressing, brushing their teeth, and eating. Using Orem's theory as a guide, the nurse develops interventions with the understanding that:

1. emphasis is on the ill person in the health-care setting.
2. nursing is concerned with promoting and restoring health.
3. people are in a constant relationship with environmental stressors.
4. self-care is a human need and self-care deficits require nursing actions.

5. The nurse is interviewing the wife of a client who died 2 weeks ago. The wife states, "I go to the cemetery every day and say several prayers." According to Engel's model of grieving, which stage of grieving is the client exhibiting?

1. Developing awareness
2. Resolving the loss
3. Idealization
4. Restitution

TEST-TAKING TIP: Identify key words in the stem that direct attention to content.

6. The health-care organization is researching how its nurses use theory combined with clinical reasoning to provide efficient and high-quality care. Knowing that theory guides all steps of the nursing process, identify how theory is used during the nursing process. **Select all that apply.**
   1. To plan and implement care
   2. To collect and organize client data
   3. To alter the provider's plan of care
   4. To describe and explain desired outcomes
   5. To understand, analyze, and interpret client's health

   TEST-TAKING TIP: Identify key words in the stem that direct attention to content.

7. The nurse is obtaining the psychosocial history of a client. When theories about stress are considered, which event generally precipitates the **highest** degree of stress?
   1. Marriage
   2. Pregnancy
   3. Relocation
   4. Retirement

   TEST-TAKING TIP: Identify the word in the stem that sets a priority. Identify the key word in the stem that directs attention to content.

8. The nurse is collecting information to prepare a teaching plan for a client with type 1 diabetes. Which question asked by the nurse is associated with collecting information in the cognitive domain of learning?
   1. "How do you inspect your feet each day?"
   2. "Can you measure a serum glucose level?"
   3. "What do you know about your diabetes?"
   4. "Are you able to perform a subcutaneous injection?"

   TEST-TAKING TIP: Identify the key word in the stem that directs attention to content. Identify the unique option. Identify the clang association.

9. The nurse is planning teaching for a newly diagnosed diabetic client who will need to self-inject insulin daily. The nurse knows that the teaching should do what? **Select all that apply.**
   1. Be taught by video and discussion
   2. Consider the client's educational level
   3. Be developed in collaboration with the health-care team
   4. Only focus on self-injection and not include lifestyle modifications
   5. Include the client but not family members since the client will be self-injecting

10. The nurse identifies that a client has been exposed to the stress of air pollution caused by a wood-burning fireplace in the home. Which classification of stress is air pollution?
    1. Physical
    2. Chemical
    3. Physiological
    4. Microbiological

11. The nurse is caring for a terminally ill teenager. The nurse's knowledge of grief theories helps them to understand the complex physical, psychological, and social reactions the client may experience. Using this knowledge, the nurse knows that which of the following is not associated with the usual process of grieving?
    1. Talking about the illness
    2. Seeking alternative therapies
    3. Becoming angry with people
    4. Attempting to commit suicide

    TEST-TAKING TIP: Identify the word in the stem that indicates negative polarity. Identify key words in the stem that direct attention to content.

12. The nurse is assessing a client coping with multiple stresses and knows that one body system has a major impact on how the client responds to stress. Which body system should the nurse assess **first** because it primarily controls the general adaptation syndrome?
   1. Endocrine
   2. Respiratory
   3. Integumentary
   4. Cardiovascular

TEST-TAKING TIP: Identify the word in the stem that sets a priority. Identify key words in the stem that direct attention to content.

13. The home health nurse is educating a new client on the plan of care to help the client achieve and maintain an optimal level of health. During the education, the client asks the nurse, "What do you mean by health?" Which concept should the nurse consider when answering the client's question?
   1. Health is the absence of disease.
   2. Health is a progressive state moving in one direction.
   3. Health is an extreme of the wellness-illness continuum.
   4. Health is individualized and relative to one's value system.

TEST-TAKING TIP: Identify key words in the stem that direct attention to content. Identify the client-centered option.

14. The nurse is planning to provide personal health-care information to several clients. The client the nurse should anticipate will be **most** motivated to learn is the:
   1. 55-year-old woman who had a mastectomy and is very anxious about her body image.
   2. 66-year-old man who had a heart attack last week and is requesting information about exercise.
   3. 22-year-old man who smokes two packs of cigarettes and is in denial about the dangers of smoking.
   4. 47-year-old woman who has a long-leg cast after sustaining a broken leg and is still experiencing severe pain.

TEST-TAKING TIP: Identify the word in the stem that sets a priority.

15. The 69-year-old diabetic client with a new below-the-knee amputation tells the nurse, "I just want to die. I can't walk, I can't go outside, I can't do anything." Based on Orem's Self-Care Theory, what should the nurse do first?
   1. Encourage the client
   2. Strategize ways to help the client with self-care
   3. Explore the client's feelings about the amputation
   4. Meet with the client's family to learn about them before the amputation

TEST-TAKING TIP: Identify the word in the stem that sets a priority.

16. A client with type 2 diabetes and restrictive airway disease comes to the emergency department of the hospital because of a productive cough and fever. The client is diagnosed with pneumonia and is admitted for treatment. During the admission health history the client tells the nurse, "I work full-time as a high school English teacher, and I am very healthy." Which is the **most** important intervention by the nurse during the client's hospitalization?
   1. Explain why the client is really not well.
   2. Identify the client's perception of the sick role.
   3. Foster client independence concerning self-care.
   4. Give the client written materials about the identified illness.

TEST-TAKING TIP: Identify the word in the stem that sets a priority. Identify the option that denies client feelings, concerns, or needs. Identify the client-centered option.

17. During a yearly physical examination, a nurse is interviewing an adolescent about preferred activities. Which activity is associated with the developmental task of adolescence? **Select all that apply.**
1. _____ Texting friends
2. _____ Reading a book
3. _____ Learning how to use a computer
4. _____ Helping parents with household chores
5. _____ Attending a high school basketball game

TEST-TAKING TIP: Identify the key word in the stem that directs attention to content.

18. Which client factor does the nurse consider relevant when assessing a client's readiness to learn about smoking cessation? **Select all that apply.**
1. _____ Perceived positive outcomes
2. _____ Lack of barriers to actions
3. _____ Internal locus of control
4. _____ Identified need
5. _____ Motivation

19. What should the nurse do to meet a client's basic physiological needs? **Select all that apply.**
1. _____ Raise the side rails
2. _____ Provide a bed bath
3. _____ Converse with the client
4. _____ Explain procedures to the client
5. _____ Ambulate the client to the bathroom

TEST-TAKING TIP: Identify the key word in the stem that directs attention to content.

20. The community health nurse is meeting with a client whose spouse recently died of cancer. The client is the sole support for a 3-year-old child who is developmentally disabled. The client complains of unexplained weight loss and ongoing stomach pain. Using the illustration below, how does the nurse best explain to the client how the concepts of stress and adaptation may be causing his symptoms?

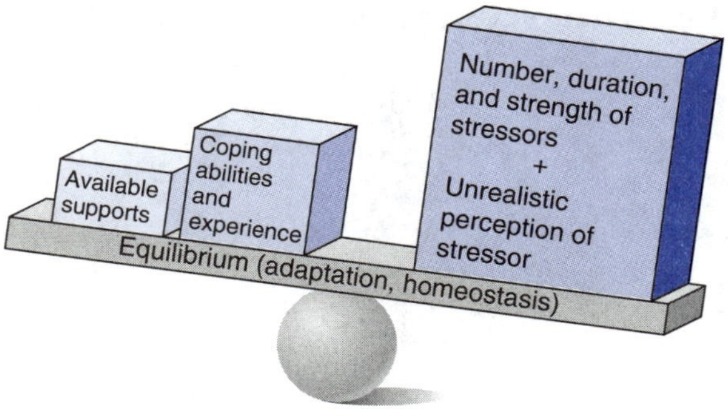

1. Adaptation is independent of a person's age or past experiences.
2. Psychological stress does not contribute to adaptation and homeostasis.
3. Coping mechanisms and support systems are independent to achieve equilibrium.
4. Response to stress depends on intensity of stress, support systems, and coping mechanisms.

TEST-TAKING TIP: Identify the word in the stem that sets a priority.

21. A mentally disadvantaged adult client is learning self-care. What should the nurse do to help the client **increase** learning? **Select all that apply.**
1. _____ Verbally recognize when goals are met
2. _____ Use demonstration as a teaching strategy
3. _____ Disregard the behavior when goals are not met
4. _____ Set one short-term objective at a time to be met
5. _____ Conduct several short teaching sessions for each skill

TEST-TAKING TIP: Identify the options that are opposites.

22. The nurse refers to Maslow's hierarchy of needs when assessing a client. Place the following client statements reflecting basic needs in order from the most to the least basic.
1. "How soon are visiting hours so that my family can visit me?"
2. "Promise me that someone will answer my call bell when I ring."
3. "I would like you to help me with the arrangements for my funeral."
4. "Can you please close the door when you help me to the bathroom?"
5. "I have been sitting here a long time, and I am very thirsty. Can I have a glass of water?"

Answer: ____________

TEST-TAKING TIP: Identify the key words in the stem that direct attention to content.

23. Lawrence Kohlberg's theory of stages of moral development is based on the ability to think at progressively higher levels as one matures. Place the following motivations for thinking in the order in which one advances from a basic to a higher level of moral development.
1. Adhering to societal standards while individualizing values and beliefs
2. Using abstract reasoning based on universal ethical principles
3. Pleasing others according to what they expect
4. Performing actions according to rules
5. Fearing negative consequences
6. Wanting positive consequences

Answer: ____________

TEST-TAKING TIP: Identify key words in the stem that direct attention to content.

24. Which of the following client levels of wellness does the nurse determine **best** represents the placement of the X on Dunn's Health Grid?

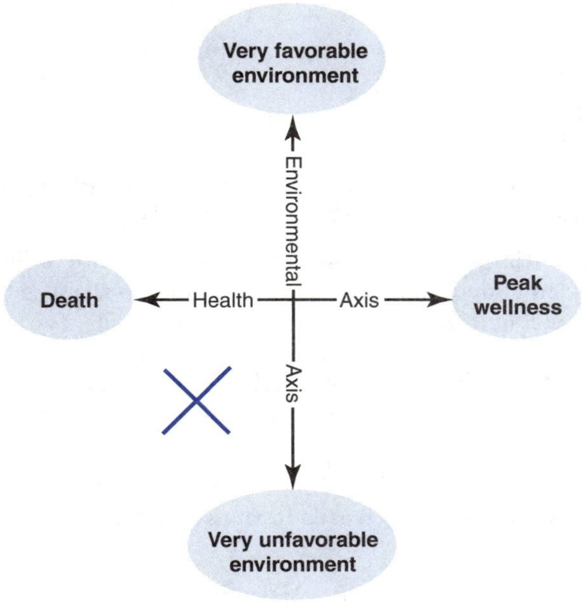

1. A person with emphysema and a history of a brain attack with left-sided weakness who lives in a nursing home while receiving respiratory rehabilitation
2. A relatively healthy person who is recovering from the birth of a stillborn and who shares a small apartment with several other unrelated individuals
3. A teenager who recently recovered from a fractured femur and lives with caring parents in a middle-class family home
4. A person who is receiving treatment at the local clinic for cirrhosis of the liver and who lives in an abandoned van

25. The nurse is caring for an 11-year-old child who was recently diagnosed with type 1 diabetes. The nurse encourages the child to practice using the equipment associated with diabetes. Which additional intervention should the nurse implement to support this client? **Select all that apply.**

1. _____ Identify non–age-appropriate behavior and gently suggest corrective actions.
2. _____ Explain that expressing feelings of sadness and anger is acceptable.
3. _____ Provide honest, concrete, and detailed answers to questions.
4. _____ Assign the client to a private room if available.
5. _____ Encourage visits from peers and siblings.

TEST-TAKING TIP: Identify client-centered options. Identify options that deny client feelings, concerns, or needs.

26. Place the following statements made by a client with a terminal illness in order according to Kübler-Ross's five stages of grief in death and dying.

1. "I will never see my grandchildren grown up and married."
2. "I will give up my cigars to see my grandchild born this summer."
3. "I'm working on a tape recording that I'm making for my grandchildren."
4. "I'm getting another opinion because I was told 3 months ago everything was fine."
5. "I cannot believe the doctor missed the tumor 3 months ago when I was last examined."

Answer: ____________

TEST-TAKING TIP: Identify key words in the stem that direct attention to content.

27. Which **most** clearly reflects a physiological need according to Maslow's hierarchy of needs? **Select all that apply.**
   1. _____ Fever
   2. _____ Trauma
   3. _____ Puberty
   4. _____ Restraints
   5. _____ Menopause
   6. _____ Dehydration

   TEST-TAKING TIP: Identify the word in the stem that sets a priority. Identify key words in the stem that direct attention to content.

28. The nurse is admitting a new resident to the long-term care facility. What steps should be included to determine the resident's ability to adapt to their new environment? **Select all that apply.**
   1. _____ Assess physical, sensory, and cognitive status.
   2. _____ Assess their beliefs and past experiences with health care.
   3. _____ Avoid discussions about family while the resident settles in.
   4. _____ Provide information on meals, visiting hours, and scheduled activities.
   5. _____ Allow the resident to decide the expected outcomes of the plan of care.

   TEST-TAKING TIP: Identify key words in the stem that direct attention to content.

29. During staff education on ethics and morals, the nurse manager is explaining Kohlberg's Theory of Moral Development. Which statement reflects components of this theory? **Select all that apply.**
   1. _____ Some people live by their own morals and ethics without conforming to societal norms.
   2. _____ If the majority follows social conventions, society can function morally and ethically.
   3. _____ The morality of the chosen action is compared to society's idea of what morality is.
   4. _____ Judgment of the morality of the action is based on its consequences.
   5. _____ People can agree to disagree while still respecting each other.
   6. _____ Treat people how you would like to be treated.

30. The nurse is caring for a variety of clients on a medical unit in the hospital. In which order should the nurse perform the following actions using Maslow's hierarchy of needs as the basis for prioritizing care?
   1. Administering 2 liters of oxygen via a nasal cannula
   2. Encouraging a family member to visit as often as desired
   3. Arranging for a minister to visit when requested by a client
   4. Asking a client about personal preferences before beginning care
   5. Placing the call bell within easy reach after a client is transferred to a chair

   Answer: ____________

   TEST-TAKING TIP: Identify key words in the stem that direct attention to content.

31. Which statement is associated with the task of generativity versus stagnation according to Erikson's developmental theory? **Select all that apply.**
   1. _____ "I want to do it myself."
   2. _____ "I will be getting married next week."
   3. _____ "I am pleased with the decisions I have made."
   4. _____ "I am volunteering at my local homeless shelter."
   5. _____ "I am teaching my children how to manage their money."

   TEST-TAKING TIP: Identify the key words in the stem that direct attention to content.

32. A nurse is completing a health history for a 90-year-old woman who is being admitted to a home health-care program. The client has Parkinson disease and stage 3 lung cancer that currently is in remission. The client says that she is able to get around all right as long as she stops frequently to catch her breath. She further explains that, other than knowing that she has cancer, she feels that "healthwise, I'm in pretty good shape." She says her children insist that she get help with bathing several mornings a week but says, "I don't feel that I need any help."

The primary health-care provider's history and physical examination states that the client's activities of daily living are significantly impaired as a result of the Parkinson disease and she may have less than 6 months to live. Where should the nurse place an X on the Health-Illness Continuum to reflect the client's perception of her health?

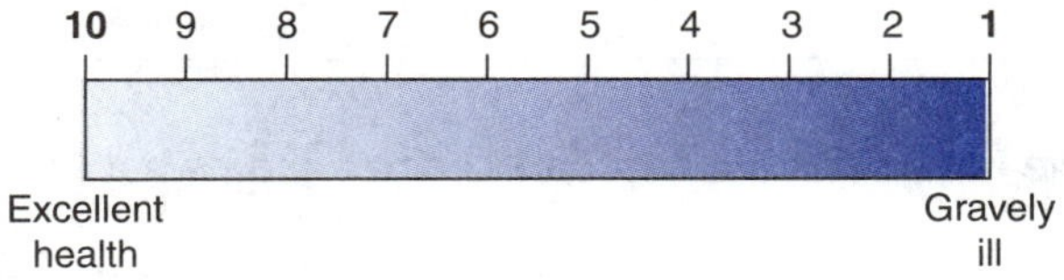

33. A nurse provides preoperative teaching for a client scheduled for surgery. What should the nurse do to ensure that the client understands the content of the teaching session? **Select all that apply.**

1. _____ Use simple vocabulary
2. _____ Obtain a return demonstration
3. _____ Ask the client what was learned
4. _____ Speak distinctly when giving directions
5. _____ Talk slowly when speaking with the client

TEST-TAKING TIP: Identify the clang association. Identify client-centered options.

34. The nurse is admitting the child in this photograph to the hospital for testing and treatment. Which should the nurse implement when caring for this child? **Select all that apply.**

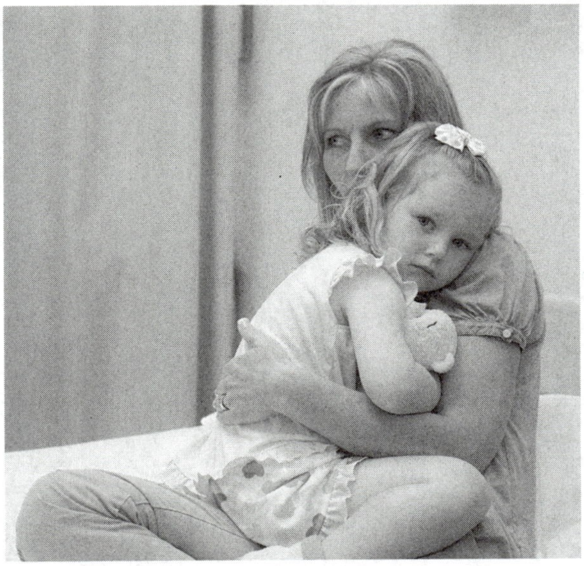

1. _____ Explain to the child that an intervention may "hurt" but that medicine can be given to make the "hurt" go away
2. _____ Use a doll to explain what is going to be done and why in terms that the child can understand
3. _____ Encourage the parent to stay with the child as much as possible
4. _____ Examine the child while she is sitting on her mother's lap
5. _____ Remind the child that she is a big girl

TEST-TAKING TIP: Identify the option that denies client feelings, concerns, or needs. Identify client-centered options.

35. The nurse is caring for a female client who is dying and her family members. The nurse has verbal interactions, listed below, with the client and several family members, who tend to hover around the client. Which is the **best** nursing action on the basis of client and family member statements?
1. Reinforce with the client the son's desire for his mother to keep on fighting.
2. Explain to the granddaughter that she should focus on her grandmother.
3. Help family members to understand the client's need to withdraw.
4. Tell the husband about bereavement counseling that is available.

Client
"I know my time is up. Everyone is hanging around and talking to me. I am so tired. I just want to rest."

Client's Husband
"We are so in love, and we have been a great team. I don't know what I am going to do when this is over."

Client's Son
"My mother was a strong independent woman all her life. I keep telling her to fight."

Client's Granddaughter
"My grandmother has been a fabulous grandmother. I am getting married in 3 weeks, and I want her at the ceremony."

TEST-TAKING TIP: Identify the word in the stem that sets a priority. Identify the unique option. Identify the central person in the question. Identify the client-centered option. Identify options with clang associations.

MON THEORIES RELATED TO MEETING CLIENTS' IC HUMAN NEEDS ANSWERS AND RATIONALES

1. **TEST-TAKING TIP: The age of the client should direct attention to content.**
   1. This is Erikson's Generativity versus Stagnation (Middle Adulthood) stage. This stage focuses on involvement with family, friends, and community and the desire to make a contribution to society. Failure to do so may cause stagnation and the client may regress to earlier levels of coping.
   2. **This is Erikson's Ego Integrity versus Despair (Older Adulthood) stage. At this stage, a person reminisces about their life to provide a sense of fulfillment and purpose. If they feel they have not achieved or cannot maintain their goals, they may experience despair. Interventions to foster fulfillment and purpose are appropriate at this stage.**
   3. This is Erikson's Initiative versus Guild (Preschool) stage. Preschoolers gain confidence and take initiative in learning. They seek out new experiences and want to understand the hows and whys of the way things work.
   4. This is Erikson's Identity versus Role Confusion (Adolescence) stage. In this stage, adolescents formulate a sense of self and decide what direction they want to proceed in life.

2. **TEST-TAKING TIP: The word *most* in the stem sets a priority. The word *learning* in the stem and the words *learner* in option 1 and *learner's* in option 4 are clang associations.**
   1. **The motivation of the learner to acquire new attitudes, information, or skills is the most important component for successful learning; motivation exists when the learner recognizes the future benefits of learning.**
   2. Although family support is important, it is not the most important factor for successful learning of a skill; some clients do not have a family support system.
   3. Although reinforcement is important, it is not the most significant factor in learning.
   4. Although a teaching program must be designed within the client's developmental and cognitive abilities, to be most successful the client should recognize the value of what is to be learned.

3. **TEST-TAKING TIP: Think about Erikson's Stages of Development and Maslow's Hierarchy of Needs for developmental theory.**
   1. **Health status influences growth and development, thus ill health negatively influences growth and development.**
   2. Developmental theory states that there are people who are orderly and predictable, starting with birth and ending with death.
   3. Developmental theorists state that there are definitive stages a person experiences with each stage helping people to learn to interact with the world.
   4. **The progress and behaviors in a stage are unique to each person. Successes and failures in each stage influence following stages.**
   5. **Heredity, individuality, life experiences, and the emotional and physical environment all influence the growth and development of a person.**

4. 1. This is Myra Levine's Theory of the Conservation Model of Nursing. The client is the center of nursing activities with care provided to conserve the client's energy and adapt to their environment.
   2. This is Jean Watson's Theory of Caring. Care is holistic and developed through interpersonal relationships.
   3. This is Betty Newman's System Model Theory stating that nursing must keep a client's system stable through assessment of environmental stressors and helping the client to adjust.
   4. **This is Orem's Self-Care Deficit Theory. This theory focuses on each client's ability to perform self-care. Nurses should develop interventions to provide self-care activities to help sustain health or recover from illness and injury.**

5. **TEST-TAKING TIP: The words *Engel's model of grieving* are key words in the stem that direct attention to content.**
   1. During the *developing awareness stage* of Engel's model of grieving, people begin to internalize the loss, and psychological pain is experienced.
   2. During the *resolving the loss stage* of Engel's model of grieving, people center their energy on thoughts and beliefs about the deceased.
   3. During the *idealization stage* of Engel's model of grieving, people initially repress negative thoughts and feelings about the deceased. Later in this stage, people tend to

incorporate some unique characteristics of the deceased into their own personalities.

4. **According to Engel's model of grieving, the wife is in the restitution stage of grieving. During the *restitution stage*, grieving people are involved with religious practices and rituals.**

6. 1. **In today's health-care environment, nurses must demonstrate efficient care within a health-care delivery system. Theory helps nurses develop nursing diagnoses to plan interventions beneficial to the client.**
   2. **Theory guides nurses to determine what client data are relevant and what should be collected during an assessment.**
   3. Altering a provider's plan of care is not within a nurse's scope of practice.
   4. **Nursing theory and concepts within theories help determine client outcomes that are client-centered and holistic.**
   5. **Four concepts common to all nursing theories are person, environment, health, and nursing. Using these concepts, nurses can analyze client data to choose interventions and outcomes that are individualized to meet client needs and to promote health.**

7. **TEST-TAKING TIP: The word *highest* in the stem sets a priority. The word *stress* is the key word in the stem that directs attention to content.**
   1. **Holmes and Rahe (1967) determined stress units for life events according to the readjustment required by individuals to adapt to the particular situations or events. The mean stress unit for marriage is 50, which is more than the unit for the other options presented.**
   2. The mean stress unit for pregnancy is 40, which is less than the unit for the correct answer.
   3. The mean stress unit for a change in residence is 20, which is less than the unit for the correct answer.
   4. The mean stress unit for retirement is 45, which is less than the unit for the correct answer.

8. **TEST-TAKING TIP: The word *cognitive* is the key word in the stem that directs attention to content. Option 3 is unique because it is the only option that is concerned with "what is" rather than "how to." Options 1, 2, and 4 all relate to the performance of a skill. The word *diabetes* in the stem and in option 3 is a clang association.**
   1. This statement focuses on the performance of a skill, inspecting the feet, which relates to the psychomotor, not the cognitive, domain.
   2. This statement focuses on the performance of a skill, measuring a serum glucose level, which relates to the psychomotor, not the cognitive, domain.
   3. **Knowledge about type 1 diabetes is in the cognitive domain because it deals with the comprehension of information.**
   4. This statement focuses on the performance of a skill, administering a subcutaneous injection, which relates to the psychomotor, not the cognitive, domain.

9. 1. The newly diagnosed diabetic needs to master certain self-care skills such as medication administration to properly manage their disease. Effective teaching for self-injection includes a teach-back demonstration to verify the client understands proper medication administration and can effectively self-inject insulin.
   2. **To be able to perform self-care activities, clients need the knowledge, attitude, and skills to maximize functioning. To maximize skills, the teaching must be at a level for the client to comprehend.**
   3. **Client education plans should include the health care team, including providers, dietitians, and pharmacists for coordination of care and ongoing follow-up.**
   4. Effective teaching is holistic and focuses on the whole disease process. Teaching is a powerful tool to help a client achieve their health goals and make informed health care decisions. It should teach knowledge about the disease process, self-care, and medication management.
   5. Family members should be included in client teaching because they may contribute to client decision making, can help improve client safety and compliance, and may need to assist the client in the future.

10. 1. Air pollution is not a physical stress; physical stresses include temperature, sound, pressure, light, motion, gravity, and electricity.
    2. **Burning wood releases toxic substances and gases into the air; these are considered chemical stresses. Acids, alkaline substances, drugs, and exogenous hormones also are considered chemical stresses.**

3. Air pollution is not a physiological stress; disturbances in the structure or function of any tissue, organ, or system of the body are considered physiological stresses.
4. Air pollution is not a microbiological stress; bacteria, viruses, molds, and parasites are considered microbiological stresses.

11. **TEST-TAKING TIP: You must identify the behavior that is not usually associated with the grieving process. The words *reactions* and *grieving* are key words in the stem that direct attention to content.**
    1. Although talking about the illness occurs throughout the grieving response, it is most expected during the early stage of disbelief (No, not me).
    2. Seeking alternative therapies occurs most often during the stage of bargaining (Yes me, but ...).
    3. Anger is expected and occurs when there is a developing awareness of the impending loss (Why me?).
    4. **Although some people who are terminally ill attempt suicide, it is not a typical or expected response to the stress of a terminal illness.**

12. **TEST-TAKING TIP: The word *first* in the stem sets a priority. The words *controls* and *general adaptation syndrome* are key words in the stem that direct attention to content.**
    1. **The general adaptation syndrome (GAS) involves primarily the endocrine system and autonomic nervous system; antidiuretic hormone, adrenocorticotropic hormone, cortisol, aldosterone, epinephrine, and norepinephrine are all involved with the fight-or-flight response.**
    2. The respiratory system does not control GAS. It is stimulated by a component of the syndrome.
    3. The integumentary system does not control GAS. It is stimulated by a component of the syndrome.
    4. The cardiovascular system does not control GAS. It is stimulated by a component of the syndrome.

13. **TEST-TAKING TIP: Option 4 is client-centered. Options 1, 2, and 3 relate to the disease process.**
    1. The World Health Organization's definition of health is "a state of complete physical, mental, and social well-being, and not merely the absence of disease or infirmity." Some people who have a chronic illness consider themselves healthy because they are able to function independently.
    2. Health fluctuates on a continuum between wellness and illness; movement can occur up or down the continuum. The nurse should consider the total person and environment to individualize nursing care.
    3. Although high-level wellness is one extreme of the wellness–illness continuum and severe illness the other, where a person plots a position on the continuum is based on the individual's value system.
    4. **A definition of health is highly individualized; it is based on each person's own experiences, values, and perceptions. Health can mean different things to different individuals; people tend to define health according to the presence or absence of symptoms, their perceptions of how they feel, and their capacity to function on a daily basis.**

14. **TEST-TAKING TIP: The word *most* in the stem sets a priority.**
    1. When a nurse is caring for a person who is coping with the diagnosis of cancer and a change in body image, the nurse should encourage the expression of feelings, not engage in teaching. High anxiety will interfere with learning.
    2. **A client who is requesting information is indicating a readiness to learn.**
    3. People in denial are not ready to learn because they do not admit they have a problem. In addition, young adults often believe they are invincible.
    4. A person who is in pain is attempting to cope with a physiological need. This client is not a candidate for teaching until the pain has been lessened; pain can preoccupy the client and prevent focusing on the information being presented.

15. **TEST-TAKING TIP: The word *first* in the stem sets a priority.**
    1. Creating an environment that promotes personal development to maintain autonomy is a key part of Orem's Self-Care Theory, but another step must be completed before doing this.
    2. Orem's theory suggests that clients recover easier and quicker if they have some independence over their self care. Strategizing interventions that can best accomplish this

are part of the planning process, not the first thing the nurse should do.

3. **Using therapeutic communication with the client develops the nurse-client relationship, which increases client participation in their care. Understanding the client's feelings provides an environment that promotes personal development.**
4. Though the nurse may meet with the client's family in the planning interventions, this is not a necessary step for the client to become autonomous.

16. **TEST-TAKING TIP: The word *most* in the stem sets a priority. Option 1 denies client feelings, concerns, or needs. The nurse is explaining that the client is "not well," whereas the client states, "I am very healthy." Option 3 is client-centered because it focuses on supporting the client's perception of being healthy, which is associated with independence.**
    1. This intervention is judgmental and argumentative and may cut off communication between the client and nurse.
    2. Although identifying the client's perception of the sick role may be done eventually by assessing the client's verbal and nonverbal interactions, it is not the priority.
    3. **The nurse should ensure that the client is as independent as possible to help the client avoid the sick role and maintain a positive self-concept. According to the Role Performance Model of Health, individuals who are able to fulfill their roles in life consider themselves healthy even though they may have an illness or disability.**
    4. Although the client may be given written materials about the identified illness, it is not the priority.

17. **TEST-TAKING TIP: The word *adolescent* is the key word in the stem that directs attention to content.**
    1. **Adolescents tend to associate with their peers as they begin to develop devotion and fidelity to others. According to Erikson's stages of psychosocial development, adolescence is concerned with Identity versus Role Confusion.**
    2. Middle childhood (6 to 12 years), not adolescence, is concerned with developing fundamental skills in reading and writing; the school-age child is very industrious.
    3. Middle childhood (6 to 12 years), not adolescence, is concerned with developing fundamental skills such as using a computer; the school-age child is very industrious.
    4. The childhood years, not adolescence, are related to helping behaviors; 3- to 5-year-olds like to imitate parents, and 6- to 12-year-olds are developing appropriate social roles.
    5. **Adolescents are concerned with developing new and more mature relationships with their peers; adolescents tend to associate with their peers rather than with their parents.**

18. 1. **When a person perceives that positive outcomes will occur as a result of learning, it provides motivation for the learning experience. It becomes a self-fulfilling prophecy.**
    2. **A person's potential for action depends on the benefits and barriers to taking action. When a person perceives that there are no barriers to change, then there is a readiness to learn.**
    3. **People who are motivated from within the self to achieve a goal (internal locus of control) are more ready to learn than people who are motivated by pressure or rewards from outside the self (external locus of control). People with an internal locus of control hold themselves responsible and believe that their actions can exert control over their lives. People with an external locus of control, who believe that control of circumstances is attributable to external factors such as other people or organizations, generally are less successful learners.**
    4. **Readiness to learn and motivation, which are closely tied together, are the two most important factors contributing to the success of any learning program. The learner must recognize that the learning need exists and that the material to be learned is valuable.**
    5. **Motivation is an essential element in readiness to learn. Motivation refers to a strong reason to engage in a specific activity to accomplish a goal. The more highly motivated a person is, the more likely the individual will have the desire, perseverance, and determination to engage in actions or make changes necessary to achieve the goal.**

19. **TEST-TAKING TIP: The word *physiological* is the key word in the stem that directs attention to content.**
   1. Raising side rails relates to the client's need for safety and security, the second level in Maslow's hierarchy of needs.
   2. **A bed bath supports the client's need to be clean and is related to physiological needs, the first level in Maslow's hierarchy of needs.**
   3. Conversing with a client relates to the need for love and belonging, the third level in Maslow's hierarchy of needs.
   4. Explaining procedures relates to the client's need for safety and security; clients have a right to know what is happening to them and why.
   5. **Elimination is a basic physiological need according to Maslow's hierarchy of needs. Basic needs relate to food, air, water, elimination, rest, sex, physical activity, temperature regulation, and cleanliness.**

20. **TEST-TAKING TIP: The word *best* in the stem sets a priority.**
   1. Adaptation is lower in the very young or very old who may not have the physiological reserves to cope. Past experiences may influence a person's perception of stress and change.
   2. Psychological stressors affect all dimensions of a person because humans want to feel loved, have a sense of belonging, feel safe and secure, and have self-esteem. To maintain well-being and health, psychological homeostasis must be maintained.
   3. Social factors, support systems, and coping mechanisms are interdependent when a person is attempting to achieve equilibrium.
   4. **Stressors for the client may include changes in family structure, feelings of helplessness and guilt, loss of control over normal routines. The client's response depends on the support system, coping mechanisms, and how long the client has been experiencing the stressors. People who have strong support systems and relationships can better adapt to stress.**

21. **TEST-TAKING TIP: Options 1 and 3 are opposites.**
   1. **Recognizing goal achievement supports feelings of self-esteem and independence; it provides external reinforcement and promotes internal reinforcement.**
   2. **Self-care requires performing skills; a demonstration and return demonstration use a variety of senses (e.g., sight, touch) that reinforce learning a psychomotor skill.**
   3. A client's behavior should never be disregarded; all behaviors should be addressed in a nonjudgmental and supportive manner.
   4. **A mentally disadvantaged person generally can focus on only one objective at a time; several may be overwhelming.**
   5. **Short sessions with a limited amount of information/practice may prevent a cognitively impaired person from becoming overwhelmed.**

22. **TEST-TAKING TIP: The words *Maslow's hierarchy of needs* are the key words in the stem that direct attention to content.**

   Answer: 5, 2, 1, 4, 3
   5. **This statement reflects the most basic level in Maslow's hierarchy of needs, which is physiological. This level is associated with concerns such as elimination, nutrition, rest and sleep, and oxygenation.**
   2. **This statement is associated with safety and security, a second-level need according to Maslow. Second-level needs are related to feeling safe from danger or risk and the need to feel secure in one's own environment.**
   1. **This statement is associated with love and belonging, a third-level need according to Maslow. Third-level needs relate to the need to feel worthy of affection and support and identification with a group.**
   4. **This statement indicates a need for privacy, which supports self-esteem, a fourth-level need according to Maslow. This level also includes the need to feel competent and respected.**
   3. **This statement indicates self-actualization, the highest-level need according to Maslow. Planning one's own funeral reflects reaching a stage of acceptance in the dying process. Acceptance is the highest level of achievement in the dying process according to Kübler-Ross. This demonstrates fulfillment of potential.**

23. **TEST-TAKING TIP: The words *Lawrence Kohlberg's theory of stages of moral***

development **are key words in the stem that direct attention to content.**

Answer: 5, 6, 3, 4, 1, 2

5. **Fearing negative consequences is the motivation for behavior that reflects the first stage of moral development—obedience and punishment.**
6. **Wanting positive consequences reflects the second stage of moral development—individualism and exchange.**
3. **Pleasing others based on what they expect reflects the third stage of moral development—interpersonal relationships.**
4. **Performing actions based on rules reflects the fourth stage of moral development—maintaining social order.**
1. **Adhering to societal standards while individualizing values and beliefs reflects the fifth stage of moral development—societal contracts and individual rights.**
2. **Using abstract reasoning based on universal ethical principles reflects the sixth stage of moral development—universal principles.**

24.

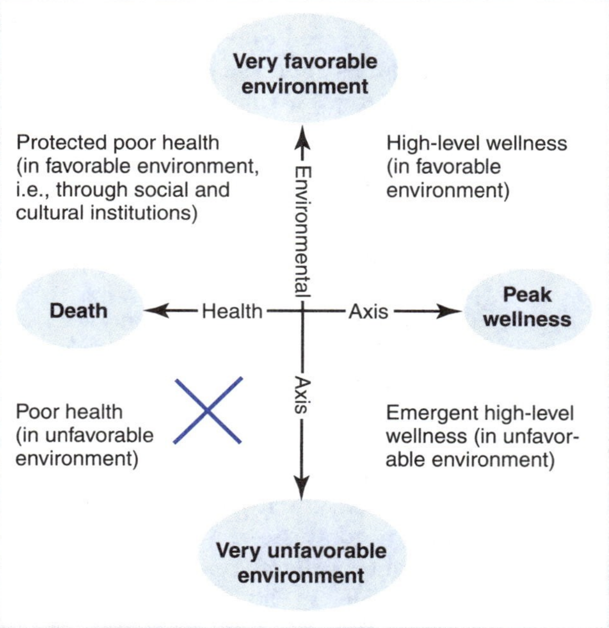

1. This client is in protected poor health and lives in a favorable environment. This person should be plotted on the upper left side of Dunn's Health Grid.
2. This person reflects emergent high-level wellness and lives in an unfavorable environment. This person should be plotted on the lower right side of Dunn's Health Grid.
3. This person reflects high-level wellness and lives in a favorable environment. This person should be plotted on the upper right side of Dunn's Health Grid.
4. **This person is in poor health and lives in an unfavorable environment. This person should be plotted on the lower left side of Dunn's Health Grid.**

25. TEST-TAKING TIP: Options 2 and 5 are client-centered options. Options 1, 3, and 4 deny client feelings, concerns, or needs.

1. The nurse should accept non–age-appropriate behaviors such as regression, resistance, or crying as long as they do not place the client or others in danger. These are features of illness in a child and should be accepted as normal reactions to hospitalization. The child needs to feel supported and accepted, not criticized.
2. **Explaining that expressing feelings of sadness and anger is acceptable gives the client permission to express these feelings in a nonjudgmental environment. These are expected reactions to grieving.**
3. Although honest and concrete answers to questions expressed by a school-age child are appropriate, too much detail can be overwhelming and should be avoided. A nurse should always ask if a client has any questions; if so, more detail can be provided on the basis of the questions asked.
4. A school-age child should be assigned to a room with an appropriate roommate when possible because socialization with peers is an important aspect of social development in this population. Also, roommates can engage in diversional activities such as crafts and board or electronic games.
5. **Encouraging visits from peers and siblings supports the client's need to maintain significant interpersonal relationships. These relationships support love and belonging needs.**

26. TEST-TAKING TIP: The words *Kübler-Ross's five stages of grief in death and dying* are key words in the stem that direct attention to content.

Answer: 4, 5, 2, 1, 3

4. **This statement indicates stage I—denial. The client is not ready to believe that something is wrong. During the denial stage, the client may be artificially cheerful, indifferent,**

or unable to deal with practical problems associated with the diagnosis or prognosis.

5. **This statement indicates stage II—anger. During the anger stage, the client may displace angry feelings onto the primary health-care provider, other caregivers, and/or loved ones. Also, clients may overreact to situations that generally would not have angered them before the loss.**
2. **This statement indicates stage III—bargaining. During the bargaining stage, the client may promise to change negative behaviors if just given more time.**
1. **This statement indicates stage IV—depression. During the depression stage, the client may withdraw and become isolated, or the client may grieve over past behavior or what will not happen.**
3. **This statement indicates stage V—acceptance. During the acceptance stage, the client has come to terms with the loss. However, that is not to say that the client is happy about the impending loss. Behaviors such as having decreased interest in supporting people or surroundings, making plans such as saying goodbye to significant others, getting financial affairs in order, or making funeral arrangements are associated with the acceptance stage.**

27. **TEST-TAKING TIP: The word *most* in the stem sets a priority. The words *Maslow's hierarchy of needs and physiological* are key words in the stem that direct attention to content.**
1. **An increase in body temperature (fever) is either the body's attempt to regain homeostasis or a response to an invading microorganism. It is a basic physiological response.**
2. **Trauma can be life threatening and can interfere with basic physiological functioning.**
3. Although physiological changes are associated with the growth spurt and the development of secondary sexual characteristics during puberty, self-identity and self-esteem often take priority at this time.
4. Restraints meet safety and security needs because they protect the client from harm.
5. Although physiological changes are associated with menopause, love, self-esteem, and self-actualization are often the priorities at this time.
6. **Loss of fluid without a significant loss of electrolytes, resulting in a hyperosmolar imbalance (dehydration), is a physiological problem. Dehydration can be caused by decreased fluid intake, loss of plasma or blood, diarrhea, vomiting, gastric decompression, sweating, adrenal insufficiency, or excessive urination (polyuria), which are all physiological issues.**

28. 1. **Methods to facilitate adaptation and reduce stress should be selected based on the resident's physical, sensory, and emotional characteristics to decrease stress and to facilitate coping.**
2. **Assessing beliefs and past experiences can help the nurse identify previously used coping mechanisms to tailor the plan of care to best support adaptation to the new environment.**
3. Plans of care should involve the resident's support systems and family to decrease anxiety and stress. Verbalizing feelings and discussing family should help decrease anxiety.
4. **Nurses use a variety of interventions to decrease stress and to facilitate coping. Providing information on meals, activities, and visiting hours are all interventions to support the resident and provide comfort.**
5. The expected outcomes for the plan of care should be mutually decided between the resident, the nurse, and the resident's support system and designed to reduce anxiety and promote adaptation.

29. 1. **According to Kohlberg's theory, some people may develop their own principles that may be different from accepted society norms. They believe their morals are right with some generally accepted societal morals wrong and even harmful.**
2. People understand their place in society and how society functions. According to Kohlberg's theory, people believe society can function as long as everyone follows accepted social conventions. Deviations place society in chaos.
3. **According to Kohlberg, this is a lower level of moral development where**

one judges their own actions by what society would think is moral.

4. **This is the lowest level of Kohlberg's theory where the judgment of the morality of the action is based on the action's consequences. Morality and judgment is based only on the consequences to themselves.**
5. **This is a higher level of moral development. People can have different opinions, rights, or values dependent on what society they live in or belong to. Even though people may have different morals and ethics, there should be a level of mutual respect.**
6. **This is midlevel development of moral reasoning, where a person begins conforming to accepted social standards and tries to do the "right thing." Persons in this level judge the morality of an action by how it affects other people and how they expect to be treated.**

30. **TEST-TAKING TIP:** **The words *Maslow's hierarchy of needs* are key words in the stem that direct attention to content.**

Answer: 1, 5, 2, 4, 3

1. **Administering 2 liters of oxygen via a nasal cannula—meeting basic physiological needs (e.g., patent airway, nutrition, elimination)—addresses first-level needs according to Maslow.**
5. **Arranging the call bell within easy reach after a client is transferred to a chair—promoting a feeling of safety and security—addresses second-level needs according to Maslow.**
2. **Encouraging a family member to visit as often as desired—maintaining support systems—provides for love and belonging needs, third-level needs according to Maslow.**
4. **Asking a client about personal preferences before beginning care—promoting self-control—supports self-esteem needs, fourth-level needs according to Maslow.**
3. **Arranging for a minister to visit when requested by a client—meeting spiritual needs—relates to self-actualization, the highest-level need according to Maslow.**

31. **TEST-TAKING TIP:** **The words *generativity versus stagnation* are the key words in the stem that direct attention to content.**

1. This statement relates to the conflict of autonomy versus shame and doubt. The 2- to 4-year-old seeks a balance between independence and dependence and attempts to achieve autonomy.
2. This statement relates to the conflict of intimacy versus isolation. The young adult, ages 20 to 30 years, seeks a partner for a life relationship.
3. This statement relates to the conflict of integrity versus despair. The person age 60 years or older struggles to feel a sense of worth about past experience and goals achieved and seeks a sense of integrity.
4. This statement relates to the conflict of generativity versus stagnation. Generativity is a concern for other people and caring for other people.
5. **This statement relates to the conflict of generativity versus stagnation. A parent is guiding children to be independent.**

32.

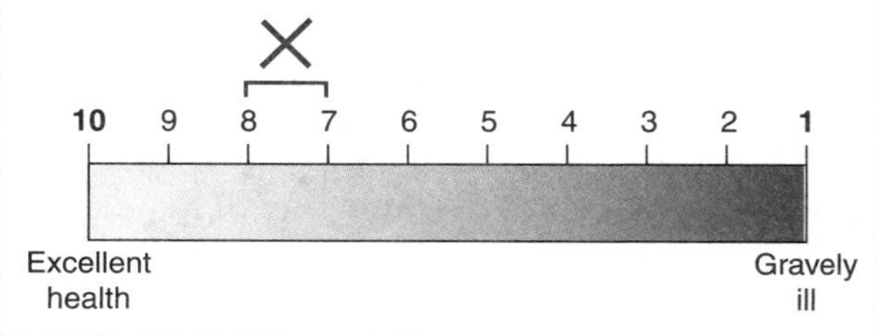

A nursing admission history and physical examination should reflect the physical and emotional status of the client and include her perception of her level of wellness. An X next to either number 7 or number 8 reflects the *client's perception of her level of wellness.* The client said that *she is able to get around alright as long as she stops frequently to catch her breath.* She went on to explain that other than knowing that she has cancer, she felt that *"healthwise, I'm in pretty good shape."* She said that the only reason she accepted home health care was because her children insisted that she get help with bathing several mornings a week, but she went on to say, *"I don't feel that I need any help."* The nurse may place the client lower on the Health-Illness Continuum; however, that would reflect the nurse's perception, not the client's perception.

33. **TEST-TAKING TIP:** **The word *understands* in the stem and the word *learned* in option 3 illustrate a covert clang association.**

Although they are different words, they have a similar meaning. Options 2 and 3 are client-centered because they are the only options that seek feedback from the client.

1. Using simple vocabulary helps to send a clearer message, but it does not inform the sender whether the receiver understood the message.
2. **When a client performs a return demonstration, the nurse can observe the exhibited technique. Incorrect actions can be corrected, and correct actions can be reinforced.**
3. **Seeking feedback enables the caregiver to know whether the message was understood as intended.**
4. Speaking distinctly when giving directions helps to send a clearer message, but it does not inform the sender whether the receiver understood the message.
5. Speaking slowly helps to send a clearer message, but it does not inform the sender whether the receiver understood the message.

34. **TEST-TAKING TIP: Option 5 denies client feelings, concerns, or needs because it is judgmental and intimidating. Option 5 denies the client's need to be a "little girl" supported by her mother. Options 1, 2, 3, and 4 are client-centered options.**

1. **Explaining that an intervention may "hurt" but that medicine can be given to make the "hurt" go away supports a trusting client-nurse rapport and reassures the child that care will be provided to support comfort.**
2. **Using a doll to explain what is going to be done and why in terms that the child can understand helps to reduce fear of the unknown.**
3. **Encouraging a parent to stay with the child as much as possible supports a child's need to feel safe, secure, and protected.**
4. **Examining the child while she is sitting on her mother's lap supports the child's need to feel safe, secure, and protected.**
5. Reminding the child that she is a big girl denies the child's potential need to regress to protect the ego.

35. **TEST-TAKING TIP: The word *best* in the stem sets a priority. Option 3 is unique because it includes all members of the family. Option 3 focuses on the needs of the client, who is the central person in the question, and is a client-centered option. All options contain clang associations; therefore, this technique is not helpful in selecting the correct answer: option 1—son, option 2—granddaughter, option 3—family members, option 4—husband.**

1. This is an inappropriate intervention. The nurse is meeting the son's needs rather than the client's needs.
2. Explaining to the granddaughter that she should focus on her grandmother is a judgmental response and may cut off further communication between the granddaughter and the nurse. The granddaughter is in the bargaining stage of grieving.
3. **Although the nurse is caring for family members as well as the client, the client must be the nurse's priority. The client is entering the acceptance stage of grieving and has decreased interest in environmental activities and people. The client needs a quiet, peaceful environment.**
4. Telling the husband about the availability of bereavement counseling at this time is premature. The nurse should first listen to the husband's feelings and concerns.

DIVERSITY AND SPIRITUALITY

This section includes questions associated with principles, concepts, and nursing care related to diversity/culture and spirituality/religion. Some questions are global in content, and others focus on specifics such as assessments of client feelings, needs, and concerns and nursing interventions supportive of clients' diversity and spirituality. Questions address topics such as caring for clients who do not accept blood transfusions, those who will accept care only from a caregiver of the same sex, and those experiencing spiritual distress. Additional questions are associated with xenophobia, racial diversity of the population of the United States, and situations related to various cultural beliefs and traditions.

QUESTIONS

1. The hospice nurse is caring for a client with stage IV ovarian cancer. The client tells the nurse, "Why is God so unfair? I thought I had a connection to God. I am being punished for not living a meaningful life." Which is the nurse's best response to this client?
   1. Tell the client that they have had a meaningful life.
   2. Call the provider to request a psychological evaluation.
   3. Request a spiritual consultation in the client's medical record.
   4. Ask the client to discuss their feelings and why they feel this way.

   TEST-TAKING TIP: Identify the priority words in the stem that direct attention to content.

2. A 6-month-old girl, who has a brother and sister who are 4 and 6 years of age, respectively, is admitted to the hospital with a diagnosis of severe combined immunodeficiency (SCID). The parents state that their religious beliefs do not allow the administration of blood but they are accepting of medical intervention. The primary health-care provider prescribes intravenous immunoglobulins (IVIGs). Which of the following should the nurse discuss with the parents?
   1. IVIG is a blood product.
   2. The older children should be tested for SCID.
   3. Administration of this drug can precipitate an infection.
   4. The siblings should not receive immunizations until their sister is cured.

   TEST-TAKING TIP: Identify the words in the stem that direct attention to content.

3. The faith community nurse (FCN) is planning a community open house to provide education on how their role works synergistically with other health-care providers. Identify roles the nurse should include in the education. **Select all that apply.**
   1. ____ Provide home health care to client
   2. ____ Serve as an advocate for community members
   3. ____ Provide education and health counseling to clients
   4. ____ Interpret and explain health-care providers' diagnoses
   5. ____ Identify resources in the community and make appropriate referrals
   6. ____ Promote client's personal responsibility for their health and wellness

   TEST-TAKING TIP: Identify words in the stem that direct attention to content.

4. The nurse is caring for a client who was just informed that her fetus has multiple congenital abnormalities and, if born, will require complex lifelong care. The client is offered the option of having an abortion. The client states, "My religion does not allow abortion, but I don't know if I have the strength to provide lifelong care for a seriously disabled child. What do you think that I should do?" What is the **best** response by the nurse?
   1. "Do you think you should get a second opinion?"
   2. "How does your husband feel about terminating the pregnancy?"
   3. "I will have your spiritual advisor visit so that you can discuss your options."
   4. "What is most important is what you think you should do. Let's talk about it."

   TEST-TAKING TIP: Identify the word in the stem that sets a priority. Identify the unique option. Identify the central person in the question. Identify the option with a clang association.

5. A mother brings her 4-day-old newborn to the well-baby clinic. The nurse finds a cloth tightly wrapped around the infant's abdomen covering the umbilical cord stump. The mother states that she tightly swaddles her infant because it is a tradition taught by her elders. Which action is appropriate when teaching the mother about cord care?
   1. Leaving the cloth off the infant after modeling cleansing of the cord site
   2. Leaving the cord site open to the air followed by swaddling the infant with the cloth
   3. Administering a topical antibiotic to the cord site before reapplying the tightly wrapped cloth
   4. Instructing the mother that tightly wrapping the cloth around the infant's abdomen and cord site is unnecessary

   TEST-TAKING TIP: Identify the options that deny the client's feelings, concerns, or needs. Identify the opposites in options.

6. The nurse is caring for a client who is dying and who practices the Muslim faith. Which is the **most** effective intervention to ensure that the client's religious needs are met in a way that minimizes the risk of spiritual distress?
   1. Discuss with the client advance directives about religious preferences concerning death and dying.
   2. Provide a prayer room that is quiet, clean, and carpeted and that has access to washing facilities.
   3. Arrange access to an imam who can read the Quran and offer comforting prayers.
   4. Assure the client that a postmortem examination will not be performed.

   TEST-TAKING TIP: Identify the word in the stem that sets a priority. Identify the global option.

7. Because of religious preferences, the client newly admitted to the labor and delivery unit prefers a female provider; however, the on-call provider is male. To provide culturally respectful care, which should the nurse do **first**?
   1. Call the client's provider to come complete the admission assessment.
   2. Tell the client the on-call provider is male and discuss options for their consideration.
   3. Have the on-call provider complete the assessment so the client does not have to wait.
   4. Explain to the client that they will need to wait until a female provider is available.

   TEST-TAKING TIP: Identify the word in the stem that sets a priority. Identify the option that considers the client's feelings, concerns, and needs.

8. The nurse is completing a spiritual assessment for a new homebound client who is unable to leave their home to attend church and bible study. From the assessment findings, the nurse is concerned the client is feeling separated from their faith community. Which nursing diagnosis is the **best** choice for this client?
   1. Spiritual Alienation
   2. Spiritual Despair
   3. Spiritual Anxiety
   4. Spiritual Pain

   TEST-TAKING TIP: Identify the priority words in the stem that direct attention to content.

9. A 32-week-old preterm infant who was born at 27 weeks gestation has a slowly dropping hemoglobin level with no evidence of bleeding. The parents refuse the primary health-care provider's recommendation of a blood transfusion because their religion prohibits this treatment. Which of the following is an acceptable alternative?
   1. Plasma
   2. Platelet cells
   3. Iron supplementation alone
   4. Erythropoietin with an iron supplement

   TEST-TAKING TIP: Identify the words in the stem that direct attention to content.

10. The nurse plans and implements care that is culturally respectful for their diverse client population. When planning care, which elements of cultural competence should the nurse consider? **Select all that apply.**
 1. ____ Encouraging a client to accept care not in alignment with their culture if it will heal them
 2. ____ Respecting a client's cultural preferences even if they do not agree with your beliefs
 3. ____ Having knowledge of a client's culturally specific definitions of health and illness
 4. ____ Educating the client that their care expectations may not be met due to their beliefs
 5. ____ Assuming that the provider's beliefs and values are in alignment with the client
 6. ____ Being self-aware to prevent influencing your own thoughts on others

 TEST-TAKING TIP: Identify the word in the stem that sets a priority. Identify the global options.

11. The nurse is caring for a client admitted with cardiovascular disease. The client tells the nurse that they use herbal supplements daily and want to continue while they are in the hospital. What is the nurse's **best** response to the client?
 1. "Good for you! Traditional medicines have so many ingredients!"
 2. "You should not take any of the supplements while in the hospital."
 3. "We need your primary care provider to approve these before you take them."
 4. "The supplements must be verified and approved by the pharmacy before taking."

 TEST-TAKING TIP: Identify the option with a specific determiner. Identify the opposites in options.

12. The nurse working in a primary care clinic identifies that a new mother's attitude toward her infant's care is inattentive and inadequate. What should the nurse do **first?**
 1. Refer her to infant care classes
 2. Teach her acceptable behaviors for infant care
 3. Assess her cultural traditions regarding infant care
 4. Encourage her to enroll her infant in a day-care program

 TEST-TAKING TIP: Identify the word in the stem that sets a priority. Identify the unique option.

13. The nurse, who is male, approaches a female client and her husband to assess the client's blood pressure. The husband moves his wife's top sheet up under her chin and raises a hand like a stop sign. What should the nurse do?
 1. Avoid eye contact with the husband, state that vital signs must be taken, and proceed with the blood pressure assessment
 2. Explain to the client what is to be done and ask permission to proceed with the blood pressure assessment
 3. State that a female nurse will be called to proceed with the blood pressure assessment
 4. Ask the husband's permission to proceed with the blood pressure assessment

 TEST-TAKING TIP: Identify the central person in the question. Identify the option that denies the client's feelings, concerns, or needs.

14. The young Hispanic mother, who speaks no English, brings her child to the emergency department for an accidental fall. The nurse caring for the child speaks no Spanish. Which is the most appropriate nursing intervention?
 1. Use facility-provided interpreter services
 2. Have the mother's adolescent child interpret for the mother
 3. Speak in short basic words to encourage client understanding
 4. Direct the client to another emergency department with Spanish-speaking nurses

 TEST-TAKING TIP: Identify the word in the stem that sets a priority. Identify the global option.

15. The nurse is caring for a client who immigrated to the United States from a country where people historically are expected to stoically cope with pain. The client received preoperative teaching before abdominal surgery and is now in the postanesthesia care unit. The client is grimacing and positioning the body in a rigid manner but states that the pain is tolerable and refuses pain medication. What should the nurse do **first?**
1. Implement nonmedicinal approaches to minimize the client's pain
2. Teach that activity can increase when there is a reduction in pain
3. Understand the client's need to be stoical in response to pain
4. Administer the opioid prescribed for pain

TEST-TAKING TIP: Identify the word in the stem that sets a priority. Identify the unique option. Identify the option that denies the client's feelings, concerns, or needs.

16. An older adult in a nursing home is talking about her life as a young woman and says, "I had no choices in life. It was expected that I was to get married and be a stay-at-home wife and mother." Which is the **best** response by the nurse?
1. "Do you feel that there were things you would have liked to have had the opportunity to do?"
2. "Times are different. Thank goodness women have so many more choices today."
3. "I can understand how frustrating that must have been. I would have rebelled."
4. "Why didn't you explain to your parents how you felt?"

TEST-TAKING TIP: Identify the word in the stem that sets a priority. Identify the option that denies the client's feelings, concerns, or needs.

17. The nurse working in a college health clinic is caring for a recent high school graduate who stated on the admission form that he is gay. Which is appropriate when collecting data to complete a nursing admission assessment? **Select all that apply.**
1. _____ Stating "Thank you for sharing that you are gay because having that information will help me take better care of you."
2. _____ Inquiring "Is there anything related to your sexuality that you believe is important to your health care?"
3. _____ Inquiring "Are you engaged in a monogamous sexual relationship?"
4. _____ Asking "Are you sexually active with men, women, both, or neither?"
5. _____ Saying "Tell me a little about yourself."

TEST-TAKING TIP: Identify the unique option.

18. After assessing the needs of a client, the nurse determines that the client is experiencing spiritual distress. Which statement by the nurse may help the client to identify beliefs and feelings that are causing the spiritual distress? **Select all that apply.**
1. _____ "How does your illness interfere with practicing your spiritual beliefs?"
2. _____ "How do your beliefs and values influence your spiritual needs?"
3. _____ "Do you think that God will forgive you for your past sins?"
4. _____ "How does your illness affect your relationship with God?"
5. _____ "What is the source of your strength?

19. The nurse manager is preparing education on culturally competent nursing care. Which examples demonstrate culturally competent nursing care? **Select all that apply.**
1. _____ Removing the client's healing and energy crystals from the windowsill
2. _____ The unlicensed health-care provider tells clients they must shower daily
3. _____ Providing the Muslim client with a special menu to select their meals
4. _____ Notifying dietary that the Jewish client requests a kosher meal tray
5. _____ Allowing the Nigerian client's family elder to make decisions
6. _____ Assigning the Muslim client to a room facing toward Mecca

TEST-TAKING TIP: Identify the words in the stem that direct attention to content.

20. The nurse is completing an assessment of a client regarding the spiritual realm. The client states that illness is caused by the intrusion of a disease-causing spirit, and a priestess must conduct a religious ritual using candles and chanting to cast out the evil spirit. Which of the following is an appropriate nursing intervention? **Select all that apply.**

1. _____ Negotiate a mutually agreeable safe alternative to the use of open flame candles during the religious ritual.
2. _____ Instruct the priestess to limit the ceremony to two or three participants so as not to disturb other clients.
3. _____ Arrange for a private space when the client has a priestess conduct the religious ritual.
4. _____ Accept the client's belief that diseases are caused by supernatural forces of evil.
5. _____ Recognize that the client's beliefs are illogical but basically harmless.

TEST-TAKING TIP: Identify the options with clang associations. Identify options that deny the client's feelings, concerns, or needs. Identify client-centered options.

21. The nurse examines the following chart, which demonstrates the changes and predictions in racial and ethnic makeup in the United States from 1990 to 2050. Which statement is accurate according to the percentages presented in the chart? **Select all that apply.**

1. _____ By 2050, the percentage of the white and non-Hispanic origin population will decline by approximately 30% from 1990.
2. _____ By 2050, the percentage of the Hispanic origin population will increase approximately 2½ times from 1990.
3. _____ By 2050, the percentage of the black origin population will increase by approximately 25% from 1990.
4. _____ By 2050, the non-Hispanic white population will decrease to a little more than 50% of the population.
5. _____ By 2050, the population other than white, non-Hispanic will be close to half the total population.

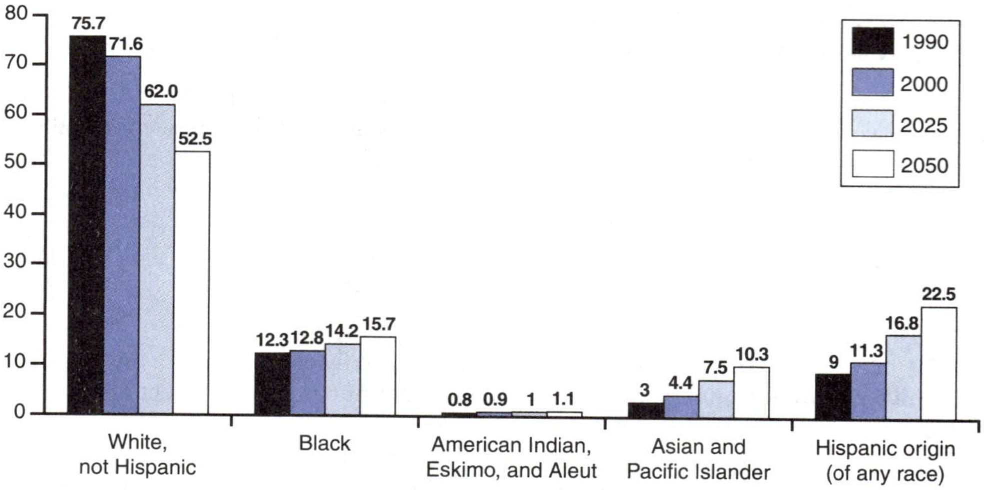

TEST-TAKING TIP: Identify the words in the stem that direct attention to content.

22. To evaluate personal biased thinking that can interfere with providing culturally competent nursing care, nurses should understand what constitutes xenophobia (i.e., fear, hatred, contempt, or mistrust of that which is foreign). Which is an example of xenophobia? **Select all that apply.**
1. _____ Violence against and rape of women
2. _____ Immigrants from Mexico being labeled as criminals
3. _____ The murder of blacks by white supremacists
4. _____ The segregation of Japanese Americans in relocation camps during World War II
5. _____ The low percentage of women in leadership positions in government and corporate America
6. _____ A man making derogatory statements about a female opponent's physical appearance

TEST-TAKING TIP: Identify the words in the stem that direct attention to content.

23. The nurse is caring for a client who recently immigrated to the United States. The client speaks limited English. Which of the following reflects culturally competent nursing care? **Select all that apply.**
1. _____ Arrange for an interpreter as necessary when interacting with the client
2. _____ Incorporate client preferences when meeting the client's daily needs
3. _____ Assess the sociocultural aspects of the client's health beliefs
4. _____ Be alert to the client's nonverbal body language
5. _____ Identify one's own cultural and health beliefs

TEST-TAKING TIP: Identify words in the stem that direct attention to content.

24. The nurse is caring for a client whose 10-year-old child recently died from leukemia. From statements made by the client, the nurse believes that the client may be suffering from spiritual distress. Which client statements do not support the nursing diagnosis of spiritual distress? **Select all that apply.**
1. _____ "I have come to the realization that I just have to depend on myself."
2. _____ "I hope that in the future I can rebuild my relationship with God."
3. _____ "I feel so vacant and hollow in my spirituality right now."
4. _____ "I am suffering because God allowed my child to die."
5. _____ "God is punishing me for not living a righteous life."

TEST-TAKING TIP: Identify the word in the stem that indicates negative polarity.

25. A 96-year-old woman who is accompanied by a grown daughter is being admitted to a nursing home. The nurse reviews the client's health history provided (below) by her primary health-care provider and interviews both the client and her daughter. Later, when she is being prepared for bed, the client says, "All my life I took care of my children, my parents, and my in-laws, and now I am discarded in a nursing home." The nurse's **best** response should be:
1. "It's sad that your sons are not able to help you."
2. "It must be difficult to feel pushed aside by your family."
3. "You now have needs that require the assistance of nurses."
4. "Your daughter feels bad that you are now in a nursing home."

Information Included in the Primary Health-Care Provider's Health History

Client is a 96-year-old woman who has a colostomy following surgery 2 years ago for cancer of the ascending colon. Recently, the client has had numerous episodes of urinary incontinence for which no cause has been identified. Client's cardiopulmonary status is stable, but she is weak and debilitated.

Client's Statements During the Admission Interview

I married young, had eight children, and took care of everyone in my family. That was a woman's job back then. I'm really OK. My mind is sharp as a tack. I just need help with my colostomy, and I occasionally make mistakes with my urine.

Daughter's Statements During the Admission Interview

My husband and I have been taking care of my mom for years now. I have seven brothers, but they will not help us. Not only does my mom have a colostomy that continuously drains, but now she can no longer control her urine. We feel bad that we are putting her in a nursing home, but we are so overwhelmed.

TEST-TAKING TIP: Identify the word in the stem that sets a priority. Identify the central person in the question. Identify the client-centered option. Identify the options that deny the client's feelings, concerns, or needs.

1. **TEST-TAKING TIP: The word "best" directs attention to the content.**
   1. This is not empathetic listening and gives the client false reassurances. The nurse should explore the client's feelings about why they feel this way.
   2. This is not the best response. The client may need some psychological counseling to cope with the diagnosis, but the nurse must first uncover why the client feels this way.
   3. This is not the best response. The nurse needs to first explore the client's feelings and then ask them if they would like a spiritual consultation. The client may not want a spiritual consultation.
   4. **This client is in spiritual distress. The nurse should assess and listen to the client first to explore why they feel this way to provide a supportive presence. After uncovering why the client feels this way, the nurse can plan interventions and outcomes to resolve the client's spiritual distress.**
2. **TEST-TAKING TIP: The words *do not allow the administration of blood* in the stem direct attention to content.**
   1. **Immunoglobulins are derived from pooled blood products. The parents should be aware that this medical intervention is a blood product.**
   2. The siblings are older. If they had SCID, they probably would have been diagnosed within the first year of life.
   3. Immunoglobulins can help fight, not precipitate, some infections.
   4. The siblings should receive all scheduled immunizations so that their sister with SCID has less risk of exposure to an infectious agent.
3. **TEST-TAKING TIP: The word *synergistically* in the stem directs attention to content.**
   1. Faith community nurses are not home health nurses and do not provide direct medical care. Though faith community nurses do not provide physical care, they should still use the nursing process to care for their clients.
   2. **Faith community nurses help bridge the emotional and spiritual support needs and advocate for clients in the hospital, the home, or long-term care facilities. They advocate on a client's behalf by coordinating care and asking for assistance from members of the faith community to provide support such as meals and visitations.**
   3. **Faith community nurses help clients understand how life transitions such as illness affect religious and spiritual beliefs. They help clients interpret and explain the relationship between faith and healing and encourage clients to engage in health promotion interventions that integrate spirituality and religious practices.**
   4. Faith community nurses do not analyze and explain providers' diagnoses to clients. This is outside the scope of nursing. They can refer clients to the provider and advocate to the provider.
   5. **Faith community nurses help with the educational and health promotion needs of the older adult population and of underserved communities.**
   6. **Faith community nurses encourage and educate clients to take responsibility for their health and wellness by teaching health promotion practices that address physical, social, and spiritual needs.**
4. **TEST-TAKING TIP: The word *best* in the stem sets a priority. Option 4 is unique. Option 4 focuses on the client, whereas options 1, 2, and 3 involve another person. The client is the central person in the question, not the husband, the spiritual advisor, or the individual who can give a second opinion. The words *think that I should* in the stem and the words *think you should* in options 1 and 4 are clang associations.**
   1. This response makes an assumption and offers unrealistic hope.
   2. At this moment, the focus should be on the client, not the husband. The client's verbalization of an inability to provide lifelong care to her disabled child is the concern that must be explored.
   3. A spiritual advisor should not be arranged without the consent of the client. In addition, this response abdicates responsibility to her spiritual advisor. The spiritual advisor may be judgmental and may impose a decision on the basis of religious laws without allowing the client an opportunity to explore her feelings and options independently.
   4. **This response places the focus on the client and her feelings. This approach is nonjudgmental and open-ended, which**

supports an exploration of feelings, concerns, and options.

5. **TEST-TAKING TIP: Options 1 and 4 deny the client's tradition of swaddling her infant. Options 1 and 4 are opposite to options 2 and 3. If you understand that traditions should be followed whenever possible, options 1 and 4 can be eliminated from consideration.**
   1. Although modeling cleansing of the cord site is an appropriate intervention, leaving the cloth off the infant after the procedure negates the mother's right to perform a cultural tradition.
   2. **Showing the mother how to expose the cord site to the air followed by swaddling of the infant acknowledges her tradition while ensuring that the cord site is cared for appropriately.**
   3. Application of a topical antibiotic to the cord site requires a prescription by a primary health-care provider and is not needed unless the cord is infected. Covering the cord site is inappropriate because it will impede healing.
   4. The mother's tradition should not be discounted. Swaddling the infant can continue as long as the nurse explains how to care for the cord site to promote healing.
6. **TEST-TAKING TIP: The word *most* in the stem sets a priority. Option 1 is the global option. The interventions in options 2, 3, and 4 can be included in the discussion about personal preferences in option 1.**
   1. **Completing advance directives supports the client's right to be in control and to have preferences regarding religious rituals implemented at the end of life and after death.**
   2. While important, providing access to a room for prayer is only one aspect of spiritual care for this client.
   3. Contacting a spiritual advisor should not be done without the consent of the client.
   4. The nurse is not in a position to ensure that a postmortem examination will not be performed. Although a postmortem examination may be refused by a Muslim family, it may be required by law.
7. **TEST-TAKING TIP: The word *first* in the stem sets a priority. Option 2 involves the client's feelings, concerns, or needs.**
   1. Notifying the client's provider to do the admission assessment is not the first thing that the nurse should do. This may be necessary if the nurse is unable to find another female provider.
   2. **Discussing the situation with the client and spouse promotes open communication with the couple and elicits their preference in the client's care. Understanding the client's culture and religious beliefs ensures culturally respectful care. Identifying actions that are acceptable to the client provides appropriate transcultural care.**
   3. Notifying the attending male provider to complete the admission assessment negates the couple's preference and rights in directing their own care. Culturally respectful care is sensitive to the needs of clients and families. Ignoring the client's request may result in the client refusing care.
   4. Waiting to be examined may place the client in danger. The nurse should consider options that are culturally respectful and safe for the client.
8. **TEST-TAKING TIP: The word *best* in the stem directs attention to content.**
   1. **Spiritual Alienation occurs when a client perceives that they are separated from their faith community. The nurse can explore alternatives and identify other spiritual options such as reading spiritual texts and arranging for the client's minister, priest, or rabbi to visit.**
   2. Spiritual despair occurs when the client feels that no one, including God, cares about them.
   3. Spiritual anxiety occurs when the client challenges their previously held belief and values system.
   4. Spiritual pain occurs when a client is unable to accept the death of a loved one.
9. **TEST-TAKING TIP: The words *their religion prohibits blood transfusions* in the stem direct attention to content.**
   1. Plasma is a by-product of whole blood and is not an acceptable medical intervention for members of a religion that prohibits blood transfusions.
   2. Platelet cells are a by-product of whole blood and are not an acceptable medical intervention for members of a religion that prohibits blood transfusions.
   3. Iron supplements act slowly and do not instigate change rapidly in an infant who is preterm.
   4. **Erythropoietin acts on bone marrow to rapidly increase production of red blood cells. The addition of an iron supplement will help sustain hemoglobin production, although it will act slowly.**

10. 1. The nurse should avoid judgmental attitudes and concepts that the traditional plan of care is the best option. Cultural imposition in health care is when health-care personnel try to impose their beliefs and practices on clients from other cultures.

2. Accepting and respecting a client's cultural differences facilitates the client's ability to make care decisions that are in alignment with their needs and beliefs.

3. The nurse should know that diverse cultures may have different acceptable definitions of health and illness. The nurse should perform a cultural assessment to identify the client's definitions.

4. Health-care professionals should not assume that a client's health-care needs will not be met because of their beliefs or assume they have the right to make decisions for these clients. Doing so may cause a client to become angry or resistant to treatment.

5. The nurse should never assume a provider's beliefs and values are in alignment with a client's beliefs as this can harm or delay client care.

6. Being open to and understanding other cultures allows nurses to grow their cultural competence. The nurse should understand client needs and adapt their care to respectfully meet those needs to provide safe and respectful care.

11. **TEST-TAKING TIP: Options 1 and 2 are opposites.**

1. Herbal supplements may contain ingredients that produce adverse effects on the cardiovascular system or have harmful interactions with prescribed medications, so they should be taken with care. They are a common method of treatment in many cultures but are not a substitute for traditional medications.

2. Telling the client not to take their herbal supplements may deny the client's right to be involved in their plan of care.

3. The primary health-care provider may determine which herbal supplements can be taken safely with prescribed medications; however, the hospital pharmacist should approve the supplements while the client is hospitalized. The client can consult with the primary health-care provider after discharge to review prescribed medications and herbal supplements.

4. Herbal supplements can negatively interact with prescribed medications or cause an adverse effect on the cardiovascular system. Because of the risks involved, the pharmacist should decide which herbal supplements are acceptable for the client to ingest. For example, garlic, feverfew, ginger, and ginkgo increase the risk of bleeding when taken concurrently with an anticoagulant, and St. John's wort reduces concentrations of digoxin. Anticoagulants and digoxin are common medications prescribed for cardiac conditions.

12. **TEST-TAKING TIP: The word *first* in the stem sets a priority. Option 3 is unique because it is the only option that attempts to obtain additional information. Options 1, 2, and 4 assume that the mother's behavior is unacceptable and provide a nursing intervention.**

1. The mother's readiness for participation in infant care classes must be determined first.

2. Teaching her how to care for her infant is premature. The nurse must first determine the underlying reason for the mother's behavior toward her infant's care.

3. More information is needed before a plan of care is formulated. It is important to assess cultural behavior, customs, traditions, and practices because they will influence infant care patterns.

4. A day-care program protects the infant only during the day, leaving the infant to the mother's inattentive and inadequate care the remainder of the day and on weekends.

13. **TEST-TAKING TIP: The client, not the husband, is the central person in the question. Option 1 denies the client's feelings, concerns, or needs. Touching the client without permission is unacceptable.**

1. Continuing with the procedure dismisses the husband's nonverbal behavior to stop. If the nurse proceeds with taking the blood pressure reading without the client's consent, the nurse can be accused of battery, which is the touching of a person without consent.

2. Explaining the blood pressure procedure supports the client's right to know what is going to be done. Asking permission to proceed with the procedure recognizes the husband's nonverbal directive to stop and supports the

client's right to make decisions about the care that is provided.

3. Responding to the behavior and identifying concerns should occur first. If it is requested that a female nurse implement the procedure, this preference should be incorporated into the plan of care whenever possible.
4. The client is the center of the health-care team and has the authority to make decisions about care. If the husband is the authority figure when it comes to making decisions about the care provided to the wife, the wife must give permission for the husband to make decisions on her behalf.

14. **TEST-TAKING TIP: The word *most* in the stem sets a priority. Option 1 is the global option.**

1. The nurse should always use the facility-provided interpreter services. Many facilities have interpreters in-house or have telephonic and electronic interpreting services. Title VI of the Civil Rights Act requires health-care facilities to provide interpreter services. Using professional medical interpreters improves client satisfaction, improves outcomes, and reduces adverse events.
2. Minors cannot serve as interpreters for their parents. Interpreting sensitive medical information for parents can be stressful for a child and there could be misinterpretation by the child. Information could be left out and the child may not understand medical jargon.
3. This is dismissive of the client. Because the client does not speak English, speaking in short basic words will not aid the client to understand what the nurse is saying.
4. **This violates the Emergency Medical Treatment and Labor Act (EMTALA), which states that all persons in an emergency department must be stabilized and treated.**

15. **TEST-TAKING TIP: The word *first* in the stem sets a priority. Option 3 is unique. It is the only option that is not an actual intervention, although one can argue that a nurse's cognitive activity is an intervention. Option 4 denies the client's feelings, concerns, or needs.**

1. Implementing nonmedicinal approaches to support comfort is something the nurse should do; however, another option takes priority.
2. Educating the client about pain management is not the first thing the nurse should do from among the options presented.
3. **Understanding the client's need to be stoical in response to pain is the first thing the nurse should do. A client has the right to refuse care even if the intervention offered supports comfort and appears to make logical sense.**
4. Providing pain medication after it has been refused by a client is battery, which is a criminal act.

16. **TEST-TAKING TIP: The word *best* in the stem sets a priority. The statement in option 2 denies the client's feelings, concerns, or needs. It focuses on the present rather than the client's past.**

1. **This therapeutic statement gently seeks clarification. It gives the lead to the client to share whatever thoughts and feelings the client may wish to express.**
2. This response focuses attention away from the client's needs and is not therapeutic.
3. The first half of the statement reflects the client's feelings of frustration, which is appropriate. However, the second half of the statement is judgmental and imposes the nurse's standards on the client, which is not therapeutic.
4. This response is a judgmental or disapproving statement and is not constructive. The client cannot change the past. In addition, *why* questions should be avoided because they can be interpreted as accusations, which can cause resentment and mistrust.

17. **TEST-TAKING TIP: Option 1 is unique. It is the only option that is not a question.**

1. **This is a supportive statement.**
2. **This is an open-ended question that invites the client to share information that believes is important.**
3. This information may not provide valuable information. The definition of *monogamous* means "having a sexual relationship with one person at a time." However, this definition depends on each person's perspective. A person may have ten sexual relationships in a year but may believe that he or she is monogamous because when sexually active with one partner, the relationship was exclusive. How many sexual partners one may have over a period of time is more valuable information.

4. **Although this question is specific, it is valuable information because risk factors increase when engaging in sexual behavior with men.**
5. **This is an open-ended question that invites the student to share information that he feels comfortable sharing.**

18. 1. **This question encourages the client to explore how the illness interferes with practicing spiritual beliefs. The nurse should work with the client to formulate a plan of care that meets self-identified spiritual needs.**
2. **This question encourages an exploration of how personal beliefs and values influence the client's spiritual needs. Beliefs and values are basic and enduring and are the foundation of one's religious/spiritual domain. This information will be valuable for the nurse to help the client minimize spiritual distress.**
3. This question is inappropriate because it introduces the subject of past sins that may not be the basis of the client's spiritual distress. Also, it is a direct question that requires only a yes or no answer.
4. **This question encourages an exploration of how the client views the illness in relation to God. How the client views the illness, such as part of life or punishment for past sins, provides the nurse with information that will facilitate meeting this client's spiritual needs.**
5. **This question encourages the exploration of sources of strength, which may empower the client. These sources can be people, communities, religious congregations, organizations, faith, personal beliefs, and so on.**

19. **TEST-TAKING TIP: Identify options that engage the nurse in cross-cultural interactions with clients.**

1. Many people believe that complementary therapy such as crystals promotes emotional and physical health. There is no scientific evidence to demonstrate that crystals heal or promote health, but they are believed to have an indirect psychological effect. Researchers have noted a placebo effect called interpersonal healing that is distinct from healing through traditional methods. Removing the client's crystals does not provide culturally competent care and can have a negative health effect on the client.
2. This is not culturally competent care. Clients should be given a choice of whether to shower or bathe, which can depend on their cultural preferences.
3. **Some clients' food preferences are determined by their religion. Muslim clients may have strict guidelines on the consumption of meat and during religious observances may have fasting requirements within a certain time window to eat. Providing a menu lets the client know that the nurse is culturally competent.**
4. **Notifying the kitchen to provide a kosher tray for a Jewish client who requests one is culturally competent. Kosher meals have strict dietary standards. If the facility is not able to provide a kosher tray, the client and the nurse can work together to find an amenable solution.**
5. **This is culturally competent nursing care as some cultures have elders who make health-care decisions. Disregarding an elder's role and providing care that is not approved by the elder may result in conflict with the client. The client may consider this a disregard for their family and cultural values. If a client has an elder, the nurse should include this person in the care planning process.**
6. **This is culturally competent nursing care. Muslim clients may pray five times a day. Once prayer begins, be cognizant and respectful, giving the client privacy and time to pray.**

20. **TEST-TAKING TIP: The words *religious ritual* in the stem and in options 1 and 3 are clang associations. Options 2 and 5 deny the client's feelings, concerns, or needs. Limiting the number of participants, as stated in option 2, may interfere with the practice of a religious ritual. When a nurse considers a client's beliefs illogical, as stated in option 5, the nurse may engage in behavior that is biased or judgmental. Options 1, 3, and 4 are client-centered because they promote the client's right to practice her religion in a safe, private, and supportive environment.**

1. **It is unsafe to have open flame candles in a hospital setting because of the risk of a fire. Negotiating a mutually agreed–upon solution is an acceptable option.**

2. Limiting the number of people participating in the religious ritual denies the client's right to practice religion. A private room can be arranged for the ceremony.
3. **Providing a private space for the religious ritual respects the client's dignity and right to privacy.**
4. **Culturally competent nursing care requires the nurse to recognize clients' rights to embrace their own beliefs and practice their religion in a nonjudgmental and supportive environment.**
5. To provide culturally competent care, the nurse must support the rights of clients to hold their own beliefs without exposure to bias, prejudice, discrimination, or judgment from members of the health-care team.

21. **TEST-TAKING TIP: The words *which statement is accurate* in the stem direct attention to content.**
1. **This is an accurate statement. According to the prediction, by 2050 the white non-Hispanic population will decline from 75.7% of the population to 52.5% of the population. This is a decline of 23.2%, which represents a decline of approximately 30% from 1990.**
2. **This is an accurate statement. The percentage of the Hispanic population is projected to increase from 9.0% in 1990 to 22.5% by 2050. This increase is approximately two and a half times the population in 1990.**
3. **This is an accurate statement. By 2050, the percentage of the population of people of black origin is predicted to increase from 12.3% in 1990 to 15.7% in 2050. This is an increase of approximately 25% from 1990.**
4. **This is an accurate statement. By 2050, the white non-Hispanic population is projected to decrease from 75.7% to 52.5% of the total population. This will be a little more than half the total population.**
5. **This is an accurate statement. By 2050, the percentage of people of Asian and Pacific Islander, American Indian, Eskimo, and Aleut descent, and people of black or Hispanic origin, is projected to represent approximately 50% of the total population.**

22. **TEST-TAKING TIP: The words *what constitutes xenophobia* in the stem direct attention to content.**
1. Violence against women and rape of women are examples of misogyny, which is hatred, dislike, mistrust, mistreatment of, or prejudice against girls and women. Misogyny is associated with behaviors that are darker, angrier, and more cynical than sexist behaviors, which represent beliefs or attitudes that one sex is inferior to another.
2. **Labeling immigrants from Mexico as criminals is an example of xenophobia, which is the fear, hatred, contempt, or mistrust of foreigners, people from different cultures, or anything foreign.**
3. **The murder of blacks by white supremacists is an example of xenophobia, which is the fear, hatred, contempt, or mistrust of foreigners, people from different cultures, or anything foreign.**
4. **The segregation of Japanese Americans in relocation camps during World War II is an example of xenophobia, which is the fear, hatred, contempt, or mistrust of foreigners, people from different cultures, or anything foreign.**
5. The low percentage of women in leadership positions in government and corporate America reflects sexist, not xenophobic, views. Because the United States initially operated as a patriarchy and because of male dominance in government and corporate America, women are underrepresented in positions of leadership. Research shows that the root cause of underrepresentation of woman in government and corporate America is sex discrimination.
6. A man making derogatory statements about a female opponent's physical appearance is an example of misogyny. Misogyny is the hatred, dislike, mistrust, or mistreatment of or prejudice against girls and women.

23. **TEST-TAKING TIP: The words *recently immigrated* and *speaks limited English* in the stem direct attention to content.**
1. **Arranging for an interpreter is necessary to ensure that the client understands what is going to be done and why. Also, it supports the client's ability to communicate concerns and requests. The ability to communicate effectively supports the emotional and physical needs of the client.**

2. **Incorporating client preferences when providing nursing care demonstrates acceptance of the client. Also, it helps to maintain the client's routine, which is reassuring and comforting.**
3. **The nurse must complete a sociocultural assessment to identify how these factors influence the client's health beliefs. This assessment is necessary for the nurse to identify the client's needs and formulate an individualized plan of care.**
4. **Assessing nonverbal body language is important for all clients but even more so when the client is not fluent in the English language. Facial expression, position of extremities, gestures, and posture convey universal messages and may communicate what a person feels and thinks more accurately than words.**
5. **Nurses must know themselves before they can help others. Nurses must identify their own cultural and health beliefs so they are aware of personal biases, stereotypes, and prejudices. These biases, stereotypes, and prejudices must be suppressed so they do not influence client care.**

24. **TEST-TAKING TIP: The words *do not support* in the stem indicate negative polarity.**
    1. **Though the client expresses loneliness, they also indicate that they want to find comfort through the help of others. If the client expressed feelings of not depending on others or God, those would be examples of spiritual alienation, one of the seven manifestations of spiritual distress.**
    2. **This statement demonstrates hope for a future relationship with God. Expressions of no hope are examples of spiritual despair, which is one of the seven manifestations of spiritual distress.**
    3. This statement, as well as expressions of temporary loss or termination of the love of God, is an example of spiritual loss, one of the seven manifestations of spiritual distress.
    4. This expression of suffering reflects spiritual pain, one of the seven manifestations of spiritual distress. The seven manifestations of spiritual distress are spiritual pain, spiritual alienation, spiritual anxiety, spiritual guilt, spiritual anger, spiritual loss, and spiritual despair.
    5. This statement indicates spiritual guilt. Expression of failure to do the things that please God during one's life is one of the seven manifestations of spiritual distress.

25. **TEST-TAKING TIP: The word *best* in the stem sets a priority. The client is the central person in the question, not the client's daughter, the daughter's husband, or the client's sons. Option 2 is client-centered because it focuses on the client's feelings. Options 3 and 4 deny the client's feelings, concerns, or needs because they focus on issues other than the client's feelings.**
    1. This statement may maximize feelings of being "discarded" in a nursing home.
    2. **This statement uses the interviewing skill known as reflective technique. It focuses on feelings and provides the client with an opportunity to further explore feelings, if desired.**
    3. This statement is not supportive and may maximize feelings of dependency and inadequacy.
    4. This statement focuses on the client's daughter rather than the client.

COMMUNICATION AND MEETING CLIENTS' EMOTIONAL NEEDS

This section includes questions related to assessing and meeting clients' psychological needs. Also, it includes questions that focus on the principles of communication, communication skills, interventions that support emotional needs, and communicating with the confused or disoriented client. Additional questions focus on patterns of behavior in response to illness, nursing interventions that help clients to adapt to illness, caring for the dying client's emotional needs, defense mechanisms, and responding to the crying client.

QUESTIONS

1. The nurse is conducting an intake interview with a client. Which should the nurse do to **best** facilitate therapeutic communication with this client?
1. Talk about expectations
2. Use probing questions
3. Ask direct questions
4. Listen attentively

TEST-TAKING TIP: Identify the word in the stem that sets a priority. Identify the unique option. Identify equally plausible options.

2. The nurse enters the room to find the client crying. The client states, "I've recently lost my son. I can't believe it. I feel so alone." Which is the most therapeutic response by the nurse?
1. "I understand, my mother felt the same way when she was grieving and ill."
2. "I know it is hard, but I am sure your son is in a better place."
3. "I am so sorry, but we need to focus on getting you better."
4. "Let's talk, what makes you feel so alone?"

TEST-TAKING TIP: Identify the word in the stem that sets a priority and has client-centered options.

3. A client is admitted to the hospital with multiple health problems. Which nursing intervention is ineffective in meeting the client's psychosocial needs?
1. Addressing the client by name
2. Assisting the client with meals
3. Identifying achievement of client goals
4. Explaining care before it is to be given to the client

TEST-TAKING TIP: Identify the word in the stem that indicates negative polarity. Identify the key word in the stem that directs attention to content. Identify the unique option.

4. The terminally ill client says to the nurse, "I was much more religious when I was young." Which is the most therapeutic response by the nurse?
1. "Do you believe in God?"
2. "Why would you say something like that?"
3. "Do you need to pray for forgiveness from God?"
4. "Would you like me to call spiritual services for you?"

TEST-TAKING TIP: Choose the option that is client-centered.

5. The nurse notices that the client newly diagnosed with rheumatoid arthritis is withdrawn and quiet during the morning assessment. Which are the most appropriate responses from the nurse? **Select all that apply.**
   1. Carry on with client care tasks
   2. Ask them if their family has come to visit
   3. Initiate small talk with the client about the weather
   4. Ask the provider to place a psychological consultation
   5. Tell the client that you notice they are quieter than usual
   6. Allow the patient to initiate conversation at their own pace

   TEST-TAKING TIP: Identify the word in the stem that directs attention to content. Identify the equally plausible options.

6. A client's spouse died 1 week ago. When reminiscing about their life together, the client begins to cry. Which is the nurse's **best** response?
   1. Stay while reorganizing the client's unit
   2. Say "Things will get better as time passes"
   3. Say "This must be a difficult time for you"
   4. Suggest that the client receive grief counseling

   TEST-TAKING TIP: Identify the word in the stem that sets a priority. Identify options that deny client feelings, concerns, or needs. Identify client-centered options.

7. A client is confused and disoriented. Which route of communication used by the nurse is **most** effective in this situation?
   1. Touch
   2. Talking
   3. Writing
   4. Pictures

   TEST-TAKING TIP: Identify the word in the stem that sets a priority. Identify the unique option.

8. The nurse is discharging a client to a long-term care facility. During the discharge teaching, the client says, "I am being sent to a nursing home to die. No one cares about me anymore." Which is the nurse's best response?
   1. "You are concerned and feel anxious that no one cares."
   2. "No one is sending you to die, everyone cares deeply for you."
   3. "Everyone is doing what is best for you. You should not be upset about that."
   4. "I know it is hard, but your family does not have the resources to care for you at home."

   TEST-TAKING TIP: Identify the word in the stem that sets a priority. Identify the clang association. Identify opposites in options. Identify the options that deny client feelings, concerns, or needs and identify the client-centered option with a specific determiner.

9. A female client talks about her children when they were young and states, "I was a very strict mother." Which response by the nurse exhibits the technique of paraphrasing?
   1. "It must have been difficult to be a disciplinarian."
   2. "Sometimes we are sorry for our past behaviors."
   3. "You don't seem like a very strict person."
   4. "You believe you were a firm parent."

   TEST-TAKING TIP: Identify the key word in the stem that directs attention to content. Identify the option that denies client feelings, concerns, or needs. Identify the client-centered option.

10. The nurse enters the room of a client. The client is crying and quietly tells the nurse, "I just found out I have cancer and I am so scared." Which nursing action is **most** therapeutic?
    1. Stands by the client's bed and says, "Try to focus on something else."
    2. Place a hand on the client's shoulder and say, "It may help to talk about it."
    3. Holds the client's hand and says, "A good cry will get this out of your system."
    4. Stands in the room and says, "Just breathe deeply and slowly to gain composure."

    TEST-TAKING TIP: Identify options that deny client feelings, concerns, or needs. Identify equally plausible options. Identify the client-centered option. Identify options that are opposites.

11. A client asks for advice regarding a personal problem. Which is the **most** appropriate response by the nurse?
    1. Explain that nurses are not permitted to give advice to a client.
    2. Encourage the client to speak with a family member.
    3. Ask the client what would be the best thing to do.
    4. Offer an opinion after listening to the client.

    TEST-TAKING TIP: Identify the word in the stem that sets a priority. Identify the option that denies client feelings, concerns, or needs. Identify opposites in options. Identify the client-centered option.

12. A newly admitted client appears upset and agitated. Which should the nurse do to assist this client?
    1. Arrange for the client to remain on bed rest.
    2. Encourage the client to share feelings.
    3. Keep the client as active as possible.
    4. Point out the behavior to the client.

    TEST-TAKING TIP: Identify key words in the stem that direct attention to content. Identify the option that denies client feelings, concerns, or needs. Identify the client-centered option. Identify opposites in options.

13. An older adult reminisces extensively and attempts to keep the nurse from leaving the room. Which nursing action is a therapeutic response?
    1. Encouraging the client to focus on the present
    2. Limiting the amount of time the client talks about the past
    3. Setting aside time to listen to the stories about the client's past
    4. Suggesting that the client reminisce with other clients of the same age

    TEST-TAKING TIP: Identify key words in the stem that direct attention to content. Identify options that deny client feelings, concerns, or needs. Identify opposites in options.

14. Several times a day, every day, a client who is experiencing short-term memory loss asks when medication is to be given. The client receives medication at the same time every day. Which is the **most** therapeutic nursing intervention?
    1. Inform the client when the time for medication has arrived.
    2. Tell the client to go to the nurse when it is time for medication.
    3. Encourage the client to remember when it is time for medication.
    4. Make the client a sign to hang on a wall indicating the times for medication.

    TEST-TAKING TIP: Identify the word in the stem that sets a priority. Identify key words in the stem that direct attention to content. Identify equally plausible options.

15. The nurse is teaching the client with a new ostomy how to change their colostomy bag. During the education, the client tells the nurse, "I am worried that I am never going to learn how to change this ostomy bag." Which communication technique could the nurse use in their response? **Select all that apply.**
1. Empathy
2. Reflection
3. Facilitation
4. Clarification

TEST-TAKING TIP: Identify the options that assist in data gathering to understand the client's feelings, concerns, or needs.

16. The nurse is completing the admission of a 2-year-old being admitted for rotavirus with excessive vomiting and diarrhea. The nurse is concerned about dehydration. Which interview technique is best to gather assessment data from the parents?
1. Assertive interview
2. Reflective interview
3. Explanatory interview
4. Clarification interview

TEST-TAKING TIP: Identify key words in the stem that direct attention to content. Identify the priority.

17. The nurse calls the provider to discuss their client's status. Which is the best response for Situation using the Situation Background Assessment and Recommendation (SBAR) format recommended by The Joint Commission?
1. "The client's urine output has decreased to less than 25 milliliters per hour."
2. "The client's urine output is continuing to decline, which is concerning."
3. "The client's urine output is less than 25 milliliters per hour for 24 hours, which is concerning."
4. "The client is not producing much urine, in fact, it has gotten worse over 24 hours."

TEST-TAKING TIP: Identify the option that provides clear communication.

18. An older adult becomes upset whenever anyone mentions an upcoming birthday and does not want to talk about age. This behavior reflects:
1. denial.
2. sorrow.
3. loneliness.
4. suppression.

19. A client has a history of verbally aggressive behavior. One afternoon, the client starts to shout at another client in the lounge. Which is an appropriate response by the nurse? **Select all that apply.**
1. _____ "Stop what you are doing."
2. _____ "Let's go talk in your room."
3. _____ "Sit down until you are calm."
4. _____ "Come with me for a walk in the hall."
5. _____ "Do not raise your voice in a hospital."

TEST-TAKING TIP: Identify key words in the stem that direct attention to content. Identify the client-centered options. Identify options that deny client feelings, concerns, or needs.

20. The nurse is caring for a teen client brought to the emergency department by their parents. The parents state that the teen has become increasingly depressed with ambivalent and labile behaviors over the last few days. During the assessment, the client tells the nurse, "Sometimes, I think it would be better if I was not around." Which is a therapeutic response by the nurse? **Select all that apply.**

1. _____ "Do you think or feel this way presently?"
2. _____ "When did you begin to have these thoughts?"
3. _____ "Has something happened to make you feel this way?"
4. _____ "Why do you feel this way? You have so much to live for."
5. _____ "Do you think you might act on these thoughts in the future?"
6. _____ "Have you told anyone about these thoughts you are having?"

TEST-TAKING TIP: Identify the key word in the stem that directs attention to content. Identify the client-centered options. Identify options that deny client feelings, concerns, or needs.

21. The nurse is performing a self-appraisal concerning the use of statements that do not support a client's needs. Which statement by the nurse is nontherapeutic? **Select all that apply.**

1. _____ "This is minor surgery."
2. _____ "You're smiling this morning."
3. _____ "A lot of people hate injections."
4. _____ "It is difficult to cope with pain."
5. _____ "You'll walk better after you have physical therapy."

TEST-TAKING TIP: Identify the word in the stem that indicates negative polarity.

22. A nurse is caring for the toddler in the photograph. Which nursing action **supports** the emotional needs of this child? **Select all that apply.**

1. _____ Demonstrating to the child how the penlight works before using it
2. _____ Maintaining a smiling expression when talking with the child
3. _____ Positioning oneself at eye level with the child
4. _____ Encouraging the child to hold a favorite toy
5. _____ Allowing the child to sit on the mother's lap

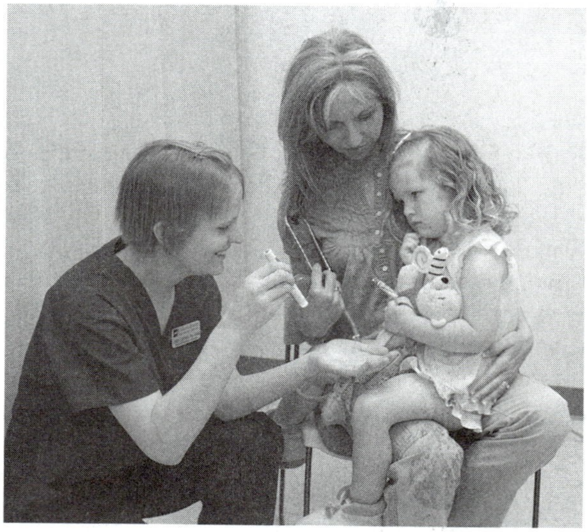

TEST-TAKING TIP: Identify client-centered options.

23. A client who is hearing-impaired tells the nurse, "I have difficulty hearing what people say to me." Which should the nurse do? **Select all that apply.**

1. _____ Speak using a lower tone of voice
2. _____ Face the client directly when talking
3. _____ Provide pencil and paper for communication
4. _____ Enunciate clearly when speaking with the client
5. _____ Ask the client questions that require a yes or no answer
6. _____ Encourage the client to use gestures and facial expressions when talking

TEST-TAKING TIP: Identify the key words in the stem that direct attention to content.

24. Nurse-client relationships happen best when the environment facilitates an easy exchange of both verbal and nonverbal communication. Which nonverbal concepts are important for the nurse to consider when interacting with clients? **Select all that apply.**

1. _____ Maintain eye contact
2. _____ Choice of clothing
3. _____ Tone of your voice as well as the client's tone of voice
4. _____ Noting your own gestures as well as the client's gestures
5. _____ Touch has various meanings for different people
6. _____ Avoid using distancing language when speaking to clients

25. The hospice nurse is completing the health history and intake assessment of their newly admitted client. The nurse notices the client and their spouse are both fearful and crying. Which behavior supports the nursing diagnosis of Anticipatory Grieving? **Select all that apply.**

1. _____ Sleeping soundly through the night
2. _____ Anger and denial of impending death
3. _____ Fear of pain during the dying process
4. _____ Statements of powerlessness and loss of control
5. _____ Worrying about the impact of the death on others
6. _____ Positive thoughts and images to prepare for a peaceful death

TEST-TAKING TIP: Identify the key word in the stem that directs attention to content.

26. A client who is dying is withdrawn and depressed. Which is a therapeutic action by the nurse? **Select all that apply.**

1. _____ Explaining that client goals still can be accomplished
2. _____ Helping the client to focus on positive thoughts
3. _____ Offering the client advice when appropriate
4. _____ Accepting the client's behavioral response
5. _____ Telling the client you are available to talk

TEST-TAKING TIP: Identify key words in the stem that direct attention to content. Identify options that deny client feelings, concerns, or needs. Identify client-centered options.

27. The nurse is assessing the client who is visually impaired. Place the communication steps in the correct order that the nurse should use while in the client's room to complete the assessment.

1. _____ Orient the client to the arrangement of their tray table and other furnishings
2. _____ Place the call bell within reach of the client
3. _____ Identify yourself by name
4. _____ Acknowledge your presence in the client's room
5. _____ Indicate to the client that you are leaving the room
6. _____ Explain the reason for touching the client before doing so

28. The nurse in the emergency department is caring for several clients who are anxious. Place the following clients in the order that reflects the levels of anxiety, progressing from mild, to moderate, to severe, and finally to panic levels.

1. Client who has vocal pitch changes, is focusing on one topic, and is exhibiting slight muscle tremors
2. Client who has normal vital signs, is asking many questions, and is exhibiting slight muscle tension
3. Client who has distorted perception, is hyperventilating, and is exhibiting erratic behavior
4. Client who has increased motor activity, is irritable, and is exhibiting dilated pupils

Answer: ___________

29. A client who is incontinent of urine becomes upset. Which is a therapeutic response by the nurse while changing the client's gown and linens? **Select all that apply.**

1. _____ "This must be difficult for you."
2. _____ "I am a nurse. This is part of my job."
3. _____ "This doesn't bother me. It often happens."
4. _____ "This occurs all the time. Try not to feel bad."
5. _____ "I am your nurse. I will change your gown and linens."

TEST-TAKING TIP: Identify the clang association. Identify options that deny client feelings, concerns, or needs. Identify client-centered options.

30. A client has difficulty communicating verbally (expressive aphasia) because of a brain attack (stroke). Which should the nurse do to help the client communicate? **Select all that apply.**

1. _____ Anticipate needs to reduce frustration
2. _____ Teach the client how to use a picture board
3. _____ Create a list of words that the client can say
4. _____ Encourage the client to elaborate with gestures
5. _____ Be patient when the client is attempting to speak
6. _____ Ask the client questions that require a yes or no response

TEST-TAKING TIP: Identify the word in the stem that directs attention to content.

31. The nurse must use specific communication techniques for older adult clients who have speech, language, and hearing disorders. Which techniques should the nurse select? **Select all that apply.**

1. _____ Demonstrate or pantomime ideas, as appropriate
2. _____ Reinforce and praise client's efforts to communicate
3. _____ Provide lengthy thorough instructions to ensure client comprehension
4. _____ Whenever possible, use open-ended questions to gather more information
5. _____ Demonstrate patience and understanding with the time needed to communicate
6. _____ Use speaking patterns that mimic childhood language for easier comprehension

TEST-TAKING TIP: Identify key words in the stem that direct attention to content. Identify opposites in options. Identify client-centered options. Identify options that deny client feelings, concerns, or needs.

32. A client verbally communicates with the nurse while exhibiting nonverbal behavior. How should the nurse confirm the meaning of the nonverbal behavior? **Select all that apply.**

1. _____ Look for similarity in meaning between the client's verbal and nonverbal behavior
2. _____ Request that family members interpret the client's nonverbal behavior
3. _____ Recognize that nonverbal behavior often is more reliable than words
4. _____ Ask the client direct questions about the nonverbal behavior
5. _____ Point out the nonverbal behavior to the client

33. The primary health-care provider prescribes alprazolam 0.5 mg PO tid for a client experiencing panic attacks. What should the nurse do when caring for this client? **Select all that apply.**

1. _____ Assess for signs of alprazolam misuse
2. _____ Ensure that naloxone is readily available
3. _____ Teach the client to provide for personal safety
4. _____ Encourage the intake of grapefruit juice during therapy
5. _____ Advise the client not to abruptly discontinue the medication
6. _____ Encourage the client to take an additional PRN dose when experiencing high-anxiety situations

TEST-TAKING TIP: Identify the clang association.

34. The health-care facility has implemented a Situation, Background, Assessment, Recommendation (SBAR) template as part of its electronic documentation to improve and increase frequency of communication among the health-care team. The nurse is giving a shift hand-off report to the oncoming nurse. Using the SBAR document provided, identify which area the following statements should be placed in the SBAR. Fill in the blank with Situation, Background, Assessment, or Recommendation.

1. The client is being monitored for a concussion __________
2. The client exhibits no signs of a concussion and is stable __________
3. The client has several bruises and three lacerations with stitches __________
4. The client is stable with no pain so should be ready for discharge __________
5. The client, a 48-year-old female, was admitted after a motor vehicle collision _______

S	**Situation** I am calling about __________ The client's code status is: __________ The problem I am calling about is: __________ Vital Signs: Blood Pressure ________ Pulse ________ Respiration ________ Temperature ________ Pulse oximeter ________
B	**Background** The client's mental status is: __________ The skin is: __________ The client is/is not on oxygen at __________ L/min.
A	**Assessment** I believe the client (state the problem) __________ The problem seems to be cardiac infection neurologic respiratory I am not sure what the problem is. The client is unstable and deteriorating.
R	**Recommendation** Provider Name __________ Transfer to __________ See client __________ Test __________ Changes in Treatment __________

35. Which level of anxiety is the client currently experiencing according to the information in the client's clinical record?
  1. Mild
  2. Moderate
  3. Severe
  4. Panic

CLIENT'S CLINICAL RECORD

Progress Note
Admitted to the coronary care unit (CCU) from the emergency department for observation because of chest pain and palpitations. On admission to the unit, the client reports the presence of a headache, dizziness, and nausea but no longer feels chest pain or palpitations. Client is asking numerous questions about the chest pain previously experienced and continually focusing on the potential for pain.

Vital Signs on Admission to the CCU
Temp: 99°F, oral route
Pulse: 120 beats/min, regular rhythm
Respirations: 32 breaths/min, deep
Pulse oximetry: 98%

Physical Assessment
Client has increased motor activity and a fearful facial expression, demonstrates a decreased ability to focus or concentrate when asked questions, and is easily distracted; client is still experiencing tachycardia and is hyperventilating.

1. **TEST-TAKING TIP: The word *best* in the stem sets a priority. Option 4 is unique because it is a receptive, nonverbal action, whereas the other options are all active verbal interventions. Options 2 and 3 are equally plausible because both involve questions.**
   1. Talking about expectations occurs later in the nurse-client relationship, after needs have been identified.
   2. Direct, not probing, questions might be asked later; probing questions violate a client's right to privacy.
   3. Asking direct questions may be done later; it is not the priority.
   4. **Reception of a message must occur before the nurse can intervene; by listening, the nurse collects information that influences future care.**

2. **TEST-TAKING TIP: The word *most* in the stem sets a priority. Options 1, 2, and 3 are not client-centered and deny the client's feelings, concerns, or needs.**
   1. The nurse should never compare their individual experiences to those of a client. This is a form of distancing where the nurse is attempting to soften the reality of the situation and may diminish the client's feelings and limit future communication.
   2. This is a communication trap of giving unwanted advice. This is an opinion and is inappropriate in this situation. The nurse should take the time to involve the client and problem-solve to help the client cope with the loss, not diminish the client's feelings.
   3. This is not therapeutic communication. This is a type of communication trap where the nurse is using authority—the provider/nurse knows best. This diminishes the client's concerns and cuts off future open communication.
   4. **This is the correct answer. This is an open-ended question asking the client for narrative information. This form of questioning is called facilitation, which is unbiased and allows the client to answer in any way they choose. It encourages the client to respond in paragraphs, rather than yes or no, and shows the client that you are interested.**

3. **TEST-TAKING TIP: The word *ineffective* in the stem indicates negative polarity. The word *psychosocial* is the key word in the stem that directs attention to content. Option 2 is unique because it is the only option that provides physical nursing care. Options 1, 3, and 4 are interventions based on psychosocial principles of care.**
   1. Calling a client by name individualizes care and supports dignity and self-esteem.
   2. **Usually, eating is an independent activity of daily living; for an adult, assistance with meals may precipitate feelings of dependence and regression.**
   3. Identifying the achievement of goals is motivating and supports independence, self-esteem, and self-actualization.
   4. Explaining care provides emotional support because it reduces fear of the unknown and involves the client in the care.

4.
   1. **This is inappropriate probing and violates the client's right to privacy or may put the client on the defensive.**
   2. This is not an appropriate response. This is considered a form of communication where the nurse uses their authority and diminishes the client's response. It could make the client feel insecure and not comfortable talking about their feelings with the nurse.
   3. This is inappropriate. This is biased language and could influence the client's response. This could make the client feel guilty and forced to answer according to what they perceive are the nurse's values.
   4. **This is a client-centered option. The nurse receives the message that the client may be asking for assistance and wanting reinforcement. Understanding this interpersonal communication will help the nurse work with a client whose negative self-talk may affect their health and selfcare.**

5. **TEST-TAKING TIP: The word *withdrawn* in the stem directs attention to content. Options 4, 5, and 6 are equally plausible because they address something that is wrong (e.g., bothering, upset).**
   1. This is not an appropriate response. Ignoring the client's behavior could make the client feel that the nurse is not interested in their feelings and further shut the client down from communication.
   2. This is a probing question that is not appropriate during the assessment. This may make the client defensive about why their family has not been to visit.

This question may be acceptable after the assessment if the client chooses to open a line of dialogue on how they are feeling and why they are quiet.

3. A good rule for nurses when assessing and gathering information on verbal and nonverbal communication messages from a client is to listen more than you talk. "Small talk" could indicate to the client that you are not interested in their feelings or concerns. Excessive talking places the focus on the nurse instead of the client.
4. This is not appropriate. There are a myriad of reasons why the client may be quieter than usual. The nurse must first investigate and analyze before deciding on such a drastic intervention.
5. **During the assessment, the nurse should gather information in both verbal and nonverbal forms. The nurse could tell the client what they notice and then ask the client if they would like to talk. This gathering of information can help the nurse to understand the subtle message the client may be sending through their silence.**
6. **Periods of silence can have important nonverbal messages. Silence allows a client to gather their thoughts and proceed at their own pace to initiate conversation.**

6. **TEST-TAKING TIP: The word *best* in the stem sets a priority. Options 1 and 2 deny the client's feelings, concerns, or needs. Options 3 and 4 are client-centered. Although encouraging grief counseling is something the nurse may do in the future, it is not the best response at this time.**
   1. Although staying at the bedside does not physically abandon the client, reorganizing the client's unit is a form of emotional abandonment. Ignoring behavior (crying) denies the client's feelings.
   2. This statement is false reassurance and denies the client's feeling.
   3. **This statement identifies feelings, focuses on the client, and provides an opportunity for the client to share feelings.**
   4. This may eventually be done, but the client needs immediate support.

7. **TEST-TAKING TIP: The word *most* in the stem sets a priority. Option 1 is unique. Touch is the only intervention that does not require higher intellectual functioning.**
   1. **Touch is a simple form of communication that is easily understood even by confused, disoriented, or mentally incapacitated individuals.**
   2. Talking requires an interpretation of words, which is a more complex form of communication than the route of communication in another option.
   3. Writing requires interpretation of symbols, which is a more complex form of communication than the route of communication in another option.
   4. Pictures require interpretation of symbols, which is a more complex form of communication than the route of communication in another option.

8. **TEST-TAKING TIP: The word *best* in the stem sets a priority. The words *no one cares* appear in the stem and option 1; this repetition is a clang association. Options 1 and 2 are opposites. Option 1 is client-centered. Options 2 and 3 deny client feelings, concerns, or needs. Option 2 contains the word *everyone,* which is a specific determiner.**
   1. **This is the communication technique of reflection where the nurse repeats some of what the client has just said. Reflection can help the client express the feelings behind their words. It can validate what the client said and encourage further communication.**
   2. This statement is an assumption that may or may not be true. This does not encourage the client to further express their feelings. This statement provides false reassurance to the client and dismisses their feelings.
   3. This statement is the communication technique of giving unwanted advice. This is inappropriate communication where the nurse assumes the role of authority figure and dismisses the client's concerns.
   4. This statement may or may not be true and does not encourage expression of feelings. This statement may make the client further shut down and avoid expressing their feelings. It is not client-centered and does not support the client's feelings.

9. **TEST-TAKING TIP: The word *paraphrasing* is the key word in the stem that directs attention to content. Although option 3 has a clang association with the word *strict,* this option denies client feelings, concerns, or needs and should be eliminated. Option 4 is the client-centered option.**
   1. This response uses reflective technique, not paraphrasing, because it identifies a feeling (difficult).

2. The client's statement does not reflect feelings of sorrow or guilt.
3. This response denies the client's feelings.
4. **This response restates the message using different words; paraphrasing focuses on content rather than the feeling or underlying emotional theme of the client's message.**

10. **TEST-TAKING TIP: Options 1, 3, and 4 deny client feelings, concerns, or needs; options 3 and 4 imply that everything will get better. These are Pollyanna-like responses that deny the client's feelings. Options 3 and 4 are equally plausible; both relate to getting emotions under control or out of the system. Option 2 is client-centered. Options 1 and 2 are opposites.**
    1. This statement denies the client's feelings. It will be impossible for the client to focus on something else after receiving this life-altering diagnosis. This is not therapeutic and does not encourage communication.
    2. **This response provides an opportunity for the client to express feelings and concerns and is client-centered.**
    3. This response is false reassurance; crying may or may not help this client. Also, use of the word *good* is a value judgment.
    4. This response implies that the client is out of control. This interferes with the client's coping mechanism—crying.

11. **TEST-TAKING TIP: The word *most* in the stem sets a priority. Option 1 denies the client's feelings, concerns, or needs. Options 3 and 4 are opposites. Option 3 is client-centered.**
    1. This approach puts the focus on the nurse and cuts off communication.
    2. Although this might eventually be done, it is not the priority. Also, the client may never want to talk about a particular concern with family members.
    3. **This response provides an opportunity for the client to explore concerns and alternative solutions without others influencing the decision making.**
    4. Offering opinions is inappropriate; opinions involve judgments that are based on feelings and values that may be different from the client's.

12. **TEST-TAKING TIP: The words *upset and agitated* are key words in the stem that direct attention to content. Option 1 denies client feelings, concerns, or needs. It is difficult for an agitated client to remain in bed. Option 2 is client-centered. Although options 1 and 3 are opposites, they are distractors in this question. More often than not, one of the options that is an opposite is the correct answer, *but not always*.**
    1. Agitated clients may not be able to lie still. They need some outlet for energy expenditure.
    2. **Agitation is a response to anxiety; the client's feelings and concerns must be addressed to help relieve the anxiety and agitation.**
    3. Keeping the client as active as possible may increase the agitation, particularly if the cause of the agitation is ignored.
    4. Pointing out the behavior to the client is confrontational and may precipitate a defensive response by the client.

13. **TEST-TAKING TIP: The words *reminisces extensively* are key words in the stem that direct attention to content. Options 1 and 2 deny client feelings, concerns, or needs. Options 1 and 3 are opposites.**
    1. Avoiding reminiscing is inappropriate; the developmental task of older adults is to perform a life review.
    2. Avoiding reminiscing is inappropriate; the developmental task of older adults is to perform a life review.
    3. **The nurse is responsible for assisting the older adult in exploring the past and dealing with the developmental conflict of integrity versus despair.**
    4. Clients should not be responsible for meeting each other's needs.

14. **TEST-TAKING TIP: The word *most* in the stem sets a priority. The words *short-term memory loss* are key words in the stem that direct attention to content. Options 2 and 3 are equally plausible because both options require the client to remember when medications are given.**
    1. Although the client might be reminded every time, it is not the most therapeutic intervention because it addresses only the next dose.
    2. The client probably is not capable of remembering. A task that is too challenging can be frustrating.
    3. The client probably will not remember when it is time for the medication. A task that is too challenging can be frustrating.
    4. **A sign promotes independence and does not demean the client; the**

client can refer to the schedule when necessary.

15. **TEST-TAKING TIP: Identify the communication techniques that demonstrate concern and caring.**
    1. **This is an appropriate communication technique. Empathy allows a person to feel accepted and strengthens rapport. It allows objective understanding of how a client views their situation. The nurse could use empathy to clarify the client's feelings.**
    2. **This is an appropriate communication technique. Reflection echoes a client's words through repeating what the person has just stated. It can help express the feelings behind the words and allow the client to elaborate on their concern or problem.**
    3. This is not appropriate for this client situation. Explanation is a communication technique where one informs and shares factual and objective information. In this situation, the nurse needs to explore the reasons why the client made this statement.
    4. This is not appropriate for this client situation. Clarification is useful when a person's word choice is confusing. In clarification, a person's words are summarized to ensure understanding by all parties involved. This does not uncover why the client made the statement.
    5. This is not appropriate for this client situation. The communication technique of confrontation clarifies inconsistent information. It can be used when a client's verbal and nonverbal behaviors are incongruent.

16. **TEST-TAKING TIP: Identify key words in the stem that direct attention to the content. Identify options to help the nurse gather information about the problem.**
    1. An assertive interview technique is not appropriate in the data-gathering phase of the client interview. This may cause the parents to exhibit defensive mechanisms and limit the assessment data gathered.
    2. The reflective interview technique is not appropriate in this client situation. The nurse needs to gather data to identify interventions for the child. Reflection helps express feelings behind words.
    3. The explanatory interview technique is not appropriate in the data-gathering phase of the interview. Explanation is when the nurse shares factual and objective information.
    4. **Clarification is the best option. The use of clarifying questions allows the nurse to gather data and gain an understanding of the client's illness. This technique can avert misunderstandings between the nurse and parents and lead to an appropriate nursing diagnosis and interventions. Clarification encourages open-ended questions for verbalization of what the parents believe to be true.**

17. **TEST-TAKING TIP: Identify the option that provides efficient and clear data. Options 1, 2, and 4 do not provide detailed, specific data.**
    1. The SBAR hand-off tool presents accurate and specific client information from one caregiver to another. This response does not give a complete objective assessment of the client. The nurse should state the timeline for the urine output decrease.
    2. The SBAR technique helps the health-care team communicate accurate data to make decisions. This statement does not include objective data of the client's current situation.
    3. **Using a standardized communication tool reduces the risk of transmitting inaccurate and incomplete information. This statement includes objective and specific data for the provider to consider.**
    4. Situation in SBAR provides background and objective information. This statement does not provide the objective data, the amount of urine output, for the provider to consider.

18.
    1. Denial is an unconscious defense mechanism; this older adult consciously and voluntarily refuses to talk about birthdays.
    2. This is an assumption; there are insufficient data to reach this conclusion.
    3. This is an assumption; there are insufficient data to reach this conclusion.
    4. **Suppression is a conscious protective mechanism in which a person actively puts anxiety-producing feelings or concerns out of the mind.**

19. **TEST-TAKING TIP: The words *verbally aggressive* and *shout* are key words in the stem that direct attention to content. Options 2 and 4 are client-centered.**

Options 1, 3, and 5 deny client feelings, concerns, or needs.

1. This statement is a command that may demean the client; it challenges the client and may precipitate more aggressive behavior.
2. **This statement interrupts the behavior and protects the other clients. Walking to another room uses energy, and talking promotes expression of feelings and concerns.**
3. This statement is judgmental; this implies the client is not calm. An agitated client has too much energy to sit quietly.
4. **This statement interrupts the behavior and protects the other clients. Walking will expend some of the client's energy. This nurse can encourage the client to express feelings and concerns while walking.**
5. This statement is inappropriate because it is challenging, which may put the client on the defensive.

20. **TEST-TAKING TIP: The words *better if I am not around* are the key words in the stem that direct attention to content. Options 1, 2, 3, 5, and 6 are client-centered. Option 4 denies client feelings, concerns, or needs.**
Suicide is the most preventable cause of death in teens and adolescents. Nurses are often the first person in the health-care setting to interact with a suicidal client, so it is important to understand how to communicate therapeutically for suicide and self-harm screening.
   1. **This is an appropriate response. To establish a therapeutic relationship and gather the appropriate assessment data, it is important to ask questions about self-harm and suicide.**
   2. **If a client feels they are a burden to others, and that their families and friends would be better off without them, the nurse should be concerned. The nurse should try to uncover the trigger for these thoughts.**
   3. **The nurse needs to identify the triggering factors for these thoughts and how the teen copes with stress. Teens have less life experience handling stress so they may be impulsive.**
   4. The nurse should avoid trying to create a cheerful and upbeat environment. Do not offer false reassurances that everything will be better with time.
   5. **When assessing the depressed or suicidal teen, the nurse should assess the level of lethality or how suicidal the client may be. Problems that may be minimal to others can be overwhelming and devastating to a teen.**
   6. **Some clients may talk about suicidal or self-harm plans with others and gauge the impact it would have on their friends and families. This can help clarify the client's feelings and suicidal or self-harm plans.**

21. **TEST-TAKING TIP: The word *nontherapeutic* in the stem indicates negative polarity. The question really is asking, Which options are examples of inappropriate statements that the nurse should avoid when interacting with clients?**
   1. **This statement implies that there is no reason to worry, which is a form of false reassurance.**
   2. This is a therapeutic response that invites the client to explore feelings.
   3. **This statement takes the focus away from the client and cuts off further communication.**
   4. This is a supportive statement that focuses on what the client may be thinking and invites an exploration of feelings and problem solving.
   5. **This statement supports an outcome that may or may not be accomplished by physical therapy; this is false reassurance.**

22. **TEST-TAKING TIP: Options 1, 2, 3, 4, and 5 are client-centered options.**
   1. **Demonstrating how equipment works before use engages the child, helps to minimize fear of the unknown, and builds trust between the child and nurse.**
   2. **Maintaining a smiling expression conveys that the nurse is friendly and approachable, communicates warmth and caring, and facilitates a connection between the nurse and child.**
   3. Positioning oneself at eye level with the child nonverbally communicates a personal interest in the child and indicates that communication is an open channel.
   4. **Encouraging the child to hold a familiar cuddly toy enhances feelings of safety and security during times of stress.**
   5. **Allowing the child to sit on the mother's lap enhances a feeling of safety and security during times of stress.**

23. **TEST-TAKING TIP: The words *hearing-impaired* are the key words in the stem that direct attention to content.**
    1. **Low-pitched sounds are easier to hear than high-pitched sounds.**
    2. **Facing the client directly allows the client to view the nurse's lips and facial expression, both of which improve the transmission and reception of a message.**
    3. **Communication can be promoted in written rather than verbal form; this reduces social isolation.**
    4. **Enunciating clearly presents a verbal message that should be clear and crisp; mumbling sends messages that can become distorted and misinterpreted.**
    5. Communication is a two-way process. The client is not having difficulty sending messages; the client is having difficulty receiving messages. This intervention is more appropriate for a client with expressive aphasia.
    6. The client is having difficulty receiving messages, not sending messages.

24. 1. **Maintaining eye contact is an important form of nonverbal communication the nurse should consider. Lack of eye contact from a client may indicate behaviors such as shyness, boredom, or depression. The nurse should maintain eye contact with clients except in cultures where direct eye contact should be avoided.**
    2. **This is an important form of nonverbal communication. Inattention to clothing and appearance may suggest a client is too sick to maintain self-care or has an emotional dysfunction. The nurse's clothing and appearance project a message of professionalism and competency.**
    3. The tone of voice is an important verbal concept that the nurse should consider.
    4. **Gestures are important forms of nonverbal communication. Gestures send messages and reinforce verbal communication.**
    5. **Touch is a form of nonverbal communication that sends a variety of messages depending on the person's culture, sex, age, past experiences, and present situation; touch also invades a person's personal space. Touch can be easily misinterpreted.**
    6. This is a form of verbal communication. Distancing language is the use of impersonal speech to place space between and threat and self. An example is when the word "the" may be used instead of "your." "The cancer is back" instead of "Your cancer is back."

25. **TEST-TAKING TIP: The words *hospice, fearful, and crying* are key words in the stem that direct attention to content. The nursing diagnosis of Anticipatory Grieving is related to the anticipated loss of physiological well-being and the perceived death of the client.**
    1. Anticipatory grieving is often evidenced by alterations in sleep patterns such as sleep disturbances and lack of sleep, changes in eating habits, and changes in communication patterns.
    2. **Anticipatory grieving is often evidenced by denial of the potential loss, anger, and repressed feelings of sadness or hurt.**
    3. **Anticipatory grieving is often evidenced by anticipated pain related to dying and fear of the dying process itself.**
    4. **Anticipatory grieving is often evidenced by powerlessness over issues related to dying and complete loss of control of their own death.**
    5. **Anticipatory grieving is often evidenced by worry and fear of the impact of the death on significant others and family members. Clients worry about being the cause of other people's grief.**
    6. Anticipatory grieving is often evidenced by negative images of death or unpleasant thoughts about upcoming events related to the death and dying process.

26. **TEST-TAKING TIP: The words *dying, withdrawn*, and *depressed* are key words in the stem that direct attention to content. Options 1, 2, and 3 deny client feelings, concerns, and needs. Options 4 and 5 are client-centered options.**
    1. Explaining that the client still can accomplish goals denies the client's feelings.
    2. Helping the client to focus on positive thoughts denies the client's feelings.
    3. It is never appropriate to offer advice; people must explore their alternatives and come to their own conclusions.
    4. **Depression is the fourth stage of dying according to Kübler-Ross; clients become withdrawn and noncommunicative when feeling a loss of control and**

recognizing future losses. The nurse should accept the behavior.

5. Clients who are dying become depressed when they realize that death is inevitable. The nurse should be available in case the client wants to talk.

27. The correct answer is 4, 3, 6, 2, 1, 5.

Nurses should always acknowledge that they are in the room and then introduce themselves using their name and position. This allows the client to know that you are present and ready to assist. Always speak directly to the client in a natural, conversational tone. Be precise and use descriptive language when assessing the client. Always let them know what areas you will be touching. After the assessment is complete, ensure they have their call bell within easy reach, orient them to other items such as IV poles or furniture they should be aware of, and let them know when you are leaving the room.

28. Answer: 2, 1, 4, 3

2. People with mild anxiety have normal or slight physiological responses (e.g., vital signs, muscle tension) because the sympathetic nervous system is barely stimulated. Their communication usually revolves around questions to obtain information.
1. People with moderate anxiety have an increase in physiological responses (e.g., tremors, slight increase in vital signs) as a result of greater stimulation of the sympathetic nervous system. Their communication is slightly impaired, as evidenced by pitch changes and tremors of the voice, selective inattention, and focusing on one topic.
4. People with severe anxiety have physiological reactions associated with the fight-or-flight response related to the sympathetic nervous system (e.g., increased motor activity, dilated pupils, elevated vital signs, headache, nausea, urgency, and frequency). Their mood reflects irritability.
3. People with a panic level of anxiety have a continuation of the physiological reactions associated with the fight-or-flight response (e.g., increased motor activity, dilated pupils, elevated vital signs, headache, nausea, urgency, and frequency). Their perception is distorted and scattered, and their motor activity can be erratic, combative, or withdrawn.

29. **TEST-TAKING TIP:** The words *gown and linens* in the stem and in option 5 is a clang association. Options 2, 3, and 4 deny client feelings, concerns, or needs. Options 1 and 5 do not minimize the client's feelings and focus on the client; they are client-centered.

1. This response focuses on feelings and is supportive.
2. This response cuts off communication and puts the focus on the nurse rather than on the client.
3. This response generalizes care rather than individualizes care. It minimizes the client's concern and may cut off communication.
4. This response generalizes care rather than individualizes care. The use of the word *bad* is an assumption.
5. This response meets the client's right to know who is providing care and what is to be done. This is a nonjudgmental, respectful response even though it does not address the client's feelings.

30. **TEST-TAKING TIP:** The words *expressive aphasia* are the key words in the stem that direct attention to content.

1. Although anticipating needs may be done occasionally, it does not increase the client's ability to communicate.
2. A picture board generally is a laminated card featuring photographs or illustrations, often with matching phrases associated with common personal needs. This device gives control of the conversation to the client, which increases independence and reduces frustration when making needs known.
3. Creating a list of words that the client can say and sharing this information with health-care team and family members broadens the group of people with whom the client can communicate.
4. Communication can be both verbal and nonverbal. The use of gestures facilitates communication.
5. Being patient while the client is attempting to speak demonstrates respect, allows the client time to form the communication, and supports self-esteem.
6. Although this may be done occasionally, it does not increase the client's ability to

communicate; a yes or no response is too limited.

31. **TEST-TAKING TIP: The words *older adult and disorders* are key words in the stem that direct attention to content. Options 3 and 6 imply the clients are not competent. Option 4 is not client-centered because it may be challenging for the client to answer many questions. Options 1, 2, and 5 are client-centered.**

1. **This is a client-centered option. The nurse should talk directly to the patient while facing them. If needed, the nurse can pantomime or demonstrate. For example, the nurse could demonstrate which button to press on the call bell.**
2. **Reinforcement and praise are client-centered. These are communication tools that recognize the work a client is doing or attempting to do as part of their care.**
3. Break down instructions into simple tasks and avoid lengthy explanations. If clients feel like they are involved in their care, they are more likely to use the nursing interventions provided. If instructions are too cumbersome, a client may choose not to complete tasks.
4. Whenever possible, avoid open-ended questions. Ask the client, "Would you like to wear the orange shirt or the blue shirt?" instead of "What would you like to wear?"
5. **The nurse should be patient and give clients time to respond. If after a time they do not respond, the nurse can repeat what was said. If necessary, provide the client with breaks so neither the nurse nor the client becomes frustrated.**
6. Communication should be simple and concrete. Speaking in childlike tones and manner implies the client is not competent and is discriminatory.

32.

1. **The client is the primary source of information. When nonverbal communication reinforces a verbal message, the client's true feelings are typically reflected because nonverbal behavior is under less conscious control than verbal statements.**
2. This abdicates the nurse's responsibility to others and obtains a response that is influenced by the family members' emotion and subjectivity.
3. **Nonverbal behaviors, rather than verbal statements, better reflect true feelings. Actions speak louder than words!**
4. **Direct questions may ultimately be necessary if the client's responses to open-ended questions do not clarify the nonverbal behavior.**
5. **Pointing out behavior is a gentle way of making the client aware of his or her behavior, which may precipitate an exploration of the client's behavior and feelings. It is an open-ended approach because the client is in control of the progression of the interaction.**

33. **TEST-TAKING TIP: The word *alprazolam* in the stem and in option 1 is a clang association.**

1. **Use of alprazolam (Xanax®) can lead to misuse and dependence; therefore, the client should be assessed for responses such as drowsiness, sedation, irritability, dizziness, blurred vision, diplopia, headache, insomnia, gastrointestinal disturbances, dry mouth, tremors, confusion, slurred speech, impaired memory, and an inability to focus.**
2. The antidote for alprazolam (Xanax®) is flumazenil, not naloxone. Naloxone is an opioid antagonist that can inhibit or reverse the effects of opioids, such as respiratory depression, sedation, and hypotension.
3. **Alprazolam (Xanax®) is a central nervous system depressant that can cause dizziness, drowsiness, lethargy, decreased level of alertness, confusion, mental depression, and blurred vision. The client should be taught ways to provide for personal safety, such as how to prevent falls and not driving until the response to the drug has been determined.**
4. Grapefruit juice should be avoided when receiving alprazolam. Grapefruit juice can interfere with intestinal enzymes that metabolize alprazolam, thus causing higher than normal levels of the drug in the blood.
5. **To avoid signs and symptoms of withdrawal, alprazolam (Xanax®) should not be discontinued suddenly. Withdrawal should be conducted under medical supervision.**
6. Alprazolam (Xanax®) should be taken only three times a day as prescribed to maintain a therapeutic blood level of the drug in the body. Extra doses can lead to toxicity or

dependence and should not be taken without medical supervision.

34. Answer: 2, 3, 1, 5, 4

2. ***Denial or disbelief* is the first stage of Kübler-Ross's grieving theory. The client is saying "No, not me." The client may be in denial, may distrust the diagnosis, or may seek multiple diagnostic opinions. The client may intellectually understand the diagnosis but not emotionally integrate it.**
3. ***Anger* is the second stage of Kübler-Ross's grieving theory. The client may ask "Why me?" The client also may cite reasons why it is impossible to have the diagnosis or may respond with anger and hostility.**
1. ***Bargaining* is the third stage of Kübler-Ross's grieving theory. The client is saying "Yes me, but" and is attempting to gain more time.**
5. ***Depression* is the fourth stage of Kübler-Ross's grieving theory. The client is saying "Yes me" as the eventual death is realized. The client may grieve future losses, talk, withdraw, cry, or feel alone.**
4. ***Acceptance* is the fifth and last stage of Kübler-Ross's grieving theory. The client is saying "OK, me." The client may have decreased interest in activities, be quiet and peaceful, and be involved in completing personal affairs or planning the funeral. Sometimes, the client will reach this stage before family members; the nurse should help family members to understand and to allow the client to withdraw.**

35. 1. **The client's responses do not support the presence of mild anxiety. Mild anxiety is associated with increased questioning, mild restlessness, increased arousal and alertness, and the absence of physiological responses.**
2. The client's responses do not support the presence of moderate anxiety. Moderate anxiety is associated with voice tremors and pitch changes, tremors and shakiness, increased muscle tension, selective inattention, slightly increased respiratory and pulse rates, and mild gastric symptoms.
3. **The client's responses are indicative of severe anxiety. Severe anxiety is associated with tachycardia, hyperventilation, headache, dizziness, nausea, increased motor activity, and inability to relax. The person's communication may be difficult to understand, and the client has difficulty concentrating and is easily distracted.**
4. The client's responses do not support the presence of a panic level of anxiety. Panic-level anxiety is associated with agitation, trembling, poor motor coordination, dyspnea, palpitations, choking, chest pain or pressure, feeling of impending doom, paresthesias, diaphoresis, distorted or exaggerated perception, and communication that may not be understandable.

PHYSICAL ASSESSMENT OF CLIENTS

This section includes questions related to various aspects of physical and psychosocial assessment. Questions focus on temperature, pulse, respirations, blood pressure, level of consciousness, level of orientation, and principles related to the collection of specimens. Questions also address assessments common to infection, the general adaptation syndrome, and the inflammatory process. Additional questions focus on whether assessment data are subjective or objective, whether sources are primary or secondary, responsibilities of the nurse regarding data collected during assessments, sources of data, and the use of common physical examination techniques.

QUESTIONS

1. The new graduate nurse is assessing the client's lung sounds with the stethoscope. The nurse is unsure of which lung sounds are heard. How should the nurse proceed?
   1. Finish the assessment and then recheck the sounds later
   2. Ask a more experienced nurse to listen and verify the sounds
   3. Notify the provider to come listen in case the sounds are worrisome
   4. Document the lung sounds according to what the nurse believes they are

   TEST-TAKING TIP: Identify the key word in the stem that directs attention to content. Identify the unique option.

2. The nurse goes to the client's room to take their temperature with an electronic oral thermometer, but the client is drinking a cup of coffee. How should the nurse proceed?
   1. Take the temperature as the sublingual pocket is not affected by drinking
   2. Obtain a rectal temperature as it will be more accurate than an oral reading
   3. Have the client take a sip of cool water to offset the temperature of the coffee
   4. Wait at least 15 minutes for the sublingual pocket to return to a stable temperature

   TEST-TAKING TIP: Identify the key word in the stem that directs attention to content.

3. The nurse is auscultating the lung sounds of a 19-year-old client and hears high-pitched, musical-like squeaking sounds, louder on expiration than inspiration. How would the nurse interpret these lung sounds?
   1. Stridor
   2. Wheezing
   3. Fine crackles
   4. Coarse crackles

   TEST-TAKING TIP: Identify the key words in the stem that direct attention to content. Identify duplicate facts among options.

4. The nurse is checking pulses during the head-to-toe assessment for a client with diabetes and peripheral artery disease. Which are the priority pulses that the nurse should palpate for this client? **Select all that apply.**
   1. Ulnar
   2. Tibial
   3. Radial
   4. Popliteal
   5. Temporal
   6. Dorsalis pedis

   TEST-TAKING TIP: Identify the key words in the stem that direct attention to content. Identify opposites in options.

5. The nurse is assessing the temperature of a client. When can the nurse expect a client's temperature to be at its lowest?
   1. 6 a.m.
   2. 10 a.m.
   3. 6 p.m.
   4. 9 p.m.

   TEST-TAKING TIP: Identify the key word in the stem that directs attention to content. Identify opposites in options.

6. As the client walks into the examination room, the nurse collects information for the general survey. Which statement best reflects the nurse's documentation that is part of a general survey?
   1. Alert, well-nourished, no deformities, good gait
   2. Alert, oriented, appears to eat well, no other concerns or issues
   3. Oriented times three, well-nourished, walks well, no deformities noted
   4. Alert and oriented times three, well-nourished, no obvious physical deformities

7. The nurse is palpating the pulse of an 82-year-old client who is resting comfortably in bed after a surgical procedure. The nurse expects the client's pulse to be within which range?
   1. 60 to 100 beats per minute and regular
   2. 40 to 70 beats per minute and irregular
   3. 80 to 110 beats per minute and regular
   4. 60 to 100 beats per minute and irregular

   TEST-TAKING TIP: Identify key words in the stem that direct attention to content. Identify duplicate facts among options.

8. The nurse obtains the rectal temperature of an adult. Which rectal temperature is within the expected range?
   1. 96.4°F
   2. 97.6°F
   3. 99.8°F
   4. 101.2°F

   TEST-TAKING TIP: Identify key words in the stem that direct attention to content.

9. The nurse is walking the client with heart disease per provider's orders. During the walk, the client becomes breathless, places a fist against their chest, and collapses into a chair. The nurse should first:
   1. walk the client back to bed.
   2. obtain the client's vital signs.
   3. administer the prescribed antacid to the client.
   4. notify the rapid response team of the client's condition.

   TEST-TAKING TIP: Identify the word in the stem that sets a priority. Identify key words in the stem that direct attention to content.

10. The nurse obtains the blood pressure reading of several clients. Which blood pressure reading is considered the **most** serious?
    1. 90/70 mm Hg
    2. 130/86 mm Hg
    3. 150/86 mm Hg
    4. 160/124 mm Hg

    TEST-TAKING TIP: Identify the word in the stem that sets a priority.

11. The nurse is assessing the client with heart failure. During inspection and palpation of the client's neck vessels, which is an unexpected finding? **Select all that apply.**
    1. Unilateral distention of the jugular veins
    2. Easily palpated and visible bilateral carotid pulses
    3. Bilateral jugular vein distention greater than 45 degrees
    4. During auscultation, the nurse hears a blowing swishing sound
    5. Unequal pulse amplitude between the left- and right-side carotid arteries

    TEST-TAKING TIP: Identify key words in the stem that direct attention to content.

12. The nurse notices on the telemetry monitor that a client's heart rate dropped from 98 beats per minute to 52 beats per minute. Which should the nurse do first?
    1. Obtain a complete set of vital signs
    2. Ask the client about recent activity
    3. Wait a half hour and retake the pulse
    4. Report the changes to the charge nurse

TEST-TAKING TIP: Identify the word in the stem that sets a priority.

13. The nurse is assessing the 25-year-old client for a 3-week follow-up after right Achilles tendon repair surgery. The client has a non–weight-bearing cast. Which assessment data require additional follow-up? **Select all that apply.**
    1. Toes are pale
    2. Right calf is red
    3. Dorsalis pedis pulse 2+
    4. Right calf tender to palpation
    5. Right calf 42 cm, left calf 38 cm
    6. Pain in right calf rated 7 out of 10

TEST-TAKING TIP: Identify the words in the stem that set a priority. Identify key words in the stem that direct attention to content. Identify expected outcomes.

14. The nurse is assessing the pulses of a diabetic client. The client has bilateral 3+ pitting edema with nonpalpable pedal pulses. How should the nurse proceed? **Select all that apply.**
    1. Assess capillary refill of the toes
    2. Assess the pulses with a Doppler device
    3. Ask the client if they have numbness or tingling
    4. Tell the client to not wear compression stockings
    5. Ask the client if they have pain in the lower extremities
    6. Have the client elevate their legs to the level of their heart

TEST-TAKING TIP: Identify the word in the stem that sets a priority. Identify key words in the stem that direct attention to content.

15. Which principle of blood pressure physiology should the nurse recall when assessing a client's cardiac function?
    1. The blood pressure reaches a peak followed by a trough.
    2. A peak pressure occurs when the left ventricle relaxes.
    3. The pulse pressure occurs during diastole.
    4. A trough pressure occurs during systole.

TEST-TAKING TIP: Identify key words in the stem that direct attention to content. Identify the clang association. Identify the unique option.

16. The nurse is monitoring the results of a culture and sensitivity report on a specimen from a wound. What does the sensitivity part of the report indicate?
    1. All of the microorganisms present in the wound
    2. Extent of the client's response to the pathogens
    3. Virulence of the organisms in the exudate
    4. Antibiotics that should be effective

TEST-TAKING TIP: Identify key words in the stem that direct attention to content. Identify the option with a specific determiner.

17. Which is an example of objective data collected during a nursing history and physical examination of a newly admitted client? **Select all that apply.**
    1. _____ Pain
    2. _____ Fever
    3. _____ Nausea
    4. _____ Fatigue
    5. _____ Pruritus

TEST-TAKING TIP: Identify the key word in the stem that directs attention to content. Identify the unique option.

18. A client has herpes zoster. Place an X over the site the nurse should assess because it is the **most** common site of herpes zoster lesions.

TEST-TAKING TIP: Identify the word in the stem that sets a priority.

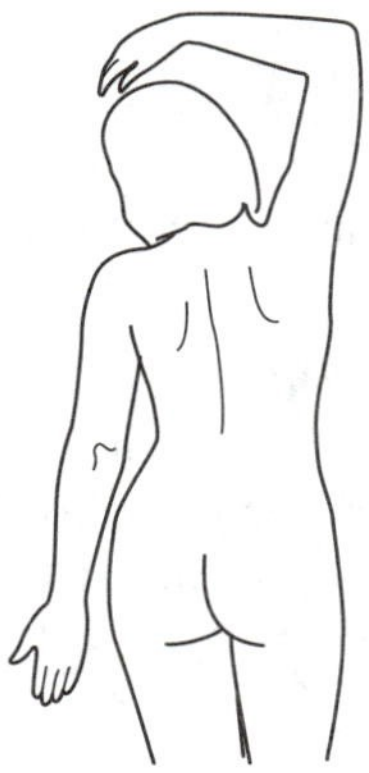

19. The nurse is assessing a client's orientation times three. Which nursing intervention should be included in this assessment? **Select all that apply.**

1. _____ Ask the client's name.
2. _____ Have the client state the time of day.
3. _____ Ascertain if the client knows the current environment.
4. _____ Determine if the client can carry out simple directions.
5. _____ Observe whether the client's eyes can follow movement.

20. The nurse is caring for a client who has an elevated temperature. Which route should the nurse use when assessing the client for a rapid change in core body temperature?

1. 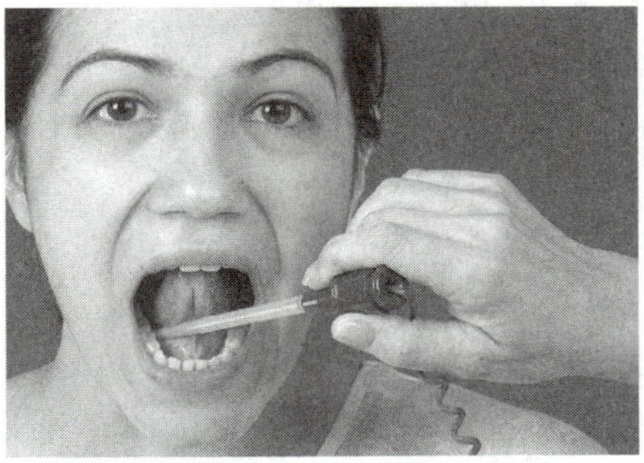

2. 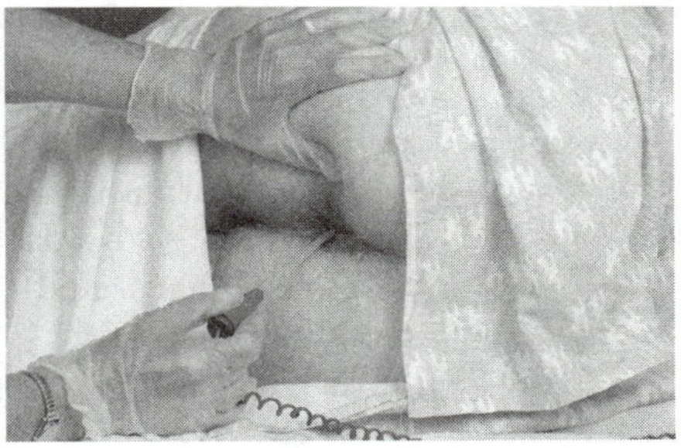

3. 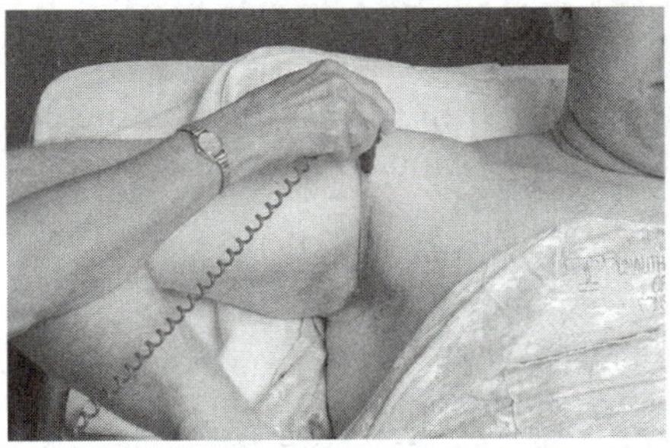

4. 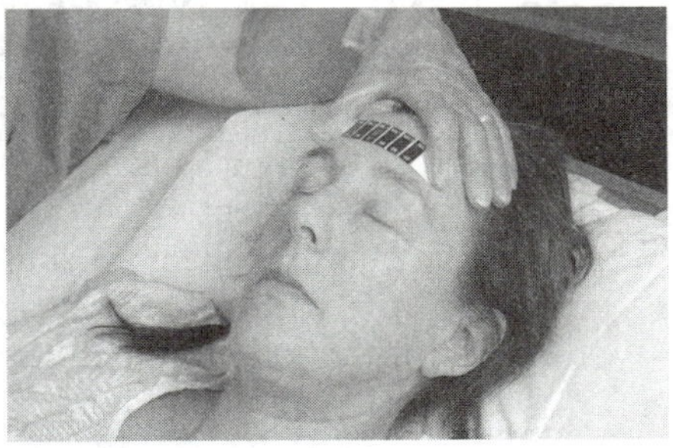

TEST-TAKING TIP: Identify key words in the stem that direct attention to content.

21. Which client reaction indicates that the local inflammatory response has entered the first phase? **Select all that apply.**
1. _____ Pain
2. _____ Heat
3. _____ Exudate
4. _____ Swelling
5. _____ Erythema

TEST-TAKING TIP: Identify key words in the stem that direct attention to content.

22. The nurse on the day shift is caring for a middle-aged adult admitted during the night with the flu. At 0800, the nurse identifies that the client is lethargic and obtains the vital signs, which are as follows: oral temperature, 103.8°F; pulse, 120 beats per minute, irregular; respirations, 34 breaths per minute, labored; oxygen saturation, 86%. The nurse compares these most recent vital signs with the values obtained previously. Which should the nurse do?

Time	0200	0400	0600
Temperature	101.8°F	102°F	102.2°F
Pulse	98 beats/min	106 beats/min	112 beats/min
Respirations	22 breaths/min	24 breaths/min	28 breaths/min
SaO_2	96%	95%	94%

1. Initiate the rapid response team
2. Administer the prescribed ibuprofen
3. Recheck the vital signs in 15 minutes
4. Change the oxygen via nasal cannula to a face mask at 6 liters

TEST-TAKING TIP: Identify opposites in options.

23. Which information about a client is classified as subjective data? **Select all that apply.**
1. _____ Describes having palpitations
2. _____ Is experiencing a headache
3. _____ States being nauseated
4. _____ Reports feeling cold
5. _____ Looks tired
6. _____ Is crying

TEST-TAKING TIP: Identify the key word in the stem that directs attention to content. Identify equally plausible options.

24. The emergency department nurse is triaging clients from a mass casualty incident. Place the following clients in the order in which they should receive care based on their triage assessment.
1. Apneic pulseless client missing right upper extremity
2. Ambulatory client with minor penetrating abdominal wound
3. Client with multiple penetrating injuries, respiratory rate of 32
4. Client with compound fracture of the arm, responds to verbal commands
5. Client with open abdominal wound, exposed bowels, responds to commands

Answer: ____________

25. An older adult reports shortness of breath, fever, coughing, and excessive mucus. The primary health-care provider diagnoses bronchitis and admits the client for IV antibiotic therapy. The nurse assesses the client's breath sounds as part of the admission assessment to the unit. Place an X over the site where the nurse should place the stethoscope when assessing for bronchial breath sounds.

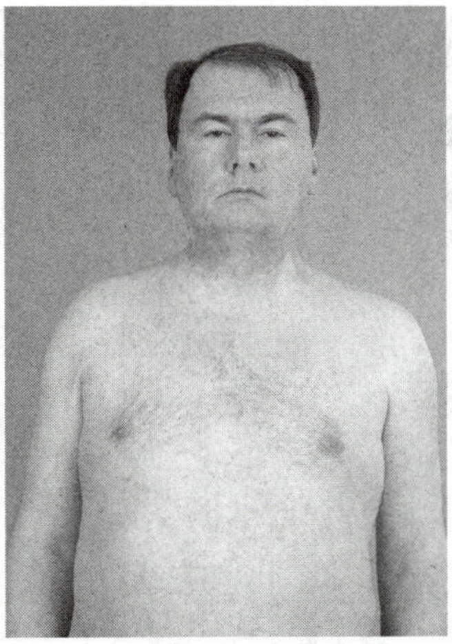

TEST-TAKING TIP: Identify the words in the stem that direct attention to content.

26. A client reports a dull ache in the calf of the left leg. Which assessment should the nurse **not** perform considering that the client is reporting a dull ache in the calf?

1. 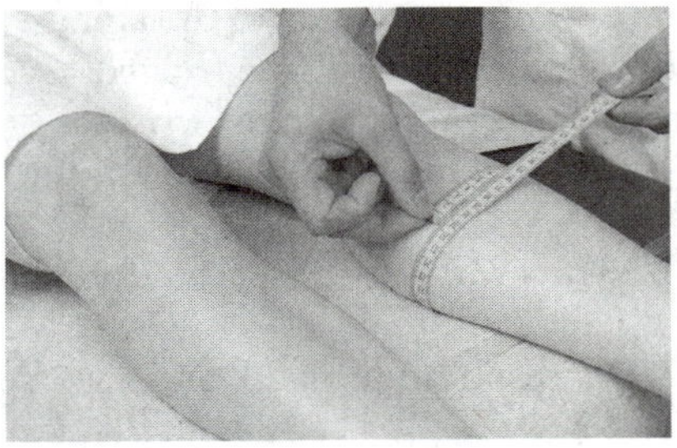

2. 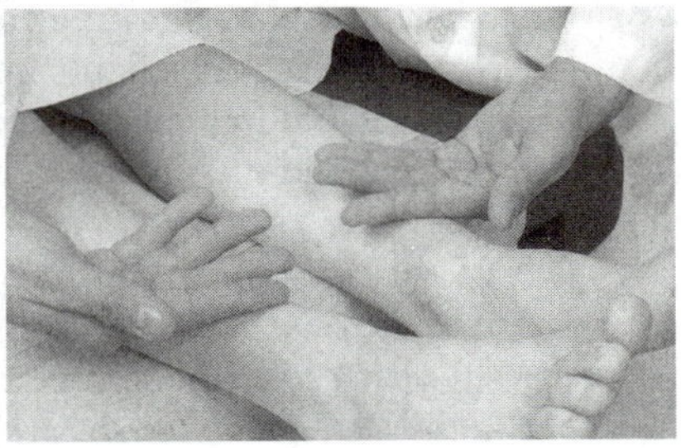

3. 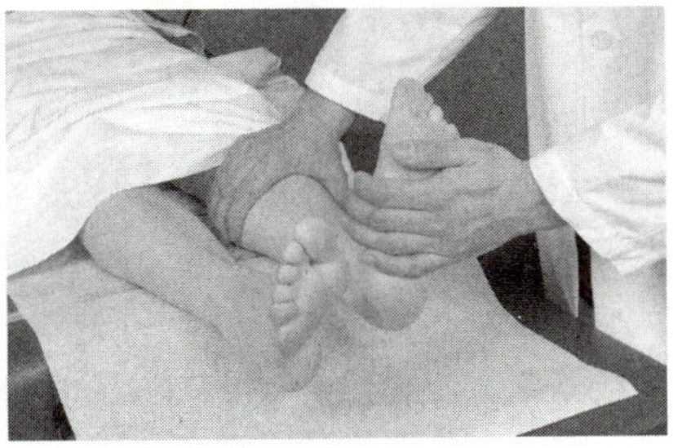

4. 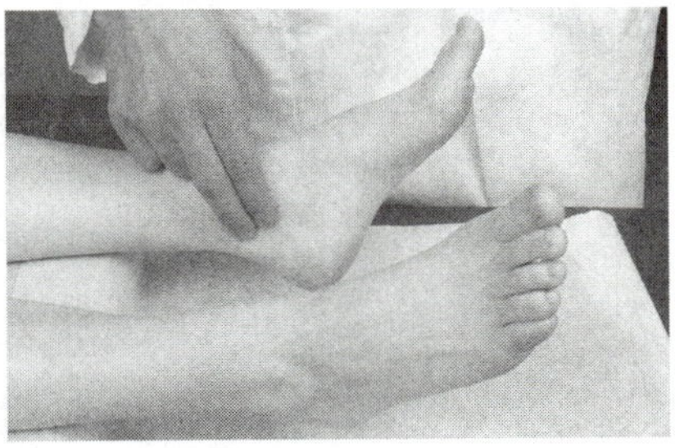

TEST-TAKING TIP: Identify the word in the stem that indicates negative polarity.

27. Which is the nurse assessing when touching the client in this manner?
   1. Appearance of reactive hyperemia
   2. Presence of sensory perception
   3. Symmetry of skin temperature
   4. Strength of the lower legs

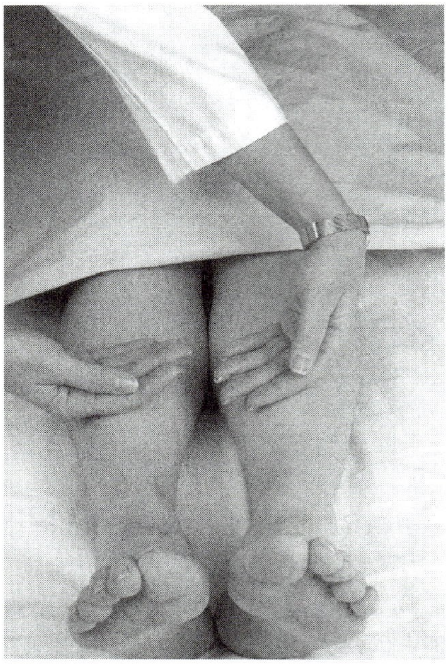

28. The triage nurse is reviewing the chief complaint of four clients in the emergency department. Place the clients in the order in which they should be triaged.
   1. A 12-year-old in a bicycle accident who reports pain in the right wrist
   2. A 30-year-old missing one-third of the right index finger, arriving with the finger on ice
   3. A 55-year-old on warfarin who fell and presents with a large painful forehead bruise
   4. A 70-year-old with a temperature of 102.4°F, respirations of 24, and a worsening cough

Answer: ___________

29. The nurse is auscultating a client's apical heart rate. Place an X on the location where the stethoscope should be placed to access the point of maximum impulse.

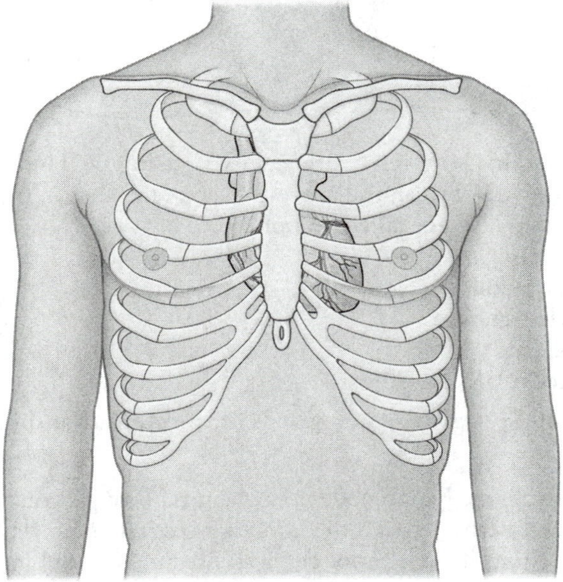

TEST-TAKING TIP: Identify the words in the stem that direct attention to content.

30. The nurse is obtaining an oral temperature with an electronic thermometer. Which must the nurse do? **Select all that apply.**

1. _____ Use the green probe
2. _____ Take it before breakfast
3. _____ Use a new probe cover for each client
4. _____ Wipe the probe with alcohol after each use
5. _____ Assess if the route is appropriate for the client

TEST-TAKING TIP: Identify key words in the stem that direct attention to content.

31. The nurse is using the equipment indicated in the illustration to assess a pedal pulse. Which step is associated with the use of this equipment? **Select all that apply.**

1. _____ Elicit the dorsalis pedis pulse.
2. _____ Tilt the end of the probe 45° to the dorsalis pedis artery.
3. _____ Use light pressure to keep the probe in contact with the client's skin.
4. _____ Apply transmission gel on the end of the probe or to the client's skin.
5. _____ Locate the groove between the great toe and first toe and move toward the top of the foot until the dorsalis pedis pulse is found.

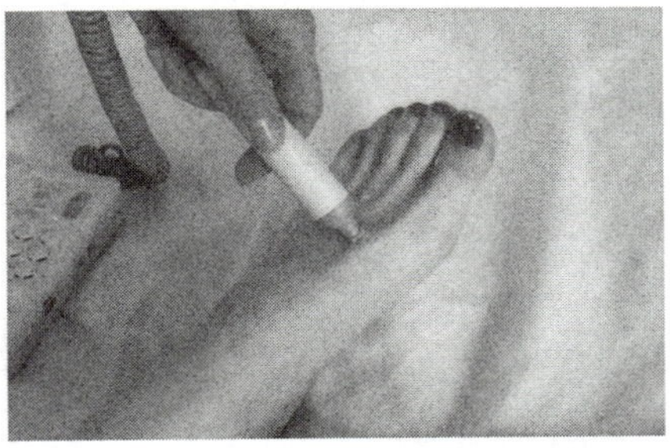

TEST-TAKING TIP: Identify the key words in the stem that direct attention to content.

32. The nurse must obtain a blood specimen from the surface of an adult's finger using a spring-loaded lancet. Place an X on the appropriate location for the skin puncture.

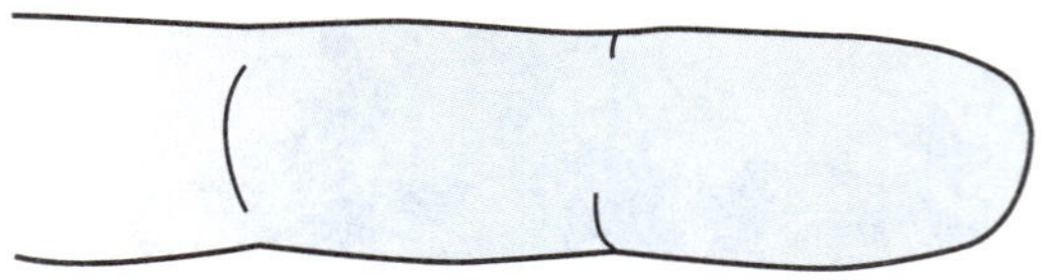

33. The nurse working in a long-term care facility is taking the blood pressures of a group of older adults. Why can the nurse expect an increase in blood pressure in this group of older adults? **Select all that apply.**
1. _____ Aging hearts
2. _____ Thicker blood
3. _____ Lifestyle stressors
4. _____ More elastic vessels
5. _____ Presence of atherosclerosis

TEST-TAKING TIP: Identify the key words in the stem that direct attention to content.

34. The nurse is assessing the lymph nodes of a client reporting a cough, sinus pressure, and body aches. Label the lymph nodes the nurse is assessing: Supraclavicular, Superficial, Deep mandibular, Tonsillar, Posterior cervical, Preauricular, Submandibular.

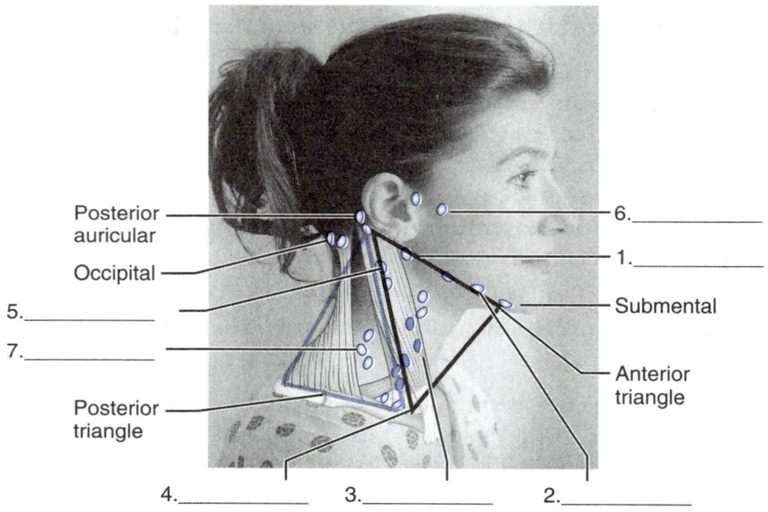

1. ______________________________
2. ______________________________
3. ______________________________
4. ______________________________
5. ______________________________
6. ______________________________
7. ______________________________

35. The nurse is caring for a client who sustained trauma in an occupational accident. The nurse makes the following client assessments: opens eyes when asked a question; speaks words but is disoriented to time, place, and person; and follows instructions when helped to change position. The nurse uses the Glasgow Coma Scale (GCS) to rate the client's level of consciousness. Which point total on the GCS should the nurse document in the client's clinical record to indicate the client's level of consciousness?
1. 9
2. 11
3. 13
4. 15

Glasgow Coma Scale

Eye Opening	Points
Eyes open spontaneously	4
Eyes open in response to voice	3
Eyes open in response to pain	2
No eye opening response	1
Best Verbal Response	**Points**
Oriented (e.g., to person, place, time)	5
Confused, speaks but is disoriented	4
Inappropriate but comprehensible words	3
Incomprehensible sounds but no words are spoken	2
None	1
Best Motor Response	**Points**
Obeys command to move	6
Localizes painful stimulus	5
Withdraws from painful stimulus	4
Flexion, abnormal decorticate posturing	3
Extension, abnormal decerebrate posturing	2
No movement or posturing	1
Total Points	**?**

36. The nurse is assessing the skin of an older adult. Which change in the client's skin should the nurse anticipate? **Select all that apply.**
1. _____ Increased pigmented spots
2. _____ Decreased thickness
3. _____ Increased elasticity
4. _____ Decreased dryness
5. _____ Increased tone

TEST-TAKING TIP: Identify key words in the stem that direct attention to content.

37. The nurse is caring for a client with a diagnosis of liver disease. Place an X over the body cavity that the nurse should assess for the presence of ascites.

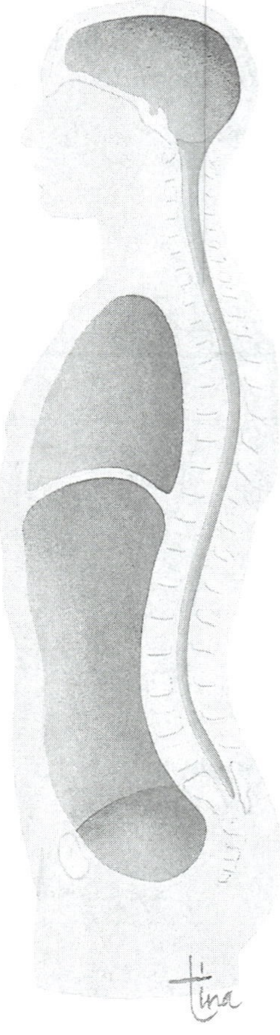

38. The nurse is palpating a client's radial pulse and determines that it can be obliterated with slight pressure. Which word should the nurse use when documenting this assessment in the client's clinical record? **Select all that apply.**

1. _____ Bounding
2. _____ Thready
3. _____ Absent
4. _____ Weak
5. _____ Full

TEST-TAKING TIP: Identify key words in the stem that direct attention to content. Identify equally plausible options. Identify opposites in options.

39. The nurse receives the following clinical record of a client being admitted to the facility from the emergency department. When the client arrives on the unit the priority nursing intervention is:

1. telemetry monitoring.
2. initiate fluid replacement.
3. medication reconciliation.
4. obtain an order for oxygen.

CLIENT'S CLINICAL RECORD

Admission History

A 75-year-old adult obtained an appointment with a primary health-care provider because of an upper respiratory infection. While entering the primary health-care provider's office, the older adult fell to the ground, and the primary health-care provider called for an ambulance. Numerous tests were performed in the emergency department, and the older adult is being admitted to the hospital for management of dehydration. The client has a 5-year history of Parkinson disease, has hypertension, has no family, and lives alone.

Vital Signs Flow Sheet

Blood pressure: 110/65 mm Hg
Pulse: 100 beats/min, thready
Respirations: 28 breaths/min, regular
Temperature: 99.6°F, orally
Oxygen saturation: 89%

Primary Health-Care Provider's Prescriptions

1000 mL 0.9% sodium chloride at 125 mL/hr
Encourage oral fluid intake
Oxygen 2 L via nasal cannula

40. The nurse assesses all the clients in a district at the beginning of a shift. Which client response requires that the nurse perform an immediate focused assessment? **Select all that apply.**
1. _____ Suprapubic distention
2. _____ Edema of 2+ in the ankles
3. _____ Difficulty sleeping at night
4. _____ Lack of a bowel movement in 3 days
5. _____ Blanchable erythema in the sacral area

TEST-TAKING TIP: Identify the word in the stem that sets a priority. Identify key words in the stem that direct attention to content.

CLINICAL JUDGMENT CASE STUDY

The home health nurse is caring for a 68-year-old client with advanced lung cancer and cardiovascular disease. The client lives alone with a small dog. The client states they are having increased difficulty breathing over the last 3 days and prefer to sleep in the chair because it "hurts too much" to walk around or sleep in the bed and that the chair is closer to the bathroom. The client is not using oxygen and states that they have never needed it before. The nurse notices the client is distressed and worried about what will happen to their dog in the future. The following vital signs were noted:

Temperature	97.6°F (36.4°C)
Pulse	102
BP	96/72
Respirations	26
Oxygen	89%
Pain	8 out of 10

STANDING ORDERS

2 L O_2 PRN to maintain above 92%
Hydrocodone 5/325 mg PRN for pain
Morphine PO PRN 12 hours for pain
Low-sodium, heart-healthy diet
Enalapril (Vasotec) 20 mg PO in morning and at bedtime
Furosemide (Lasix) 20 mg PO in morning and at bedtime

THORAX AND LUNGS FOCUSED ASSESSMENT

Sitting in chair holding hands over chest
Observed respiratory distress when talking
Breathing regular and shallow with prolonged expiration
AP to transverse diameter—wide costal angle
Facial expressions indicate pain, client appears anxious
Skin color—some cyanosis present, skin is pale and dry
Diminished and moist breath sounds on auscultation
Productive cough
No clubbing of nails noted

41. **Recognize cues—What matters most?** The nurse understands that which of the following should be done first for this client?
1. Discuss concerns about pet
2. Oxygenation status
3. Pain medication
4. Comfort client

42. **Analyze cues—What could it mean?** The client states that they have difficulty breathing and prefer to sleep in the chair. The nurse recognizes the client may need education on which topics? **Select all that apply.**
1. Low-sodium diet
2. Care of oxygen tank
3. Sitting in the tripod position
4. Use of pursed-lip breathing
5. Elevating the legs above the heart
6. Timing of blood pressure medications

43. **Prioritize hypotheses—Where do I start?** The nurse reviews the standing orders for the client. Place an X on the orders that the nurse should clarify with the provider.

STANDING ORDERS

2 L O_2 PRN to maintain above 92%	
Hydrocodone 5/325 mg PRN for pain	
Morphine PO PRN 12 hours for pain	
Low-sodium, heart-healthy diet	
Enalapril (Vasotec) 20 mg PO in morning and at bedtime	
Furosemide (Lasix) 20 mg PO in morning and at bedtime	

44. **Generate solutions—What can I do?** The nurse notices that the client's blood pressure has decreased and the pain level has increased from the prior home health visit. Which is the best course of action for the nurse?
1. Give the client the hydrocodone and reevaluate pain in 6 hours
2. Give the furosemide but hold the enalapril until provider notified
3. Hold the blood pressure medications until reviewed with provider
4. Hold pain and blood pressure medications until reviewed with provider

45. **Take action—What will I do?** The nurse identifies nursing diagnoses and develops interventions to make the client more comfortable and improve their breathing. Choose the most appropriate "related to" for the client's nursing diagnoses.

Nursing Diagnosis	Related To
Ineffective Airway Clearance	1. r/t change in health status
Insomnia	2. r/t to change in health status
Activity Intolerance	3. r/t dyspnea
Anxiety	4. r/t bronchial secretions and obstruction

1. _____ Ineffective Airway Clearance
2. _____ Activity Intolerance
3. _____ Insomnia
4. _____ Anxiety

46. **Evaluate outcomes—Did it help?** The nurse visits the client three days later. Which items in the nursing note indicate the client is compliant with the education and interventions? **Select all that apply.**

NURSING NOTE

Client appears rested and states that they plan to try to sleep in the bed soon. Client was in a tripod position in a chair and using pursed-lip breathing. Blood pressure is 122/88. Pain is still 8/10. Cigarettes noted on the coffee table. Nasal cannula around client's neck. O_2 is 90%. Client became tearful when stating that she is putting her dog up for adoption. Client has 2+ edema.

1. _____ Nasal cannula around neck
2. _____ Placing dog up for adoption
3. _____ Plan to sleep in bed soon
4. _____ Pursed-lip breathing
5. _____ Tripod position
6. _____ O_2 90%

1. **TEST-TAKING TIP: The word *unsure* is the key word in the stem that directs attention to content. Option 4 is unique. Options 1, 3, and 4 are not competent, safe client care.**
   1. Rechecking the lung sounds later is not a correct option. Client care and safety is paramount. Returning to check lung sounds later could be detrimental and dangerous for client care.
   2. **When unsure of a sound while assessing, the nurse should get the opinion of a more experienced nurse to ensure accurate sounds are documented. Auscultation is challenging to master and the new graduate nurse should know that sound identifications come with practice.**
   3. This is not an appropriate choice. The provider expects the nurse to be competent and skilled to care for clients. Once the correct sounds are identified, it may be appropriate to notify the provider if the lung sounds are concerning.
   4. The nurse should never assume to know and document inaccurate sounds. The nurse should first verify that they have eliminated any confusing sounds, such as the television or other room noise, and are listening on direct skin. The nurse should also ensure that they eliminate their own artifact sounds such as their own breathing. Once the nurse has recognized what is considered "normal" breath sounds, abnormal sounds can be distinguished.

2. **TEST-TAKING TIP: The word *oral* is the key word in the stem that directs attention to content.**
   1. The sublingual pocket has a rich blood supply that quickly responds to changes in the body's inner core temperature. Hot fluids cause these tissues to dilate and heat, so will cause an inaccurate increase in the temperature reading.
   2. The oral temperature is the most convenient and accurate site. Rectal temperatures are the most accurate but are also the most invasive. The risks and benefits must be weighed for clients, though it is the preferred route when other routes are not practical.
   3. This is unnecessary and will not adjust the temperature to an accurate reading.
   4. **It takes at least 15 minutes for the vessels in the mouth and the mucous membranes of the sublingual pocket to recover from the hot fluid and for the client's mouth to return to the previous temperature.**

3. **TEST-TAKING TIP: The words *high-pitched* and *squeaking* are the key words in the stem that direct attention to content.**
   1. Crepitus is a coarse, crackling sound that is usually heard when palpating over the skin's surface, not auscultating. It is often found in clients with subcutaneous emphysema when air from the lungs escapes to the subcutaneous tissue.
   2. **Wheezing is high-pitched, musical squeaking sounds that can occur in both inspiration and expiration. The sound is made from air squeezing through a narrow or compressed airway passage.**
   3. Fine crackles are discontinuous, high-pitched, short popping sounds heard during inspiration that cannot be cleared with coughing.
   4. Coarse crackles are loud, low-pitched bubbling and gurgling sounds. They usually start early in inspiration but can also be heard on expiration. These sounds may disappear or diminish with suctioning or coughing but typically reappear shortly after.

4. **TEST-TAKING TIP: The words *diabetes* and *peripheral artery disease* are the key words in the stem that direct attention to content. The radial site is the most common site for assessing the heart rate.**

   Diabetes causes arterial dysfunction in both the upper and lower extremities. Occlusions from peripheral artery disease are caused by atherosclerosis, the gradual accumulation of fat in the arteries, causing calcification of the vessel wall and thrombus formations. Diminished or absent pulses in the various arteries examined may indicate impaired blood flow. When assessing pulses, the intensity, rate, rhythm, tortuosity, and nodularity should be noted.
   1. The ulnar artery is deeper and often more difficult to feel than the pulse from the radial artery. It is usually not necessary to palpate the ulnar pulses.
   2. **Obesity or edema may prevent successful detection of the posterior tibial pulse, but palpation should be attempted by the nurse.**

3. **The radial pulse is just medial to the radius in the wrist. It is shallow and easier to palpate than the ulnar pulse.**
4. The popliteal pulse can be difficult to palpate and localize. A client can be turned prone and the lower leg lifted. On many clients, the popliteal is impossible to palpate.
5. The temporal artery is palpated anteriorly to the ear. It is typically only palpated in a client with visual changes, severe headaches, or suspected temporal arteritis.
6. **The dorsalis pedis is usually not difficult to palpate and only requires a light touch. Edema may make palpation more difficult. This pulse should be palpated but it is congenitally absent in 10% of people.**

5. **TEST-TAKING TIP: The words *temperature* and *lowest* are the key words in the stem that direct attention to content. Options 1 and 3 are opposites.**
   1. **A person's body temperature is at its lowest in the early morning. Core body temperatures vary with a predictable pattern over 24 hours (diurnal or circadian rhythms) because of hormonal variations.**
   2. Body temperature is not at its lowest at 10 a.m.; body temperature steadily increases as the day progresses.
   3. Body temperature peaks between 5 and 7 p.m.
   4. Body temperature is not at its lowest at 9 p.m.; body temperature is still decreasing from its peak.

6. **TEST-TAKING TIP: The general survey is the first part of an overall health assessment. The nurse is gathering "general" data before beginning the head-to-toe assessment. The general survey includes level of consciousness, nutritional status, posture, deformities, gait, and mobility.**
   1. This does not address if the client is oriented to time, place, or situation. The word "good" should be avoided in legal medical documentation unless using a direct quote from a client.
   2. This statement does not indicate if the client is oriented to time, place, and situation. It also uses inferences such as "appears." The assessment is just beginning so the nurse does not yet know if there are any issues or concerns.
   3. This statement does not indicate alertness. "Walks well" is not a concise and clear statement; rather, it is an opinion.
   4. **This is the correct answer. The client is described concisely with relevant data necessary for documentation.**

7. **TEST-TAKING TIP: The words *pulse*, *resting*, *older adult*, and *expects* are key words in the stem that direct attention to content. Options 2 and 4 relate to an irregular pulse. Options 1 and 3 relate to a regular pulse. If you know that a pulse should be regular, then focus attention on options 1 and 3 and eliminate options 2 and 4. If you know that the expected range for a pulse is 60 to 100 beats per minute, focus on options that are within that range.**
   1. **The expected heart rate of an older adult is between 60 and 100 beats per minute and is regular. This client is resting comfortably in bed, so the nurse would expect the pulse to be regular and within the expected range.**
   2. A rate below 60 is below the expected range of a pulse rate in an older adult. The rhythm should be regular, not irregular.
   3. The expected heart rate of an older adult is between 60 and 100 beats per minute and regular, not 80 to 110 beats per minute.
   4. 60 to 100 beats per minute is within the expected range, but this pulse is also expected to be regular.

8. **TEST-TAKING TIP: The words *rectal temperature* and *expected range* are key words in the stem that direct attention to content.**
   1. A temperature of 96.4°F is below the expected range for a rectal temperature.
   2. A temperature of 97.6°F is below the expected range for a rectal temperature.
   3. **A temperature of 99.8°F is within the expected range of 98.5°F to 100.5°F for a rectal temperature.**
   4. A temperature of 101.2°F indicates a fever.

9. **TEST-TAKING TIP: The word *first* in the stem sets a priority. The words *history of heart disease* are key words in the stem that direct attention to content.**
   1. Activity at this time is unsafe because it will increase the demands on the heart.
   2. **A further assessment is necessary; vital signs reflect the cardiopulmonary status of the client. The client may be experiencing a cardiac event.**
   3. The nurse does not have enough information to conclude that the problem is gastritis.
   4. At this time, the nurse does not have sufficient information to initiate the rapid response team.

10. **TEST-TAKING TIP: The word *most* in the stem sets a priority.**
   1. A blood pressure reading of 90/70 mm Hg reflects hypotension because the systolic pressure is less than 100 mm Hg.
   2. A blood pressure of 130/86 mm Hg is considered high-stage 1 hypertension. High-stage 1 hypertension parameters are a systolic pressure of 130 to 139 mm Hg or a diastolic pressure of 80 to 89 mm Hg. Although this blood pressure is elevated, it is not as serious as the blood pressure in another option.
   3. A blood pressure of 150/86 mm Hg is considered high-stage 2 hypertension. High-stage 2 hypertension parameters are a systolic pressure of 140 to 179 mm Hg or a diastolic pressure equal to or higher than 90 mm Hg. Although this blood pressure is elevated, it is not as serious as the blood pressure in another option.
   4. **A blood pressure of 160/124 mm Hg is considered crisis hypertension. The parameters for crisis hypertension are a systolic pressure higher than 180 mm Hg and/or a diastolic pressure higher than 120 mm Hg. This is the most elevated and serious blood pressure of the options presented.**

11. **TEST-TAKING TIP: Key words include inspection and palpation. First distinguish expected findings in a healthy client, then the unexpected can be identified. A cardiovascular assessment includes assessment of the vascular structures in the neck (the carotid arteries and jugular veins) to assess the efficiency of cardiac function.**
   1. **The jugular veins carry deoxygenated blood directly to the superior vena cava. There is no cardiac valve between the superior vena cava and the right atrium, allowing the jugular veins to provide information on the right side of the heart. The jugulars reflect volume changes and filling pressures so when the heart is not pumping efficiently, the jugular veins become distended. Unilateral distention is usually caused by a local cause such as kinking of the vein or an aneurysm.**
   2. The carotid artery is a central artery close to the heart. Its pulsation coincides with the ventricular systole and is typically easy to palpate.
   3. **Bilateral jugular vein distention greater than 45 degrees is an indication of heart failure and signifies increased central venous pressure.**
   4. **A bruit is a blowing swishing sound that indicates blood flow turbulence. A bruit is usually caused by local vascular disease and is an indicator for atherosclerotic disease.**
   5. **Inequality between the left- and right-side carotid pulse typically reflects atherosclerosis but can also indicate aortic dissection, arteritis, or embolus.**

12. **TEST-TAKING TIP: The word *first* in the stem sets a priority.**
   1. **Corroborative data should be obtained; the vital signs reflect cardiopulmonary functioning. When there is an alteration in one vital sign, there usually is a change in another.**
   2. Activity will increase, not decrease, the heart rate.
   3. Waiting is unsafe. The change in pulse may indicate an impending problem.
   4. Alerting the nurse in charge might be necessary after other, more appropriate interventions.

13. **TEST-TAKING TIP: First identify the expected outcomes from surgery, then identify issues of concern for the client.**
   1. **Pale toes may indicate that the cast has been applied too tightly, compressing the veins and arteries.**
   2. **Wearing a cast for several weeks slows the blood flow through the veins, increasing the risk of a blood clot (thrombus). Redness and warmth are both indicators of a deep vein thrombosis.**
   3. A dorsalis pedis pulse of 2+ is an expected finding.
   4. **The right calf tender to palpation is an indication of a deep vein thrombosis. The client is 3 weeks postsurgery and should not be experiencing tenderness. Tenderness and warmth of the skin may also indicate a wound infection or too much pressure from the cast.**
   5. **Swelling immediately following surgery is expected, but if it continues 3 weeks out, this indicates that the cast is too tight.**
   6. **The client should not continue to have pain 3 weeks out from surgery. Significant pain is an unexpected finding and can indicate a DVT or that the cast is too tight.**

14. **TEST-TAKING TIP: The words *edema* and *nonpalpable* in the stem set a priority. The words *pedal pulse* are key words in the stem that direct attention to content. Although the function of the heart can be assessed any time an arterial pulse is monitored, pedal pulses generally are monitored to assess adequacy of blood flow to the feet.**
    1. **The capillary refill should be assessed. When assessing the capillary refill, the nurse should observe if the skin blanches and immediately returns to normal or if there is a delay. A delayed cap fill can indicate perfusion issues and should be used in conjunction with a thorough assessment.**
    2. **Using a handheld Doppler is a noninvasive method to verify pedal pulses. It is not a diagnostic tool but can help verify pulses are present. It must be used in conjunction with a complete assessment that incorporates the client's clinical history and clinical presentation.**
    3. **This question should be asked as part of the complete assessment. The presence or absence of pedal pulses should prompt further assessment. Limb circulation should be assessed, though it is not uncommon for diabetics to complain of numbness and tingling in the extremities.**
    4. The nurse should obtain an order for compression stockings. Compression stockings keep pressure on the extremities to prevent further fluid from collecting in the tissues.
    5. **Pain is part of a complete assessment. Swelling of the lower extremities can cause pain and the client may have a low tolerance for the touching and probing when assessing the legs. The skin may also be stretched and seeping serous fluid with edema.**
    6. **As long as a DVT is not suspected, clients should elevate their limbs above the level of the heart. Elevation helps circulate fluid back toward the heart.**

15. **TEST-TAKING TIP: The words *cardiac function* are key words in the stem that direct attention to content. The word *blood* in the stem and in option 1 is a clang association. Options 2, 3, and 4 each identify one factor related to blood pressure and when it occurs. Option 1 is unique because it identifies two factors related to blood pressure and does not contain the words *pressure occurs*.**
    1. **Peak pressures occur when the ventricles contract, and trough pressures occur when the ventricles relax; these occur with each contraction and relaxation of the heart.**
    2. Peak pressures occur when the ventricles contract.
    3. Pulse pressure is the difference between the systolic and diastolic pressures.
    4. Peak pressures, not trough pressures, occur during systole.

16. **TEST-TAKING TIP: The words *sensitivity* and *indicate* are key words in the stem that direct attention to content. Option 1 contains the word *all*, which is a specific determiner. This option can be eliminated from consideration.**
    1. Examination of a specimen under a microscope, not the sensitivity part of a culture and sensitivity test, identifies the microorganisms present.
    2. The clinical manifestation of the disease process reflects the extent of the client's response to the microorganism present.
    3. The ability to produce disease (virulence) is not determined by the sensitivity portion of a culture and sensitivity test; virulence is determined by statistical data concerning morbidity and mortality associated with the microorganisms.
    4. **Areas lacking growth of microorganisms surrounding an antibiotic on a culture medium indicate that the microorganism is sensitive to the antibiotic and the antibiotic is capable of destroying the microorganism.**

17. **TEST-TAKING TIP: The word *objective* is the key word in the stem that directs attention to content. Option 2 is unique because it is the only option that can be measured quantitatively. Options 1, 3, 4, and 5 are similar because these responses can be described only by the client.**
    1. Pain is a subjective clinical indicator; subjective data are a client's perceptions, feelings, sensations, or ideas.

2. **Fever is an objective clinical indicator because it can be measured quantitatively with a thermometer.**
3. Nausea is a subjective clinical indicator based on a client's feelings or perceptions.
4. Fatigue is a subjective clinical indicator based on a client's feelings or perceptions.
5. Pruritus (itching sensation that makes one want to scratch) is a subjective clinical indicator based on a client's feelings or perceptions.

18. **TEST-TAKING TIP: The word *most* in the stem sets a priority.**

The site indicated by the X is the most common site for herpes zoster lesions. Herpes zoster is a disease related to activation of the latent human herpesvirus 3. It is also known as *shingles*. Lesions most commonly occur along affected nerves, causing crops of vesicles over the related dermatome.

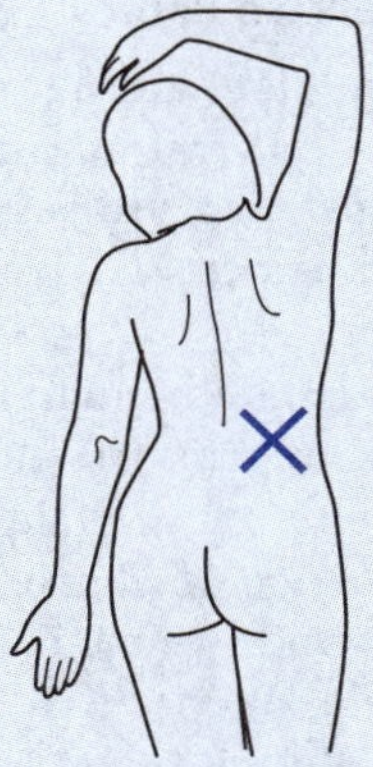

19.
1. **Questions related to orientation times three include "person." When oriented, clients should know their names (person).**
2. **Questions related to orientation times three include "time." When oriented, clients should know the time of day (time).**
3. **Questions related to orientation times three include "place." When oriented, clients should know where they are (place).**
4. Confused, disoriented clients are typically able to carry out simple directions.
5. Confused clients can typically follow movement with their eyes.

20. **TEST-TAKING TIP: The words *rapid change* and *core body temperature* are key words in the stem that direct attention to content.**

1. **This is the oral route. It is the best route when assessing a rapid change in a client's core body temperature. When an oral thermometer is placed posteriorly into the sublingual pocket, it is close to the sublingual artery, which reflects a rapid change in core body temperature.**

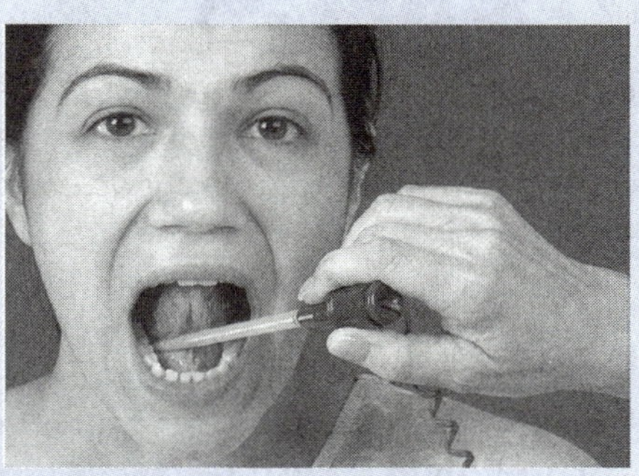

2. This is the rectal route. Although the rectal route is an accurate route for measuring core body temperature, it is not the best route to assess for a rapid change in core body temperature.

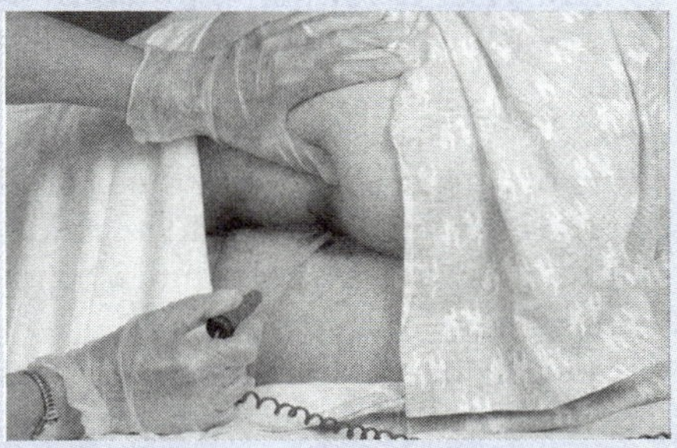

3. This is the axillary route. Although it is noninvasive and easily accessible, it is not the best route for this client because the axillary temperature lags behind the core temperature during a rapid change in core temperature.

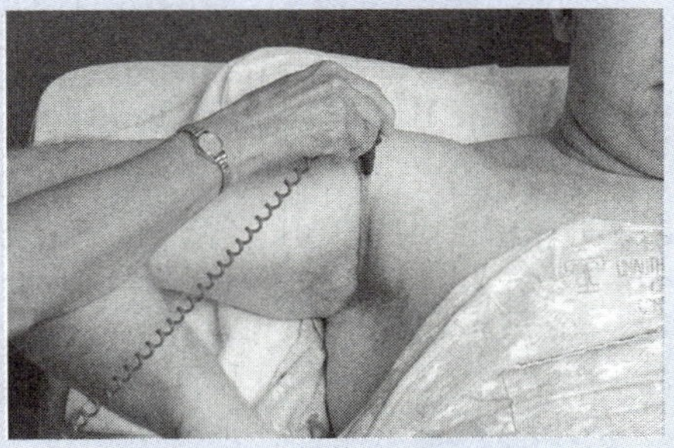

4. This is the skin route. This route indicates only body surface temperature. This is the least accurate and reliable route for obtaining a core body temperature.

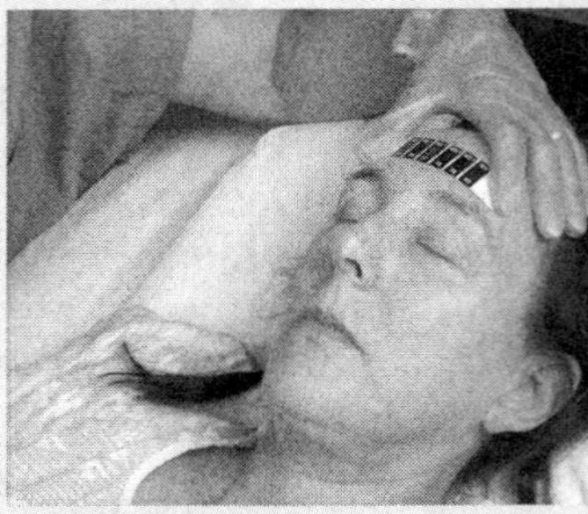

21. **TEST-TAKING TIP: The words *local inflammatory response* and *first phase* are the key words in the stem that direct attention to content.**
   1. **Pain occurs during the first phase of the inflammatory response in reaction to the release of histamine at the injury site. Histamine promotes vessel permeability, which increases edema, causing pressure on nerve endings.**
   2. **Heat occurs during the first phase of the inflammatory response in reaction to the release of histamine at the injury site. Histamine causes dilation of capillaries, resulting in blood flooding the area, which makes it warm to the touch.**
   3. Exudate is fluid consisting of a combination of cellular debris and fluids produced at the local site of injury. Exudate occurs during the second, not the first, phase of the inflammatory process.
   4. **Swelling occurs during the first phase of the inflammatory process. Swelling (abnormal enlargement of a body part) occurs because of the increased permeability of blood vessels and the migration of fluids, proteins, and white blood cells to the site of tissue damage.**
   5. **During the first phase of the inflammatory response, histamine is released, resulting in increased blood flow to the area. Dilation of capillaries causes the area to be flooded with blood, which makes the area appear red.**

22. **TEST-TAKING TIP: Options 1 and 3 are opposites. The intervention in option 1 does something immediately, whereas the intervention in option 3 involves waiting 15 minutes.**
   1. **The client's status indicates the need for immediate medical intervention. The client's condition continually deteriorated over the past 6 hours.**
   2. Although ibuprofen may be administered, another option is the priority.
   3. It is unsafe to waste 15 minutes considering the client's deteriorating condition. Another option is the priority.
   4. Changing from oxygen via a nasal cannula to a face mask at 6 liters should be done after the priority option has been implemented. Taking the time to gather equipment to change the nasal cannula to a face mask will delay the primary action.

23. **TEST-TAKING TIP: The word *subjective* is the key word in the stem that directs attention to content. Options 1, 2, 3, and 4 are similar because the client is the only one who can describe palpitations, nausea, headache, and feeling cold. Options 5 and 6 are similar because they include assessments that can be observed by another person. The options within each group are equally plausible. You have to identify which group of options you should choose on the basis of your understanding of the concept of objective versus subjective data.**
   1. **Subjective data are data that can be described or verified only by the client. Palpitations are the subjective symptom of an excessively rapid, irregular heart rate.**
   2. **Experiencing a headache is subjective information that can be described or verified only by the client.**
   3. **The presence of nausea is subjective information because it can be described only by the client.**
   4. **Reports of feeling cold are subjective information because they can be described only by the client.**
   5. Looks tired is a conclusion based on an observation and therefore is objective information.
   6. Crying is an objective datum because it can be observed by another person.

24. Answer: 3, 5, 4, 2, 1
   3. **This client is a priority for triage. The bleeding needs to be controlled and the respiratory rate lowered. The client cannot maintain a respiratory rate of 32 and is in a life-threatening situation.**
   5. **This client is responsive to commands. They need urgent treatment for the open wound and it may be life-threatening, but the client with the respiratory rate of 32 should be attended to first.**
   4. **This client will need treatment and surgery to their arm, but the clients**

with airway, breathing, and circulation issues should be attended to first.

2. **This client is ambulatory and responsive. They are not the priority.**
1. **This client is in the expectant or dead category. They still require resources, which may be focused on comfort measures, but clients with a greater chance of survival should be attended to first.**

25. **TEST-TAKING TIP: The words *bronchial breath sounds* are the words in the stem that direct attention to content.**

Bronchial breath sounds are heard in the anterior neck and nape of the neck posteriorly. They are loud, high-pitched, hollow sounds with a short inspiratory phase and a long expiratory phase.

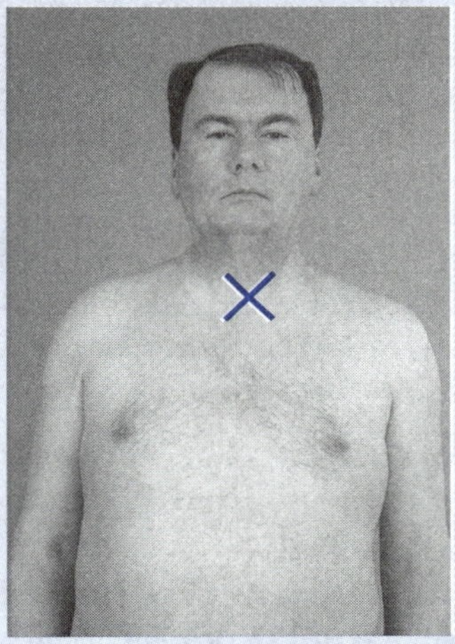

26. **TEST-TAKING TIP: The words *not perform* in the stem indicate negative polarity.**

1. This photograph depicts measuring the circumference of the calf. This is an acceptable objective assessment of edema or inflammation of the calf.
2. This photograph depicts assessing skin temperature using the backs of the hands, which are more sensitive to skin temperature than the palms of the hands. The nurse is assessing the symmetry of skin temperature. This is an acceptable assessment technique in this situation.
3. **This photograph depicts supporting the client's leg while dorsiflexing the foot. Dorsiflexion of a foot that precipitates calf pain (Homan's sign) indicates the presence of a deep vein thrombosis. Eliciting the Homan's sign in the presence of calf pain is contraindicated because this action increases the risk of causing a thrombus to dislodge, which can migrate to the lung, resulting in a life-threatening pulmonary embolism.**
4. This photograph depicts assessment of the posterior tibial pulse. This is an acceptable assessment technique in this situation.

27. 1. The nurse is not testing for the appearance of reactive hyperemia. Reactive hyperemia is the transient increase in blood flow following a short period of ischemia. Hyperemia is often associated with the response of tissue over a bony prominence after relief of pressure accompanying a change in a person's position.

2. The nurse is not testing for the presence of sensory perception. In an extremity, sensory perception is commonly tested for pain, vibration, and position sense, along with other tests using stimuli such as cotton balls and pointy and dull objects while the client's eyes are closed.
3. **The nurse is testing the client's skin temperature to determine whether circulation is the same in both legs. If circulation is impaired in one leg, it will feel cooler than the leg with more adequate circulation. The backs of the hands, rather than the palms, are more sensitive when assessing changes in skin temperature.**
4. The nurse is not testing the strength of the client's legs. When testing for strength in the legs, the nurse may flex the client's knee while supporting the client's lower leg and then ask the client to press the sole of the foot against the nurse's hand.

28. **Answer: 3, 2, 4, 1**

3. **The client taking warfarin (Coumadin®) should be attended to first because the risk of bleeding internally as a result of the fall can be life-threatening. Once the client's vital signs are assessed and it is determined that the client is not bleeding internally, another client can be attended to next.**
2. **The 30-year-old client missing one-third of the right index finger should be attended to second. It is essential that reconstructive surgery occur quickly if the severed finger is to remain viable. Although this client's condition is serious, a client with a potentially life-threatening situation should be attended to first.**
4. **The 70-year-old with a temperature of 102.4°F, respirations of 24, and a worsening cough should be attended to**

third. The vital signs are not elevated enough to indicate imminent danger. Two other clients require more immediate attention. This client should be attended to before the last client because the older adult has a reduced compensatory reserve.

1. Although the 12-year-old may have a fractured wrist, this situation is least serious compared with the other situations.

29. **TEST-TAKING TIP: The words *point of maximum impulse* are the words in the stem that direct attention to content.**

To assess the apical heart rate, the nurse should position a stethoscope over the site of maximum impulse, the apex of the heart. Two-thirds of the heart extends to the left of the midline of the body. The widest part is called the *base* and is located just below the second rib. The base is where the great vessels enter and leave the heart. The blunt pointed end is called the *apex* and is located to the left of the client's sternum just over the diaphragm.

To find the apex of the heart, find the angle of Louis (the bump below the sternal notch where the manubrium and sternum meet) and slide a finger into the second intercostal space on the left side of the sternum. Place one finger in each intercostal space, moving down to the fifth intercostal space. Slide a finger to the midclavicular line over the apex of the heart. This is the location indicated by the X.

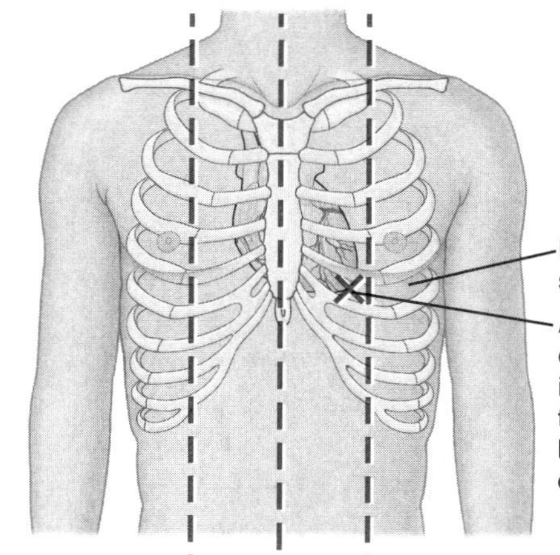

30. **TEST-TAKING TIP: The words *oral* and *electronic thermometer* are key words in the stem that direct attention to content.**

1. **A green probe is used for an oral temperature, and a red probe is used for a rectal temperature.**
2. Taking the temperature before breakfast is unnecessary; however, daily temperatures should be taken at the same time for comparison purposes. Temperatures usually are lowest in the early morning and highest between 5 and 7 p.m.
3. **Because an electronic thermometer is used for multiple clients, a probe cover is used as a medical aseptic barrier to prevent the spread of microorganisms.**
4. Wiping the probe with alcohol after each use is unnecessary because the probe is fitted with a new probe cover before each use, which is discarded after it is used. If the probe is accidentally contaminated, it must be decontaminated by wiping it with alcohol.
5. **The oral route should not be used for individuals who are unconscious, are mouth breathers, cannot follow directions, or have just consumed cold or hot liquids or food.**

31. **TEST-TAKING TIP: The words *pedal pulse* are the key words in the stem that direct attention to content.**

1. **When a Doppler probe is used, the presence of the dorsalis pedis pulse indicates the presence of arterial circulation to the distal portion of the extremity. A Doppler machine accentuates the sounds of blood flowing through an artery.**
2. **Tilting the probe at a 45° angle to the dorsalis pedis artery helps to access the signal (e.g., pulsing, rhythmic hissing sound), indicating the presence of the dorsalis pedis pulse.**
3. **Using light pressure to keep the probe in contact with the client's skin is appropriate; too much pressure can stop blood flow and obliterate the signal.**
4. **Transmission gel ensures optimal contact between the probe and the client's skin, is an excellent conducting agent, and has a gliding property that facilitates movement of the probe without loss of contact with the skin.**
5. **This is the best action to find the dorsalis pedis pulse. Place the Doppler**

probe in the groove between the great toe and first toe, and move along the top of the foot toward the ankle until the dorsalis pedis pulse is located.

32. **An X within either of the two shaded areas toward the fingertip is a correct answer. The area off-center toward the lateral aspect of a finger has fewer nerve endings compared with the center of the pad of the distal end of a finger.**

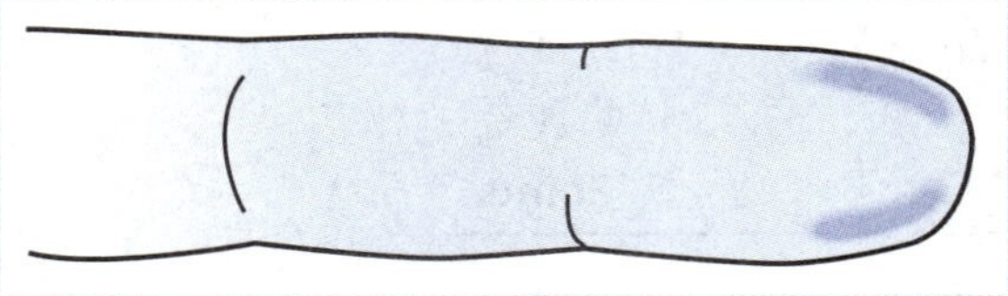

33. **TEST-TAKING TIP: The words *blood pressure* and *older adults* are key words in the stem that direct attention to content.**
   1. In aging hearts, there is decreased contractile strength of the myocardium, which results in decreased cardiac output. The body compensates for this by increasing the heart rate, not the blood pressure.
   2. Aging does not cause thicker blood. However, polycythemia (greater concentration of erythrocytes to plasma), a pathological condition, can cause higher viscosity of the blood, resulting in hypertension.
   3. This is a generalization that may or may not be true. An older adult may have physical, cognitive, and social changes, and how the person perceives them and adapts to them determines whether one's lifestyle is stressful and whether it influences blood pressure.
   4. As people age, vascular changes and the accumulation of sclerotic plaques along the walls of vessels occur, making them more rigid, not more elastic. Vascular rigidity increases vascular resistance, which increases blood pressure.
   5. **As people age, yellowish plaques containing cholesterol, lipoid material, and lipophages build up in the intima and inner media of large and medium-sized arteries (atherosclerosis); this pathological process narrows the lumen of vessels, increasing the pressure within the vessels.**

34. Using a gentle circular motion with the pads of the fingers, palpate the lymph nodes. Many lymph nodes are close to each other so the examination should be systematic and thorough. Lymph nodes are best examined using both hands to compare symmetry of both sides of the neck. For the deep cervical chain, turn the client's head toward the side being examined to enable examination under the muscle. Note any palpable nodes for mobility, consistency, and tenderness.
   1. **Submental**
   2. **Submandibular**
   3. **Deep mandibular**
   4. **Supraclavicular**
   5. **Superficial**
   6. **Tonsillar**
   7. **Posterior cervical**

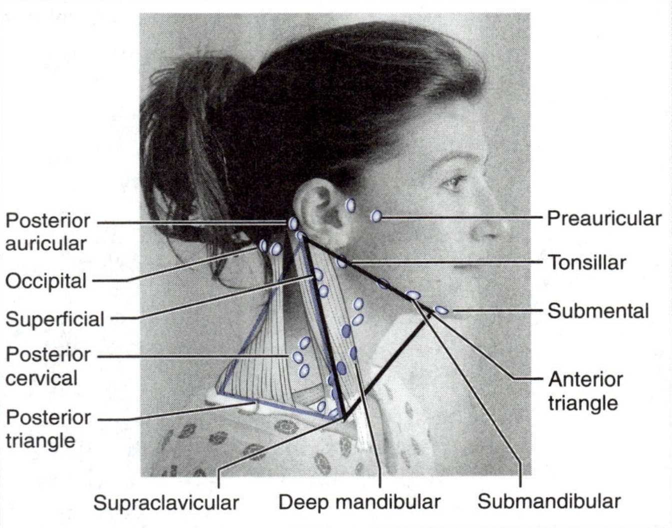

35. 1. The number 9 does not reflect the client's total points on the GCS.
   2. The number 11 does not reflect the client's total points on the GCS.
   3. **The number 13 reflects the client's total points on the GCS as demonstrated in the scale shown below.**
   4. The number 15 does not reflect the client's total points on the GCS.

Eye Opening	**Points**
Eyes open spontaneously	4
Eyes open in response to voice	**3**
Eyes open in response to pain	2
No eye-opening response	1
Best Verbal Response	**Points**
Oriented (e.g., to person, place, time)	5
Confused, speaks but is disoriented	**4**
Inappropriate but comprehensible words	3
Incomprehensible sounds but no words are spoken	2
None	1
Best Motor Response	**Points**
Obeys command to move	**6**
Localizes painful stimulus	5
Withdraws from painful stimulus	4
Flexion, abnormal decorticate posturing	3
Extension, abnormal decerebrate posturing	2
No movement or posturing	7
Total Points	**13**
Major head injury	**≤8**
Moderate head injury	**9–12**
Minor head injury	**13–15**

36. **TEST-TAKING TIP: The words *older adult* and *skin* are key words in the stem that direct attention to content.**

1. **The size of pigment-containing cells (melanocytes) increases as one ages, particularly on skin exposed to the sun.**
2. **The skin of the older adult decreases in thickness because of loss of dermal and subcutaneous mass. These losses occur in response to a flattening of the dermal-epidermal junction, reduced thickness and vascularity of the dermis, and slowing of epidermal proliferation.**
3. As a person's skin ages, it decreases, not increases, in elasticity because collagen fibers become coarser and more random and there is a degeneration of elastic fibers in the dermal connective tissue.
4. As a person's skin ages, it increases, not decreases, in dryness because of reductions in moisture content, sebaceous gland activity, and circulation to the skin.
5. As a person's skin ages, it decreases, not increases, in tone because of loss of dermal mass. This occurs because of flattening of the dermal-epidermal junction, reduced thickness and vascularity of the dermis, and slowing of epidermal proliferation.

37. **Venous return from the stomach, small intestine, colon, spleen, and pancreas flows via veins to the portal vein (hepatic portal circulation). The portal vein transports blood to the liver, where blood is detoxified. Blood then exits the liver via hepatic veins to the inferior vena cava and eventually to the right atrium of the heart. With advanced liver disease, there is increased pressure in liver blood flow, which in turn results in an increase in pressure in the hepatic portal circulation (portal hypertension). In addition, an impaired liver is unable to produce adequate amounts of albumin, the principal protein in blood,**

which is necessary to maintain blood volume. The increase in venous pressure in the hepatic portal circulation and decrease in albumin are responsible for fluid moving from the hepatic portal circulation, a high-pressure space, to the abdominal cavity, a low-pressure space, resulting in ascites. See Figure B for an illustration of hepatic portal circulation.

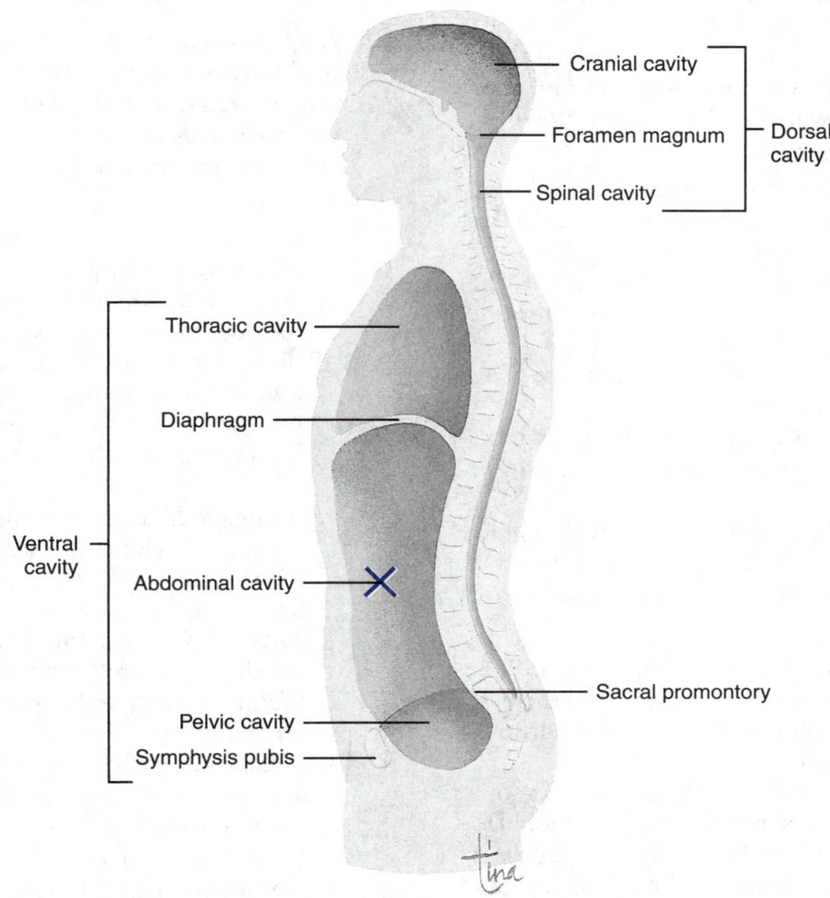

A: Abdominal cavity

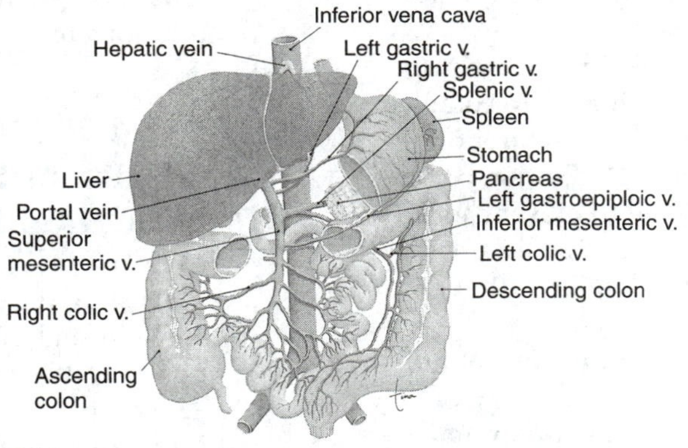

B: Hepatic portal circulation

38. TEST-TAKING TIP: The words *obliterated with slight pressure* are key words in the stem that direct attention to content. The words *Bounding* and *Full* are equally plausible. The words *Thready* and *Weak* are equally plausible. The words *Bounding* and *Full* are opposites of the words *Thready* and *Weak*. More often than not, a correct answer is one of the opposites. Either *Bounding* and *Full* are correct answers or *Thready* and *Weak* are correct answers.

1. A bounding pulse is strong when palpated. The pulse is not obliterated when moderate pressure is applied to the artery.
2. **A thready pulse is difficult to feel when palpated and is obliterated with slight pressure.**
3. An absent pulse is the nonexistence of a detectable pulse.
4. **A weak pulse is difficult to feel when palpated and is obliterated with slight pressure.**
5. A full pulse is strong and easily counted when palpated. The pulse is not obliterated when moderate pressure is applied to the artery.

39. 1. This is not the priority intervention. The client may need monitoring, but there are other options that need immediate intervention.
2. The client needs fluids but there is another option that is the priority. Crystalloid IV fluids are typically used for older adults if admitted to a facility with a diagnosis of dehydration. The fluids may contain glucose or dextrose and electrolytes such as potassium. They always contain sodium to help restore hydration.
3. Medication reconciliation is not the priority, though the nurse will need to complete this once the client's oxygen saturation is within expected limits. Medication reconciliations are completed to prevent adverse events and provide correct medications to a client at all transition points within the health-care system.
4. **The client's oxygen saturation rate of 89% is below the expected range of 95% to 100% in a healthy older adult. The primary health-care provider should be informed when the oxygen saturation level decreases below a parameter preset by the primary health-care provider or agency protocol (frequently 92% for a client without a history of obstructive airway disease; 88% for a client with a history of obstructive airway disease because the oxygen saturation level is chronically low), as a change in the oxygen prescription may be necessary to meet the oxygen needs of the client.**

40. TEST-TAKING TIP: The word *immediate* in the stem sets a priority. The words *response requires* and *focused assessment* are key words in the stem that direct attention to content.

1. **Suprapubic distention may indicate urinary retention; an immediate focused assessment is required.**
2. **Dependent edema is a response related to problems such as hypervolemia, decreased cardiac output, or impaired kidney functioning. The client should be assessed further immediately because these conditions can be life-threatening.**
3. Although difficulty sleeping at night should be explored further, it is not a life-threatening problem and therefore is not a priority.
4. Although lack of a bowel movement should be explored further, it is not a life-threatening problem and therefore is not a priority.
5. Blanchable erythema in an area at risk for a pressure ulcer indicates that the area has been exposed to pressure. However, circulation to the area is not impaired. Pressure that produces nonblanchable erythema signals a potential ulceration and meets the criterion for a stage I pressure ulcer. The client should be assessed further, but it is not a priority.

CLINICAL JUDGMENT CASE STUDY ANSWERS AND RATIONALES

41. 1. Discussing the client's pet demonstrates empathy and caring from the nurse; however, it is not the priority.
2. The client's oxygen level is at 89%. This is the priority. The client should be encouraged to take deep breaths and a nasal cannula with oxygen at 2 L/min should be initiated. The client should be educated on the nasal cannula and why they are receiving oxygen.
3. **The client's pain level is 8 out of 10 so this will need to be addressed, but**

oxygenation status is the priority intervention.

4. The client will need comfort once they are stabilized, and vital signs are within normal limits as defined by the facility.

42. 1. Education on a low-sodium diet is not appropriate education for the client to improve breathing. The client may follow a low-sodium diet to control their heart disease. There is not enough information provided to warrant this education.

2. The client has an order for PRN oxygen. The client should be instructed on how to assess their oxygen level and when to use a nasal cannula. The client should also be provided with education on the safe use of oxygen and how to properly store oxygen.

3. The client should be educated on using the tripod position. This position is used to increase chest and lung expansion and decrease a client's work of breathing. The client should be instructed to sit with their arms propped on an overbed table or place their hands on their knees and lean slightly forward.

4. Pursed-lip breathing is an easy way for the client to control their breathing and lower their respiratory rate. This method of breathing releases air trapped in the lungs and prolongs exhalation to slow the respiratory rate. The client should inhale with their mouth closed, pucker their lips, and exhale very slowly.

5. Elevating the legs above the heart may improve circulation for the client with cardiovascular disease but there is not enough information in the client record to indicate this is warranted at this time.

6. The client indicated that the chair was closer to the bathroom. This topic should be explored further because she does take a diuretic and may be using the bathroom frequently during the night. The timing of her medications could be revised to an earlier time.

43.

2 L O_2 PRN to maintain above 92%	x
Hydrocodone 5/325 mg PRN for pain	x
Morphine PO PRN 12 hours for pain	x
Low-sodium, heart-healthy diet	
Enalapril (Vasotec) 20 mg PO in morning and at bedtime	x
Furosemide (Lasix) 20 mg PO in morning and at bedtime	x

Hydrocodone 5/325 PRN for pain and morphine PO PRN 12 hours for pain should be clarified. A complete medication order should include the name of the medication, the ordered dosage, the form of the medication, the route, and the time or frequency of administration. Both orders are missing parts of a complete medication order.

The nurse should also clarify the blood pressure medications with the provider as the client's blood pressure is 96/72 so giving these medications may further lower the blood pressure. Additionally, the client mentions one of the reasons for sleeping in the chair is because it is closer than the bed to the bathroom. Adjusting the timing of the furosemide may be needed.

44. 1. The nurse must first clarify the pain medication orders as they are incomplete.

2. The client's blood pressure is low so before the nurse gives either medication, they should contact the provider to review the client's vital signs.

3. Both the blood pressure medications and the pain medications should be reviewed with the provider before administering. The client's blood pressure is low, and the pain medication orders are not complete.

4. All medications should be reviewed with the provider before administering. If the client was administered the blood pressure medications, their blood pressure could drop further. The nurse would be operating out of their scope of practice by administering the pain medications without a complete order.

45. 1. 4 Ineffective Airway Clearance
2. 3 Activity Intolerance
3. 1 Insomnia
4. 2 Anxiety

1. Ineffective Airway Clearance related to bronchial secretions and obstruction as evidenced by diminished and moist breath sounds and a productive cough
2. Activity Intolerance related to dyspnea as evidenced by the client reporting increased difficulty breathing and sleeping in a chair
3. Insomnia related to pain and medications as evidenced by the client reporting it hurts too much to sleep in the bed and that they prefer the chair because it is closer to the bathroom
4. Anxiety related to change in health status as evidenced by the client being distressed over who will care for their dog

1. The nasal cannula around the client's neck indicates that they are not wearing the cannula properly and not getting oxygen delivered to their tissues as needed.
2. Placing the dog up for adoption indicates that the client is experiencing despair and may need some spiritual or emotional counseling.
3. The client is still not sleeping in their bed. Sleeping in a chair is not conducive to a good night's sleep and indicates the client is not compliant with interventions.
4. The client is using pursed-lip breathing to help prolong expiration and to decrease the respiratory rate.
5. The client is using the tripod position to help open the airways and decrease the work of breathing.
6. An oxygen level of 90% indicates the client is not compliant with the prescribed oxygen order.

46.
_____ 1. Nasal cannula around neck
_____ 2. Placing dog up for adoption
_____ 3. Plan to sleep in bed soon
__X__ 4. Pursed-lip breathing
__X__ 5. Tripod position
_____ 6. O_2 90%

MEETING CLIENTS' PHYSICAL SAFETY AND MOBILITY NEEDS

This section includes questions related to maintaining clients' physical safety and mobility needs. In relation to clients' safety needs, this section emphasizes concepts regarding the use of restraints, issues associated with smoking and fire, prevention of injury, electrical safety, protection of a client experiencing a seizure, and safety related to oxygen use. In relation to clients' mobility needs, this section includes questions addressing the maintenance and restoration of musculoskeletal function and the prevention of musculoskeletal complications. These questions focus on knowledge, principles, and devices related to the prevention of pressure (decubitus) ulcers, contractures, and other hazards of immobility. Additional questions test principles associated with body alignment, transfer, range of motion, ambulation, positioning, and dressing.

QUESTIONS

1. The legal nurse is reviewing the primary causes of accidental injuries and traumas for hospitalized clients. Which should the nurse conclude is the priority intervention to prevent accidental injuries and trauma to these clients?
1. Keeping client rooms clean and decluttered
2. Screening clients for dementia and confusion
3. Document according to policy and facility guidelines
4. Avoid giving clients antianxiety or hypnotic medications

TEST-TAKING TIP: Identify the word in the stem that sets a priority. Identify the priority option that all health-care staff can support.

2. The nurse identifies that a client sitting in a wheelchair is having a tonic-clonic (formerly called *grand mal*) seizure. The nurse should **first:**
1. transfer the client to an empty room to provide privacy.
2. return the client to bed to provide a soft surface.
3. move the client to the floor to prevent injury.
4. secure the client to prevent falling.

TEST-TAKING TIP: Identify key words in the stem that direct attention to content.

3. The confused and disoriented client, in restraints for safety concerns, continues to struggle against the restraints. When developing the care plan for this client, the nurse identifies that the primary reason for this behavior is:
1. a response to discomfort.
2. an attempt to gain control.
3. an effort to manipulate the staff.
4. the inability to understand what is occurring.

TEST-TAKING TIP: Identify the word in the stem that sets a priority. Identify key words in the stem that direct attention to content. Identify the clang association.

4. The nurse is teaching a parenting class about methods to safeguard the home to prevent the accidental poisoning of children. Which should the nurse include in the teaching? **Select all that apply.**
1. Administer syrup of ipecac to induce vomiting.
2. Have the number of poison control readily available.
3. Administer home remedies first, then call poison control.
4. Bring the child to the emergency department for gastric lavage.
5. Medications can be stored anywhere if they are in childproof containers.
6. Activated charcoal is the most effective agent to prevent toxin absorption.

TEST-TAKING TIP: Identify key words in the stem that direct attention to content. Identify options that are client-centered and emphasize safety.

5. The nurse is responding to a fire alarm within the hospital. Which should be done when transporting a fire extinguisher to a fire scene on a different level of the building than the one on which the nurse is working?
   1. Use the stairs
   2. Pull the safety pin
   3. Keep it from touching the floor
   4. Always run as quickly as possible

   TEST-TAKING TIP: Identify key words in the stem that direct attention to content. Identify the option with a specific determiner.

6. The nurse is admitting a postsurgical client with a right knee replacement to the nursing unit. When orienting the client to the unit, which is the priority education?
   1. Providing contact information for the charge nurse
   2. Educating the family on the potential date of discharge
   3. Demonstrating how to use the call bell and placing it with the client
   4. Orienting the client to their physical and occupational therapy schedule

   TEST-TAKING TIP: Identify the word in the stem that sets a priority. Use Maslow's hierarchy of needs to help identify the most important information that the client should know from among the options presented.

7. The nurse on the evening shift in the hospital is caring for a slightly confused client. Which is the **most** effective nursing intervention to help prevent disorientation at night?
   1. Check on the client regularly
   2. Place a call bell in the client's bed
   3. Turn on a night-light in the client's room
   4. Describe the physical environment to the client

   TEST-TAKING TIP: Identify the word in the stem that sets a priority. Identify key words in the stem that direct attention to content. Identify the unique option. Identify equally plausible options. Identify the clang association.

8. While walking, a client becomes weak and the knees begin to buckle. Which should the nurse do?
   1. Hold up the client
   2. Walk the client to the closest chair
   3. Call for assistance to help the client
   4. Lower the client to the floor carefully

   TEST-TAKING TIP: Identify key words in the stem that direct attention to content. Identify opposites in options.

9. The nurse identifies that the electrical cord on a client's cell phone charger is frayed. Which should the nurse do?
   1. Report the problem to the supervisor
   2. Unplug it and put it in the client's closet
   3. Remove it from the client's room and send it home with a family member
   4. Ask the maintenance department to apply nonconductive tape to the damaged section

10. The nurse is caring for an older adult who is on bed rest. Which should the nurse provide to **best** prevent a pressure (decubitus) ulcer in this client?
    1. An air mattress
    2. A daily bed bath
    3. A high-protein diet
    4. An indwelling urinary catheter

    TEST-TAKING TIP: Identify the word in the stem that sets a priority. Identify key words in the stem that direct attention to content.

11. Which is the **most** therapeutic exercise that can be done by a client confined to bed?
   1. Isometric exercise
   2. Active-assistive exercise
   3. Active range-of-motion exercise
   4. Passive range-of-motion exercise

   TEST-TAKING TIP: Identify the word in the stem that sets a priority. Identify opposites in options.

12. The nurse is transferring a client from the bed to a chair using a mechanical lift. As the nurse begins to raise the lift off the bed, the client begins to panic and scream. Which should the nurse do?
   1. Immediately lower the client back onto the bed
   2. Say "Relax" and slowly continue the procedure
   3. Quickly continue and say "Be calm; it's almost over"
   4. Stop the lift from rising until the client regains control

   TEST-TAKING TIP: Identify key words in the stem that direct attention to content. Identify opposites in options. Identify options that deny client feelings, concerns, or needs. Identify the client-centered option.

13. While a client is lying in the dorsal recumbent position, the legs externally rotate. Which equipment should the nurse use to prevent external rotation?
   1. Bed cradle
   2. Trochanter roll
   3. Elastic stockings
   4. High-top sneakers

   TEST-TAKING TIP: Identify key words in the stem that direct attention to content.

14. A client is afraid of falling when it is time to get out of bed to a chair. Which is the **best** action by the nurse to reduce the client's fear?
   1. Permit the client to set the pace of the transfer
   2. Transfer the client using a mechanical lift
   3. Inform the client that a fall will not occur
   4. Allow the client to decide when to get up

   TEST-TAKING TIP: Identify the word in the stem that sets a priority. Identify key words in the stem that direct attention to content. Identify the clang association. Identify the option that denies client feelings, concerns, or needs. Identify client-centered options.

15. A client who had a brain attack (stroke, cerebrovascular accident) 3 days earlier has left-sided hemiparesis. Which should the nurse plan to do when dressing the client?
   1. Put the client's left sleeve on first
   2. Encourage the client to dress independently
   3. Instruct the client to wear clothes with zippers
   4. Tell the client to get clothes with buttons in the front

   TEST-TAKING TIP: Identify key words in the stem that direct attention to content. Identify the clang association. Identify equally plausible options. Identify the unique option. Identify the option that denies client feelings, concerns, or needs.

16. The home health nurse is developing the plan of care for an 82-year-old client just released from the hospital after falling at home. When completing a safety evaluation of the home, the nurse knows which of the following are modifiable risk factors to prevent falls? **Select all that apply.**
   1. Advanced age
   2. Postural dizziness
   3. Lower body weakness
   4. Gait and balance issues
   5. Improper use of assistive devices
   6. Use of psychoactive medications

   TEST-TAKING TIP: Identify the word in the stem that sets a priority. Identify key words in the stem that direct attention to content.

17. Warm, dry heat to be applied via an aquathermia pad to a client's lower back is prescribed to ease muscle spasms resulting from a fall. Which should the nurse do? **Select all that apply.**
1. _____ Set the pad at 110°F to 115°F
2. _____ Apply the pad directly to the client's skin
3. _____ Remove the pad 20 to 30 minutes after it is applied
4. _____ Moisten the liner between the pad and the cover of the pad
5. _____ Put the pad under the client after the client is placed in the supine position

TEST-TAKING TIP: Identify the key words in the stem that direct attention to content.

18. A client with one-sided weakness (hemiparesis) has a prescription to be transferred out of bed to a chair twice a day. Which should the nurse plan to do? **Select all that apply.**
1. _____ Arrange the client's feet a shoulder width apart
2. _____ Place rubber-soled shoes on the client's feet
3. _____ Position the hands on the client's scapulae
4. _____ Support the client on the affected side
5. _____ Pivot the client on the unaffected leg

TEST-TAKING TIP: Identify key words in the stem that direct attention to content.

19. When the home care nurse places an egg crate pad under a client, the spouse asks, "What is the purpose of that pad?" Which is the purpose of an egg crate pad that should be included in the response to the spouse? **Select all that apply.**
1. _____ Absorbs moisture
2. _____ Limits perspiration
3. _____ Provides for comfort
4. _____ Supports the body in alignment
5. _____ Distributes pressure over a larger area

TEST-TAKING TIP: Identify the key words in the stem that direct attention to content.

20. The nurse identifies the illustrated ulcer when completing a skin assessment for a newly admitted client. Which stage ulcer should the nurse indicate on the pressure ulcer flow sheet?

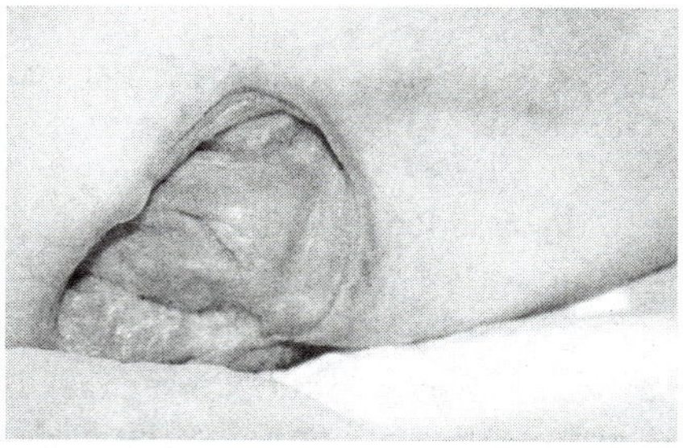

1. Stage I
2. Stage II
3. Stage III
4. Stage IV

21. The nurse is planning a turning schedule for a client with limited mobility. Which position that will contribute to the development of a pressure ulcer in the sacral area should be avoided in this client's plan of care? **Select all that apply.**
1. _____ Semi-prone
2. _____ Prone
3. _____ Contour
4. _____ High Fowler
5. _____ Dorsal recumbent

TEST-TAKING TIP: Identify the word in the stem that indicates negative polarity. Identify key words in the stem that direct attention to content.

22. The nurse assumes care for an 88-year-old client admitted with urosepsis. After reviewing the client's clinical record, the nurse notes a change in the client's behavior from their baseline assessment. Which is the priority intervention for the client?
1. Place the client on a bed alarm
2. Administer the prescribed sedative
3. Place the client in a vest restraint and notify the provider
4. Assign a staff member to stay with the client and notify the provider

CLIENT'S CLINICAL RECORD

Progress Note

Nursing Note 1800: 88-year-old adult with mild dementia admitted to the hospital for urosepsis at 1300. On admission, the client was alert and answering and asking questions appropriately. Over the past several hours, the client has become confused and is attempting to pull out the IV line and urinary catheter and climb over the bed rail. The client's eyes are darting about the room, and intermittently the client will wring the hands and pick at the bedding.

Vital Signs Flow Sheet

Blood pressure: 160/95 mm Hg
Pulse: 110 beats/min
Respirations: 28 breaths/min
Temperature: 99.6°F

Primary Health-Care Provider's Prescriptions

IV 1000 mL 0.9% sodium chloride every 12 hours
Urinary retention catheter
Vital signs every 4 hours
Zolpidem 10 mg PO hs

23. The wound care nurse is assessing several clients on the unit. Which client would the nurse recognize as being at risk for impaired skin integrity? **Select all that apply.**
1. _____ The paraplegic client
2. _____ The ambulatory confused client
3. _____ The client with a new colostomy
4. _____ The ambulatory incontinent client
5. _____ The client with imbalanced nutrition
6. _____ The client on bed rest who can still move

TEST-TAKING TIP: Identify key words in the stem that direct attention to content.

24. The nurse is caring for a terminally ill client who reports increasing episodes of pain while ambulating. The client states, "I am just going to lay in bed until I die." Knowing that end-of-life pain is one of the most reported symptoms of terminally ill clients, which should the nurse include in the plan of care to encourage mobility? **Select all that apply.**
1. _____ Administer pain medications after ambulation
2. _____ Assess pain for intensity and alleviating factors
3. _____ Assess the effectiveness of pain relief measures frequently
4. _____ Minimize irritants from heat or cold, wetness, and pressure
5. _____ Provide complementary and alternative therapies as needed
6. _____ Administer medications in a timely manner to provide constant relief

25. The nurse is caring for a client positioned in the left lateral position. Place an X over the bony prominence that the nurse should be **most** concerned about regarding development of a pressure ulcer.

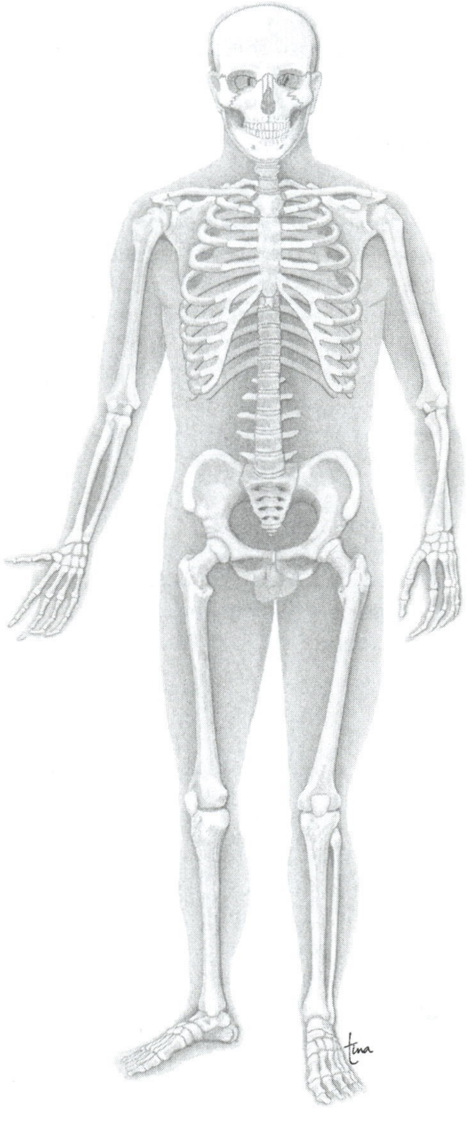

26. The nurse is caring for a client who was recently diagnosed with a latex allergy. Which information should the nurse include in the teaching plan? **Select all that apply.**
1. _____ Wear clothing labeled hypoallergenic.
2. _____ Carry injectable epinephrine or keep it within easy reach.
3. _____ Avoid clothing with spandex because spandex contains rubber.
4. _____ Examine tags on clothing to ensure that they do not contain latex.
5. _____ Have someone remove plants such as poinsettias, ficus, and rubber tree plants from the home.

27. A primary health-care provider prescribes crutches for a person who has a left lower leg injury. The nurse is teaching the person how to rise from a chair without bearing weight on the left leg. Place the following steps in the order in which they should be implemented.
1. Put one crutch under each arm.
2. Slide the buttocks toward the edge of the chair.
3. Hold both crutches together on the hand bars with the left hand.
4. Push down on the arm of the chair on the unaffected side while bearing weight on the hand bars of the crutches.
5. Extend the left leg while keeping the right foot flat on the floor, elevate the body to a standing position, and then check balance.

Answer: ____________

28. The nurse is positioning a client in a lateral position. Which action by the nurse contributes to the client's functional alignment? **Select all that apply.**
1. _____ Putting a pillow under the upper leg
2. _____ Placing a small pillow under the waist
3. _____ Using a pillow to support the upper arm
4. _____ Keeping the lower hip and knee extended
5. _____ Positioning a pillow behind the client's back

TEST-TAKING TIP: Identify key words in the stem that direct attention to content.

29. Which knot should the nurse use when attaching the strap of a restraint to a bed frame?

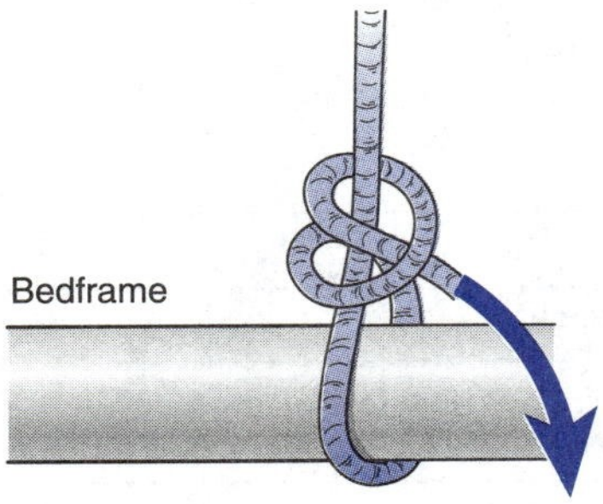

1.

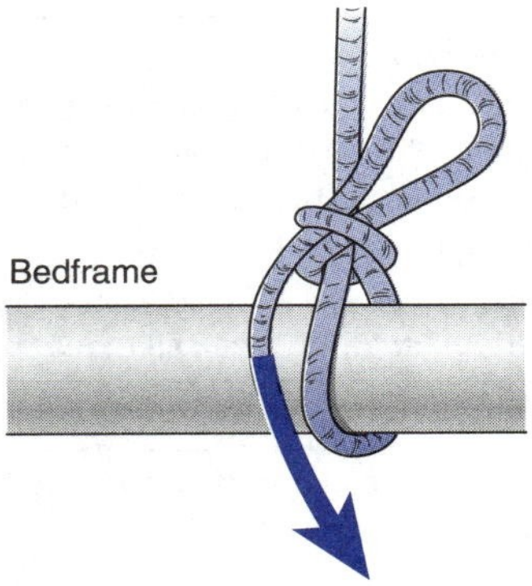

2.

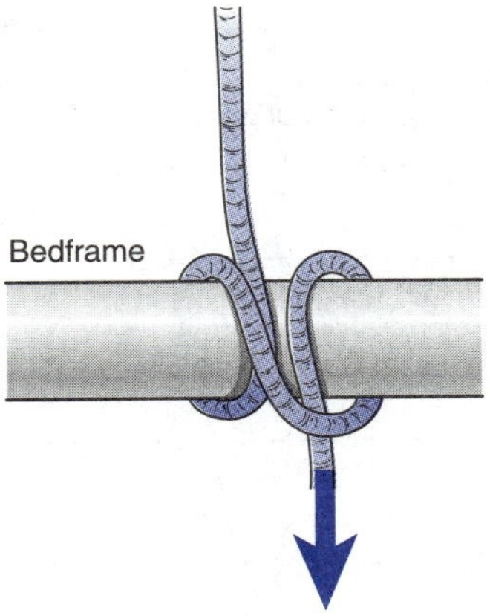

3.

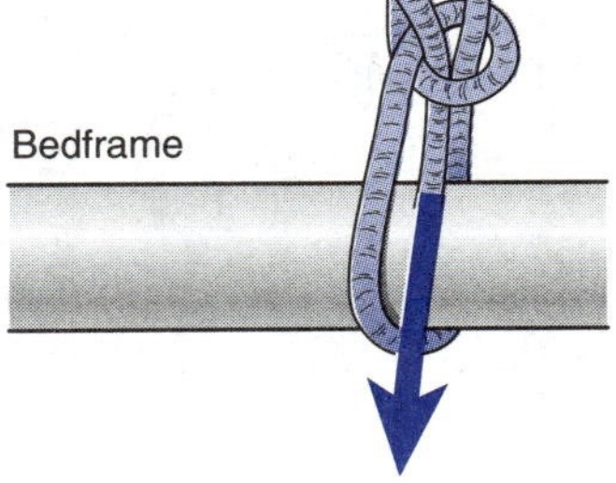

4.

30. The nurse left a bedside rail down for a client who was premedicated with an opioid in preparation for surgery. The client was found on the floor. The client was examined by the rapid response team, and no injury was identified as a result of the fall. The client was returned to bed. The nurse inserted a brief description of the event on the Unusual Occurrence Report. Place a check in the box in front of the most appropriate category in the "Occurrence Category" section of the Unusual Occurrence Report that relates to this event.

Unusual Occurrence Report

Date of Event: __________ **Time of Event:** __________ **Department:** ________________

Client Last Name:	**First Name:**	**MI:**
Client #:	**Attending Physician:**	
Visitor Last Name:	**First Name:**	**Phone #:**
Employee Name:	**Dept:**	
Physician Name:	**Specialty:**	
Occurrence Category (Check most appropriate)		
☐ Agency nurse-related	☐ AMA	☐ Delay in treatment
☐ Diet-related	☐ HIPAA compliance	☐ Loss of personal property
☐ Medication-related	☐ Narcotics-related	☐ Order not executed
☐ Client injury	☐ Peer-review related	☐ Restraint-related
☐ Staff injury	☐ Supplies/Equipment	☐ Visitor injury
☐ Fall		
☐ Other (please explain):		

Description of Occurrence:
A client was medicated with an opioid. The client's bedside rail was left in the down position. The client was found on the floor. The client was examined by the rapid response team. No injury was identified as a result of the fall. The client was returned to bed.

Contributing Factors (Check all that apply)	
☐ Individual:	☐ System:
Knowledge, skills, and/or experience (please list): ☐ Unclear ☐ Incomplete	Policies/procedures not in place (please list): ☐ Unclear ☐ Outdated
Standard of care or practice (please list): ☐ Non-adherence	Environmental: ☐ Staffing ☐ Client acuity ☐ Congestion
Documentation (please list): ☐ Incomplete ☐ Inadequate	Communications and work flow: ☐ Intradepartmental ☐Interdepartmental ☐ Equipment failure
Other (please explain):	

Submitted by:	**Dept:**	**Date:**

31. Which is a reason why restraints are used when caring for clients? **Select all that apply.**

1. _____ Support joints
2. _____ Reduce agitation
3. _____ Immobilize clients
4. _____ Prevent client injury
5. _____ Prohibit a client from hurting others

32. Which event requires a nurse to complete an incident report? The clinical documentation specialist is discussing incidents that occurred within the facility during the weekend. Which of these events requires the filing of an incident report? **Select all that apply.**

1. _____ The client who fell in their room but was not injured
2. _____ The nurse who refused to be floated to a different unit
3. _____ The visitor who fainted when seeing an ill family member in the intensive care unit
4. _____ The provider who is angry when awakened during the night to examine a client
5. _____ The unlicensed assistive personnel who applied medication to a client's perineal area

33. Identify the illustration that indicates flexion and extension of the ankle.

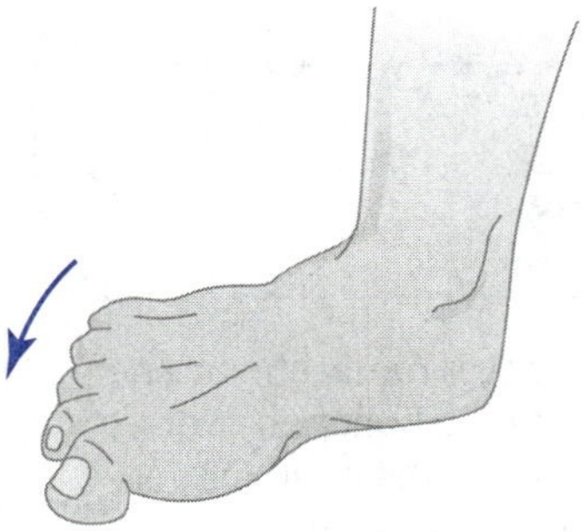

1.

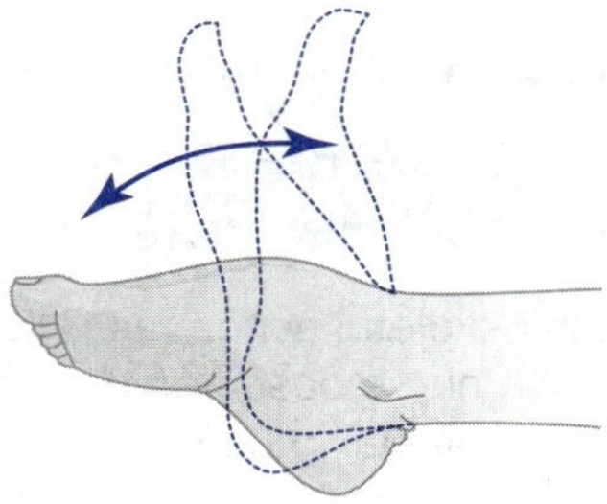

2.

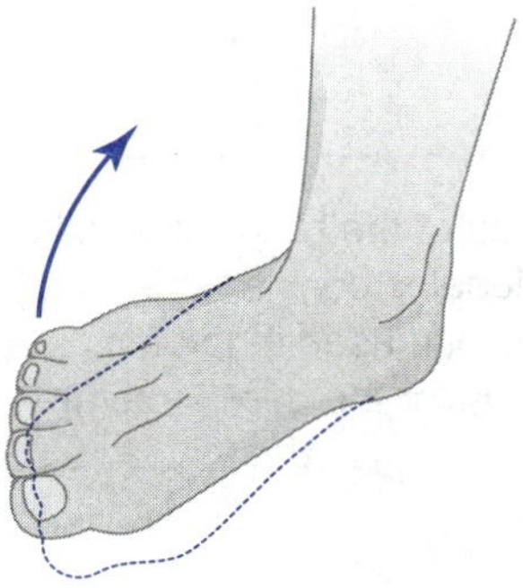

3.

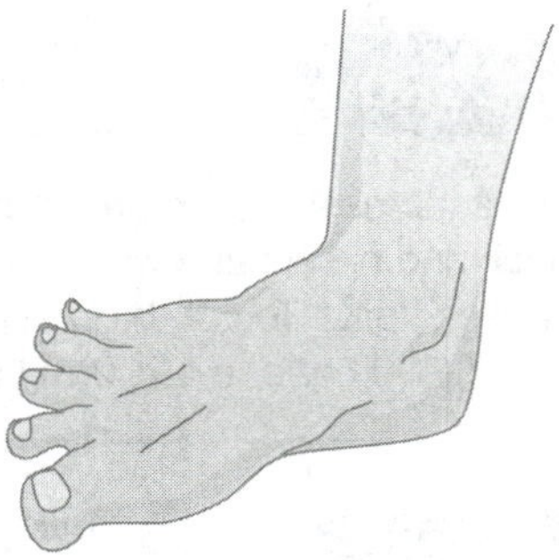

4.

34. The nurse manager has noticed an increase in the use of restraints on the medical-surgical unit during the night shift, so an educational session on restraint use is being planned for all unit staff. Which should the manager include in the education? **Select all that apply.**
1. _____ Restraint use decreases the need for additional staff
2. _____ Restraint use decreases incontinence, depression, and delirium
3. _____ Physical restraints reduce the risk of serious injury due to a fall
4. _____ Medications used to control behavior are not considered a restraint
5. _____ Restraints should only be used to protect the client, staff, and others
6. _____ Negative outcomes of restraint use include skin breakdown and contractures

TEST-TAKING TIP: Identify key words in the stem that direct attention to content.

35. An older adult has been taking 20 mg of furosemide by mouth twice a day along with an antihypertensive medication. The client's blood pressure has progressively decreased, and the client has experienced several episodes of light-headedness. The primary health-care provider changes the furosemide prescription to 15 mg by mouth twice a day. An oral solution is prescribed because the client has difficulty swallowing pills. The furosemide solution states that there are 10 mg/1 mL of solution. How many milliliters of furosemide should the nurse administer over 24 hours? **Record your answer using a whole number.**

Answer: __________ mL

CLINICAL JUDGMENT CASE STUDY

A 47-year-old male client comes to an outpatient clinic.

REASON FOR SEEKING CARE

Ongoing musculoskeletal aches not relieved by over-the-counter medications such as ibuprofen. The nurse observes the client has a wobbled gait, hunched over at the shoulders, and facial grimaces while the client is getting on the examination table. Client also reports mild tinnitus that usually goes away on its own.

MEDICAL RECORD

The client reports increasing joint and muscle pain on both sides of the body, especially in the lower back and hands and wrists. The client works at a loading dock and reports "lifting heavy boxes daily." To get through the day, the client has increased ibuprofen intake to between 800 mg and 1200 mg every 4 to 6 hours daily for the past 4 months.

MEDICAL HISTORY

High blood pressure; two deep vein thromboses (DVTs), one in the left leg 10 years ago and one in the right leg 2 years ago; family history of cardiovascular disease and diabetes.

MEDICATIONS

Furosemide 40 mg daily
Omeprazole 20 mg daily
Warfarin 3 mg daily
Ibuprofen 800 mg to 1200 mg as needed

36. **Recognize cues—What matters most?** After reviewing the client's medical record, which question should the nurse ask first?
    1. Have you had any accidents or trauma that affected your bones, muscles, or joints?
    2. Is your pain aggravated by movement, rest, position, or the weather?
    3. Have you noticed any unexplained bruising or bleeding?
    4. Do you smoke or use alcohol and if so, how often?

37. **Analyze cues—What could it mean?** The nurse assesses the client's musculoskeletal system by having the client perform several range-of-motion exercises. The client reports pain when pronating and supinating the wrists on both hands and when rotating the spine. Based on the client's history and results from the range-of-motion exercises, the nurse develops a plan of care based on:
    1. an undiagnosed autoimmune disease.
    2. degenerative changes due to aging.
    3. overuse and repetitive motions.
    4. episode of acute gout.

38. **Prioritize hypotheses—Where do I start?** The nurse discusses the client with the provider. Which laboratory tests does the nurse anticipate will be ordered by the provider? **Select all that apply.**
    1. BUN (blood urea nitrogen) and creatinine
    2. T_3 (triiodothyronine) and T_4 (thyroxine)
    3. INR (international normalized ratio)
    4. Platelet and liver function tests
    5. Lipase and amylase
    6. K^+ (potassium)

39. **Generate solutions—What can I do?** The nurse is educating the client on proper body mechanics to help alleviate pain and reduce injury. Which teaching should the nurse provide to the client? **Select all that apply.**
    1. Stand with feet together
    2. Hold loads away to your body
    3. Keep knees straight when lifting
    4. Move torso from shoulder to hips
    5. Tighten abdominal muscles when lifting

40. **Take action—What will I do?** The nurse reviews the client's vital signs and computed tomography (CT) scan. The client's blood pressure is 110/62 mm Hg and the heart rate is 102 beats/min. The CT scan of the abdomen notes changes to the mucosal membrane of the upper gastrointestinal tract. The x-ray of the lumbar spine notes narrowed disc space alignment. Based on these findings, the nurse develops several interventions. For each potential nursing intervention, select whether the intervention is **indicated, not indicated,** or **contraindicated.**

Intervention	Indicated	Not Indicated	Contraindicated
Educate the client that aspirin is a better choice than ibuprofen			
Encourage the client to eat small amounts of food every hour			
Encourage physical and psychosocial lifestyle modifications			
Educate the client to eat a diet rich in creams and milk			
Encourage bed rest when the client is not at work			
Sleep in a semi-Fowler's position			

41. **Evaluate outcomes—Did it help?** The client comes to the clinic for a follow-up visit. For each assessment finding, place an X indicating if the client has **improved,** has had **no change,** or has **declined.**

Assessment Finding	Improved	No Change	Declined
Intestinal pain			
Ongoing tinnitus			
Steady gait			
No pain after eating			
Weight loss of 10 lb.			

1. **TEST-TAKING TIP: The word *primary* in the stem sets a priority. All health-care staff can help keep rooms clean and decluttered to prevent accidental falls and injury.**
   1. **Falls are the most common cause of accidental injury and trauma for hospitalized clients; therefore, hospital rooms should always be kept free of clutter. IV poles and other equipment should be placed so the client can safely move.**
   2. Though clients should be screened for confusion and other neurological impairments that can influence safety, this is not the priority intervention.
   3. Nurses should always document according to policy and facility guidelines; however, this is not a priority intervention to prevent injury to clients.
   4. If a client has an order for an antianxiety or antihypnotic, it is not within the nurse's scope of practice to decide to not give the medication to prevent accidental injury.
2. **TEST-TAKING TIP: The words *wheelchair* and *tonic-clonic seizure* are key words in the stem that direct attention to content.**
   1. The need for privacy is not the priority. Transporting a client in a wheelchair during a tonic-clonic (grand mal) seizure can cause muscle strain, bone fractures, or other injury and is unsafe.
   2. Attempting to return a client to bed during a tonic-clonic (grand mal) seizure can cause muscle strain, bone fractures, or other injury. The client should be returned to bed after the seizure is over.
   3. **Moving the client to the floor is the safest action; it provides free movement on a supported surface.**
   4. Securing a client in a wheelchair during a tonic-clonic (grand mal) seizure can cause muscle strain, bone fractures, or other injury and is an unsafe action.
3. **TEST-TAKING TIP: The word *primary* in the stem sets a priority. The words *confused* and *struggle* are key words in the stem that direct attention to content. The word *confused* in the stem and the words *inability to understand* in option 4 reflect an obscure clang association.**
   1. A restraint should not cause discomfort if it is applied correctly and checked frequently.
   2. Clients who are confused, are disoriented, and are restrained may become agitated and respond in a reflex-like way; attempts to gain control require problem solving, which they usually are unable to perform.
   3. A client usually struggles against a restraint to get free, not to manipulate staff.
   4. **Disoriented and confused clients do not always have the cognitive ability to understand what is happening to them and often struggle against restraints.**
4. **TEST-TAKING TIP: Identify the key words in the stem that set priorities and direct attention to content.**
   1. Syrup of ipecac is no longer recommended because vomiting a toxic substance may be more hazardous and dangerous coming up than when it was initially swallowed.
   2. **All households should have the phone number of poison control readily available to not delay treatment and interventions aimed at reducing accidental injury and death from poisoning.**
   3. Poison control should be called immediately for guidance before giving any home remedies or treatments.
   4. Gastric lavage is not routinely used for treatment because it may move the poison into the small intestine, where absorption will occur, and the amount of poison removed by gastric lavage is negligible.
   5. Childproof containers are primarily responsible for the marked reduction in accidental deaths of children by poisoning. Even though children should not be able to access these childproof containers, they should still be stored out of reach of children.
   6. **Activated charcoal is the most effective agent to prevent absorption of ingested poisons. It can be administered in the emergency department for serious poisonings after the medical provider has determined risks and benefits. The focus of emergency treatment is to stabilize body functions, prevent absorption, and encourage excretion of the poison.**
5. **TEST-TAKING TIP: The words *different level* are key words in the stem that direct attention to content; they should direct the test taker to the word *stairs* in option 1. The word *always* in option 4 is a specific determiner.**
   1. **Using the stairs during a fire is safe practice; elevators must be avoided because they may break down and trap a person.**

2. The safety pin is pulled only when the extinguisher is going to be used.
3. Often extinguishers are dragged along the floor en route to a fire because they are heavy; this is an acceptable practice.
4. Running should be avoided; it can cause injury and panic.

6. **TEST-TAKING TIP: Identify the priority for the client. Learning how to use the call bell system for immediate assistance is a necessary safety issue and takes priority over the other options according to Maslow's hierarchy of needs.**
   1. Although the client should be told the name of the nurse in charge of the unit, this is not the priority intervention.
   2. Identifying the potential date of discharge is the client's health-care provider's responsibility, not the nurse's.
   3. **Explaining the use of a call bell meets basic safety and security needs; the client must know how to signal the staff for help.**
   4. Although orienting the client about their daily schedule of physical and occupational therapy is important and should be done, it is not the priority among the options presented in the question.

7. **TEST-TAKING TIP: The word *most* in the stem sets a priority. The words *slightly confused* and *prevent disorientation at night* are key words in the stem that direct attention to content. Option 3 is the only option that states an action that is unique to nighttime. Options 1, 2, and 4 are equally plausible and are implemented regardless of the time of day or orientation of the client. The word *night* in the stem and in option 3 is a clang association.**
   1. Although checking on the client regularly is something the nurse should do, it will not prevent disorientation.
   2. The client has to be oriented enough to be aware of the presence of the call bell before it can be used.
   3. **A small night-light in the room provides enough light for visual cues for a slightly confused client, which should help prevent or limit disorientation when the client awakens at night.**
   4. The client may not remember the description of the environment on awakening and may become disoriented in the dark.

8. **TEST-TAKING TIP: The words *knees begin to buckle* are key words in the stem that direct attention to content. Options 1 and 4 are opposites.**
   1. Trying to hold up the client may injure the nurse and cause both the nurse and the client to fall.
   2. The client is already falling; walking the client to the closest chair is not an option.
   3. By the time help arrives, the client may already be on the floor; calling out can scare the client and others.
   4. **Lowering the client to the floor is the safest action; guiding the client to the floor helps to break the client's fall and minimize injury, particularly to the head.**

9. 1. Reporting the frayed wire is ineffective in preventing the risk of injury.
   2. Putting the cell phone charger in the client's closet does not preclude that it may be taken out and used again.
   3. **Removing the cell phone charger from the room and sending it home with a family member is the safest option; this action removes it from use.**
   4. Attempting to repair an electrical cord with nonconductive tape is unsafe; it should be repaired properly by a trained person.

10. **TEST-TAKING TIP: The word *best* in the stem sets a priority. The words *bed rest, prevent,* and *pressure ulcer* are key words in the stem that direct attention to content.**
    1. **An air mattress distributes body weight over a larger surface and reduces pressure over bony prominences.**
    2. Although bathing removes secretions and promotes clean skin, a daily bath can be drying, which can compromise skin integrity.
    3. Protein does not prevent pressure (decubitus) ulcers. Protein is the body's only source of nitrogen and is essential for building, repairing, or replacing body tissue. It requires a primary health-care provider's prescription.
    4. An indwelling urinary catheter should never be used to prevent a pressure (decubitus) ulcer; however, a catheter may be used to prevent contamination of a pressure (decubitus) ulcer after it is present in a client who is incontinent of urine. It requires a primary health-care provider's prescription.

11. **TEST-TAKING TIP: The word *most* in the stem sets a priority. Options 3 and 4 are opposites.**
    1. Isometric exercise involves contracting and relaxing a muscle without moving the

joint; this improves muscle tone but does not put joints through the full range of motion.

2. In active-assistive exercise, the client attempts active exercise and receives some support and assistance from the nurse. Active-assistive range-of-motion exercise does not provide as much isotonic exercise as does the exercise presented in another option.
3. **Active range-of-motion exercise is preferable because it is an isotonic exercise that causes muscle contraction and increases joint mobility, circulation, and muscle tone as the client actively moves joints through their full range of motion.**
4. Passive range-of-motion exercise occurs when a joint is moved by a source other than the muscles articulating to the joint. Passive range-of-motion exercise puts a joint through the full range and prevents contractures but does not increase muscle tone because the muscles are not contracted.

12. **TEST-TAKING TIP: The words *panic* and *scream* are key words in the stem that direct attention to content. Options 1 and 3 are opposites. Options 2, 3, and 4 deny the client's feelings of fear. Option 1 is client-centered.**

1. **Lowering the client onto the bed recognizes the cause of the fear and responds to the source.**
2. Continuing with the transfer ignores the client's concern. Telling a person to relax will not necessarily precipitate a relaxation response.
3. Continuing with the transfer denies the client's concerns. Also, it can intensify the client's fearful response.
4. Leaving the lift up in the air can intensify the client's fearful response.

13. **TEST-TAKING TIP: The words *prevent external rotation* are key words in the stem that direct attention to content.**

1. A bed cradle keeps linen off the feet and legs; it supports client comfort, but it does not prevent external rotation of the legs.
2. **A trochanter roll prevents the hip and leg from externally rotating by maintaining the leg in functional alignment. It is a cylindrical device placed against the lateral aspect of the thigh that extends from the hip to the knee.**
3. Elastic stockings do not prevent external rotation of the legs; they are used to increase venous return in the lower legs.
4. High-top sneakers prevent plantar flexion, not external rotation of the legs.

14. **TEST-TAKING TIP: The word *best* in the stem sets a priority. The words *afraid* and *reduce* are key words in the stem that direct attention to content. The words *falling* in the stem and *fall* in option 3 are clang associations; however, this option is a distractor. More often than not, an option with a clang is the correct answer, *but not always*. Eliminate option 3 because it clearly denies the client's feelings. Options 1 and 4 are client-centered.**

1. **Allowing the client to set the pace of the transfer supports the client's need to be in control; the client's concerns generally are reduced in proportion to an increase in control.**
2. Using a mechanical lift may contribute to feelings of dependence and loss of control. The question identifies a fearful client, not an immobile client.
3. Informing the client that a fall will not occur is false reassurance and denies the client's fears.
4. Waiting and thinking about the transfer can increase fear, not reduce fear; the client may decide never to get out of bed.

15. **TEST-TAKING TIP: The words *3 days earlier* and *left-sided hemiparesis* are key words in the stem that direct attention to content. The word *left* in the stem and in option 1 is a clang association. Options 3 and 4 are equally plausible. Options 2, 3, and 4 are similar because they contain the verbs *encourage*, *instruct*, and *tell*, all of which require verbal interaction with the client. Option 1 is unique because it is the only option in which the nurse is actually dressing the client. Option 2 denies the client's need for assistance during the acute phase of this illness.**

1. **The left upper extremity on the affected side should be dressed first to avoid unnecessary strain; the unaffected side generally has greater range of motion.**
2. It is unreasonable to expect self-sufficiency during the acute phase.
3. Zippers are difficult to close with one hand. Velcro closures may be more appropriate.

4. Buttons are difficult to close with one hand. Velcro closures may be more appropriate.

16. **TEST-TAKING TIP: Identifying the key words of *safety evaluation* in the stem direct attention to content.**

1. Advanced age is not a modifiable risk factor though older adults are not the only population at high risk of falling. The nurse should assess and encourage fall risk reduction behaviors.
2. **Postural dizziness may be a modifiable risk factor. The nurse must first identify contributing factors such as medications that may be causing dizziness. The nurse should educate the client to rise slowly and how to manage and monitor hypotension. The nurse can also consult with the client's provider to modify medications.**
3. **Lower body weakness is a modifiable risk factor. The client can be referred to physical therapy to enhance functional mobility and improve strength and balance.**
4. **Gait and balance issues are modifiable risk factors. The client can be referred to physical therapy to enhance functional mobility and improve strength and balance.**
5. **The nurse must assess the client's use of assistive devices and educate or refer to physical therapy for education on proper use.**
6. **Psychoactive medications can contribute to the risk of falling. The nurse must educate the client and family on the proper use of these medications and if necessary, consult with the provider on medication modifications.**

17. **TEST-TAKING TIP: The words *warm, dry heat* are key words in the stem that direct attention to content.**

1. Setting the pad at 110°F to 115°F is too high and may cause a burn. The aquathermia pad should be set at 98°F to 104°F for the application of warm, dry heat. This is warm enough to cause capillary dilation without resulting in a burn.
2. A covering or towel should be placed between the pad and the client to prevent burns.
3. **This prevents the rebound phenomenon. Heat produces maximum vasodilation in 20 to 30 minutes; if left on beyond this, the blood vessels constrict, limiting the dissipation of heat via blood circulation.**
4. Placing a moist liner between the pad and the cover of the pad provides for moist, not dry, heat.
5. Placing the pad under the client generally is not suggested by manufacturers because the heat cannot dissipate and may burn the client.

18. **TEST-TAKING TIP: The words *one-sided weakness* and *hemiparesis* are key words in the stem that direct attention to content.**

1. **Arranging the client's feet at shoulder-width apart widens the base of support, which increases stability.**
2. **Rubber-soled shoes provide traction between the client's feet and the floor, supporting safety.**
3. **Positioning the hands on the client's scapulae prevents pulling on the client's arms and shoulders, which can injure the structures of the client's upper extremities and shoulders.**
4. When transferring this client, the nurse should stand in front of, not next to, the client's affected side.
5. **When the client is transferred, pivoting avoids unnecessary movement while the client supports body weight on the unaffected leg.**

19. **TEST-TAKING TIP: The words *purpose* and *egg crate* are the key words in the stem that direct attention to content.**

1. The purpose of an egg crate pad is not to absorb moisture. When an egg crate pad becomes wet, it should be removed because moisture against the skin can contribute to skin breakdown.
2. The opposite may be true. Because egg crate pads are made of synthetic materials, they can promote, rather than limit, perspiration.
3. Although a client may feel more comfortable using an egg crate pad, this is not the purpose of an egg crate pad in the prevention of pressure ulcers.
4. Pillows and wedges, not an egg crate pad, are used to keep the body in functional alignment.
5. **Intermittent raised areas on the egg crate pad help to distribute body weight evenly over the entire body surface that is in contact with the pad.**

20. 1. This is a stage I pressure ulcer: nonblanchable erythema of intact skin.

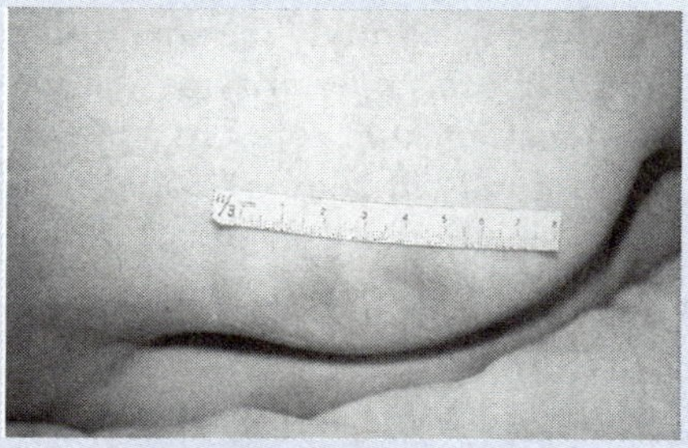

2. This is a stage II pressure ulcer: superficial partial-thickness loss involving the epidermis and dermis. It is a shallow crater and looks like an abrasion or blister.

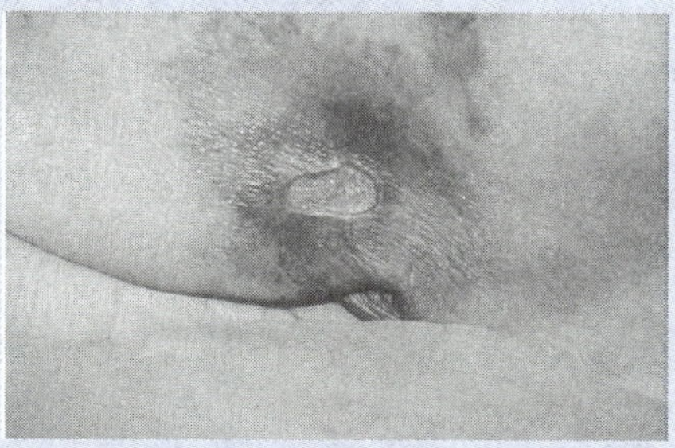

3. This is a stage III pressure ulcer: full-thickness involvement of subcutaneous tissue. It is a deep crater that may extend to but not through the fascia as well as include undermining of adjacent tissue.

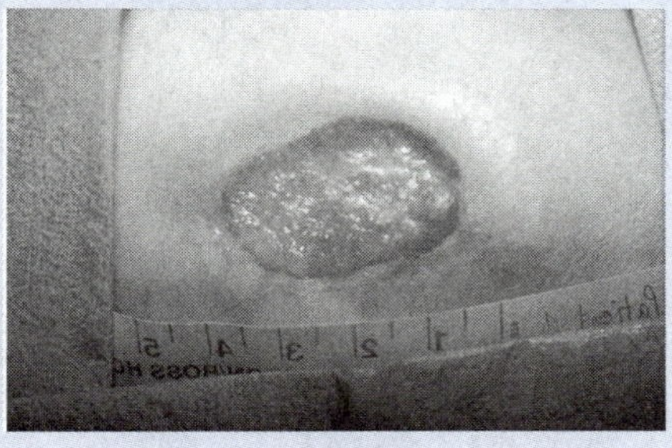

4. The question presents a stage IV pressure ulcer: full-thickness involvement that includes muscle, bone, or supporting structures. Also, it may include sinus tracts and undermining of adjacent tissue.

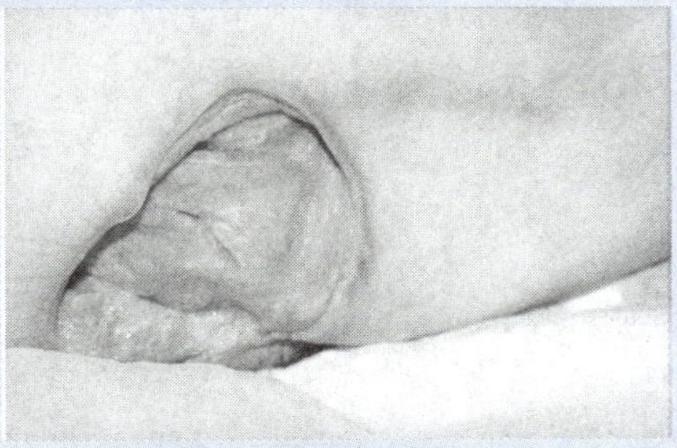

21. TEST-TAKING TIP: The word *avoided* in the stem indicates negative polarity. The words *pressure ulcer* and *sacral area* are key words in the stem that direct attention to content.

1. The semi-prone position avoids pressure on the sacral area; weight is on the anterior ilium, humerus, and clavicle.
2. The prone position avoids pressure on the sacral area; prone is lying on the abdomen.
3. **The contour position is a sitting position that places pressure on the sacral area; it should be avoided when trying to prevent a sacral pressure ulcer.**
4. **In the high Fowler position, most of the weight is placed on the sacral area; this causes sacral pressure.**
5. **In the dorsal recumbent (supine) position, the majority of the weight is on the sacral area; other areas affected include the back of the head, scapulae, and heels of the feet.**

22. 1. Although a bed alarm will alert the nurse when a client attempts to get out of bed, it will not prevent the client from pulling out catheters.

2. Zolpidem (Ambien®) is a sedative/hypnotic used for the induction of sleep. It is only 6 p.m., which is too early to administer the zolpidem. A sedative/hypnotic-antianxiety agent such as lorazepam (Ativan®) may be necessary to calm the client's behavior, which requires a prescription from a primary health-care provider. This behavior is associated with confusion and disorientation that increases during the late afternoon/evening in a client with a history of dementia (sundowning).

3. In this situation, a vest restraint will not fully protect the client from self-injury. A vest restraint will not prevent the client from pulling out the IV line or urinary retention catheter. Although a vest restraint may be used in an emergency without a prescription, the client must be evaluated by a primary health-care provider within a predetermined time (as per protocol/state legal requirements) to rescind or provide a written prescription for the restraint.

4. Assigning a staff member to provide constant reassurance, reorientation, and monitoring is the most effective and least restrictive intervention to provide for the client's safety. These interventions often will reassure and calm a client experiencing sundown syndrome (confusion and disorientation that increases during the afternoon and evening hours in a client with dementia). The primary health-care

provider should be notified of the client's change in behavior because the primary health-care provider may want to prescribe additional interventions.

23. **TEST-TAKING TIP:** The words *risk* and *impaired skin integrity* are key words in the stem that direct attention to content.
    1. Paralysis of the lower extremities (paraplegia) increases the risk of pressure injuries because the client may remain in the same position for prolonged periods. This can be prevented if a routine turning schedule is followed and skin care provided.
    2. A confused ambulatory client can walk and therefore relieve pressure on bony prominences.
    3. A colostomy does not increase the risk of pressure injuries. However, it may increase the risk of excoriation around the stoma if special skin care is not performed.
    4. As long as a person can move, positioning can be changed to relieve pressure. Though the client can ambulate, they are still at risk for maceration and excoriation due to incontinence.
    5. Clients with imbalanced nutritional states are at risk for impaired skin integrity. Clients with severe protein depletion and an albumin level of less than 2.5 g/dL, clients with wound exudates because the exudate generates protein loss, clients with obesity, and clients with dehydration are all at increased risk for impaired skin integrity.
    6. As long as a client on bed rest can move, pressure can be relieved by shifting the body weight or changing positions.

24. 1. Pain should be managed around the clock for terminally ill clients rather than waiting until the pain may be unbearable and difficult to relieve.
    2. Pain should be continually assessed and treated. Knowing what alleviates it can help the nurse develop the plan of care and may encourage mobility.
    3. Assessing the effectiveness of pain relief measures frequently ensures that the client is on a correct and adequate medication and complementary therapy regimen.
    4. Minimizing irritants is part of a pain relief care plan for clients. Irritants can cause or intensify pain.
    5. Complementary and alternative therapies such as guided imagery, massage, and relaxation techniques can minimize pain.
    6. Treating pain and administering medications in a timely manner and on a regular basis may provide consistent and manageable relief to a client. Terminally ill clients should never have pain relief measures delayed or denied.

25. When a client is in the left lateral position, the site over the left greater trochanter is most vulnerable to pressure because it bears the most body weight. Also, there is little body tissue between the bone and the epidermis. Additional sites at risk include the side of the head (parietal and temporal bones), ear, shoulder (acromial process), knee (medial and lateral condyles), and malleolus (medial and lateral).

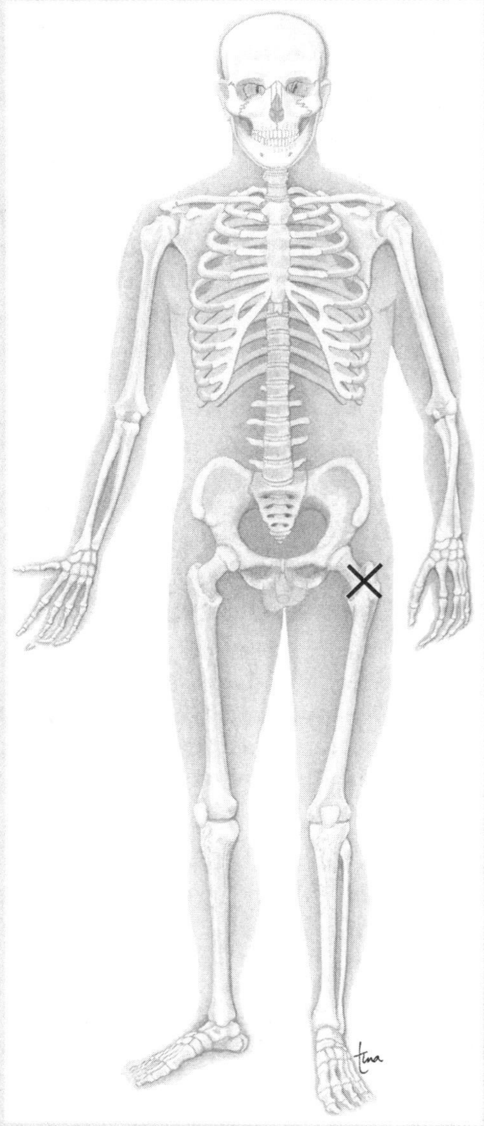

26. 1. A "hypoallergenic" label does not mean a product is latex free. A person must examine packaging or tags to ensure that the product is free of latex.

2. Injectable epinephrine, such as an EpiPen®, is used to manage severe allergic reactions to latex, insect bites, or foods. Its therapeutic effects are bronchodilation and maintenance of heart rate and blood pressure.

3. Spandex (generic name) was developed in 1959 by the DuPont Company and was trademarked as Lycra. Spandex fibers are rubber-free fibers that are alternatives to latex and can be worn by a person with a latex allergy. Spandex can stretch; can return to its original shape; is stronger than latex rubber fibers; is comfortable, soft, smooth, and supple; is resistant to perspiration, lotions, and body oils; blends with other fabrics; and does not pill or create static. Most important, it does not contain latex protein allergens.

4. Latex rubber is used in the manufacture of many types of clothing to give them stretch, comfort, and freedom of movement. It is used in clothing such as leotards, athletic wear, bodysuits, bathing suits, socks, stockings, and elastic waistbands. Latex contains 57 allergenic proteins, and more than 200 different chemicals used during its manufacture are known allergens. For this reason, a person with a latex allergy must examine the tags of clothing to ensure that items do not contain latex.

5. These three houseplants contain latex protein allergens and should be removed from the home of a person with a latex allergy.

27. **3. This frees the right hand for the next step in the procedure.**

2. Moving the buttocks toward the edge of the chair allows room for the right knee to bend so that the unaffected right foot and leg are under the center of the body's mass when standing.

4. Pushing off the right arm of the chair with the right hand and extending the elbow use an upper extremity to assist the client to a standing position.

5. Extending the left leg and keeping the right foot flat on the floor while elevating the body uses the unaffected lower extremity to assist the client to a standing position. Once standing, the client must ensure that balance is maintained. The unaffected leg can be supported against the edge of the chair while holding the hand bars of the crutches.

1. Transferring the crutches to under the arms prepares a person for crutch walking.

28. **TEST-TAKING TIP: The words *lateral* and *functional alignment* are key words in the stem that direct attention to content.**

1. Putting a pillow under the upper leg positions the upper leg and hip in functional alignment and reduces stress and strain on the hip joint.

2. A pillow under the waist is used when a client is positioned in the supine, not the lateral, position.

3. Supporting the upper arm on a pillow helps to keep the shoulder in functional alignment.

4. Keeping the lower hip and knee extended promotes functional alignment.

5. A pillow behind the back will help maintain the client in the lateral position.

29. 1. This is a two-half hitch knot. This knot cannot be released easily and should not be used to secure a restraint strap to a bed frame.

2. This is a quick-release slip knot. The knot will immediately release when the loose end of the strap is pulled. This is the appropriate knot to secure a restraint strap to a bed frame because it permits quick release in an emergency.

3. This is a clove hitch knot. This knot cannot be released easily and should not be used to secure a restraint strap to a bed frame.

4. This is a bowline knot. This knot cannot be released easily and should not be used to secure a restraint strap to a bed frame.

30. **The client fell out of bed but did not sustain an injury. Therefore, the section titled "Fall" is the most appropriate section to check in the Occurrence Category.**

Unusual Occurrence Report

Date of Event: __________ **Time of Event:** __________ **Department:** ____________________

Client Last Name:	**First Name:**	**MI:**
Client #:	**Attending Physician:**	
Visitor Last Name:	**First Name:**	**Phone #:**
Employee Name:	**Dept:**	
Physician Name:	**Specialty:**	

Occurrence Category (Check most appropriate)

☐ Agency nurse-related	☐ AMA	☐ Delay in treatment
☐ Diet-related	☐ HIPAA compliance	☐ Loss of personal property
☐ Medication-related	☐ Narcotics-related	☐ Order not executed
☐ Client injury	☐ Peer-review related	☐ Restraint-related
☐ Staff injury	☐ Supplies/Equipment	☐ Visitor injury
☑ Fall		
☐ Other (please explain):		

Description of Occurrence:

A client was medicated with an opioid. The client's bedside rail was left in the down position. The client was found on the floor. The client was examined by the rapid response team. No injury was identified as a result of the fall. The client was returned to bed.

Contributing Factors (Check all that apply)

☐ Individual:	☐ System:
Knowledge, skills, and/or experience (please list): ☐ Unclear ☐ Incomplete	Policies/procedures not in place (please list): ☐ Unclear ☐ Outdated
Standard of care or practice (please list): ☐ Non-adherence	Environmental: ☐ Staffing ☐ Client acuity ☐ Congestion
Documentation (please list): ☐ Incomplete ☐ Inadequate	Communications and work flow: ☐ Intradepartmental ☐ Interdepartmental
	☐ Equipment failure
Other (please explain):	

Submitted by:	**Dept:**	**Date:**

31. 1. The purpose of restraints is not to support joints.

2. Restraints can increase agitation; when used on a client who is severely agitated, they can cause injury.

3. Immobilization is not the purpose of restraints. Restraints should be snug, yet loose enough for some movement.

4. The primary reason for the use of restraints is to prevent client injury;

restraints are used only as a last resort.

5. **In an emergency, restraints can be used when a client's activity threatens the safety of others.**

32. 1. **Anytime a person falls in a facility, even if not injured, an incident report must be completed. Documentation of the possible causes of falls collectively may help to identify trends and initiate potential corrective action.**
2. A nurse who refuses to float to another unit is a management problem that is handled by a nurse manager. It does not require the initiation of an incident report.
3. **When a visitor faints, an incident report must be initiated. Collectively, this information may help to identify trends and initiate potential corrective action.**
4. An angry provider who has been awakened to examine a client does not require the completion of an incident report. If the individual's anger impinges on the ability to provide safe and effective client care, the nurse should step in as a client advocate and immediately report the event to the nursing supervisor. The nursing supervisor would then intervene, which may include an incident report if anyone was harmed. However, this scenario does not indicate that anyone was harmed or client care was jeopardized.
5. **The application of medication is outside the job description of an unlicensed assistive personnel (UAP). A violation of standards of nursing practice requires the initiation of an incident report. In some limited settings, a UAP may be trained and certified to administer medications that do not require an assessment of the client. Assessment of the client before and after a medication is administered is the function of the nurse, who has the educational preparation to determine the significance of the client's status.**

33. 1. This illustration indicates flexion of the toes. Flexion of the toes occurs when the joints of the toes are curled downward. Extension of the toes occurs when the toes are straightened.
2. **This illustration indicates flexion and extension of the ankle. Flexion of the ankle occurs when the toes of the foot are pointed upward toward the head. Extension of the ankle occurs when the toes are pointed downward, away from the head.**
3. This illustration indicates eversion and inversion of the foot. Eversion of the foot occurs when the sole of the foot is turned outward (laterally). Inversion of the foot occurs when the sole of the foot is turned inward (medially).
4. This illustration indicates abduction of the toes. Abduction of the toes occurs when the toes are moved out to the side and spread apart. Adduction of the toes occurs when the toes are moved toward each other and brought together.

34. **TEST-TAKING TIP: *Increase*, *restraints*, and *education* are all key words that direct attention to content.**
1. The adverse health consequences from restraint use increase the need for additional staff because the clients' conditions can deteriorate rapidly in facilities where restraints are routinely employed.
2. Restraint use increases incontinence, depression, and delirium, especially in older adults. Clients with dementia have the highest risk of being restrained.
3. Physical restraints increase the potential for serious injuries due to a fall because they can worsen agitation and confusion.
4. Medications used to control behavior that are not part of a client's normal medication regimen can be considered a chemical restraint.
5. **Federal and state mandates and The Joint Commission recommend restraints be used only as a last resort and that in all settings, the primary responsibility is to protect and promote client rights and can only be used to protect the client, staff, or others. Restraints must be discontinued at the earliest possible time.**
6. **Restraint use may cause skin breakdown and contractures, anxiety, aspiration, respiratory distress, and even death. Clients must be monitored frequently to prevent serious injury.**

35. **Answer: 3 mL**
Solve the problem using the formula for ratio and proportion.

$$\frac{\text{Desire}}{\text{Have}} \quad \frac{0.5 \text{ mg}}{1 \text{ mg}} = \frac{x \text{ ml}}{1 \text{ mL}}$$

$$10x = 15$$

$$x = 15 \div 10$$

$$x = 1.5 \text{ mL for each dose}$$

$$\text{Multiply } 1.5 \times 2 = 3 \text{ mL over 24 hours.}$$

CLINICAL JUDGMENT CASE STUDY ANSWERS AND RATIONALES

36. 1. For client-centered care, the nurse will need to ask subjective and objective questions about the client's musculoskeletal system, but there is another question that is the most important.

2. These are questions on the musculoskeletal system that the nurse will need to ask the client, but there is another question that is the priority.

3. Based on the client's reported medical history of two deep vein thromboses, increased use of ibuprofen exceeding the recommended daily dose of 3200 mg, reports of tinnitus, use of warfarin, and use of furosemide, this is the priority question to ask the client. The client may be overdosing on ibuprofen, placing the client at increased risk for bleeding or stomach or intestinal perforation. Additionally, the use of furosemide with higher doses of ibuprofen can cause kidney failure. Tinnitus is a side effect of ibuprofen overdose. The nurse should also question why the client takes omeprazole as heartburn is often reported with too much ibuprofen use.

4. Clients should be asked about their smoking and drinking habits every time they visit a medical provider to educate them on the relationship between these habits and poor health outcomes, though this is not the priority question.

37. 1. There is no definitive test for diagnosis of autoimmune diseases. They are usually diagnosed based on symptoms, blood tests, and sometimes tissue biopsies. The range-of-motion exercises do not indicate an undiagnosed autoimmune disease.

2. Diagnosis of degenerative changes due to aging is based on symptoms, x-rays, a physical examination, and a thorough health history. Though range-of-motion exercises can contribute to the diagnosis, the healthcare providers will need more information.

3. Based on the client's reported symptoms, pain during the range-of-motion exercises, and the client's reported work environment, the nurse may develop a plan of care based on overuse or repetitive motions. The client reports continual lifting of heavy boxes daily, indicating overuse.

4. There is nothing in the medical history of assessment of the client to indicate an episode of acute gout.

38. 1. Urea nitrogen is a normal waste product in the blood that comes from the breakdown of protein from food and metabolism. It is normally removed from the blood by the kidneys, but when kidney function slows down, the BUN level rises. Creatinine is a waste product in the blood that comes from muscle activity. It is removed from the blood by the kidneys, but if kidney function slows down, the creatinine level rises. Furosemide and overuse of ibuprofen can both impact kidney function.

2. T_3 (triiodothyronine) and T_4 (thyroxine) are thyroid tests. There is no indication that this client needs thyroid function testing.

3. Because the client is on warfarin and may potentially have an NSAID-induced ulcer, the client's INR level should be checked. The client is at high risk of bleeding due to warfarin use combined with overuse of ibuprofen. Checking the INR level identifies if the blood is clotting normally. The higher the INR, the greater the risk of bleeding.

4. Platelet testing is needed because of the client's increased risk of bleeding due to warfarin use and from taking more than the recommended dosage of ibuprofen. Cortisol is not indicated for this client. Cortisol tests for adrenal function, and there is no indication to test for adrenal abnormalities with this client.

5. Lipase and amylase are digestive enzymes that should be checked when suspicious of a peptic ulcer. If there is a perforation, lipase and amylase may spill from the digestive tract into circulation.

6. Potassium should always be checked in clients taking loop diuretics such as furosemide. These medications remove potassium through the loop of Henle and can cause hypokalemia.

39. 1. Standing with the feet apart creates good posture. Standing with the feet too close together over extended periods of time places abnormal stress on the spine that can lead to degeneration of spinal structures.

2. Holding loads close to the body minimizes the effect of their weight.
3. Keeping the knees bent when lifting makes the legs work harder and reduces the stress on the back.
4. **Moving the torso from the shoulder to the hips as one solid unit helps to prevent twisting injuries.**
5. **Tightening the abdominal muscles when lifting helps to support movement and maintain balance.**

40.

Intervention	Indicated	Not Indicated	Contraindicated
Educate the client that aspirin is a better choice than ibuprofen			X
Encourage the client to eat small amounts of food every hour		X	
Encourage physical and psychosocial lifestyle modifications	X		
Educate the client to eat a diet rich in creams and milk			X
Encourage bed rest when the client is not at work			X
Sleep in a semi-Fowler's position		X	

1. **Contraindicated: Aspirin is an anticoagulant and should be avoided when a client is also taking warfarin.**
2. **Not indicated: Encourage the client to eat regularly spaced meals with dietary modifications such as avoiding acid-inducing foods.**
3. **Indicated: Reducing environmental stress includes both physical and psychosocial modifications.**
4. **Contraindicated: Diets rich in creams and milk, as well as alcohol, coffee, tea, and other caffeinated beverages, should be avoided if a nonsteroidal antiinflammatory drug (NSAID)–induced ulcer is suspected.**
5. **Contraindicated: Reassure clients that musculoskeletal pain is normal but can have an impact on functioning and work. Simple exercises and remaining as active as possible can minimize pain. Clients should remain as active as possible as bed rest can further contribute to the pain.**
6. **Not indicated: Sleeping position should be dependent on what is comfortable for the client. If the client is having nighttime heartburn, a semi-Fowler's position may help, but this is not essential.**

41.

Assessment Finding	Improved	No Change	Declined
Intestinal pain			X
Ongoing tinnitus			X
Steady gait	X		
No pain after eating			X
Weight loss of 10 lb.			X

1. Reports of intestinal pain may indicate further development of an NSAID-induced peptic ulcer. Stomach acid may make the pain from a peptic ulcer worse.
2. Ongoing tinnitus is a symptom of overuse/overdose of ibuprofen. The client initially reported intermittent tinnitus so ongoing tinnitus may indicate a worsening of the side effects of taking too much ibuprofen.
3. A steady gait is an improved symptom of the client's musculoskeletal pain.
4. Pain that dissipates after eating is often a symptom of peptic ulcer disease. Eating certain foods may buffer the stomach acid temporarily, but once the food is digested, the pain may come back.
5. Stomach pain may cause a decrease in appetite. A weight loss of 10 pounds within 1 month without trying to lose weight is a warning sign that should not be ignored.

MEETING CLIENTS' MICROBIOLOGICAL SAFETY NEEDS

This section includes questions on concepts and principles related to topics such as medical asepsis, surgical asepsis, types of isolation, and the chain of infection. Particular emphasis is placed on nursing actions that protect the nurse and the client from microorganisms, including questions about hand hygiene and disposal of contaminated equipment and linens. The questions also address risk factors for infection, common clinical findings related to infection, and client education about infection control practices.

QUESTIONS

1. The nurse is teaching a client about ways to prevent infection. Which **best** increases a client's defense against microorganisms?
1. Bathing daily
2. Maintaining intact skin
3. Changing bed linens daily
4. Using an antiseptic mouthwash

TEST-TAKING TIP: Identify the word in the stem that sets a priority. Identify the word in the stem that directs attention to content.

2. The nurse delegates care of an obese client with a fungal infection in the skin folds to the unlicensed assistive personnel (UAP). Which is the priority intervention when caring for this client?
1. Thoroughly drying the client's skin folds
2. Applying moisturizer to the client's skin
3. Providing a daily bath for the client
4. Keeping the client's room cool

3. The nurse is assessing a client's wound. Which characteristic of the wound's exudate indicates to the nurse that the wound may be infected?
1. Serosanguineous
2. Sanguineous
3. Purulent
4. Serous

TEST-TAKING TIP: Identify the unique option.

4. A client who has a respiratory infection and a mild productive cough is admitted to the hospital for IV antibiotic therapy. The primary health-care provider orders droplet precautions. The nurse should **first:**
1. don a gown, gloves, and face shield when entering the client's room.
2. wear a particulate filter mask when providing direct client care.
3. assign the client to an airborne infection isolation room.
4. place a surgical mask on the client during transport.

TEST-TAKING TIP: Identify the words in the stem that direct attention to content.

5. The nurse educator working in the acquired immunodeficiency syndrome (AIDS) specialty clinic is preparing training for nurses on caring for AIDS clients when hospitalized. When developing the training, which complications does the nurse know these clients are at risk for? **Select all that apply.**
1. Secondary pneumonias
2. Secondary cancers
3. Pressure injuries
4. Disorientation
5. Liver disease
6. Thyroiditis

TEST-TAKING TIP: Identify the key word in the stem that directs attention to content.

6. The nurse is admitting a client with a postsurgical site infection. Which is the priority assessment for this client?
   1. Obtain vital signs to establish a baseline
   2. Evaluate the client's nutritional status
   3. Encourage early ambulation
   4. Treat the client's pain

TEST-TAKING TIP: Identify the word in the stem that sets a priority. Identify the key word in the stem that directs attention to content.

7. The infection control nurse is teaching a group of nursing students about the risks for infection in hospitalized or ill clients. The nurse knows that the susceptibility of the host for an infectious agent depends on what? **Select all that apply.**
   1. The pH levels of the gastrointestinal and genitourinary tracts
   2. The number of the client's white blood cells
   3. Integrity of skin and mucous membranes
   4. Fatigue, nutrition, and general health
   5. Age, sex, race, and heredity
   6. Stress level

TEST-TAKING TIP: Identify equally plausible options.

8. An adult man is admitted to the hospital with a medical diagnosis of fever of unknown origin. Which laboratory result should the nurse report to the primary health-care provider?
   1. White blood cell count of 20,000 cells/mcL
   2. Urine specific gravity of 1.020
   3. Hemoglobin of 14.5 g/dL
   4. Hematocrit of 42%

9. The nurse observes the unlicensed assistive personnel (UAP) violating aseptic technique when removing personal protective equipment. Which did the UAP do that was incorrect?
   1. Remove the respirator inside the doorway to the client's room
   2. Remove goggles by holding the headband and pulling away from the face
   3. Touches inside of gown, pulls away from the body, and turns inside out for disposal
   4. Grasp outside of glove with opposite gloved hand turning inside out when pulling off

TEST-TAKING TIP: Identify words in the stem that indicate negative polarity.

10. When removing protective gloves that were worn to start an IV infusion, a female nurse notices that there is a small amount of the client's blood on two sections of her forearm. Which should the nurse do **first?**
    1. Wash blood-exposed areas with warm water and soap
    2. Clean soiled areas with gauze moistened with alcohol
    3. Flush from the elbow to the fingers with hot water
    4. Soak the forearm in a dilute bleach solution

TEST-TAKING TIP: Identify the word in the stem that sets a priority. Identify the option with a clang association.

11. Blood leaked onto the client's bed linens when the nurse started a new IV, so the nurse is changing the soiled linens. Which is correct when changing soiled bed linens? **Select all that apply.**
    1. Bagging and placing the linens in the soiled linen hamper
    2. Placing the linens in an infectious waste bag for disposal
    3. Holding the soiled linens away from the body
    4. Placing the soiled linens in the laundry chute
    5. Placing the linens on the overbed table
    6. Placing the linens on a chair

TEST-TAKING TIP: Identify the clang association. Identify equally plausible options.

12. In which environment do bacteria rapidly multiply?
   1. Hot
   2. Cool
   3. Cold
   4. Warm

   TEST-TAKING TIP: Identify opposites in options.

13. Linens that are still clean are often reused by the same client. Which article of linen is **least** likely to be reused by the nurse when making the bed?
   1. Top sheet
   2. Bedspread
   3. Pillowcase
   4. Cotton blanket

   TEST-TAKING TIP: Identify the word in the stem that indicates negative polarity. Identify the unique option.

14. A client on contact precautions needs a blood pressure reading taken every shift. Which practical intervention by the nurse will keep the sphygmomanometer from spreading microorganisms?
   1. Placing it in a protective bag
   2. Keeping it in the client's room
   3. Soaking it in a germicidal solution
   4. Storing it in the dirty utility room

   TEST-TAKING TIP: Identify the key word in the stem that directs attention to content.

15. Which has the **highest** impact on limiting the spread of microorganisms?
   1. Disposable equipment
   2. Double-bagging
   3. Wearing gloves
   4. Hand hygiene

   TEST-TAKING TIP: Identify the word in the stem that sets a priority.

16. The nurse is cleaning an emesis basin containing purulent material. The nurse should **first:**
   1. spray the basin with a disinfectant.
   2. wash the basin with hot, soapy water.
   3. rinse the basin with cold running water.
   4. clean the basin with an antiseptic agent.

   TEST-TAKING TIP: Identify the word in the stem that sets a priority.

17. The client with methicillin-resistant *Staphylococcus aureus* (MRSA) in an open wound is placed in precautions. Which interventions are appropriate for the nurse when caring for this client? **Select all that apply.**
   1. _____ Do not wash hands before client contact
   2. _____ Wear shoe covers for client care
   3. _____ Wash hands after client contact
   4. _____ Wear goggles for client care
   5. _____ Wear a gown for client care
   6. _____ Wear gloves for client care

   TEST-TAKING TIP: Identify the key words in the stem that direct attention to content. Identify the clang association. Identify the unique option.

18. One dose of penicillin 2.4 million units IM is prescribed for a client with an infection. The medication comes in the form of a powder with 5 million units per vial and instructions for reconstitution. The directions state that 3.2 mL of sterile diluent should be added to yield 3.5 mL of solution. How many milliliters should the nurse administer? **Record your answer using one decimal place.**

Answer: ___________ **mL**

19. The nurse is observing a student nursing assistant practice activities associated with exiting the room of a client on contact isolation. Which photograph indicates that further teaching is necessary?

1.
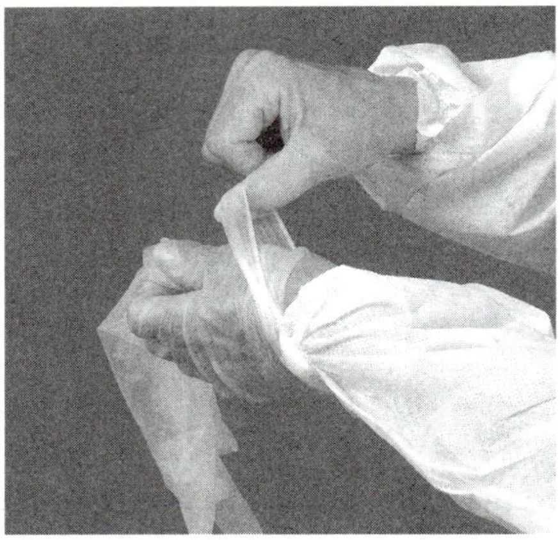

2.
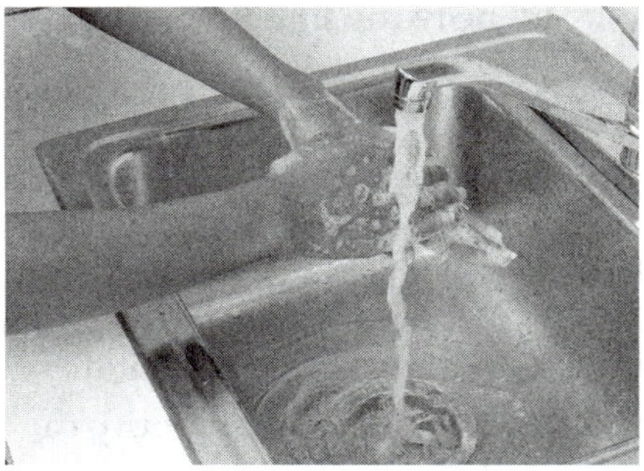

3.
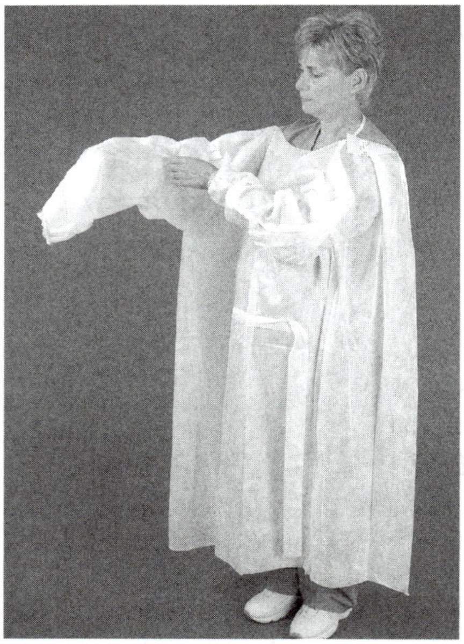

4.
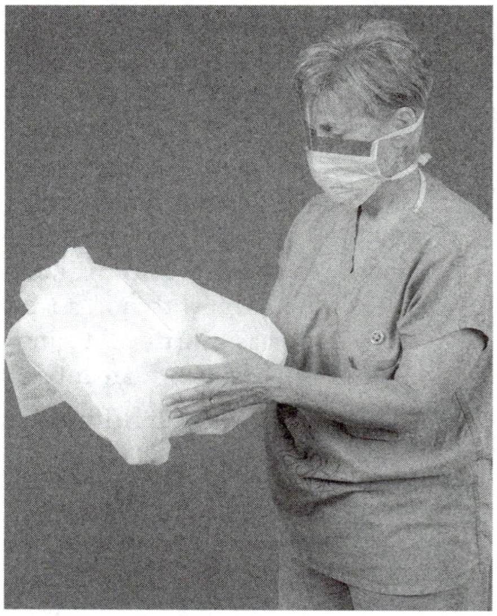

20. Which action breaks the chain of infection from a portal of exit from a reservoir? **Select all that apply.**

1. _____ Washing the hands
2. _____ Disposing of soiled linen
3. _____ Disinfecting used equipment
4. _____ Covering the mouth when coughing
5. _____ Swiping the skin with alcohol before administering an injection

TEST-TAKING TIP: Identify key words in the stem that direct attention to content.

21. Airborne precautions are ordered for a client with the diagnosis of tuberculosis. Which nursing action is specific to caring for a client on airborne precautions? **Select all that apply.**

1. _____ Keeping the client's door closed
2. _____ Donning a gown when administering medications
3. _____ Wearing disposable gloves when delivering a meal
4. _____ Wearing a high-efficiency particulate air filter respirator
5. _____ Instructing the client to wear a mask when receiving care

TEST-TAKING TIP: Identify key words in the stem that direct attention to content.

22. The nurse must change a client's sterile dressing. Place the following steps in the order in which they should be performed.

1. Don the first glove with the fingers held downward toward the floor.
2. Open the outer glove package, grasp the inner package, and lay it on a waist-high, clean surface.
3. Interlock the fingers of both hands to ensure that the gloves and their fingers are securely in place.
4. Grasp the inside cuff of the glove of the dominant hand with the thumb and first two fingers of the nondominant hand.
5. Pick up the glove for the nondominant hand from the outside of the cuff with the gloved dominant hand and insert the nondominant hand.

Answer: ____________

23. The charge nurse is rounding on clients on the medical-surgical unit and identifies the following sources of infection. Which situation requires the nurse to intervene to reduce the risk of infection? **Select all that apply.**

1. _____ IV tubing used for normal saline that was changed 2 days ago
2. _____ A urinal with urine inside hanging from the side rail of the client's bed
3. _____ Blood transfusion tubing hung 36 hours ago that currently has blood infusing
4. _____ A urinary catheter collection bag containing 1500 mL of urine sitting on the floor
5. _____ An opened pudding container on the bedside table being saved for an afternoon snack

TEST-TAKING TIP: Identify the words in the stem that indicate negative polarity.

24. Postoperatively, a client has an order for cleansing of an incision with normal saline and application of a dry sterile dressing. Which stroke should the nurse perform **first** when cleansing the wound?

1. A
2. B
3. C

TEST-TAKING TIP: Identify the word in the stem that sets a priority.

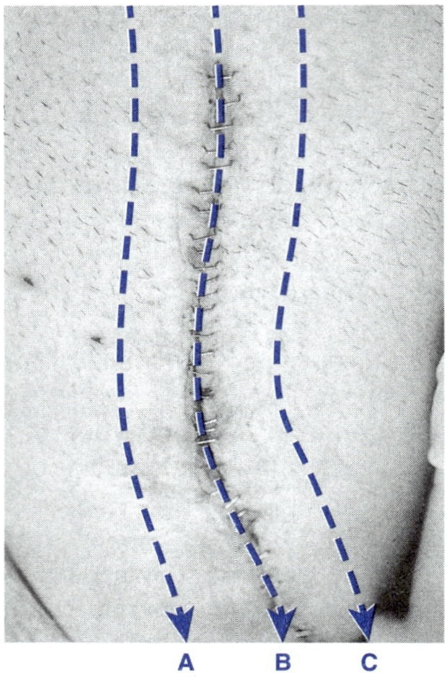

25. A 75-year-old man is transferred from a nursing home to the emergency department of the hospital. Which type of isolation precautions should the nurse initiate after reviewing the transfer form supplied by the nursing home and the results of the initial physical assessment in the hospital?

1. Droplet
2. Contact
3. Airborne
4. Protective

CLIENT'S CLINICAL RECORD

Laboratory Results
RBC: 4.8 cells/mcL
WBC: 18,000 cells/mcL
Hb: 16 g/dL
Hct: 45%

Client History
MRSA positive
Type 1 diabetes
Brain attack with residual left hemiparesis

Physical Assessment
Full-thickness skin loss including subcutaneous tissue in the sacral area; area is 3 x 4 cm with a small amount of yellow drainage. Vital signs: temperature, 100°F (oral); pulse, 92 beats per minute; respirations, 22 breaths per minute. Incontinent of urine and feces.

26. A client with a vertical abdominal wound that is healing by secondary intention has a prescription for the wound to be irrigated with 0.9% sodium chloride twice a day. The nurse places the client in the low Fowler position. Indicate with an arrow where the nurse should start the stream of solution when irrigating the client's wound.

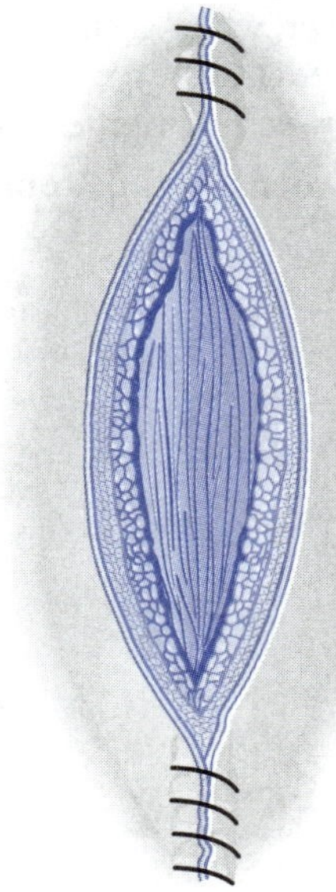

27. A client with gonorrhea is to receive ceftriaxone 250 mg IM STAT. The vial contains 1 gram of ceftriaxone with instructions to add 3.5 mL of diluent to yield 4 mL of solution. How much solution of ceftriaxone should the nurse prepare for administering the prescribed dose? **Record your answer using a whole number.**

Answer: ___________ mL

28. The nurse is teaching inexperienced staff about hand hygiene opportunities to prevent transmission of potentially harmful organisms to clients. Which opportunity should the nurse include in the teaching? **Select all that apply.**

1. _____ After touching a client
2. _____ Before touching a client
3. _____ After a body fluid exposure risk
4. _____ After touching client surroundings
5. _____ Before a clean or aseptic procedure
6. _____ Before touching client surroundings

TEST-TAKING TIP: Identify the options with clang associations.

29. The nurse is caring for several patients on a medical-surgical unit. When planning care for these clients, the nurse knows which client is at high risk for developing a health-care–acquired infection? **Select all that apply.**

1. _____ 58-year-old client who has smoked three packs of cigarettes daily for 40 years
2. _____ 27-year-old IV drug user admitted with a white blood cell count of 7500/mm^3
3. _____ 63-year-old client who has had an indwelling urinary catheter for 4 days
4. _____ 54-year-old client admitted receiving radioactive iodine treatment
5. _____ 42-year-old client receiving medications through a central line
6. _____ 84-year-old client admitted with heart dysrhythmias

TEST-TAKING TIP: Identify the word in the stem that sets a priority. Identify the obscure clang association.

30. The nurse is caring for a client who is on contact precautions because of an infected wound. Which nursing action is appropriate when caring for this client? **Select all that apply.**
1. _____ Maintaining the client in a private room
2. _____ Donning goggles when irrigating the wound
3. _____ Wearing a disposable gown when giving care
4. _____ Washing the hands immediately after removing soiled gloves
5. _____ Dedicating certain client-care equipment to be kept in the room

TEST-TAKING TIP: Identify key words in the stem that direct attention to content.

ING CLIENTS' MICROBIOLOGICAL SAFETY NEEDS
SWERS AND RATIONALES

1. **TEST-TAKING TIP: The word *best* in the stem sets a priority. The word *increases* in the stem directs attention to content.**
   1. Bathing daily removes sebum from the skin. Sebum lubricates the skin and prevents drying and skin tears. Tears in the skin provide a portal of entry for microorganisms.
   2. **The skin is a barrier to pathogens; if pierced or broken, it serves as a portal of entry for microorganisms.**
   3. Although changing bed linens daily may reduce the number of microorganisms present, it does not best protect the client from microorganisms.
   4. Although using an antiseptic mouthwash may reduce the number of microorganisms present, it does not best protect the client from microorganisms.

2. 1. **Fungi multiply rapidly in places where moisture content is high, such as in skin folds. Careful drying of skin folds, especially under the breasts and arms, between the toes, and in the perineal area, helps prevent the development of fungal infections.**
   2. This is not the priority intervention. Moisturizers soften the skin; they do not protect the skin from fungal infections.
   3. Although bathing daily is helpful in preventing infection, it is not the priority intervention or the best way to prevent the growth of fungi.
   4. A cool room may reduce perspiration; however, it is not the best way to prevent the growth of fungi.

3. **TEST-TAKING TIP: Option 3 is unique because it begins with the letter "P." Options 1, 2, and 4 all begin with the letter "S."**
   1. Serosanguineous exudate consists of clear and blood-tinged drainage, as seen in healing surgical incisions.
   2. Sanguineous exudate indicates damage to capillaries that allows the escape of red blood cells from plasma.
   3. **Purulent exudate contains materials such as dead and living bacteria and dead tissue; it indicates the possibility of an infection.**
   4. Serous exudate is watery in appearance, is composed of mainly serum, and does not indicate an infection.

4. **TEST-TAKING TIP: The words *droplet precautions* in the stem direct attention to content.**
   1. Wearing a gown, gloves, and face shield is necessary only when providing direct care for a client on droplet precautions when the client has substantial respiratory secretions or when splashing of body fluids is anticipated.
   2. A particulate filter mask (N95 respirator) is worn when the client is on airborne precautions, not droplet precautions. Airborne precautions are based on the concept that droplet nuclei smaller than 5 mcg can remain suspended in the air and travel via air currents.
   3. An airborne infection isolation room (AIIR) with the door closed and with negative pressure air flow of 6 to 12 air exchanges per hour via HEPA filtration or discharge to outside air is necessary when a client is on airborne precautions, not droplet precautions.
   4. **Droplet precautions are ordered according to the concept that microorganisms larger than 5 mcg within 3 feet of the client can be transmitted to others through direct contact with the client or via contaminated objects. Therefore, clients must wear a surgical mask when transported outside their rooms. Personal protective equipment does not have to be worn by the nurse when the nurse is farther than 3 feet from the client or when not touching anything in the client's room.**

5. **TEST-TAKING TIPS: The words *hospitalized* and *complications* are key words in the stem that direct attention to content. The correct answers must address something that is common to all clients with AIDS. HIV damages the immune system, making it difficult to fight infections.**
   1. **Pneumocystis pneumonia is a fungal infection caused by AIDS and is the most common cause of pneumonia in people with AIDS.**
   2. **Clients with AIDS are at risk for developing lymphoma, a cancer in the white blood cells and Kaposi's sarcoma, a tumor in the walls of blood vessels that can also affect the digestive tract and the lungs.**

3. Having AIDS does not necessarily place the client at risk for pressure injuries. These types of skin complications usually occur in clients who are bedbound or cachectic.
4. Not all clients who have AIDS have central nervous system involvement that can cause cognitive impairments such as disorientation.
5. **Liver disease is a complication of AIDS, especially in clients with hepatitis B or C.**
6. Thyroiditis is the swelling of the thyroid gland usually caused by either high or low levels of thyroid hormones in the blood. Though some AIDS clients may have thyroid dysfunction, it is typically not a complication associated with AIDS.

6. **TEST-TAKING TIP: The words *postsurgical site infection* are key words in the stem that set a priority.**
   1. **Establishing baseline vitals helps the nurse identify any physiological changes. Fever is the most common response of the hypothalamus (thermoregulatory center) to pyrogens that are released when phagocytic cells respond to the presence of pathogens. Blood pressure, pulse, and respiration also help identify any rapidly changing hemodynamic stability of the client.**
   2. Nutritional status contributes to a client's wound healing after surgery, but another option is priority.
   3. Early ambulation after surgery reduces complications and promotes oxygen and blood flow through the body, but this is not the priority for this client. Another choice is better.
   4. The client's pain will need to be treated, but first vital signs should be assessed to establish a baseline.

7. **TEST-TAKING TIP: Identify all options that provide opportunities for a pathogen to enter a host. Identify key words of susceptibility and infectious agent to help determine correct responses.**
   1. **Maintaining normal pH levels in the gastrointestinal and genitourinary tracts helps to counter potential microbial invasion by determining proper immune cell activity.**
   2. **The integrity and number of the host's white blood cells help provide resistance to some potential pathogens.**
   3. **The skin is the body's first line of defense against pathogens. Intact skin and mucous membranes protect against microbial invasion.**
   4. **A person's general health and nutritional status along with their level of fatigue contribute to susceptibility to infections. Sensible nutrition, adequate rest, and good personal health habits contribute to reducing susceptibility to infection.**
   5. **Age, sex, race, and heredity all play a part in susceptibility with the very young and the very old being more vulnerable to infection.**
   6. **Stress levels influence susceptibility. Increased stress can inhibit a person's normal defense mechanisms and make a person more vulnerable to a potential pathogen.**

8. 1. **A white blood cell count of 20,000 cells/mcL is higher than the expected range of 4500 to 11,000 cells/mcL in an adult male and generally indicates the presence of an infection.**
   2. This is within the expected range of urine specific gravity of 1.001 to 1.029 and is unrelated to infection.
   3. This is within the expected range for hemoglobin in an adult male, which is 13.2 to 17.3 g/dL; hemoglobin is unrelated to infection.
   4. This is within the expected range for a hematocrit in an adult male, which is 37% to 49%; hematocrit is unrelated to infection.

9. **TEST-TAKING TIP: The words *violating* and *incorrect* in the stem indicate negative polarity. The question really is asking which action is *not an acceptable practice* when removing soiled gloves.**
   1. **You should always remove the respirator after leaving the client's room and closing the door. Removing the respirator inside the doorway exposes the nurse to potentially infectious and airborne agents.**
   2. You should handle goggles by the headband and lift them away from the face, placing them in the appropriate receptacle for cleaning or disposing of them in the appropriate waste container.
   3. Unfasten gown ties at the neck and waist and allow the gown to fall away from the body. Touch only the inside of the gown and pull away, keeping hands on the inside of the gown. Pull the gown away from the arms, tuck it inside out and dispose of it in the proper receptacle.

4. Grasp the outside of one gloved hand with the opposite gloved hand and peel off, turning the glove inside out as you pull off. Hold the removed glove in the remaining gloved hand, slide fingers of the ungloved hand under the wrist of the remaining gloved hand, avoiding touching the outside of the glove, and remove the glove at the same time as the other glove. Dispose in appropriate receptacle.

10. **TEST-TAKING TIP: The word *first* in the stem sets a priority. The word *blood* in the stem and option 1 is a clang association.**
   1. **Washing includes the action of wetting, rubbing, and rinsing. Soap reduces the surface tension of water, friction mechanically disturbs microorganisms, and rinsing flushes microorganisms from the skin.**
   2. The disinfectant isopropyl alcohol can kill bacteria but cannot kill spores, viruses, or fungi.
   3. Hot water does not disinfect and is unnecessary; it also may injure the tissue.
   4. Water and bleach in a 1 to 10 ratio should be used to cleanse a blood or body fluid spill in the environment, not on the skin.

11. **TEST-TAKING TIP: The words *soiled linens* in the stem and option 1 are clang associations. Options 4 and 5 are equally plausible because they are both furniture in the room and one is not better than the other.**
   1. **Depositing soiled linen in a soiled linen hamper is a safe and acceptable way to contain microorganisms.**
   2. The Occupational Health and Safety Administration (OSHA) states that blood-stained linens are not considered infectious waste and should not be placed in an infectious waste bag for disposal. Countless linens that could be washed are thrown away each year because of this, contributing to waste and increased costs for health-care facilities. OSHA emphasizes the importance of proper handling of soiled linens to prevent cross-contamination.
   3. Holding linens away from the body helps reduce the risk of cross-contamination of clothing.
   4. Placing soiled linen in a laundry chute without first placing it in a soiled linen laundry bag is an undesirable practice because it will contaminate the chute. Soiled linen must be bagged to contain microorganisms before it is deposited in a laundry chute.
   5. Placing soiled linen on the overbed table contaminates the overbed table and is an undesirable practice; the overbed table is considered a clean surface and should not be used to hold soiled linen.
   6. Placing soiled linen on a chair contaminates the chair and is an undesirable practice; a chair is considered a clean surface and should not be used to hold soiled linen.

12. **TEST-TAKING TIP: Options 1 and 3 and options 2 and 4 are opposites. Unfortunately, the test-taking tip "identify opposites in options" is not helpful in eliminating options in this question.**
   1. Hot temperatures are used to destroy bacteria (e.g., sterilization).
   2. Bacteria do not multiply rapidly in cool environments.
   3. Bacteria do not multiply rapidly in cold environments.
   4. **Bacteria grow most rapidly in dark, warm, moist environments, particularly when the environment is close to body temperature (98.6°F).**

13. **TEST-TAKING TIP: The word *least* in the stem indicates negative polarity. Options 1, 2, and 4 are all similar because they are articles of linen that are generally placed over the client. Option 3 is unique because it is the only article of linen in the options that is positioned under the client.**
   1. A top sheet often is used again if it is still clean.
   2. A bedspread often is used again if it is still clean.
   3. **The pillowcase comes in contact with the client's hair, exudate from the eyes, mucus from the nose, and saliva from the mouth. A pillowcase is easily soiled and usually needs to be replaced more often than other linen.**
   4. A cotton blanket often is used again if it is still clean.

14. **TEST-TAKING TIP: The word *practical* is the key word in the stem that directs attention to content.**
   1. Placing it in a protective bag is unsafe. The outer surface of the bag also is contaminated and, if taken out of the room, will contaminate any surface on which it is placed.
   2. **Keeping it in the client's room is the most practical action; when isolation is**

discontinued, all of the equipment can be terminally disinfected.

3. Soaking it in a germicidal solution is impractical and will harm the sphygmomanometer.
4. The sphygmomanometer is contaminated and must be disinfected before it is removed from the client's room.

15. **TEST-TAKING TIP: The word *highest* in the stem sets a priority.**
   1. Using disposable equipment is not the most effective method to reduce the spread of microorganisms; not all equipment is disposable.
   2. Although double-bagging limits the spread of microorganisms, it is not the most effective method to reduce the spread of microorganisms.
   3. Although gloves protect the nurse and limit the spread of microorganisms, this is not the most effective method to reduce the spread of microorganisms.
   4. **Hand hygiene is the most effective measure to reduce the spread of microorganisms because it helps to remove them from the hands before they come in contact with other clients and objects.**

16. **TEST-TAKING TIP: The word *first* in the stem sets a priority.**
   1. Spraying the basin with a disinfectant is unnecessary.
   2. Washing the basin in hot, soapy water should not be the initial intervention. Hot water coagulates the protein of organic material and causes it to stick to a surface.
   3. **Rinsing the basin with cold running water is a correct action because it does not coagulate the protein of organic material, permitting it to be flushed from the surface of the basin.**
   4. Antiseptics are used to limit bacteria on the skin or in wounds, not for cleaning objects.

17. **TEST-TAKING TIP: The words *MRSA* and *open wound* are key words in the stem that direct attention to content. Option 1 is unique because it is the only option that presents an intervention from the negative perspective (i.e., do not).**
   1. According to the Centers for Disease Control and Prevention (CDC), soap and water or alcohol-based hand rub should always be used before and after client care or contact with the client-care environment. Cleansing hands before and after care decreases MRSA transmission and decreases health-care–associated infections.
   2. Shoe covers are not needed for clients with MRSA infections. Shoe covers should be worn if fluid-based transmissions may occur.
   3. **According to the CDC, soap and water or alcohol-based hand rub should always be used before and after client care or contact with the client-care environment. Cleansing hands before and after care decreases MRSA transmission and decreases health-care–associated infections.**
   4. Eye protection is not necessary for clients with MRSA.
   5. **Contact precautions (gloves and gowns) are used during clinical encounters with patients who are colonized or infected with MRSA and may help reduce the spread of MRSA in a health-care facility.**
   6. **Gloves are considered contact precautions and should be worn for this client. Gloves should always be worn when contact with potentially infectious material occurs.**

18. **Answer: 1.7 mL**
   Solve the problem by using ratio and proportion.

$$\frac{\textbf{Desire}}{\textbf{Have}}\ \frac{\textbf{2.4 million units}}{\textbf{5 million units}} = \frac{x\ \textbf{mL}}{\textbf{3.5 mL}}$$

$$5x = 2.4 \times 3.5$$

$$5x = 8.4$$

$$x = 8.4 \div 5$$

$$x = 1.68\text{; round 1.68 up to 1.7 mL}$$

19. 1. Once the first soiled glove has been removed, the photograph reflects the correct way to remove the soiled glove from the other hand. The clean hand is touching the inside of the soiled glove and not the contaminated outside of the soiled glove.
   2. Once protective equipment has been removed, the hands are washed again before the caregiver leaves the client's room.
   3. **Clean hands should not touch the contaminated outer surface of the gown as it is being removed. The illustration indicates how the nurse should peel the gown from one shoulder and then the other in the direction of the**

hands while keeping the hands inside the gown. Doing so will turn the gown inside out. While keeping the hands inside the gown, the gown should be rolled so that the exterior of the gown is wrapped inside the rest of the gown and the clean inner surface encircles and contains the contaminated outer surface.

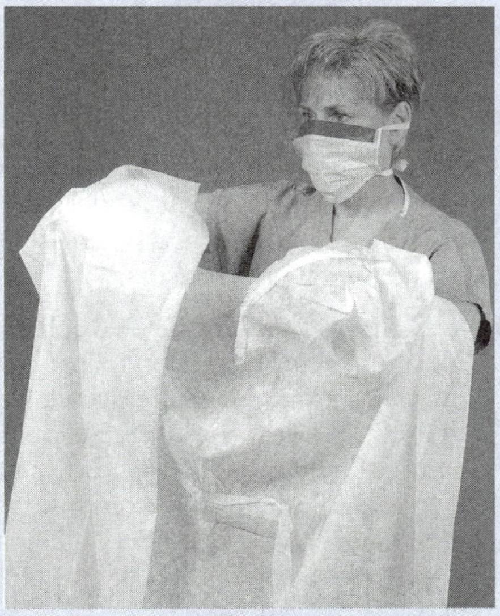

4. The photograph demonstrates the correct way to hold a contained soiled gown away from the body so as not to contaminate the uniform. The rolled gown is then discarded into the appropriate waste receptacle. The mask can be removed at any time during the disrobing procedure as long as the hands are washed first.

20. TEST-TAKING TIP: The words *portal of exit* are key words in the stem that direct attention to content.

1. Hand hygiene is an important means of controlling the transmission of microorganisms from one person or object to another; it does not limit the number of microorganisms directly exiting from a reservoir.
2. Disposing of soiled linen is an important means of controlling the transmission of microorganisms from one person or object to another; it does not limit the number of microorganisms directly exiting from a reservoir.
3. Disinfecting used equipment is an important means of controlling the transmission of microorganisms from one person or object to another; it does not limit the number of microorganisms directly exiting from a reservoir.
4. **Covering a cough limits the number of microorganisms that exit from the respiratory tract. The respiratory tract is one portal of exit from the human reservoir (source of microorganisms). Other human portals of exit include the gastrointestinal, urinary, and reproductive tracts and blood and body fluids.**
5. Swiping the skin with alcohol before administering an injection prevents the introduction of microorganisms into a puncture site. A puncture site is a portal of entrance, not exit, to the body.

21. TEST-TAKING TIP: The words *specific to* and *airborne precautions* are key words in the stem that direct attention to content.

1. **Keeping the door closed prevents the spread of microorganisms that can be transmitted via air currents. The client should be in a room with negative air pressure.**
2. It is not necessary for a nurse to wear a gown when administering medications to a client who has airborne precautions.
3. It is not necessary for a caregiver to wear gloves when delivering a meal tray to a client who has airborne precautions.
4. **Wearing a high-efficiency particulate air (HEPA) filter respirator prevents transmission of droplet nuclei less than or equal to 5 μm or dust particles containing a pathogen; these particles remain suspended in the air for extended periods of time.**
5. The nurse, not the client, wears an HEPA filter respirator for self-protection.

22. Answer: 2, 4, 1, 5, 3

2. **Touching the outside package of sterile equipment with ungloved hands is an acceptable practice. A clean, dry surface prevents contamination of the wrapper; objects below the waist are considered contaminated.**
4. **The ungloved hand is permitted to touch the inner surface of a sterile glove; both surfaces are considered contaminated.**
1. **Donning the gloves with the fingers facing downward prevents the fingers of the sterile glove from folding over onto the ungloved hands and becoming contaminated.**
5. **Putting on the second glove by inserting the gloved fingers under the everted cuff**

of the second glove maintains sterile to sterile contact.

3. **Sterile to sterile contact maintains sterility of the gloves. Interdigital pressure ensures that the fingers of the gloves are fully in place over the fingers.**

23. **TEST-TAKING TIP: The words *intervene to reduce the risk of infection* indicate negative polarity.**

1. This is not unsafe. Most protocols require that IV tubing be changed every 72 to 96 hours. Extending use beyond the time indicated in a protocol places the client at risk for infection. Inflammation of a vein (phlebitis) can progress to an infection.
2. **Urinals should be emptied as soon as they are used. Clean urinals should be stored in the lowest drawer of a bedside table or in a designated area in a client's bathroom. The urinal should be labeled with the client's initials.**
3. **According to the Centers for Disease Control and Prevention (CDC), tubing used to administer blood, blood products, or lipid emulsions should be replaced within 24 hours of initiating the infusion. Many health-care facilities require blood tubing to be replaced much earlier than 24 hours.**
4. **A urinary collection bag sitting on the floor contaminates the bag and may contaminate the tube used to empty the urine from the collection bag. Although 1500 mL is a large amount of urine, most urinary collection bags can hold 2000 mL of urine. Ideally urinary collection bags should be emptied when half full to minimize stress on the tubing that can cause tension on the catheter entering the urinary meatus. Catheter bags should always be placed off the floor.**
5. **Uncovered food should not be kept at the bedside because it can spoil and/or attract insects. Some health-care facilities will permit a piece of fruit wrapped in plastic or a snack in a labeled, covered container to be kept at the bedside for a short period of time.**

24. **TEST-TAKING TIP: The word *first* in the stem sets a priority.**

1. Cleansing the skin on the left side of the incision first may drag microorganisms on the skin into the incision, possibly contaminating the incision.
2. **The first cleansing stroke should be over the center of the incision following line "B." The next stroke can be either on the left or right side of the incision, with the final stroke being the side of the incision that has not already been cleansed. Cleaning the center of the incision first follows the concept of clean to dirty. The incision is considered "clean," whereas the skin is considered "dirty." Cleaning the skin first will draw microorganisms on the skin into the incision, possibly contaminating the incision.**
3. Cleansing the skin on the right side of the incision first may draw microorganisms on the skin into the incision, possibly contaminating the incision.

25. 1. There is no sputum culture result indicating a respiratory infection that requires droplet precautions. Increased vital signs indicate an infection, but there are no clinical findings (e.g., dyspnea, cough, increase in respiratory secretions, labored breathing, crackles/rhonchi) indicating a respiratory infection that requires droplet precautions.

2. **The client must have contact precautions instituted because of the client's history of being methicillin-resistant *Staphylococcus aureus* (MRSA) positive, experiencing urine and fecal incontinence, and having a wound with yellow drainage. Contact precautions prevent the spread of pathogens from the client to the nurse and others. The white blood cell (WBC) count is increased above the expected range, indicating an infectious process.**

   Clients with diabetes are at risk for infection because of a decreased immune response and a high glucose level in the tissues, which support the growth of microorganisms. Yellow drainage from a pressure ulcer is suggestive of an infection. The increase in vital signs above the expected range reflects the stimulation of the general adaptation syndrome in response to the presence of a pathogen (e.g., MRSA).
3. There is no sputum culture result indicating a respiratory infection that requires airborne precautions. The increased vital signs indicate an infection, but there are no clinical findings (e.g., dyspnea, cough, increase in respiratory secretions, labored

breathing, crackles/rhonchi) indicating a respiratory infection that requires airborne precautions.

4. Protective precautions are unnecessary. Protective precautions would be necessary if the WBC count was low, not high, putting the client at risk for infection.

26. The irrigating solution should begin flowing from the top inside edge of the wound. Initiating the flow of solution inside the wound prevents microorganisms on the skin from being carried into the wound, possibly contaminating the wound. This follows the principle of clean to dirty. The wound itself is considered "clean," and the skin is considered "dirty." By beginning at the top of the wound, the solution will flow by gravity into a container held by the nurse at the bottom of the wound.

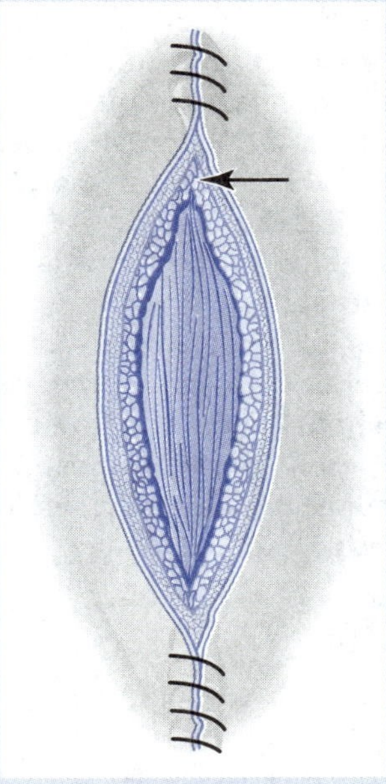

27. Answer: 1 mL

To answer the question, first convert milligrams to grams.

$$\frac{\text{Desire}}{\text{Have}}\ \frac{250\text{ mg}}{1{,}000\text{ mg}} = \frac{x\text{ gram}}{1\text{ gram}}$$

$$1000\,x = 250$$

$$x = 250 \div 1000$$

$$x = 0.25 \text{ gram is equal to } 250 \text{ mg}$$

Next use ratio and proportion to determine the amount of solution to administer.

$$\frac{\text{Desire}}{\text{Have}}\ \frac{0.25\text{ gram}}{1\text{ gram}} = \frac{x\text{ mL}}{4\text{ mL}}$$

$$1x = 0.25 \times 4$$

$$x = 1\text{ mL}$$

28. TEST-TAKING TIP: Examine options 1, 2, 3, 4, and 5 carefully. Proper hand hygiene is a key element in preventing the spread of infection, but there are still significant compliance issues in health care. If hands are not visibly soiled, alcohol-based rubs are recommended and are proven to reduce bacterial counts on hands.

1. The Centers for Disease Control and Prevention (CDC) recommends hand hygiene before and after direct contact with a client.
2. The CDC recommends hand hygiene before and after direct contact with a client.
3. Hand hygiene should always be performed after contact with body fluids, mucous membranes, nonintact skin, wounds, and wound dressings.
4. Hand hygiene should always be performed after touching a client's surroundings. People frequently touch their eyes, nose, and mouth without even realizing it, potentially transferring bacteria to themselves. They may also touch other clients, transferring bacteria to them. Potentially harmful agents from unwashed hands can also be transferred to other objects, such as handrails or tabletops, or toys and then transferred to someone else.
5. Hand hygiene before a clean or aseptic procedure helps to protect the client from harmful germs, including the client's own germs, from entering their body.
6. It is not required to perform hand hygiene before touching a client's surroundings but may be a personal preference. According to the CDC and the World Health Organization, hand hygiene should always be performed after touching client surroundings.

29. TEST-TAKING TIP: The words ***high risk*** in the stem set a priority.

1. Cigarette smoking is a substantial risk factor for bacterial and viral infections contracted outside of the health-care facility; but not necessarily health-care–acquired infections (HAIs). HAIs are infections a client gets because of treatment in a health-care facility, whether from the treatment itself or from a health-care provider or from another client.
2. The IV drug user with a low white blood cell count is at high risk for developing a

community-acquired infection, which is an infection contracted outside of a health-care facility or diagnosed within 48 hours of admission.

3. **This client is at risk for an HAI because of the indwelling catheter. An HAI from an indwelling catheter is called a catheter-associated urinary tract infection (CAUTI). Prolonged use of an indwelling catheter is the most important risk factor for developing a CAUTI, so catheters should be removed as soon as possible.**
4. Radioactive iodine for treatment of thyroid disorders does not place a client at a higher risk for hospital-acquired infections.
5. **Any clients receiving medications through a central line are at high risk for developing a central line–associated bloodstream infection (CLABSI). Central lines access major veins close to the heart so can easily introduce germs and bacteria to the bloodstream. A CLABSI is a hospital-acquired infection that can be prevented by health-care workers using stringent infection control practices and closely monitoring the site.**
6. Some scientists are studying links between some types of dysrhythmias such as atrial fibrillation and biomarkers of infection; however, heart dysrhythmias are not known to increase the risk for hospital-acquired infections.

30. **TEST-TAKING TIP: The words *contact precautions* are key words in the stem that direct attention to content.**

1. **A client on contact precautions should be kept in a private room to prevent the exposure of other clients to the infectious agent. Clients infected with the same infectious agent may be kept together in the same room (cohorted) after consultation with infection control personnel.**
2. **When a client has a condition that requires contact precautions, the nurse should wear additional personal protective equipment, such as goggles, when splashing of body fluids can occur.**
3. **The nurse should wear a gown to provide a barrier when caring for a client who has a condition requiring contact precautions. The gown will protect the nurse's clothing from being a source for cross-contamination.**
4. **Hands should be washed before donning gloves and immediately after removing them.**
5. **Everything in the room is considered contaminated. Therefore, equipment that is used routinely, such as a thermometer and sphygmomanometer, should remain in the room. Some equipment can be disposed of in an appropriate container, and others can be disinfected.**

MEETING CLIENTS' HYGIENE, PAIN, COMFORT, REST, AND SLEEP NEEDS

This section includes questions related to meeting clients' hygiene, comfort, rest, and sleep needs. Questions focus on theories of pain; assessment of pain; pain relief measures; rest and sleep; the back rub; making a bed; the use of heat and cold; principles associated with bed baths; preventing skin breakdown; perineal care; and care of the hair, feet, and oral cavity.

QUESTIONS

1. Which temperature should the water be when the nurse gives a client a bed bath?
1. 80°F to 85°F
2. 90°F to 95°F
3. 100°F to 105°F
4. 110°F to 115°F

2. Why should the nurse rinse the client's skin after using soap and water during a bed bath?
1. Increases circulation
2. Minimizes pressure ulcers
3. Removes residue and debris
4. Promotes comfort and relaxation

3. The home health nurse noticed the client with upper dentures has foul-smelling breath and is concerned about the client's oral hygiene. Interventions for oral hygiene include all the following except: **Select all that apply.**
1. Eat high sugar carbohydrate meals
2. Eat foods that do not generate odors
3. Brush teeth at least two times per day
4. Have a dental examination at least once per year
5. Remove dentures every other day for cleaning
6. Rinse mouth with antiplaque mouthwash daily

TEST-TAKING TIP: Identify the word in the stem that indicates negative polarity. Identify the options with a specific determiner. Identify equally plausible options.

4. The nurse is changing the bed linens of a client on bed rest. Which should the nurse do to prevent pressure injuries from the linens for this client?
1. Always use a draw sheet
2. Complete a full linen change daily
3. Make a toe pleat with the bottom sheet
4. Secure the bottom sheet at all corners of the mattress

TEST-TAKING TIP: Identify key words in the stem that direct attention to content. Identify the option with a specific determiner.

5. The school nurse is educating a group of high school students about healthy sleep habits. The nurse should recommend all the following to the students to promote healthy sleep habits except:
1. avoid daytime naps.
2. avoid caffeine all day.
3. do not use a bedroom clock.
4. eat a light carbohydrate snack before bed.

TEST-TAKING TIP: Identify the word in the stem that indicates negative polarity.

6. A client has a nasogastric tube. Which is a daily nursing intervention that contributes to hygiene?
   1. Instilling the system with 1 ounce of water
   2. Replacing the fixation device
   3. Suctioning the oral pharynx
   4. Lubricating the nares

TEST-TAKING TIP: Identify key words in the stem that direct attention to content.

7. The client with atherosclerosis and diabetes reports cold feet at night. Which is the most appropriate intervention that the nurse should teach the client?
   1. Wear socks to bed
   2. Keep feet elevated
   3. Apply a heating pad
   4. Use a hot water bottle

TEST-TAKING TIP: Identify key words in the stem that direct attention to content. Identify equally plausible options.

8. The nurse is planning to give a client a back rub to promote comfort and rest. Which is the reason why a back rub promotes comfort and rest?
   1. Causes vasodilation
   2. Stimulates circulation
   3. Relieves muscular tension
   4. Increases oxygen to tissues

TEST-TAKING TIP: Identify key words in the stem that direct attention to content. Identify the unique option. Identify equally plausible options.

9. A client asks the nurse why cold compresses were ordered to treat a recent muscle sprain. Which statement explains why cold is effective in reducing the discomfort associated with a local inflammatory response and should be included in the nurse's response?
   1. Anesthetizes nerve endings and causes vasoconstriction
   2. Stimulates nerve endings and causes vasoconstriction
   3. Anesthetizes nerve endings and causes vasodilation
   4. Stimulates nerve endings and causes vasodilation

TEST-TAKING TIP: Identify duplicate facts among options.

10. The nurse uses a cotton blanket when bathing a client. Which principle is the basis for using a blanket to prevent the loss of body heat during a bed bath?
    1. Evaporation
    2. Conduction
    3. Diffusion
    4. Osmosis

11. The hospitalized client has a nursing diagnosis of Disturbed Sleep Pattern. Which nursing interventions are most appropriate for this diagnosis? **Select all that apply.**
    1. Decrease evening fluid intake
    2. Maintain home sleep schedule
    3. Encourage a short daytime nap
    4. Assess side effects of medication
    5. Encourage use of sleep medications
    6. Wake client to take scheduled medications

TEST-TAKING TIP: Identify the word in the stem that sets a priority.

12. An order is written to apply a warm soak to a client's extremity. Which information should the nurse include when teaching the client about how a warm soak reduces discomfort at a local inflammatory site?
    1. Decreases local circulation and limits capillary permeability
    2. Decreases tissue metabolism and increases local circulation
    3. Increases local circulation and promotes muscle relaxation
    4. Provides local anesthesia and decreases local circulation

TEST-TAKING TIP: Identify duplicate facts among options.

13. The nurse is providing oral hygiene for a client with dentures. Which should the nurse do to **support** the client's dignity?
1. Supply a container for the client's teeth
2. Pull the curtain around the client's bed
3. Place the client in the high Fowler position
4. Resist looking at the client while the teeth are out

TEST-TAKING TIP: Identify the key word in the stem that directs attention to content. Identify the client-centered option.

14. The nurse is providing a client with a back rub after a bed bath. Which technique is **most** effective in promoting relaxation?
1. Tapotement
2. Effleurage
3. Pétrissage
4. Friction

TEST-TAKING TIP: Identify the word in the stem that sets a priority. Identify the key word in the stem that directs attention to content.

15. The nurse is changing the bed linens for their hospice client with limited mobility. What is the priority when changing the linens of an occupied bed?
1. The least possible disturbance to the client
2. So the client does not have to exercise
3. To help the client's caregiver
4. To assess the client's skin

TEST-TAKING TIP: Identify the word in the stem that sets a priority. Identify the unique option. Identify the client-centered option.

16. The nurse in a long-term care facility is assessing clients for foot and nail problems. Which clients does the nurse know are at high risk for these complications? **Select all that apply.**
1. The client with a BMI of 32
2. The client with a BMI of 22
3. The client with type 2 diabetes
4. The client who picks at their nails
5. The client with peripheral artery disease
6. The client with rheumatoid arthritis

TEST-TAKING TIP: Identify the word in the stem that sets a priority. Identify clang associations. Identify opposites.

17. Which factor has the **most** significant influence on pain perception and is important for the nurse to consider when assessing a client's pain?
1. Duration of the stimulus
2. Activity of the cerebral cortex
3. Characteristics of the stimulus
4. Level of endorphins in the blood

TEST-TAKING TIP: Identify the word in the stem that sets a priority.

18. On the day after surgery, a client states that the pain is unbearable no matter how many times the button is pushed on the patient-controlled analgesia pump. After ensuring accurate placement and functioning of the catheter, the nurse should:
1. provide a back rub.
2. reposition the client for comfort.
3. inform the anesthesiologist about the situation.
4. increase the dosage of medication delivered per hour.

19. When providing physical hygiene, the nurse identifies that a client's long hair is tangled and matted. Which should the nurse do? **Select all that apply.**
   1. _____ Braid the hair in sections
   2. _____ Use a comb instead of a hairbrush
   3. _____ Comb a small section of the hair at a time
   4. _____ Encourage the client to get a shorter haircut
   5. _____ Brush the hair starting from the roots progressing toward the ends

TEST-TAKING TIP: Identify the key words in the stem that direct attention to content.

20. Which should the nurse do to provide emotional comfort when administering perineal care to a client? **Select all that apply.**
   1. _____ Drape areas that are not being washed
   2. _____ Place the client in the supine position
   3. _____ Pull a curtain around the bed
   4. _____ Use warm water for washing
   5. _____ Call the client by name

TEST-TAKING TIP: Identify key words in the stem that direct attention to content.

21. The nurse assumes care of a client recently admitted to the medical-surgical unit. After reviewing the client's clinical record, which interventions should the nurse implement for this client? **Select all that apply.**
   1. Offer client a bedpan
   2. Allow client to eat in bed
   3. Approach client on their left side
   4. Involve the client in dressing activities
   5. Place meal tray on right side of the client's visual field
   6. Place call bell on the left side of the client's visual field

CLIENT'S CLINICAL RECORD

Progress Note

A female client with left-sided hemiparesis from a cerebrovascular accident (CVA) 2 years ago. The client is currently admitted for right flank pain with tests scheduled to rule out renal calculus. Client is incontinent of urine and stool.

Braden Scale

Score: 16. Client responds to verbal commands and has no sensory deficit. Skin is constantly moist as assessed when the client is turned and positioned. Needs assistance transferring from bed to a chair, makes frequent shifts in position, and requires assistance to turn or move up in bed. Generally eats most of every meal.

Physical Assessment

Client is incontinent of urine and stool and is damp where skin surfaces touch (under the arms, perineal area, and under the breasts). Client is alert and responding appropriately and reports that flank pain is a level 2 since pain medication was administered 30 minutes ago. IV is running at 125 mL as prescribed; IV catheter insertion site is dry and intact with no signs of infiltration or thrombophlebitis.

TEST-TAKING TIP: Identify key words in the stem that direct attention to content. Identify duplicate facts in options.

22. The nurse is caring for a client who is coping with chronic pain. Which psychological reaction to chronic pain may occur? **Select all that apply.**
1. _____ Dyspnea
2. _____ Depression
3. _____ Self-splinting
4. _____ Hypertension
5. _____ Compromised relationships

TEST-TAKING TIP: Identify key words in the stem that direct attention to content.

23. The nurse is caring for a client who is experiencing lower back pain. The muscle relaxant cyclobenzaprine (Amrix®) 10 mg three times a day by mouth is prescribed. Cyclobenzaprine is available in 5-mg tablets. How many tablets of cyclobenzaprine will the client be taking in 24 hours? **Record your answer using a whole number.**

Answer: ___________ tablets

24. The nurse is cleansing the perineal area of an uncircumcised male client. Which is an important action by the nurse when performing this procedure? **Select all that apply.**
1. _____ Handling the penis with a firm touch
2. _____ Washing the shaft of the penis before the scrotum
3. _____ Repositioning the foreskin after washing the penis
4. _____ Cleansing the length of the penis down the shaft from the glans toward the scrotum
5. _____ Washing the glans of the penis with a circular motion from the urinary meatus outward

25. A client comes to the emergency department reporting pain, nausea, vomiting, and a low-grade fever. Rovsing's sign is elicited when the primary health-care provider palpates the client's left lower quadrant. Place an X over the site where the client felt an **increase** in pain.

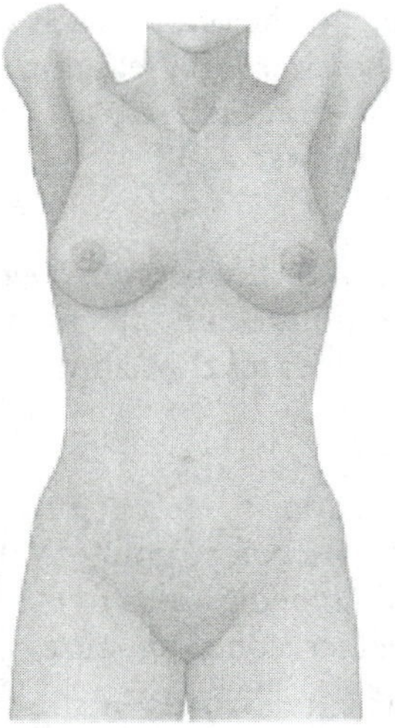

TEST-TAKING TIP: Identify the words in the stem that direct attention to content.

26. The nurse is assessing a client who is experiencing pain. Which factor associated with the pain indicates that it is acute pain, rather than chronic pain? **Select all that apply.**
1. _____ Rapid onset
2. _____ Pressured speech
3. _____ Constricted pupils
4. _____ Increased heart rate
5. _____ Decreased blood pressure
6. _____ Slow, monotonous speech

TEST-TAKING TIP: Identify key words in the stem that direct attention to content. Identify the options that are opposites.

27. A nurse is caring for a client who has a fungal infection of the feet. Which is an independent action that the nurse should teach the client to use to care for the fungal infection of the feet? **Select all that apply.**
1. _____ Wear flip-flops to protect the feet when walking in a locker room.
2. _____ Soak the feet in a medicated solution during hygiene care.
3. _____ Apply body lotion to the feet to avoid cracks in the skin.
4. _____ Increase circulation to the feet by encouraging exercise.
5. _____ Dry well between the toes of the feet after bathing.

28. The nurse is admitting a new resident to the long-term care facility. The fully independent client is concerned about their sleep schedule being interrupted and maintaining their personal hygiene. Which intervention should the nurse plan to provide client-centered care? **Select all that apply.**
1. _____ Provide privacy for the client
2. _____ Assist the client with dressing
3. _____ Assist the client with hair care
4. _____ Provide oral care every 2 hours
5. _____ Keep the door unlocked in case of emergency
6. _____ Allow client to use prepackaged disposable bath products

TEST-TAKING TIP: Identify the option with a specific determiner. Identify the obscure clang association.

29. A client has had difficulty sleeping, and the nurse secures a prescription for zolpidem (Ambien) extended-release tablets 12.5 mg PO at bedtime. The medication supplied by the pharmacy is 6.25 mg/tablets. How many tablets should the nurse administer? **Record your answer using a whole number.**

Answer: ____________ **tablets**

30. The nurse is providing perineal care for a female client. Which should the nurse do during this procedure? **Select all that apply.**
1. _____ Use a new area of the washcloth for each stroke
2. _____ Wash from the pubis toward the rectum
3. _____ Use a circular motion with each stroke
4. _____ Wash the cleanest area first
5. _____ Use warm tap water

31. The nurse knows that hospitalized clients often have a nursing diagnosis of disturbed sleep patterns. Which interventions should the nurse implement to promote rest and sleep in hospitalized clients? **Select all that apply.**
1. _____ Quiet, darkened room
2. _____ Administer a sedative
3. _____ Reduce environmental noise
4. _____ Encourage client to void before going to sleep
5. _____ Reschedule all evening medications to the morning
6. _____ Keep head of bed flat to reduce pressure on neck and spine

TEST-TAKING TIP: Identify the key words in the stem that direct attention to content.

32. A client is experiencing interrupted sleep. For which response associated with shortened non–rapid eye movement (NREM) sleep should the nurse assess the client? **Select all that apply.**
1. _____ Fatigue
2. _____ Anxiety
3. _____ Hyperactivity
4. _____ Delayed healing
5. _____ Aggressive behavior

33. A nurse is performing oral care for a client. Place the following illustrations in the order in which they should be performed.

1. 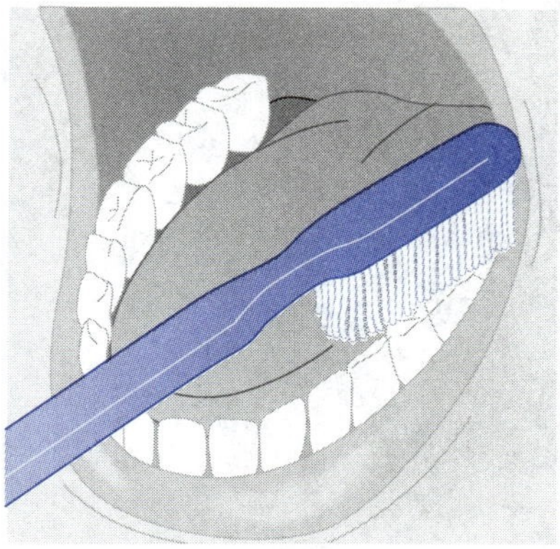

2. 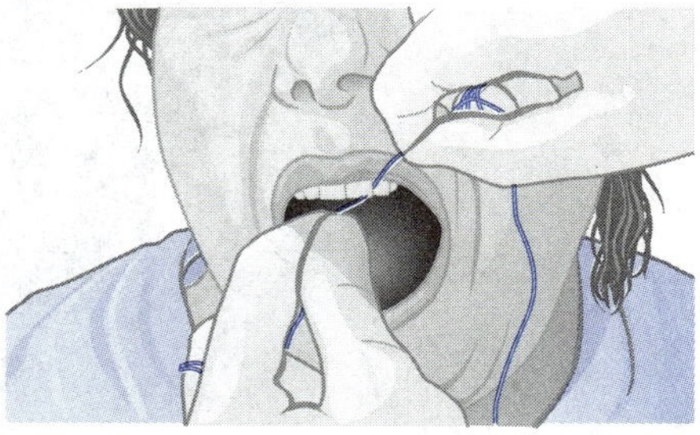

3. 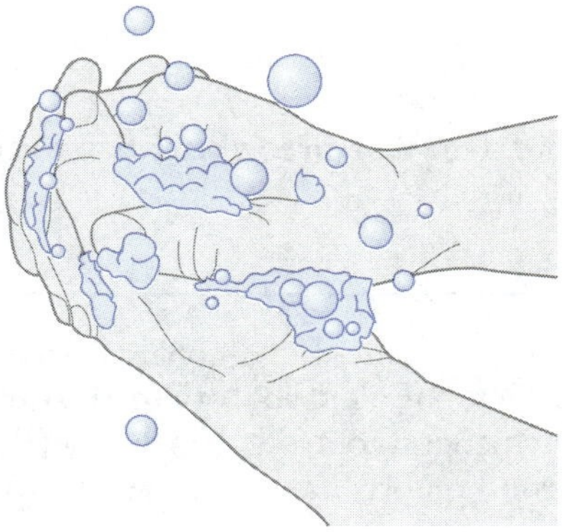

4. 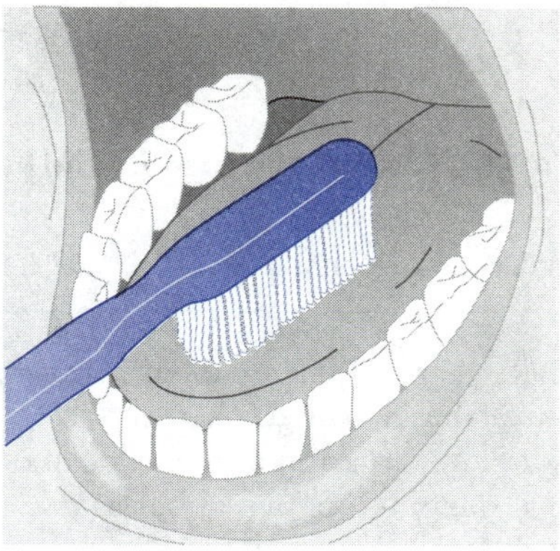

Answer: ____________

34. The nurse in charge delegates the application of a cold pack to a client. Place the following steps in the order in which they should be performed.

1. Review the order for the application of the cold pack.
2. Assess the site 5 minutes after application of the cold pack.
3. Place a protective barrier between the cold pack and the client.
4. Explain the details of the application of the cold pack to the client.
5. Assess the condition of the site where the cold pack is to be applied.

Answer: ____________

35. The nurse is caring for a client diagnosed with pediculosis *(Pediculus humanus capitis)*. Lindane Shampoo is prescribed to treat this condition. Which grooming device should the nurse use after washing the client's hair and scalp with Lindane Shampoo?

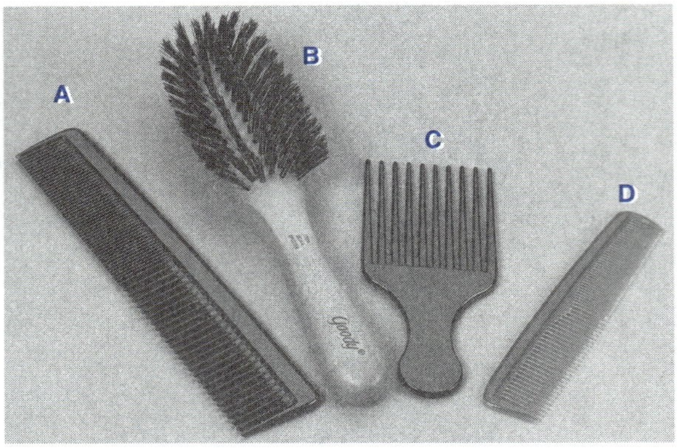

1. A
2. B
3. C
4. D

TEST-TAKING TIP: Identify the key word in the stem that directs attention to content.

CLINICAL JUDGMENT CASE STUDY

Dorothy, a 48-year-old female client, is admitted to the surgical unit after an open abdominal hysterectomy. She arrives to the unit at 1800 and is groggy but alert and oriented to time, place, person, and situation and is educated on use of the patient-controlled analgesia (PCA) pump. She is sleeping on arrival but as the night progresses, reports an increasing amount of pain in the abdominal region.

PAIN MEDICATION ORDERS

PCA pump: 1 mg—client demand dose

Lockout q10 min, no continuous infusion

ADDITIONAL ORDERS

Vitals signs q4 hours, per protocol. Notify physician if systolic blood pressure greater than 140 or less than 100

Cefazolin 2 g IV @ 2200 and 0200

LR at 125 mL/hr, Saline lock when tolerating fluids & stable vital signs

Remove urinary catheter when alert and oriented and able to ambulate to bathroom

Ambulate 2 times shift

Advance diet as tolerated

NURSING NOTES

2000. Client sleeping. Bandage dry and intact. No edema noted. Vitals WNL. Blood pressure 122/78.

2200. Client awake but still groggy. Reports pain of 4 out of 10 in abdominal region. Describes as dull ache. Bandage dry and intact. Blood pressure 100/60. IV left forearm, WNL, flushed and antibiotic started.

0030. Client awake, reports pain of 6 out of 10 in abdominal region. Cannot localize pain to any specific quadrant. Client educated on use of PCA pump. Bandage dry and intact. Reports mild nausea, unable to ambulate, left arm appears puffy. Blood pressure 96/58.

0200. Client is alert and oriented × 4. Client reports unrelenting pain in abdominal region, 8 out of 10, but cannot localize to specific quadrant. No use of PCA pump. Client educated on how to use PCA pump when admitted to the unit and again at 0030. Sanguineous fluid noted on bandage. Still refuses to ambulate, left arm edematous. Blood pressure 92/58.

36. **Recognize cues—What matters most?** After reviewing this client's clinical record, the nurse calls the surgeon. Which is the **priority** concern that the nurse should address with the provider?
1. Request bolus dosing for PCA pump
2. Client's decreasing blood pressure
3. Client's refusal to ambulate
4. Client's unrelenting pain

37. **Analyze cues—What could it mean?** The nurse notes that the client's blood pressure continues to drop throughout the evening and that the client's left arm becomes edematous. Which should the nurse be concerned about? **Select all that apply.**
1. Phlebitis
2. Infiltration
3. Extravasation
4. Hypervolemia

38. **Prioritize hypotheses—Where do I start?** The client's pain continues to increase as she wakes from anesthesia. After reviewing the client's description of her pain, which does the nurse believe is the source of the client's increasing pain?
1. Surgical pain
2. Somatic pain
3. Visceral pain
4. Incisional pain

39. **Generate solutions—What can I do?** The client is not using the PCA pump though the nurse has educated her on how to receive an on-demand morphine dose. Which should the nurse do to develop a plan of care for the client's pain control? **Select all that apply.**
1. Explore understanding of equipment
2. Assess past experiences with pain control
3. Ask the provider to increase the on demand dose
4. Identify the client's expectations for pain control
5. Identify if the client had any preoperative PCA teaching
6. Request a change from morphine to fentanyl to help with pain

40. **Take action—What will I do?** Based on the client's clinical record, the nurse knows the client is at the greatest risk for 1. ________ as evidenced by 2. ___________. The priority intervention is 3. _____________. **Choose from the options provided.**
1. hypovolemic shock, high blood pressure, pulmonary embolism, pulmonary edema
2. increase in pain, decrease in blood pressure, refusal to ambulate, continual IV fluids
3. fluid replacement, ambulation, use of incentive spirometer, diuretic administration

41. **Evaluate outcomes—Did it help?** The nurse knows that pain is a significant barrier to surgical recovery. The client's assessments also identify other concerns that may delay recovery. Place an X by the indicators that the nurse should anticipate and request to be included in the client's plan of care for pain control and postsurgical recovery. **Select all that apply.**
1. _____ Fluid replacement
2. _____ Self-report of pain
3. _____ Incentive spirometer
4. _____ Maintain IV site in left forearm
5. _____ Multiple modalities of pain control
6. _____ Communicating pain management plans to incoming staff

ENE, PAIN, COMFORT, REST, WERS AND RATIONALES

1. 1. A temperature range of 80°F to 85°F is too cool; this will promote chilling.
2. A temperature range of 90°F to 95°F is too cool; this will promote chilling.
3. A temperature range of 100°F to 105°F is too cool; this will promote chilling.
4. **The temperature of bath water should be between 110°F and 115°F to promote comfort, dilate blood vessels, and prevent chilling.**

2. 1. **Friction from firm, long strokes used during bathing increases circulation; it is not the reason for rinsing.**
2. Local back rub and repositioning every 2 hours, not rinsing, prevent pressure ulcers.
3. **Rinsing flushes the skin with clean water, which removes debris and soap residue.**
4. A back rub and positioning in functional alignment, not rinsing, promote rest and comfort.

3. TEST-TAKING TIP: The word *except* indicates negative polarity. Options 3 and 6 are equally plausible.

1. **Clients with impaired dentition should limit their intake of sugary, starchy food and drink. In poor dental hygiene, there is an excess of bacteria in the mouth, which metabolizes the sugar into acids that demineralize tooth enamel.**
2. Although some foods can cause halitosis, it is more often caused by inadequate oral hygiene, a local infection, or a systemic disease. With proper dental hygiene, clients can continue to eat these foods.
3. Brushing teeth at least two times per day and after meals helps to limit the buildup of plaque and bacteria, promoting good dental health.
4. **Regular dental checkups, at least twice a year, can help prevent potential dental problems because they identify problems early.**
5. **Dentures should be removed and cleaned every night. Regular cleaning of dentures helps prevent mucosal irritation.**
6. Rinsing with mouthwash as a supplement to good teeth brushing and denture care promote good oral hygiene and help prevent the buildup of plaque.

4. TEST-TAKING TIP: The words *prevent, pressure injuries,* and *bed linens* are key words in the stem that direct attention to content. The word always in option 1 is a specific determiner.

1. A drawsheet is an additional sheet that can add to the number of wrinkles; the purpose of a drawsheet is to keep the bottom sheet clean or to use it to lift and move the client.
2. A complete linen change does not need to be made daily unless the sheets are wet or soiled.
3. A toe pleat should be placed in the top sheet and spread, not in the bottom sheet. A toe pleat prevents foot drop.
4. **Wrinkles exert pressure and friction against the skin, promoting the formation of pressure injuries. Securing the bottom sheet tightly at the top and bottom corners helps remove wrinkles.**

5. TEST-TAKING TIP: The word *except* in the stem indicates negative polarity.

1. Teens need 8 to 10 hours of sleep a night. Avoiding daytime naps or keeping to a minimum of 20 minutes helps promote melatonin release at night to keep the teen on a regular circadian rhythm.
2. **Teens should avoid caffeine, but they especially should avoid it in the late afternoon and evening because caffeine can cause insomnia and restlessness. It may be difficult to have a teen avoid all caffeine intake.**
3. Bedroom clocks emit blue light, which can be disruptive to sleep. Rooms should be kept dark with minimal artificial light.
4. Eating a light carbohydrate snack before bed may help stabilize blood glucose and initiate sleep.

6. TEST-TAKING TIP: The words *contributes to hygiene* are key words in the stem that direct attention to content.

1. After placement is verified, instillation of solution may be done to promote catheter patency, not hygiene.
2. This is not necessary; the fixation device should be replaced only if the nares become irritated or the device becomes soiled. An alternative fixation device should be used if the area is irritated.
3. Suctioning is not necessary; cleaning the oral cavity when necessary with a toothbrush, dental floss, and mouthwash followed by application of a lubricant to the lips is sufficient.
4. **Lubricating the nares keeps the skin supple and prevents drying, which limits the development of encrustations.**

7. **TEST-TAKING TIP: The words *atherosclerosis* and *diabetes* are key words in the stem that direct attention to content. Options 3 and 4 are equally plausible.**
   1. **Wearing socks is the safest way to keep the feet warm; socks contain the heat generated by the body.**
   2. Elevation will not alter the temperature of the feet.
   3. External heat produced by a heating pad may burn the feet of older adults, who have reduced peripheral sensation.
   4. External heat produced by a hot water bottle may burn the feet of older adults, who have reduced peripheral sensation.

8. **TEST-TAKING TIP: The words *comfort and rest* are key words in the stem that direct attention to content. Option 3 is unique because it addresses muscles and what is decreased (relieves) rather than what is increased ("causes" in option 1, "stimulates" in option 2, "increases" in option 4). Options 1, 2, and 4 are equally plausible because they all refer to the circulatory system.**
   1. Although a back rub causes vasodilation, which improves circulation and brings oxygen and nutrients to the area, vasodilation does not promote comfort and rest.
   2. Stimulation of circulation brings oxygen and nutrients to the area, but it does not promote comfort and rest.
   3. **Applying long, smooth strokes while moving the hands up and down the back without losing contact with the skin has a relaxing and sedative effect. Its effect may be related to the gate-control theory of pain relief; rubbing the back stimulates large muscle fiber groups, which close the synaptic gates to pain or uncomfortable stimuli, permitting a perception of relaxation.**
   4. Although a backrub ultimately does increase oxygen and nutrients to the area, oxygen and increased nutrients do not promote comfort and rest.

9. **TEST-TAKING TIP: Four hypotheses are being tested in this question: cold anesthetizes nerve endings, causes vasoconstriction, stimulates nerve endings, and causes vasodilation. If you know just one of these hypotheses is correct, then you can eliminate two distractors. If you know just one of these hypotheses is wrong, then you can eliminate two distractors.**
   1. **Cold slows the nervous conduction of impulses, thereby anesthetizing nerve endings, which relaxes muscle tension and relieves pain. Vasoconstriction decreases the flow of blood to the affected area; this limits the development of edema, which puts pressure on nerve endings, resulting in pain.**
   2. Cold anesthetizes rather than stimulates nerve endings; it causes vasoconstriction.
   3. Although cold does anesthetize nerve endings, it causes vasoconstriction, not vasodilation.
   4. Cold anesthetizes, rather than stimulates, nerve endings and causes vasoconstriction.

10. 1. **Evaporation (vaporization) is the transfer of heat through the conversion of water to a gas. This occurs when there is fluid on the skin from either perspiration or bath water.**
    2. Conduction is the transfer of heat from one molecule to another while in direct physical contact.
    3. Diffusion is a process whereby molecules move through a membrane from an area of higher concentration to an area of lower concentration without the expenditure of energy.
    4. Osmosis is the movement of water across a membrane from an area of lesser concentration to an area of greater concentration.

11. **TEST-TAKING TIP: The word *most* in the stem sets a priority.**
    1. **Too much fluid intake in the evening can cause excess voiding during the night. Educate the client on the reasons to limit fluid intake to promote restful sleep.**
    2. **Keeping the same sleep pattern encourages the body's natural circadian rhythms and adhering to this schedule as much as possible for the hospitalized client promotes relaxation and sleep.**
    3. Daytime napping should be avoided or kept to no more than 20 minutes to not disrupt the body's natural circadian rhythm.
    4. **Many medications cause side effects that interfere with sleep. Evaluate the client's medications, such as diuretics, and consult with the provider about rescheduling to earlier times to avoid waking at night to void or other things that could wake the client.**
    5. Sleep aides should only be administered when indicated and on an as-needed basis.

The limitations of these medications should be explained to the client. Other self-care strategies such as healthy sleep and lifestyle behaviors should be encouraged.

6. Nursing care should be scheduled to avoid unnecessary interruptions. Try to provide care when the client is normally awake and avoid awakening during REM sleep.

12. **TEST-TAKING TIP: The words *increases local circulation* in options 2 and 3 and *decreases local circulation* in options 1 and 4 are examples of duplicate facts among the options. If you know that one or the other is true, the chances of selecting the correct answer have improved to 50%.**

1. Heat increases, rather than decreases, local circulation, capillary vasodilation, and capillary permeability.
2. Although heat increases local circulation, it increases, rather than decreases, tissue metabolism. Heat causes vasodilation, facilitating the exchange of nutrients and waste products and increasing cellular metabolism.
3. **Heat increases circulation because of its vasodilating effect. Heat is known to relax muscle spasms and the discomfort associated with muscle spasms; this mechanism is unknown.**
4. Cold, not heat, provides local anesthesia and decreases local circulation.

13. **TEST-TAKING TIP: The word *dignity* is the key word in the stem that directs attention to content. Option 2 is client-centered.**

1. A container is used to store the dentures when the client is sleeping and addresses the client's safety and security needs.
2. **This provides privacy while the dentures are out of the mouth and supports the client's dignity and self-esteem.**
3. This supports the client's physical needs.
4. This is unsafe; the nurse must look at the client to inspect the oral cavity.

14. **TEST-TAKING TIP: The word *most* in the stem sets a priority. The word *relaxation* is the key word in the stem that directs attention to content.**

1. The technique of *tapotement* is gentle rhythmic tapping or percussion over tense muscles. The technique of tapotement is not as relaxing as another back rub technique.
2. **The technique of *effleurage* uses long, smooth, circular strokes that slide over the skin to produce muscle relaxation. The French word effleurage means "to touch lightly." It is performed at the beginning of a back rub before pétrissage and again at the end of the back rub.**
3. The technique of *pétrissage* kneads the skin and underlying muscles. This technique targets specific muscles to reduce muscle tension and promote circulation to peripheral capillaries. The technique of pétrissage is not as relaxing as another back rub technique.
4. The technique of *friction* uses small circular strokes that move the surface of the skin as well as underlying tissue. This stroke is used to promote circulation to peripheral capillaries. The technique of friction is not as relaxing as another back rub technique.

15.
1. **The priority when changing the linens of an occupied bed is to provide the least possible disruption for the client who may have limited mobility.**
2. This is not a priority reason to change an occupied bed. If the client is unable to perform active range of motion exercises, passive exercises should be attempted to avoid contractures and other musculoskeletal problems.
3. Though the nurse may be helping the client's caregiver when changing an occupied bed, this is not the priority.
4. The nurse should be consistently assessing the client's skin. Though this can be done when changing the bed linens, it is not the priority.

16. **TEST-TAKING TIP: The words *high risk* in the stem set a priority. The word *nails* in the stem and option 2 is a clang association.**

1. **The client with a BMI of 32 is considered obese and research correlates obesity with toenail fungus, known as onychomycosis. Obesity also puts unnecessary strain on the feet, causing dry skin and potential decreased circulation.**
2. A BMI of 22 is within normal range and does not place a client at high risk for foot and nail problems.
3. **Diabetes can cause peripheral neuropathy leading to tingling and pain in the feet. Over time you may lose feeling in**

your feet predisposing a person to cuts, bruises, and other serious complications leading to amputation.

4. **Clients who pick their nails, either the hands, feet, or both, potentially damaging the skin around the nail and increasing the risk of infection.**
5. **Poor circulation inhibits nail growth. Peripheral artery disease also causes a thickening of the nails and the presence of sores on the feet that do not heal.**
6. **Rheumatoid arthritis causes thickening, yellowing, and development of ridges in the nails. It can also cause splinter hemorrhages in nails, which are not painful but may be unsightly.**

17. **TEST-TAKING TIP: The word *most* in the stem sets a priority. All of the options address factors that influence pain perception, but option 2 is the "most" significant.**

1. Although the duration of pain is one component associated with the perception of pain, it is not as important as the information in another option.
2. **The cerebral cortex controls the higher levels of the perceptual aspects of pain. Each individual perceives pain in a unique way.**
3. Although the characteristics of the stimulus that precipitates pain are associated with the perception of pain, this is not as important as the information in another option.
4. Although endorphin levels influence pain perception, this is not the most influential factor that affects the perception of pain.

18.
1. A back rub is ineffective for severe pain; it may be effective for mild pain.
2. Repositioning may be effective for mild to moderate pain, not severe, unbearable pain.
3. **The pain-control plan is ineffective, and the primary health-care provider or anesthesiologist should be notified to reassess the situation. The analgesic dose may be increased, the analgesic may be changed, or an alternative delivery route may be selected.**
4. Increasing the dose is not within the scope of nursing practice. A prescription from a primary health-care provider is required.

19. **TEST-TAKING TIP: The words *tangled* and *matted* are the key words in the stem that direct attention to content.**

1. Braiding the hair in sections should be done after the hair is combed and untangled. Not all clients want their hair to be braided.
2. Either a comb or a hairbrush can be used.
3. **Separating the hair into small sections promotes ease in combing/brushing and limits discomfort.**
4. This intervention is inappropriate because it meets the nurse's need, not the client's need. Also, clients have a right to wear their hair as they please.
5. The opposite should be done. When removing tangles, the hair should be grasped at the scalp and the loose ends combed/brushed; each stroke should progress higher up the shafts of hair strands than the preceding stroke.

20. **TEST-TAKING TIP: The words *perineal* and *emotional comfort* are key words in the stem that direct attention to content.**

1. **All areas of the body below the neck that are not being washed should be covered with a bath blanket to provide privacy and to avoid chilling.**
2. Correct positioning provides for physical, not emotional, comfort.
3. **Perineal care is a private activity, and measures should be taken to provide for privacy.**
4. Warm water provides physical, not emotional, comfort.
5. **Calling the client by name is a respectful, individualized approach that provides emotional support during invasive care.**

21. **TEST-TAKING TIP: The key words in the scenario are *incontinent of urine and stool, constantly moist skin, requires assistance to turn,* and *pain level 2.* If you know that a person who is incontinent of urine and stool and has constantly damp skin surfaces needs interventions to prevent skin breakdown, option 1 is a good option. If you know that individuals with tolerable pain and the ability to engage in some movement generally prefer to be as independent as possible, then you know that option 4 is a good choice. Options 2, 3, and 6 do not account for the client's left-sided deficits and can be eliminated.**

1. **A regular toileting time should be established for this client. Their voiding pattern should be assessed, and a bedpan offered frequently dependent on their voiding schedule. Offering a**

bedpan can reduce moisture and the potential for skin breakdown.

2. A client with a history of stroke should never eat in bed. They should always sit upright, preferably in a chair, when eating and drinking. With paralysis, there is a risk of coughing and food or drink dribbling out of the mouth or pooling in one side of the mouth.
3. Clients with left-sided hemiparesis should be approached from their unaffected side. They may not notice a person if approached on the affected side so approach from the side where visual perception is intact.
4. **Active participation in personal hygiene activities should be encouraged. Remind the person of the affected side and encourage them to turn and look in the direction of the visual deficits when performing self-care.**
5. **Meals should be placed on the unaffected side to encourage proper nutrition.**
6. The call bell should be placed on the right side of the client's visual field. The client has left-side deficits and may not see or be able to use the call bell if it is placed on the left side.

22. **TEST-TAKING TIP: The words *psychological* and *chronic* are key words in the stem that direct attention to content.**

1. Dyspnea is a physiological, not a psychological, response to stress.
2. **Clients with chronic pain commonly experience depression; this is a psychological response to lack of control over relentless pain.**
3. Self-splinting is a behavioral attempt to minimize pain.
4. Hypertension is a physiological, not a psychological, response to stress.
5. **Compromised interpersonal relationships may occur as the client with chronic pain depletes emotional energy and resources needed to sustain relationships.**

23. **Answer: 6 tablets**

Solve the problem using ratio and proportion.

Desire/Have $\frac{10\text{ mg}}{5\text{ mg}} = \frac{x\text{ tablets}}{1\text{ tablet}}$

Cross-multiply $5x = 10$

Divide each side by $\frac{5}{5} = \frac{10}{5}$

$x = 2$ **tablets**

Multiply 2 tablets by three times a day = 6 tablets in 24 hours.

24. 1. **A firm but gentle touch should be used. A light touch is stimulating and may precipitate a penile erection.**
2. **Washing the shaft of the penis before the scrotum reflects the principle of working from clean to dirty. The tip of the penis at the urethral meatus should be washed first; then the nurse should progress down the shaft of the penis toward the perineum and then the scrotum.**
3. **Repositioning the foreskin protects the head of the penis and prevents drying and irritation; if it is allowed to remain retracted, it may cause local edema and discomfort.**
4. **Cleaning the penis should start at the urinary meatus and then progress down the shaft of the penis away from the urinary meatus. This action follows the principle of "clean to dirty."**
5. **Cleaning with a circular motion beginning at the urinary meatus and moving outward moves secretions and debris away from the urinary meatus; this lessens potential contamination of the urinary tract.**

25. **TEST-TAKING TIP: The words *site* and *increase in pain* are the words in the stem that direct attention to content.**

Palpation of the left lower quadrant in a client with appendicitis precipitates pain at McBurney's point (Rovsing's sign). McBurney's point is in the lower right quadrant, half the distance from the anterior iliac crest to the umbilicus.

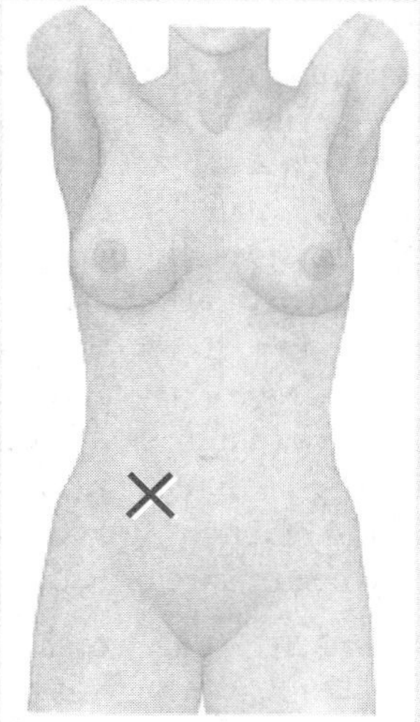

26. **TEST-TAKING TIP:** **The words *acute pain* are the key words in the stem that direct attention to content. Options 2 and 6 are opposites.**

1. **Pain that has a rapid onset is associated with acute pain. The pain is related to potential or actual tissue damage. Chronic pain usually has a gradual onset.**
2. **The general adaptation syndrome stimulates the sympathetic branch of the autonomic nervous system, which results in speech that is accelerated, hurried, and sometimes erratic (pressured speech).**
3. Constricted pupils occur with chronic pain because of the effects of the parasympathetic branch of the autonomic nervous system. Dilated pupils occur with acute pain as a result of the effects of the sympathetic branch of the autonomic nervous system.
4. **The general adaptation syndrome stimulates the sympathetic branch of the autonomic nervous system, which results in an increase in heart rate and an increase in respirations.**
5. Chronic pain is associated with a decrease in blood pressure because of the effects of the parasympathetic branch of the autonomic nervous system. An increase in blood pressure occurs with acute pain because the general adaptation syndrome stimulates the sympathetic branch of the autonomic nervous system.
6. Slow, monotonous speech is associated with chronic pain because of the effects of the parasympathetic branch of the autonomic nervous system.

27.
1. **Fungi grow and are transmitted to others in areas where there is moisture, and the feet are not protected.**
2. Medicated foot baths generally are prescribed for ingrown toenails, not fungal infections. A medicated footbath requires a primary health-care provider's prescription; this is a dependent, not an independent, nursing action.
3. Moisturizers should be avoided between the toes because they keep the area moist, which supports fungal growth.
4. Exercise does not minimize fungal growth.
5. **Moist, dark, warm areas facilitate the growth of microorganisms, especially fungi in the area of the feet.**

28. **TEST-TAKING TIP:** ***Fully independent* are key words. Option 4 contains the word *every*, which is a specific determiner. Examine options 2 and 3 carefully.**

1. **Independent clients who can safely shower or bathe independently should be given privacy, though a call bell should be within reach if the client requires assistance.**
2. Clients who can care for themselves should be capable of dressing and maintaining their personal hygiene independently. Maintaining Erikson's Integrity versus Despair is important for these clients as they transition from home care to long-term care environments.
3. Independent clients should be able to care for their hair independently, though they should know that if they want assistance, the nurse or aide can provide it.
4. This client does not need oral care every 2 hours. Clients at risk for impaired oral mucous membrane integrity, malnutrition, or dehydration, or who cannot care for themselves, should have oral care every 2 hours.
5. **Doors should remain unlocked so health-care personnel can enter if the client needs help. Privacy signs can be used to allow the client privacy and independence.**
6. Prepackaged, disposable bath products should be reserved for clients who are bedbound and cannot independently wash themselves.

29. **Answer: 2 tablets**
Solve the problem using ratio and proportion.

$$\frac{\text{Desire}}{\text{Have}} \qquad \frac{12.5\text{ mg}}{6.25\text{ mg}} = \frac{x\text{ Tab}}{1\text{ Tab}}$$

$$6.25x = 12.5$$

$$x = 12.5 \div 6.25$$

$$x = 2\text{ tablets}$$

30.
1. **This is a basic principle of medical asepsis. This should be done so that contaminated material will not be carried by the washcloth to another area of the perineum.**
2. **Cleaning from the pubis toward the rectum prevents contaminating the urinary meatus and vagina with fecal material.**
3. A circular motion should not be used because it will move debris from more soiled areas to less soiled areas.
4. **The area closest to the urinary meatus and vagina is cleaned first because it**

is considered the cleanest area of the perineum.

5. **Warm water should be used to clean the perineal area; cool water will feel uncomfortable, and hot water can injure the perineal area.**

31. **TEST-TAKING TIP: The words *promote rest* and *sleep for hospitalized clients* are the key words in the stem that direct attention to content.**
    1. **A quiet and darkened room with privacy helps promote sleep, though a small night-light may be needed to promote safety if the client awakens at night.**
    2. Medications may be prescribed to address sleep disturbances for hospitalized clients, though nonpharmacological methods should be tried first. Sedatives are used to initiate and maintain sleep but can cause residual drowsiness in the morning. If used, these medications should only be given short-term and client safety should be considered. These medications should be used as a last resort.
    3. **Environmental noise should be kept to a minimum. This includes people entering and leaving the room, sounds of elevators, and talking at the nurse's station. Environmental noises often bring complaints from clients and their families. Many health-care facilities have quiet times on the units to create a supportive environment to encourage rest.**
    4. **Clients should be encouraged to void before going to sleep. The need to void is one of the greatest deterrents to sleep. Hospitalized clients are often on IV fluids and other medications that increase the need to void.**
    5. Evening medications should be reviewed to assess side effects that may cause sleep disturbances, but not all evening medications should be rescheduled to the morning. Many medications work better if taken before bedtime.
    6. **Proper body alignment should be maintained and is conducive to sleep; however, unless ordered by the provider, the head of the bed does not need to remain flat. Unless the client has specific orders for bed elevation, it should be client preference.**

32.
    1. **During non–rapid eye movement (NREM) sleep, the parasympathetic nervous system dominates. Heart rate, respirations, and blood pressure decrease as the body physically restores and regenerates itself. NREM sleep accounts for 75% to 80% of sleep. When NREM sleep is interrupted, a person experiences fatigue and lethargy.**
    2. Rapid eye movement (REM), not NREM, sleep is essential for maintaining mental and emotional equilibrium and, when interrupted, results in anxiety, irritability, excitability, confusion, and suspiciousness.
    3. Interrupted REM, not NREM, sleep is associated with hyperactivity and excitability.
    4. **During NREM sleep, growth hormone is consistently secreted, which provides for protein synthesis, anabolism, and tissue repair. A lack of NREM sleep results in delayed wound healing and immunosuppression.**
    5. Interrupted REM, not NREM, sleep is associated with excitability, emotional lability, and suspiciousness. Interrupted NREM sleep is associated with apathy, withdrawal, and hyporesponsiveness.

33. Answer: 3, 1, 4, 2
    3. **The hands must be washed before performing any direct client care. This limits the presence of microorganisms on the nurse's hands and prevents cross-contamination.**
    1. **All teeth surfaces should be brushed, such as the biting and chewing surfaces of teeth and the inner and outer surfaces of teeth, including the gum line.**
    4. **Brushing the tongue removes accumulated debris and dried mucus, which provide a reservoir for bacteria and produce bad breath.**
    2. **Moving dental floss up and down between teeth removes food particles. The mouth should be rinsed with water at the end of the procedure. Oral suction may be necessary if the client is at risk for aspiration or is unconscious.**

34. Answer: 1, 4, 5, 3, 2
    1. **The application of a cold pack is a dependent function of the nurse. The order will include the type of cold delivery device to be used, the site where it should be applied, and the length of time it should remain in place.**
    4. **Clients have a right to know the details of a procedure to be performed and**

by whom. They also have the right to accept or refuse the treatment.

5. **Assessing the condition of the site (appearance of the skin, such as color, edema, and temperature; integrity of the skin; and the presence of discomfort or pain) provides baseline information for comparison with the client's response to the procedure. The primary health-care provider should be notified if a contraindication (e.g., sensory impairment) to the procedure exists.**
3. **Placing a protective barrier (e.g., washcloth, towel, fitted cloth sleeve) between the cold device and the client limits the intensity of the cold application, preventing tissue trauma.**
2. **Five minutes after the application of the cold pack, the site should be assessed for signs such as pallor and mottling and to check whether the client feels it is too cold. The ice pack should be removed if these signs occur to prevent the progression to frostbite.**

35. **TEST-TAKING TIP: The word *pediculosis* is the key word in the stem that directs attention to content.**
   1. The distance between the teeth of this comb is appropriate for combing thin, straight, or slightly curly hair, not for removing nits (eggs) associated with head lice *(Pediculus humanus capitis)*.
   2. This brush is appropriate for grooming thick or thin, straight, or slightly curly hair, not for removing nits (eggs) associated with head lice *(Pediculus humanus capitis)*.
   3. This comb is not appropriate to use after shampooing with Lindane to remove nits (eggs). The distance between the teeth of this comb is appropriate for thick, very curly hair because it allows the comb to gently detangle this type of hair.
   4. **This comb is appropriate for removing nits (eggs) attached to hair shafts close to the scalp after shampooing for head lice infestation (pediculosis). The teeth are extremely close together, which uses friction to loosen nits attached to hair shafts.**

CLINICAL JUDGMENT CASE STUDY ANSWERS AND RATIONALES

36. 1. The nurse may want to request bolus dosing for the client's pain, but this is not the priority. Another choice is the priority answer.
   2. **The client's decreasing blood pressure is the priority concern. The nurse should address this with the provider to determine the underlying cause for the continual decrease.**
   3. The nurse should document the client's refusal to ambulate and assess to determine why the client does not want to ambulate.
   4. Addressing the client's unrelenting pain is important for the nurse; however, uncovering the reason for the decreasing blood pressure is the priority.

37. 1. Phlebitis is inflammation of the vessel where an IV is cannulated. Clinical signs include pain, inflammation, redness, and warmth.
   2. **Infiltration is when nonvesicant fluid or medicine leaks into the tissue surrounding a cannulated vein. Swelling and puffiness around the sight is a clinical sign.**
   3. Extravasation is when a vesicant and irritating fluid or medicine leaks into the tissue surrounding a cannulated vein. Extravasation can cause extensive tissue damage to the area surrounding the vein.
   4. Hypervolemia is excess fluid volume in the extracellular compartments in the body. This client only has edema in the left arm indicating infiltration.

38. 1. Surgical pain is from a surgical procedure and is caused by tissue damage at the incision, the surgical procedure itself, the closing and healing of the wound, and force or pressure used during the procedure. Surgical pain is a form of somatic pain.
   2. Somatic pain is localized to the injury and incisional site. It can be intermittent or constant and can be described as achy or throbbing.
   3. **Visceral pain is vague and usually characterizes pain in the abdomen and intestinal area. Damage to internal organs and tissues causes this type of pain. Visceral pain is difficult for the client to describe because of poor localization.**
   4. Incisional pain is a form of somatic pain because it is localized to the incisional site.

39. 1. **The client may not understand the directions or may be frightened by the equipment. Exploring the client's understanding of what the equipment is used for can help the nurse discern why the client is not using the PCA pump for pain control.**

2. **Pain assessment should include the client's past experiences with pain and how past pain was treated and controlled. Any education the client received preoperatively should also be assessed.**
3. Before asking for an increase in the demand dose, the nurse should first ask for a basal dose. The client is not using on-demand dosing so basal dosing may be appropriate for this client's pain relief.
4. **The client's understanding of visceral pain should be assessed and the client should be educated that visceral pain is challenging to treat. Identifying the client's expectations can also identify any misconceptions about pain and pain relief, providing the nurse with a basis for teaching. Nonpharmacological methods of pain relief such as relaxation, imagery, and distraction can also be taught.**
5. **The nurse should identify what preoperative teaching the client had. She may have received education on how to use the PCA pump, but she may not have understood when or why she should use it. The nurse should also identify if the client is avoiding using the PCA pump because she wants to avoid pain medication due to the negative connotations associated with opioids.**
6. The nurse must first educate the client to use the current medication prescribed before requesting a change to a more potent medicine.

40. 1. **Hypovolemic shock**
2. **Decrease in blood pressure**
3. **Fluid replacement**

Hypovolemic shock occurs when the body suddenly loses blood or fluids, resulting in a drop in blood volume circulating in the body. If the blood volume drops too low, organs cannot function. A drop in blood volume causes a decrease in blood pressure. This client had abdominal surgery so the nurse should be concerned about internal bleeding. Treatment for hypovolemic shock is fluid replacement and uncovering the root cause.

41. 1. **Fluid replacement is necessary for this client to address the ongoing drop in blood pressure. Once the underlying cause is identified and blood pressure is stabilized, the fluids may be discontinued per provider's orders.**
2. **Clients should be taught to self-report pain, how the pain will be managed, and the treatment plan shared during hand-off report. Identifying other causes of pain besides incisional pain is important. For example, if the client's Foley catheter is removed, they may have a full or distended bladder that masks itself as pain.**
3. **Incentive spirometers should be given to all postoperative clients to encourage deep breathing and lung expansion. Incentive spirometers help prevent alveolar collapse and help move respiratory secretions to the larger airways for secretion.**
4. This client's IV site should be relocated. The nursing note describes swelling and edema around the IV site, which may indicate infiltration.
5. **An appropriate pain control plan includes multiple modalities including pain medication and behavioral modifications such as distraction and guided imagery.**
6. **Reviewing the client's pain and pain control options should be discussed in the hand-off report. Continual education and treating pain before it becomes too severe help with pain control.**

MEETING CLIENTS' FLUID, ELECTROLYTE, AND NUTRITIONAL NEEDS

This section includes questions related to basic fluid balance and nutrition. Questions focus on principles associated with therapeutic diets, enteral feedings, fluid and electrolyte balance, intake and output (I&O), dehydration, feeding clients, vitamins, parenteral nutrition, intralipids, and medications associated with meeting clients' nutritional needs.

QUESTIONS

1. The nurse is caring for a client who is obese and is receiving a 1000-calorie diet per day. Which is nontherapeutic when providing nursing care?
   1. Telling the client about low-calorie snacks that can be eaten
   2. Teaching the client to avoid starches on the meal tray
   3. Encouraging the client to eat meals slowly
   4. Praising the client when weight is lost

   TEST-TAKING TIP: Identify the word in the stem that indicates negative polarity. Identify the unique option.

2. The nurse is monitoring a client's intake and output. Which is an accurate way for the nurse to measure the amount of urine from the client's urinary retention catheter?
   1. With a urometer
   2. With a marked graduate
   3. By emptying it into a bedpan
   4. By the markings on the collection bag

3. The nurse is planning for the nutritional needs of clients and is concerned about the influence of age on energy requirements. Which age group has the **highest** energy requirement?
   1. Birth to 1 year of age
   2. 3 to 5 years of age
   3. 13 to 19 years of age
   4. Older than 65 years of age

   TEST-TAKING TIP: Identify the word in the stem that sets a priority.

4. Which should the nurse do to prevent trauma to the oral mucous membranes from hot food being served to a cognitively impaired client?
   1. Request a menu that includes mostly cold foods
   2. Touch the food to test its temperature
   3. Wait for hot food to cool slightly
   4. Mix hot food with cold food

   TEST-TAKING TIP: Identify options that deny client feelings, concerns, or needs.

5. The nurse is caring for a confused client with a nursing diagnosis of risk for impaired nutrition. To meet the nutritional needs of this client, the priority interventions for this client include all of the following except: **Select all that apply.**
   1. Feed the client at every meal
   2. Promote proper positioning
   3. Ask for an order for parenteral nutrition
   4. Provide supervision when the client eats
   5. Explain to the client everything on the tray
   6. Encourage family members to take turns feeding the client

   TEST-TAKING TIP: Identify the words in the stem that sets a priority.

6. The client with atherosclerotic plaques had a myocardial infarction (MI) 1 week ago. The client is beginning a cardiac rehabilitation program that includes healthy lifestyle teaching. The cardiac rehab nurse should include all except ________ in the nutritional counseling.
   1. Avoid drinking whole milk
   2. Increase saturated fat intake
   3. Incorporate legumes into the diet
   4. Increase the amount of complex carbohydrates in the diet

   TEST-TAKING TIP: Identify the word in the stem that indicates a negative polarity. Identify the key words in the stem that direct attention to content.

7. The nurse is caring for a client with a stage 4 pressure injury that is draining fluid, exudate, and pus. Which is the nurse most concerned about when caring for this client?
   1. Loss of fluid
   2. Loss of weight
   3. Loss of protein
   4. Loss of leukocytes

   TEST-TAKING TIP: Identify the word in the stem that sets a priority. Identify key words in the stem that direct attention to content.

8. The client has been receiving enteral tube feedings. Before the nurse provides a feeding to the client, which intervention should the nurse implement? **Select all that apply.**
   1. Check the external tube marking to verify placement
   2. Verify tube placement with an x-ray
   3. Check gastric residual
   4. Use sterile gloves
   5. Lay the bed flat

   TEST-TAKING TIP: Identify key words in the stem that direct attention to content. Identify equally plausible options.

9. Which client response occurs when the amount of calories ingested is not sufficient for the client's basal metabolic rate?
   1. Loss of weight
   2. Thready pulse
   3. Dependent edema
   4. Need for more sleep

10. The client admitted with dehydration has orders for fluid replacement protocol with both oral and IV therapy and accurate intake and output (I&O). Which should the nurse do immediately after the client drinks 8 ounces of oral fluid?
    1. Document the intake in the medical record
    2. Assess the client's skin turgor
    3. Offer the client a bedpan
    4. Provide oral hygiene

    TEST-TAKING TIP: Identify the word in the stem that sets a priority.

11. The home health nurse is educating the newly diagnosed heart failure client on foods to include in a low-sodium diet. Which foods should the nurse encourage the client to eat?
    1. Milk
    2. Fruit
    3. Bread
    4. Vegetables

    TEST-TAKING TIP: Identify key words in the stem that direct attention to content.

12. A client has a pressure injury. Which breakfast food should the nurse encourage the client to eat?
   1. French toast and oatmeal
   2. Oatmeal and orange juice
   3. French toast and poached eggs
   4. Poached eggs and orange juice

   TEST-TAKING TIP: Identify duplicate facts among options.

13. A client has a medical diagnosis of anemia. Which vitamin should the nurse expect the primary health-care provider to prescribe?
   1. Ascorbic acid
   2. Riboflavin
   3. Folic acid
   4. Thiamin

   TEST-TAKING TIP: Identify the key word in the stem that directs attention to content.

14. How should the nurse administer intralipids when a client also is receiving total parenteral nutrition (TPN)?
   1. Give after the TPN infusion is completed
   2. Administer the intralipids via an infusion pump
   3. Give piggybacked into the proximal port of the TPN catheter
   4. Administer the intralipids through a separate intravenous line

   TEST-TAKING TIP: Identify key words in the stem that direct attention to content. Identify opposites in options. Identify clang associations.

15. Which responses can occur if a client's prescribed flow rate of total parenteral nutrition (TPN) solution is administered faster than the prescribed rate?
   1. Osmotic diuresis and hypoglycemia
   2. Hypoglycemia and dumping syndrome
   3. Electrolyte imbalance and osmotic diuresis
   4. Dumping syndrome and electrolyte imbalance

   TEST-TAKING TIP: Identify duplicate facts among options.

16. The nurse is caring for a group of clients. Which group of clients has the **most** need for supplemental iron?
   1. Menstruating women
   2. School-age children
   3. Active adolescents
   4. Older men

   TEST-TAKING TIP: Identify the word in the stem that sets a priority.

17. The dietitian is teaching a group of newly diagnosed type 2 diabetics about the importance of eating a healthy diet. Which nutrient does the dietitian include as the most important to maintain the body's metabolic functions?
   1. Carbohydrates
   2. Vitamins
   3. Proteins
   4. Fluids

   TEST-TAKING TIP: Identify the word in the stem that sets a priority.

18. Which group of individuals has the **highest** need for calcium?
   1. Postmenopausal women
   2. School-age children
   3. Pregnant women
   4. Working men

   TEST-TAKING TIP: Identify the word in the stem that sets a priority. Identify the key word in the stem that directs attention to content.

19. Which can the nurse expect the client to do when urine output is less than fluid intake?
   1. Experience nausea
   2. Become jaundiced
   3. Void frequently
   4. Gain weight

20. The nurse is completing a nutritional assessment on a new admission. Which client statement indicates a misconception about health and vitamins? **Select all that apply.**
   1. "I don't need to take vitamins until I am older."
   2. "I don't need vitamins because I eat a balanced diet."
   3. "Vitamins do not interact with food or medications."
   4. "Vitamins can be taken without the fear of side effects."
   5. "Since my body produces some vitamins, I only need ones it can't produce."
   6. "I should increase my vitamin intake as I age since my metabolism slows down."

TEST-TAKING TIP: Identify the word in the stem that indicates negative polarity.

21. Iron supplements are prescribed for a client with the diagnosis of anemia. The nurse teaches the client that the absorption of iron is facilitated by the ingestion of foods high in a particular vitamin. Which vitamin should the nurse include in this discussion?
   1. D
   2. C
   3. A
   4. K

TEST-TAKING TIP: Identify key words in the stem that direct attention to content.

22. A client with lung cancer is concerned about having had rapid weight loss and asks why this occurred. When answering this client's question, which information should the nurse use as a basis for a response?
   1. Anabolism exceeds catabolism.
   2. Nutrients are unable to be absorbed.
   3. Cell division causes an altered nitrogen balance.
   4. Cancer increases the body's metabolic demands.

TEST-TAKING TIP: Identify the clang association.

23. The nurse is assessing a client's pulse. Which should the nurse do if the client's pulse is full and bounding? **Select all that apply.**
   1. _____ Reduce the flow rate of the client's intravenous fluids
   2. _____ Measure the client's urine specific gravity
   3. _____ Monitor the client's serum glucose level
   4. _____ Lower the head of the client's bed
   5. _____ Obtain the client's blood pressure

TEST-TAKING TIP: Identify key words in the stem that direct attention to content.

24. A client who is receiving chemotherapy is nauseated. Which should the nurse include in the plan of care when addressing the nutritional needs of this client? **Select all that apply.**
   1. _____ Seek a prescription for chamomile, ginger, or peppermint tea
   2. _____ Encourage the intake of bananas, rice, applesauce, and toast
   3. _____ Suggest the avoidance of extremely hot or cold foods
   4. _____ Serve the ordered diet in small quantities often
   5. _____ Provide oral liquid supplements frequently
   6. _____ Teach avoidance of fluids with meals

TEST-TAKING TIP: Identify the key word in the stem that directs attention to content.

25. The postsurgical client drinks 9 ounces of cranberry juice along with one 3-ounce container of pudding, one 4-ounce container of Jell-O, and one 4-ounce popsicle for lunch. Knowing that 1 ounce equals 30 milliliters, what should the nurse document for liquid intake in the client's medical record? Record your answer using a whole number.

Answer: ____________ mL

26. The nurse is caring for a client with a vitamin K deficiency. For which response should the nurse monitor the client? **Select all that apply.**

1. _____ Anemia
2. _____ Bruising
3. _____ Tarry stool
4. _____ Cardiac dysrhythmias
5. _____ Increased temperature
6. _____ Heavy menstrual flow

TEST-TAKING TIP: Identify key words in the stem that direct attention to content. Identify options that are equally plausible.

27. Intermittent enteral feedings are prescribed for a client with a percutaneous endoscopic gastrostomy tube in place. Place the following steps in the order in which they should be performed.

1. Provide privacy.
2. Cleanse the hands.
3. Raise the head of the bed.
4. Collect all appropriate equipment.
5. Explain the procedure to the client.
6. Verify the accuracy of the formula, amount, and times to be administered.

Answer: ____________

28. The nurse is feeding a client with left hemiparesis as the result of a brain attack. Which intervention by the nurse is important when feeding this client? **Select all that apply.**

1. _____ Provide food that requires chewing.
2. _____ Place food in the center of the mouth.
3. _____ Offer fluids with each mouthful of food.
4. _____ Elevate the head of the bed during the feeding.
5. _____ Allow time to empty the mouth between spoonfuls.

TEST-TAKING TIP: Identify the key words in the stem that direct attention to content. Identify the option with a clang association.

29. Based on the information on the client's clinical record and the electrocardiogram, the nurse should **first:**
1. initiate the rapid response team.
2. discontinue the intravenous infusion.
3. remove the milk from the client's lunch tray.
4. encourage the client to use salt to season food on the lunch tray.

CLIENT'S CLINICAL RECORD

Nurse's Progress Note

1200: Client receiving IV 1000 mL of 0.9% sodium chloride with 40 mEq of KCl at 125 mL/hr.
IV insertion site dry and intact with no signs or symptoms of infiltration or thrombophlebitis.
Pulse: 70 beats/min, irregular
Client had two episodes of diarrhea and is irritable and slightly confused.

Electrocardiogram

T waves are narrow and peaked; ST segment shows depression; QT interval is shortened.

Laboratory Findings

Serum sodium: 140 mEq/L
Serum potassium: 6.9 mEq/L
Total serum calcium: 9.0 mg/dL

30. A client is experiencing diarrhea and needs to replace potassium. Which nutrient selected by the client indicates that additional teaching is necessary regarding nutrients high in potassium? **Select all that apply.**
1. _____ Beef bouillon
2. _____ Orange juice
3. _____ Poached egg
4. _____ Warm tea
5. _____ Bananas
6. _____ Raisins

TEST-TAKING TIP: Identify the words in the stem that indicate negative polarity.

31. A client is receiving a full-liquid diet. Which of the following should the nurse expect will be on the client's tray? **Select all that apply.**
1. _____ Ice cream
2. _____ Prune juice
3. _____ Cream of wheat
4. _____ Mashed potatoes
5. _____ Raspberry gelatin

TEST-TAKING TIP: Identify key words in the stem that direct attention to content.

32. The nurse is caring for a client who is receiving chemotherapy that is nephrotoxic. The primary health-care provider prescribes 1000 mL of IV fluid in the immediate 4 hours before the infusion of the chemotherapeutic agent. At how many milliliters per hour should the nurse set the infusion pump? **Record your answer using a whole number.**

Answer: __________ **mL/hr**

33. Which can the nurse expect to identify when a client had a fluid intake of only 500 mL over 48 hours? **Select all that apply.**
1. _____ Small amounts of urine at each voiding
2. _____ Development of an atonic bladder
3. _____ Decreased tissue turgor
4. _____ Low specific gravity
5. _____ Rapid pulse

34. The nurse reviews a client's clinical record to gather data that will influence the choice of sleeping position that the client should assume. Which position should the nurse encourage the client to assume when going to sleep?
1. Left side-lying with head slightly elevated
2. Prone with a small pillow under the abdomen
3. Semi-prone with the upper leg supported on a pillow
4. Supine with a small pillow under the small of the back

CLIENT'S CLINICAL RECORD

Nurse's Progress Notes
Reports frequent episodes of epigastric discomfort, slight difficulty swallowing, and excessive salivation. States the presence of a persistent cough, sore throat, and hoarseness.

Vital Signs Flow Sheet
Temp: 99°F, oral route
Pulse: 84 beats/min, regular
Respirations: 18 breaths/min, unlabored

Primary Health-Care Provider's Prescriptions
Dietitian consultation
Esomeprazole 20 mg PO once daily
Magnesium/aluminum hydroxide 20 mL PO, four times a day between meals and at bedtime

35. The nurse is caring for a client who is diagnosed with an IV fluid overload and hyponatremia. For which clinical indicator of hyponatremia should the nurse assess the client? **Select all that apply.**
1. _____ Thirst
2. _____ Headache
3. _____ Muscle weakness
4. _____ Increased temperature
5. _____ Dry mucous membranes

TEST-TAKING TIP: Identify the key word in the stem that directs attention to content.

36. The client was admitted to the telemetry unit because of excessive laxative use. During the nursing assessment, the client reports increasing muscle weakness, muscle twitching, and fatigue. The client's electrocardiogram (ECG) tracing is below. Which additional client response does the nurse expect to find during the assessment?
1. Thirst
2. Tremors
3. Weak, rapid pulse
4. Severe constipation

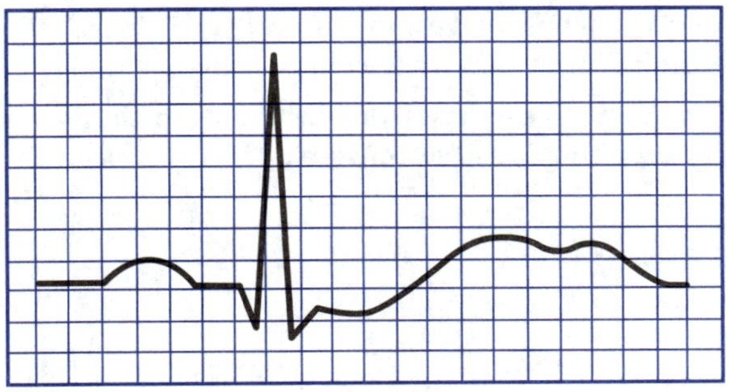

37. The nurse is working in a nursing home with a large population of older adults. Which factor related to aging influences the nutritional status of older adults and should be considered by the nurse? **Select all that apply.**

1. _____ Decreased ability to absorb calcium
2. _____ Decline in saliva production
3. _____ Less activity in older adults
4. _____ Reduced sense of smell
5. _____ Atrophy of taste buds

TEST-TAKING TIP: Identify key words in the stem that direct attention to content. Identify the clang association.

38. Which photograph illustrates a technique that will elicit information about a client's hydration status?

1.
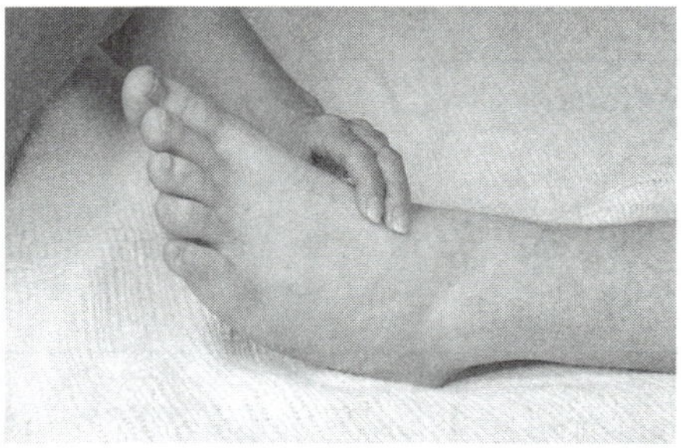

2.
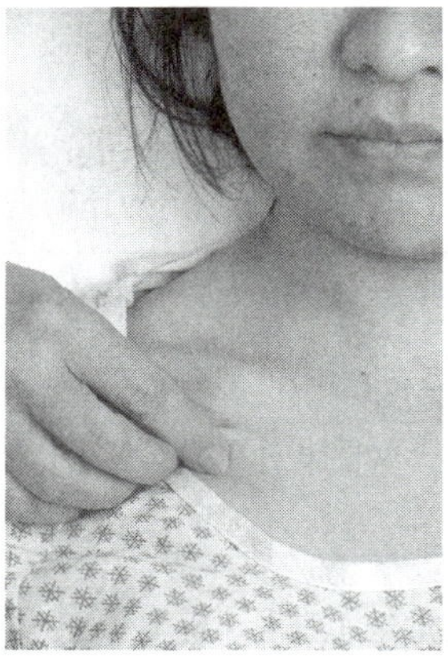

3.
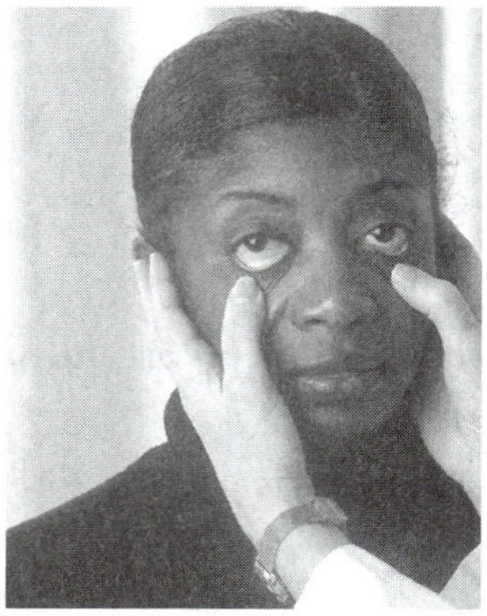

4.
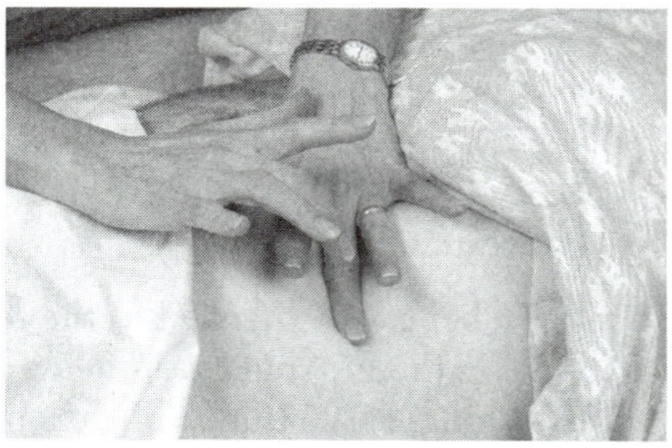

39. An order is written to keep a client NPO. Which is an important action by the nurse? **Select all that apply.**

1. _____ Allow the client to sip clear fluids with medication
2. _____ Remove the water pitcher from the client's bedside
3. _____ Give the client mouth care every 4 hours
4. _____ Measure the client's intake and output
5. _____ Permit the client to suck on ice chips

TEST-TAKING TIP: Identify the key word in the stem that directs attention to content. Identify equally plausible options.

40. The nurse is caring for a client who has a history of gastroesophageal reflux and reports burning pain in the epigastric region after eating spicy food brought to the hospital by a relative. Place an X on the location that the nurse expects the client to identify as the site of the pain.

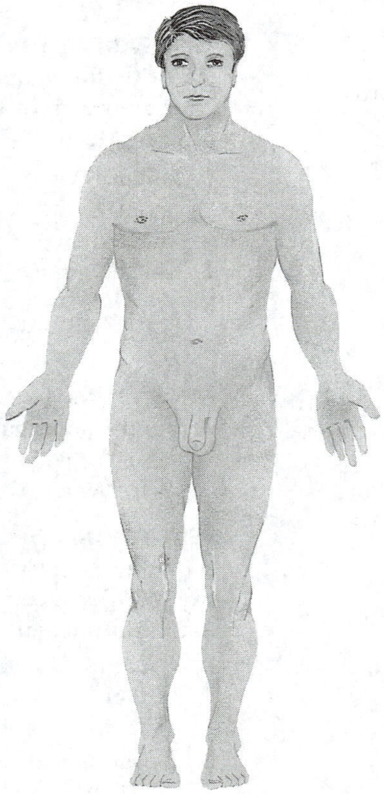

ENTS' FLUID, ELECTROLYTE, AND NUTRITIONAL ERS AND RATIONALES

1. **TEST-TAKING TIP: The word *nontherapeutic* in the stem indicates negative polarity. Option 2 is the unique option; it is the only option that tells the client to avoid something. The other options are positive statements.**
   1. Identifying low-calorie snacks helps reduce caloric intake.
   2. **The client is receiving a special diet that is carefully calculated, and all food on the tray should be eaten.**
   3. Encouraging the client to eat meals slowly allows more time for the body to feel full.
   4. Progress should be identified to provide motivation.
2.
   1. A urometer is used to measure the specific gravity of urine, not the volume of urine.
   2. **A graduate is a special container with volume markings on the side for measuring fluid; of all the options presented, it is the most accurate way to measure urine.**
   3. Bedpans are designed to collect excreta when a person cannot use a toilet or commode, not to measure urine volume.
   4. Using the markings on a urine collection bag is not accurate because the plastic that the bag is made of often stretches.
3. **TEST-TAKING TIP: The word *highest* in the stem sets a priority.**
   1. **During the first year of life, the infant grows at a faster pace than at any other developmental stage; infants double their birth weight by 6 months and triple their birth weight during the first year.**
   2. The preschool (3- to 5-year-old) child's growth rate is slower than the age presented in another option. A child gains four times the birth weight during the first 3 years of life. Then, during the 3- to 5-year (preschool) span the child gains only 7 to 12 additional pounds. This growth rate is not as spectacular as the growth rate reflected by an age group presented in another option.
   3. Although the adolescent goes through a dramatic physical growth spurt that reflects significant changes in height, weight, dentition, and skeletal and sexual development, it is not as spectacular as the growth rate reflected by individuals presented in another option.
   4. No physical growth occurs when a person is older than 65 years; different parts of the body begin to degenerate and function more slowly.
4. **TEST-TAKING TIP: Options 1 and 4 deny client feelings, concerns, or needs. The client has a right to ingest foods of different temperatures.**
   1. Clients have a right to a variety of foods, textures, and temperatures within the ordered diet.
   2. Touching the client's food will contaminate it.
   3. **Waiting for hot foods to cool slightly is the safest and most practical action; to be safe to eat, food should be warm rather than hot.**
   4. Foods should not be mixed; they should be served separately so that they retain their own flavor, texture, and temperature.
5. **TEST-TAKING TIP: Key words in the stem include *risk for impaired nutrition*. Identify priority interventions to establish and maintain normal nutrition.**
   1. **Feeding the client when this level of assistance is not necessary contributes to feelings of dependence.**
   2. Elevating the head of the bed or feeding the client in a chair aids in swallowing and reduces the risk for aspiration when eating.
   3. **A confused client does not necessarily mean they need parenteral nutrition. Patients who have trouble absorbing nutrients, have an obstruction of the bowel, or other diagnoses that prevent them from adequate food intake may need parenteral nutrition.**
   4. Supervision keeps the client focused on the task of eating while supporting independence.
   5. Although this is something the nurse may do to orient the client, the client may forget or not understand the explanation.
   6. Although family members can be helpful, it is the responsibility of the staff, not the family members, to care for the client.
6. **TEST-TAKING TIP: The word *except* in the stem indicates a negative polarity. The words *atherosclerotic plaques* and *myocardial infarction* are key words in the stem that direct attention to content.**
   1. Whole milk contains fat, which contributes to arterial plaque formation associated with atherosclerosis.

2. **Eating higher amounts of saturated fat increases the levels of low-density lipoproteins, or the bad cholesterol, that increases risks associated with heart disease.**
3. Of the options presented, legumes, such as beans, peas, and lentils, contain the least amount of cholesterol and fat and are high in protein, which is necessary for tissue regeneration.
4. Complex carbohydrates such as whole grains include a variety of plant-based foods. Brown rice, whole wheat pasta, and whole grain bread are examples of complex carbohydrates that should be incorporated into a heart-healthy diet. Complex carbohydrates decrease inflammation, which aids in decreasing plaque buildup in the arteries.

7. **TEST-TAKING TIP: The word *most* in the stem sets a priority. The words *loss* and *draining* are key words in the stem that direct attention to content.**

1. Although fluid is lost from a draining pressure injury, this does not have the most serious implication.
2. Weight loss is related to inadequate caloric intake, not the presence of a draining pressure injury.
3. **A client can lose as much as 50 g of protein daily from a draining pressure injury; this is a large percentage of the usual daily requirement of 60 g of protein for women and 70 g of protein for men. Clients with a draining pressure injury should ingest two to four times the usual daily requirements of protein to rebuild epidermal tissue.**
4. When a pressure injury is infected, the leukocyte count increases, not decreases.

8. **TEST-TAKING TIP: The words *enteral tube feeding* are key words in the stem that direct attention to content.**

1. **Tube placement should always be checked before administering any fluids, medications, or feedings. After initial placement verification with an x-ray, tube placement can be checked by the external tube length marking.**
2. This is not an initial tube feeding so an x-ray is not needed.
3. **Gastric residual should always be checked before each feeding or every 4 to 6 hours depending on facility policy. Residual volumes of more than 200 mL may cause aspiration.**
4. The nurse should perform hand hygiene and put on nonsterile gloves before preparing or handling any part of the feeding. This is not considered a sterile procedure.
5. The client should be upright during feedings. The head of the bed should be elevated 30 to 45 degrees at all times during enteral feedings and for 1 hour afterward to prevent reflux and aspiration unless it is contraindicated for the client.

9. 1. **When calories are insufficient to meet metabolic needs, the body catabolizes fat, resulting in weight loss.**
2. A thready pulse occurs with dehydration and hemorrhage. Dehydration occurs when fluid, not caloric, intake is insufficient.
3. Dependent edema occurs with decreased cardiac output.
4. Sleeping is not related directly to a decreased caloric intake; however, a client who is anemic may tire easily from an inadequate intake of iron or folic acid.

10. **TEST-TAKING TIP: The word *immediately* in the stem sets a priority.**

1. **Nursing care should be documented immediately after it is provided. There are 30 mL in each ounce; therefore, the client ingested 240 mL.**
2. Assessing skin turgor immediately after a client drinks 8 ounces of fluid is too early to evaluate the response to the fluid intake.
3. Expecting a client to void immediately after drinking 8 ounces of fluid is premature. Offering a bedpan immediately after a client drinks 8 ounces of fluids is too early to expect the client to void.
4. Mouth care usually is not required after drinking fluids; mouth care should be provided routinely on awakening, after meals, and at bedtime.

11. **TEST-TAKING TIP: The words *low-sodium* are the key words in the stem that direct attention to content.**

1. Depending on the brand, whole milk has approximately 130 mg of sodium per 8 oz.
2. **Fresh fruits contain the least amount of sodium per serving compared with the nutrients in the other options presented; most fresh fruits such as apples, pears, bananas, peaches, and cantaloupe contain less than 10 mg of sodium per serving.**

3. Depending on the brand, white bread has 55 to 225 mg of sodium per slice.
4. Fresh vegetables, such as peas, beans, carrots, broccoli, cauliflower, corn, and celery, contain approximately 40 mg of sodium per serving.

12. **TEST-TAKING TIP: Four different foods that contribute to healing are presented. If you can identify one food that most contributes to healing (eggs or orange juice), you can narrow the correct answer to two options. If you can identify one food that is least beneficial to the healing process (oatmeal or French toast), you can narrow the correct answer to two options.**

1. Although French toast contains some egg coating, which has protein, it does not contain the greatest amount of protein compared with the nutrients presented in the other options. Oatmeal does not contain protein or vitamin C.
2. Although orange juice contains vitamin C, which contributes to wound healing, oatmeal does not contain protein or vitamin C.
3. Each poached egg contains 6 to 8 g of protein, and French toast contains some egg coating; both contain the amino acids necessary for building cells and therefore for wound healing. However, neither contains vitamin C.
4. **This is the best combination of foods in the options presented. Each egg contains 6 to 8 g of protein; protein contains the amino acids necessary for building cells and therefore for wound healing. Orange juice contains vitamin C, which promotes collagen formation, enhances iron absorption, and maintains capillary wall integrity.**

13. **TEST-TAKING TIP: The word *anemia* is the key word in the stem that directs attention to content.**

1. Ascorbic acid (vitamin C) is not used to treat anemia. Ascorbic acid promotes collagen formation, enhances iron absorption, and maintains capillary wall integrity.
2. Riboflavin (vitamin B_2) is not used to treat anemia. Riboflavin functions as a coenzyme in the metabolism of carbohydrates, fats, amino acids, and alcohol.
3. **Folic acid (vitamin B_9, folate) promotes the maturation of red blood cells. When red blood cells decrease below the expected range of 4.2 million/mm^3 for women and 4.7 million/mm^3 for men, a person is considered anemic.**
4. Thiamin (vitamin B_1) is not used to treat anemia. Thiamin performs as a coenzyme in the metabolism of carbohydrates, fats, amino acids, and alcohol.

14. **TEST-TAKING TIP: The words *intralipids* and *total parenteral nutrition (TPN)* are key words in the stem that direct attention to content. Options 3 and 4 are opposites. Examine these options carefully. The word *intralipids* in the stem and in options 2 and 4 are clang associations. *TPN* in the stem and options 1 and 3 are clang associations. Unfortunately, because all four options have a clang association, the test-taking tip "identify clang associations" will not help you to arrive at the correct answer.**

1. The solutions can be run at the same time.
2. Because an intralipid solution is a concentrated source of nonprotein kilocalories, it is desirable that an infusion pump be used; however, an infusion pump does not have to be used because the solution can flow via gravity.
3. If an intralipid solution is mixed with a dextrose/amino acid solution, the fat emulsion breaks down; the solutions must not be administered through the same line.
4. **Administering intralipids through a separate IV line ensures that the intralipid solution is NOT mixed with a dextrose/amino acid solution. If they are mixed, the fat emulsion breaks down.**

15. **TEST-TAKING TIP: Four clinical findings are presented as undesirable results from an increase in the flow rate of TPN above the prescribed rate: osmotic diuresis, hypoglycemia, dumping syndrome, and electrolyte imbalance. If you can identify one response that is unrelated to an increased TPN rate, you can eliminate two distractors. If you can identify one response that is related to an increase in a TPN rate above the prescribed rate, you can narrow the correct answer to two options.**

1. Although osmotic diuresis does occur, hyperglycemia, not hypoglycemia, may result.
2. Hyperglycemia, not hypoglycemia, may result. Dumping syndrome, the rapid entry of food from the stomach into the jejunum, can occur with an intermittent enteral feeding, not TPN.

3. **The hypertonic TPN solution pulls intracellular and interstitial fluids into the intravascular compartment; the increased blood volume increases circulation to the kidneys, raising urinary output (osmotic diuresis). Potassium and sodium imbalances are common among clients receiving TPN. Therefore, TPN rates must be controlled carefully.**
4. Potassium and sodium imbalances are common among clients receiving TPN. However, dumping syndrome can occur with an intermittent enteral feeding, not TPN.

16. **TEST-TAKING TIP: The word *most* in the stem sets a priority.**
1. **Iron is essential to the formation of hemoglobin, a component of red blood cells that is lost in menstrual blood.**
2. Supplemental iron is unnecessary in growing children (1 to 13 years of age). However, infants (birth to 1 year old) who are breastfed need some iron supplementation from 4 to 12 months of age, and formula-fed infants need iron supplementation throughout the first year of life.
3. Supplemental iron is unnecessary for active adolescents.
4. Supplemental iron is unnecessary for healthy older men.

17. **TEST-TAKING TIP: The word *most* in the stem sets a priority.**
1. Although carbohydrates are important, the body can survive longer without this nutrient than it can without the nutrient presented in the correct answer.
2. Although vitamins are important, the body can survive longer without this nutrient than it can without the nutrient presented in the correct answer.
3. Although proteins are important, the body can survive longer without this nutrient than it can without the nutrient presented in the correct answer.
4. **The most basic nutrient needed is water because all body processes require an adequate fluid balance.**

18. **TEST-TAKING TIP: The word *highest* in the stem sets a priority. The word *calcium* is the key word in the stem that directs attention to content.**
1. Although postmenopausal women can benefit from an increase in calcium to prevent osteoporosis, the need is not as high as for the individuals in the correct answer.
2. School-age children do not have the highest need for calcium. An adequate intake of milk and dairy products meets minimum daily requirements of calcium for school-age children.
3. **Calcium should be increased 50% to an intake of 1.2 grams per day to provide calcium for fetal tooth and bone development; this is essential during the third trimester when fetal bones are mineralized.**
4. Working men do not have the highest need for calcium. An adequate intake of milk and dairy products meets the minimum daily requirement of calcium for working men.

19.
1. Nausea is not a common symptom of excess fluid volume.
2. Jaundice is related to impaired liver and biliary function, not excess fluid volume.
3. The opposite is true; the client will void infrequently.
4. **Fluid weighs 1 kg (2.2 lb) per liter. A client can gain 6 to 8 lb before edema can be identified through inspection.**

20. **TEST-TAKING TIP: The word *misconception* in the stem indicates negative polarity. This question is asking which option contains inaccurate information.**
1. **Vitamins are needed for the metabolism of carbohydrates, protein, and fat and are only present in food in small amounts. Everyone should take vitamins regardless of age. Infants, adolescents, pregnant or lactating women, smokers, alcoholics, chronically ill, and poor eaters should especially supplement their diet with vitamins.**
2. **Vitamins are needed for the metabolism of carbohydrates, protein, and fat. They are essential in the diet because most are not synthesized in the body or are made in insufficient quantities. Vitamins are present in foods in only small amounts and may be destroyed by light, heat, air, and during preparation—fresh foods are usually higher in vitamins than processed foods.**
3. **Food interactions can happen with vitamins. Some vitamins can affect the way the body metabolizes food and**

medicine, causing either issues with absorption or elimination. Vitamin A should be avoided if a person eats excess amounts of liver. Taking too much folic acid can hide a vitamin B_{12} deficiency.

4. **Megadoses of vitamins can cause hypervitaminosis and result in toxicity. Also, various vitamins and supplements are known to have negative consequences when they interact with prescribed medications.**
5. **A proper balance and an adequate level of essential nutrients and vitamins are important for many of our body's processes. When taken as supplements, vitamins are introduced into the body at levels that cannot be achieved by even eating the most healthy of diets.**
6. As people age, their basal metabolic rate (BMR) decreases, they lose lean body mass, and their energy expenditure decreases, decreasing their caloric needs. The need for vitamins and nutrients, however, increases, especially protein, B vitamins, and calcium.

21. TEST-TAKING TIP: The words *absorption of iron is facilitated by* are key words in the stem that direct attention to content.

1. Vitamin D is essential for adequate absorption and utilization of calcium for bone and tooth growth; it does not facilitate the absorption of iron.
2. **Ascorbic acid (vitamin C) helps to change dietary iron to a form that can be absorbed by the body.**
3. Vitamin A is essential for the growth and maintenance of epithelial tissue, maintenance of night vision, and promotion of resistance to infection; it does not facilitate the absorption of iron.
4. Vitamin K is essential for the formation of prothrombin, which prevents bleeding; it does not facilitate the absorption of iron.

22. TEST-TAKING TIP: The word *cancer* in both the stem and option 4 is a clang association.

1. With cancer, catabolism exceeds anabolism.
2. The ability to absorb nutrients is not impaired with lung cancer. The absorption of nutrients may be impaired with cancer of the gastrointestinal system.
3. The by-products of cell breakdown, not cell division, cause a negative nitrogen balance.
4. **The energy required to support the rapid growth of cancerous cells increases the metabolic demands 1.5 to 2 times the resting energy expenditure.**

23. TEST-TAKING TIP: The words *full and bounding* are key words in the stem that direct attention to content.

1. Reducing the flow rate of a client's IV fluids is a dependent function of the nurse and requires a prescription from the primary health-care provider. If the IV flow rate is excessive, it will cause a full, bounding pulse related to hypervolemia. If the full, bounding pulse is caused by an excessive flow rate of the IV fluids, the nurse should secure a prescription from the primary health-care provider to change the flow rate.
2. The specific gravity of urine reflects the concentrating ability of the kidneys, not the cardiovascular system.
3. A full, bounding pulse is not related to hyperglycemia or hypoglycemia; a weak, thready pulse is a late sign of diabetic ketoacidosis.
4. A full, bounding pulse may indicate hypervolemia; in this compromised client, lowering the head of the bed may impede respirations and is therefore contraindicated.
5. **The blood pressure (BP) reading reflects the pressure within the arteries during the contraction of the ventricles of the heart (systolic BP) and between the contractions of the heart (diastolic BP). Both the systolic and diastolic results will be increased when the intravascular volume is increased. A full, bounding pulse indicates an increase in the intravascular volume.**

24. TEST-TAKING TIP: The word *nauseated* is the key word in the stem that directs attention to content.

1. **These herbal teas have natural antinausea properties such as relaxing smooth muscles of the stomach, which has a calming effect on the digestive system. However, herbs have medicinal properties that may interact with prescribed medications; therefore, the nurse should seek a prescription for an herbal tea before encouraging the client to ingest it.**
2. **The BRAT (bananas, rice, applesauce, and toast) diet is bland, low in fiber,**

and easy to digest and is less likely to precipitate nausea.

3. **Extremely hot or cold foods can precipitate nausea.**
4. **Small quantities of food that are offered frequently establish small, realistic goals for the client without being overwhelming.**
5. Supplements may interfere with the intake of regularly scheduled meals.
6. **Fluids with meals can excessively fill the stomach, which can precipitate nausea.**

25. One ounce is equal to 30 mL. Foods that require minimal digestion and leave minimal residue are considered liquids in a hospital. This includes clear broth, coffee, tea, clear fruit juices, gelatin, and popsicles.

Cranberry juice 9 oz × 30 mL = 270 mL
Jell-O 4 oz × 30 mL = 120 mL
Popsicle 4 oz × 30 mL = 120 mL
270 mL + 120 mL + 120 mL = 510 mL of liquid intake

26. **TEST-TAKING TIP: The words *vitamin K deficiency* are key words in the stem that direct attention to content. Options 1, 2, 3, and 6 all have to do with bleeding and are equally plausible. Options 4 and 5 have nothing to do with bleeding. Options 1, 2, 3, and 6 are either all correct answers or they are all incorrect answers.**

1. **Anemia can be caused by bleeding that occurs with vitamin K deficiency. Vitamin K is essential for prothrombin formation and blood clotting; a vitamin K deficiency can prolong clotting time resulting in bleeding.**
2. **Bruising (ecchymosis) is caused by blood leaking from microscopic tears in the capillaries under the skin due to trauma. Bruising easily is a common sign of vitamin K deficiency. Vitamin K is essential for prothrombin formation and blood clotting; a vitamin K deficiency can lead to a prolonged clotting time resulting in bleeding.**
3. **Tarry stools indicate bleeding in the upper gastrointestinal tract. Vitamin K is essential for prothrombin formation and blood clotting; when a client is deficient in vitamin K, prolonged clotting time can result in bleeding.**
4. Vitamin K deficiency is unrelated to cardiac dysrhythmias. A deficiency of vitamin B_1 (thiamin) can result in tachycardia; deficiencies in calcium, magnesium, and potassium also can contribute to cardiac problems.
5. A deficiency in vitamin K does not contribute to the occurrence of infection, which will cause an increase in temperature. Vitamins A and C help build resistance to infection.
6. **Vitamin K is essential for prothrombin formation and blood clotting. When deficient in vitamin K, a prolonged clotting time can lead to bleeding. A client who has a deficiency in vitamin K and who is experiencing a heavy menstrual flow is at risk for excessive bleeding.**

27. **Answer: 6, 5, 2, 4, 1, 3**

6. **Administering a tube feeding is a dependent function of the nurse. The primary health-care provider's prescription must be verified.**
5. **The procedure should be explained to the client before equipment is brought to the bedside. Bringing equipment to the bedside without a prior explanation may cause anxiety.**
2. **Hand hygiene (e.g., washing with soap and water or using an alcohol-based gel) removes microorganisms from the nurse's skin that may contaminate clean equipment.**
4. **Collecting all equipment at the same time avoids the need to interrupt the procedure to collect forgotten equipment.**
1. **Privacy should be provided (e.g., pulling the curtain, closing the door) to maintain client confidentiality and emotional comfort. A tube feeding is an invasive procedure.**
3. **Raising the head of the bed helps to keep the formula in the stomach via gravity; it limits the risks of formula passing into the esophagus and trachea, resulting in aspiration.**

28. **TEST-TAKING TIP: The words *left hemiparesis* are the key words in the stem that direct attention to content. The word *feeding* in the stem and in option 4 is a clang association.**

1. This may be unsafe and possibly unreasonable because the client has reduced ability to move the muscles necessary for chewing on one side of the face. A mechanical soft diet may be necessary.
2. This action may be unsafe because the facial muscles on the client's left side are weak. Food should be placed in the right

side of the client's mouth. The facial muscles on the client's right side are stronger than the facial muscles on the client's left side.
3. Fluids with each mouthful will increase the risk of aspiration; fluid is more difficult to control than food when swallowing.
4. **Elevating the head of the bed reduces the risk of aspiration.**
5. **Allowing time to empty the mouth of food between spoonfuls minimizes food buildup in the mouth; also it does not rush the client.**

29. 1. **The electrocardiogram tracing indicates hyperkalemia (e.g., peaked T waves, depressed ST segments, and shortened QT intervals). The client's clinical responses are signs of hyperkalemia (e.g., irregular pulse, diarrhea, irritability, and confusion). The client's serum potassium level indicates hyperkalemia because 6.9 mEq/dL is more than the expected value of 3.5 to 5 mEq/dL. The client is experiencing medication-induced hyperkalemia, which can cause a life-threatening cardiac dysrhythmia. Initiating the rapid response team is the priority.**
2. If the nurse discontinues the IV infusion, IV access will not be available for emergency medications. After initiating the first action, which has priority, the nurse should replace the IV bag that is hanging with 0.9% sodium chloride as the second action.
3. Removing milk from the client's lunch tray is unnecessary. The client's total serum calcium level is within the expected range of 8.5 to 10.5 mg/dL.
4. Encouraging the client to use salt to season food on the lunch tray is unnecessary. The client's serum sodium level is within the expected range of 135 to 145 mEq/L.

30. **TEST-TAKING TIP: The words *additional teaching is necessary* in the stem indicate negative polarity. This question is asking which food or drink contains the least amount of potassium.**
1. **One cup (one package) of beef bouillon contains approximately 27 mg of potassium and is not a good choice because it is low in potassium. Beef bouillon is high in sodium.**
2. One cup of orange juice is a good choice because it contains approximately 475 mg of potassium.
3. **A poached egg contains approximately 65 mg of potassium and is not a good choice because it is low in potassium.**
4. **One cup of tea contains approximately 35 mg of potassium and is not a good choice because it is low in potassium.**
5. One banana is a good choice because it contains approximately 450 mg of potassium.
6. One ounce ($\frac{1}{8}$ cup) of raisins is a good choice because it contains approximately 200 mg of potassium.

31. **TEST-TAKING TIP: The words *full-liquid diet* are key words in the stem that direct attention to content.**
1. **Ice cream changes its state from a solid to a liquid at room temperature and is permitted on a full-liquid diet.**
2. **Prune juice is a fluid and is permitted on a full-liquid diet.**
3. Cream of wheat is considered solid food and is not permitted on a full-liquid diet.
4. Mashed potatoes are considered solid food and are not permitted on a full-liquid diet.
5. **Raspberry gelatin changes its state from a solid to a liquid at room temperature and is permitted on a full-liquid diet.**

32. Answer: 250 mL/hr
Infusion pumps are set at milliliters per hour.
1000 mL ÷ 4 hr = 250 mL/hr

33. 1. The bladder still fills to the client's usual capacity before there is a perceived need to void. Passing small amounts of urine at each voiding is associated with urinary retention with overflow.
2. An atonic bladder is caused by a neurological problem; it is a loss of the sensation of fullness that leads to distention from overfilling.
3. **As fluid in the intravascular compartment decreases, fluid is pulled from the intracellular and interstitial compartments in an attempt to maintain cardiac output.**
4. Reduced fluid intake produces a concentrated urine with a specific gravity greater than 1.030. The expected range for urine specific gravity is 1.001 to 1.029.
5. **The heart rate increases when hypovolemia occurs in an attempt to increase cardiac output.**

34. 1. **The client is receiving esomeprazole (Nexium®) and magnesium/aluminum hydroxide (Mylanta®) for upper gastrointestinal issues. The client's clinical manifestations indicate**

gastroesophageal reflux disease. The respiratory signs and symptoms are most likely due to respiratory aspiration of gastric contents, causing mucosal irritation and inflammation and the resulting cough, sore throat, and hoarseness. A left side-lying position with the head slightly elevated uses gravity to keep gastric contents in the stomach as well as facilitate esophageal emptying along the normal left to right anatomic curve into the stomach. In a home, the head of the bed can be raised on 4- to 6-inch blocks. Gravity helps to keep gastric contents in the stomach when sleeping.

2. The client's responses indicate gastroesophageal reflux disease. The prone position increases intraabdominal pressure, which increases the risk of gastroesophageal reflux and aspiration of gastric contents.
3. The client's responses indicate gastroesophageal reflux disease. The semi-prone position will increase intraabdominal pressure, which will increase the risk of gastroesophageal reflux and aspiration of gastric contents.
4. The client's responses indicate gastroesophageal reflux disease. The supine position allows gastric contents to reflux easily into the esophagus and pharynx, placing the client at risk for aspiration.

35. TEST-TAKING TIP: The word *hyponatremia* is the key word in the stem that directs attention to content.

1. Thirst is a clinical indicator of hypernatremia, which is not associated with an IV fluid overload.
2. **An IV fluid overload precipitates hyponatremia. Hyponatremia can cause a headache because of the central nervous system's response to a low level of sodium in the brain. Sodium is an integral component of the sodium-potassium pump.**
3. **An IV fluid overload precipitates hyponatremia. Hyponatremia can cause muscle weakness because of the neuromuscular system's response to a low level of sodium. Sodium is an integral component of the sodium-potassium pump.**
4. An increased temperature is a clinical indicator of hypernatremia, which is not associated with an IV fluid overload.
5. Dry mucous membranes are a clinical indicator of hypernatremia, which is not associated with an IV fluid overload.

36.
1. Thirst is associated with hypernatremia, which is not this client's clinical situation as indicated by the ECG tracing. In addition, hypernatremia is associated with an elevated temperature, tachycardia, elevated blood pressure, nausea and vomiting, increased reflexes, restlessness, and seizures.
2. Tremors are associated with hyponatremia, which is not this client's clinical situation, as indicated by the ECG tracing. In addition, hyponatremia is associated with anorexia, nausea, vomiting, headache, lethargy, nonelastic skin turgor, confusion, and seizures as a result of increased intracranial pressure.
3. **A weak, rapid pulse is associated with hypokalemia, which is confirmed by the ECG tracing; with hypokalemia, there is ST-segment depression, a flattened T wave, and the presence of a U wave. In addition to the characteristic ECG tracing, a weak, rapid pulse, muscle weakness, and fatigue, a client with hypokalemia may experience nausea and vomiting, decreased gastrointestinal motility, decreased reflexes, abdominal distention, and dysrhythmias. Excessive laxative use causes diarrhea, which can deplete the body's potassium.**

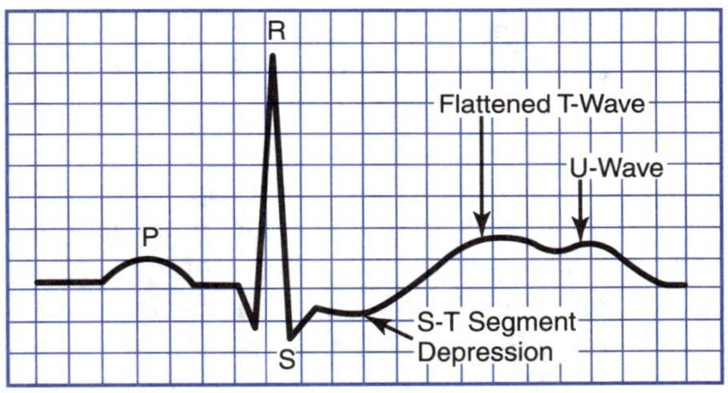

4. Severe constipation is associated with hypercalcemia, which is not this client's clinical situation as indicated by the ECG tracing. In addition, hypercalcemia is associated with deep bone pain, flank pain from renal calculi, vomiting, decreased reflexes, increased urine calcium, osteoporosis, increased hyperparathyroid hormone (PTH) levels, and decreased PTH levels with malignancy.

37. TEST-TAKING TIP: The words *aging* and *nutritional status* are key words in the stem that direct attention to content. The words *older adults* in the stem and in option 3 are clang associations.

1. **Aging skin is thinner and less able to produce vitamin D. This in turn limits the body's ability to absorb calcium. Vitamin D and calcium are necessary to prevent bone loss associated with aging.**
2. **Saliva production decreases by approximately 66% when one ages. Salivary ptyalin decreases, interfering with the breakdown of starches.**
3. **The need for kilocalories decreases because of a lower metabolic rate and reduction in physical activity associated with older adults.**
4. **Practically all body systems decline slightly with aging, including the senses. The sense of smell is interrelated to the sense of taste.**
5. **Taste perception decreases because of atrophy of the taste buds; sweet and salty tastes are lost first.**

38. 1. In this photograph, the nurse is palpating the client's dorsalis pedis pulse. This assessment provides information about the client's distal arterial circulation, not hydration status.
2. **In this photograph, the nurse is testing the client's skin turgor. The nurse gently pinches the client's skin and assesses how long it takes to return to its prepinched state. If it takes more than several seconds to return to its prepinched state (tenting), the client may be dehydrated.**
3. In this photograph, the nurse is assessing the client's conjunctiva for a blue discoloration (cyanosis—blue discoloration from excessive deoxyhemoglobin in the blood) or yellow discoloration (jaundice—yellow discoloration from deposition of bile pigments). Normally, the conjunctiva are pink. This assessment does not elicit information about a client's hydration status.
4. In this photograph, the nurse is performing indirect palpation. This technique elicits a sound when one of the nurse's fingers strikes another finger positioned over a site. The sound elicited may indicate that air, fluid, or solid tissue is under the area that is being tapped. This assessment does not elicit information about a client's hydration status.

39. TEST-TAKING TIP: ***NPO*** **is the key term in the stem that directs attention to content. Options 1 and 5 are equally plausible. Both are either correct answers or incorrect answers.**

1. Fluids of any kind are contraindicated when a client is NPO; *NPO* means *nil per os,* which means "nothing by mouth."
2. **Removing the water pitcher from the client's bedside prevents the client from accidentally drinking fluid.**
3. **When people are NPO, they tend to have dry mucous membranes and thick secretions on the tongue and gums; mouth care cleans the oral cavity.**
4. **A client who is NPO generally is receiving IV fluids. The intake and output should be measured when a client is NPO to ensure that the client is receiving adequate fluid intake via the IV route and is in fluid balance.**
5. Ice chips are considered fluids; fluids of any kind are contraindicated when a client is NPO. *NPO (nil per os)* means "nothing by mouth."

40. The epigastric region is over the stomach, liver, pancreas, and right and left kidneys. A client who has burning pain indicative of gastroesophageal reflux generally will point to the epigastric region as the site of the pain, indicated by the X.

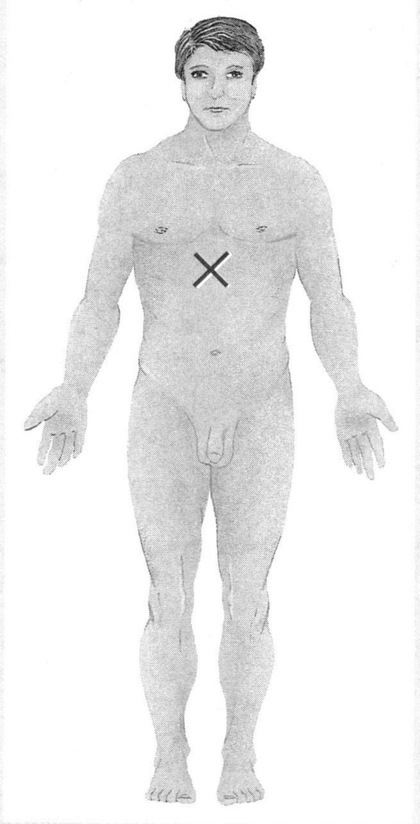

MEETING CLIENTS' ELIMINATION NEEDS

This section includes questions related to intestinal and urinary elimination. Topics associated with intestinal elimination include incontinence, constipation, diarrhea, enemas, bowel retraining, and medications. Questions also focus on client needs associated with urinary elimination and on topics such as incontinence, bladder retraining, toileting, and external and indwelling urinary catheters.

QUESTIONS

1. The UAP transfers the client safely from the bed to the bedside commode. The UAP reports to the nurse that the client had a small, dark, tarry bowel movement. The nurse understands that this is a common finding in which diagnosis?
   1. Lower gastrointestinal bleeding
   2. Gastrointestinal infection
   3. Upper gastrointestinal bleeding
   4. Pancreatic dysfunction

   TEST-TAKING TIP: Identify the key words in the stem that direct attention to content.

2. A client scheduled for bowel surgery asks the nurse why a tap-water enema was ordered. Which information is important for the nurse to include in a response to the client's question?
   1. Minimizes intestinal gas
   2. Cleanses the bowel of stool
   3. Reduces abdominal distention
   4. Decreases the loss of electrolytes

   TEST-TAKING TIP: Identify the key word in the stem that directs attention to content. Identify equally plausible options. Identify the clang association.

3. A client living with advanced Alzheimer's disease asks for assistance ambulating to the toilet. The client was assisted to the toilet 30 minutes earlier. Which of the following is the nurse's most appropriate action?
   1. Remind the client that they just returned from the toilet
   2. Obtain an order to insert a Foley catheter
   3. Explain that clients are only assisted to the toilet once per hour
   4. Assist the client to the bathroom or delegate this task

   TEST-TAKING TIP: Identify words that set a priority. Identify options that deny client feelings, concerns, or needs. Identify the client-centered option. Identify specific determiners.

4. The nurse is assessing a client for the presence of dysuria. Which question should the nurse ask the client?
   1. "Does pain or burning occur when you urinate?"
   2. "Can you start and stop the flow of urine with ease?"
   3. "Do you pass a little urine when you cough or sneeze?"
   4. "Are you able to empty your bladder fully each time you void?"

5. The nurse is caring for four clients with gastrointestinal diagnoses. Which of the following clients is at greatest risk for constipation?
   1. The client receiving metronidazole to treat a *Clostridium difficile* infection
   2. The client preparing to discharge after an uncomplicated laparoscopic appendectomy
   3. The older adult client with an NPO order and poorly controlled pain
   4. The older adult client receiving IV hydration and being treated for ulcerative colitis

   TEST-TAKING TIP: Identify words in the stem that set a priority.

6. The nurse is caring for a client who is constipated and unable to tolerate a large volume of enema solution. Which solution should the nurse anticipate that the primary health-care provider will prescribe?
   1. Hypertonic fluid
   2. Normal saline
   3. Soapy water
   4. Tap water

   TEST-TAKING TIP: Identify the key words in the stem that direct attention to content.

7. In which position should a nurse place a client when administering an enema?
   1. Dorsal recumbent
   2. Right lateral
   3. Back lying
   4. Left semi-prone

   TEST-TAKING TIP: Identify equally plausible options. Identify opposites in options.

8. The nurse is teaching a client with a newly formed colostomy about dietary changes that reduce gas production. Which of the following is an appropriate recommendation?
   1. Consume milk with each meal
   2. Increase the consumption of green vegetables
   3. Take over-the-counter fish or cod liver oil
   4. Avoid carbonated beverages

   TEST-TAKING TIP: Identify words that indicate negative polarity and identify opposites in options.

9. An 80-year-old female client states, "I'm a bit embarrassed to need help from someone else to go to the bathroom—especially a handsome young man." What is the nurse's **best** action?
   1. Ignore the comment and assist the client
   2. Offer to find a female nurse or UAP to assist
   3. Explain that assistance walking to the toilet promotes safety
   4. Explain that the client doesn't need to feel embarrassed

   TEST-TAKING TIP: Identify solutions that deny client needs.

10. The nurse is caring for a client diagnosed with stress incontinence. Which is the common underlying cause of stress incontinence that the nurse should consider when caring for this client?
    1. Response to a specific volume of urine in the bladder
    2. Results from an increase in intraabdominal pressure
    3. Results from a urinary tract infection
    4. Response to an emotional strain

    TEST-TAKING TIP: Identify the key words in the stem that direct attention to content.

11. The nurse is planning to insert a rectal tube to manage diarrhea in a critically ill client. In what order does the nurse complete the following activities? Place the following procedure steps in order.
    1. Position the client on the left side
    2. Obtain vital signs, auscultate bowel sounds, and assess tissue integrity
    3. Perform peri-care
    4. Insert the lubricated rectal tube
    5. Remove the rectal tube

    Answer: ____________

    TEST-TAKING TIP: Use the If-Then technique to order the steps according to the nursing process.

12. Which aspect of urine should the nurse evaluate when assessing the patency of a urinary retention (Foley) catheter?
 1. Color
 2. Clarity
 3. Volume
 4. Constituents

TEST-TAKING TIP: Identify the key word in the stem that directs attention to content. Identify the unique option.

13. Which should the nurse anticipate as the **most** common concern of clients who have a colostomy?
 1. Maintenance of skin integrity
 2. Frequency of defecation
 3. Consistency of feces
 4. Presence of odor

TEST-TAKING TIP: Identify the word in the stem that sets a priority. Identify the unique option.

14. The nurse is caring for a neonate and notes sticky, greenish-black stools that are becoming more yellow in color with each bowel movement. What is the nurse's most appropriate action?
 1. Continue to monitor and document the stools
 2. Increase the water mixed into the formula
 3. Notify the provider
 4. Ask the infant's breastfeeding mother about dietary patterns

TEST-TAKING TIP: Identify words in the stem that set a priority. Identify opposites in options.

15. A culture and sensitivity test of a client's urine is ordered. To ensure accurate results of the urine culture and sensitivity test, the nurse should:
 1. obtain two urine specimens.
 2. collect a midstream urine sample.
 3. use only the first urine voided in the morning.
 4. use a 24-hour urine collection schedule.

TEST-TAKING TIP: Identify key words in the stem that direct attention to content. Identify the option with a specific determiner.

16. A 750-mL tap-water enema is ordered for a client. Which should the nurse do to promote acceptance of the volume ordered? **Select all that apply.**
 1. _____ Interrupt the flow of fluid when the client has an intestinal spasm
 2. _____ Encourage the client to take slow, deep breaths
 3. _____ Place the client in the left lateral position
 4. _____ Instill the fluid at body temperature
 5. _____ Administer the fluid slowly

17. The nurse on the previous shift instructed the client to increase fiber in the diet to lower the risk for constipation. While ordering lunch, the client asks which foods on the menu are high in fiber. The nurse correctly identifies which of the following as foods high in fiber? **Select all that apply.**
 1. _____ Chicken
 2. _____ Broccoli
 3. _____ Legumes
 4. _____ Fresh fruit
 5. _____ Plain yogurt
 6. _____ Whole-grain bread

TEST-TAKING TIP: Identify the key word in the stem that directs attention to content.

18. The nurse is caring for a client who has to go home with an indwelling urinary catheter (Foley catheter). Which should the nurse teach the client about the urine collection system? **Select all that apply.**
    1. _____ Apply an antiseptic ointment to the insertion site daily.
    2. _____ Prevent dependent loops in the tubing.
    3. _____ Keep it below the level of the pelvis.
    4. _____ Carry it at waist level when walking.
    5. _____ Change it at least once a week.
    6. _____ Clamp it when out of bed.

19. The nurse is applying a condom catheter (external catheter) after perineal care for an uncircumcised client. Which should the nurse do? **Select all that apply.**
    1. _____ Replace the foreskin over the glans
    2. _____ Secure the condom directly behind the glans
    3. _____ Retract the foreskin behind the head of the glans
    4. _____ Dry the shaft of the penis and the area around the glans
    5. _____ Leave an inch space between the condom sheath and the tip of the glans

TEST-TAKING TIP: Identify key words in the stem that direct attention to content. Identify opposites in options.

20. The nurse is caring for a client who has an order for insertion of a catheter for continuous bladder irrigation. Identify the catheter that should be inserted by the nurse.

1. 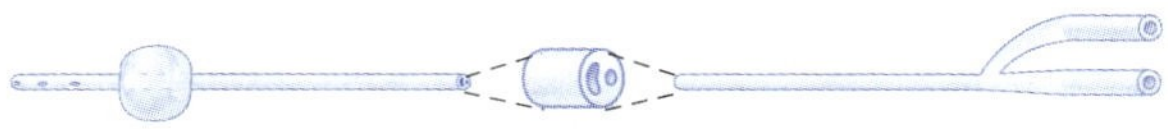

2. 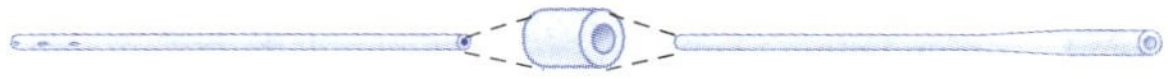

3. 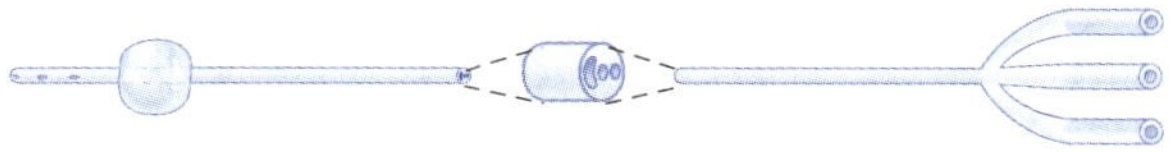

21. A urinary retention catheter is prescribed for a female client. Place an arrow that points to the area where a urinary retention catheter should be inserted.

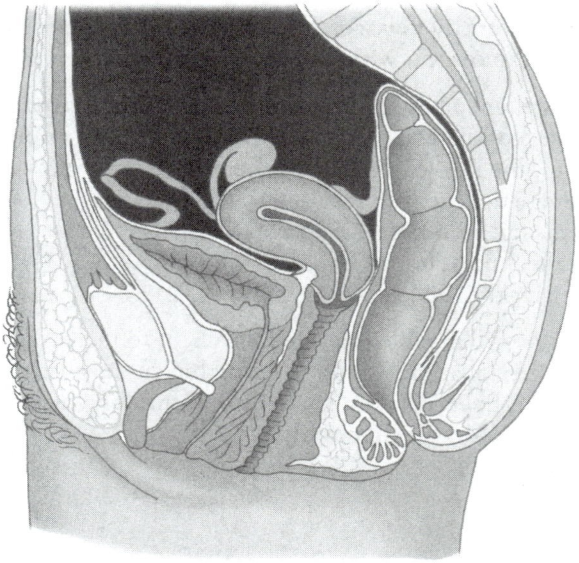

22. A primary health-care provider prescribes 400 mg of ciprofloxacin via intravenous piggyback (IVPB) method to a client with urosepsis. The medication is delivered to the nursing unit from the pharmacy in 250 mL 5% dextrose. To administer this IVPB over 1 hour, at what rate should the nurse set the IV pump? **Record your answer using one decimal place.**

Answer: ___________ mL/hr

23. A client has a health history of an enlarged prostate. The nurse makes the inference that the client is experiencing urinary retention. Which client clinical manifestation **supports** this inference? **Select all that apply.**
1. _____ Painful micturition
2. _____ Concentrated urine
3. _____ Abdominal distention
4. _____ Functional incontinence
5. _____ Frequent urination of small amounts

24. The nurse is providing education to a mother of a 4-year-old experiencing nocturnal enuresis. Which of the following are appropriate education points for managing nocturnal enuresis? **Select all that apply.**
1. _____ Nocturnal enuresis will not go away on its own, intervention is necessary
2. _____ Increase fluid intake to prevent dehydration
3. _____ Cover the child's mattress with a plastic-backed pad
4. _____ A thorough medical evaluation to rule out disease processes is required
5. _____ Bathe the child in the morning

25. The nurse is caring for a client who had general anesthesia for surgery 6 hours ago. Place an X over the area of the abdomen that the nurse should palpate when determining whether the urinary bladder is distended with urine.

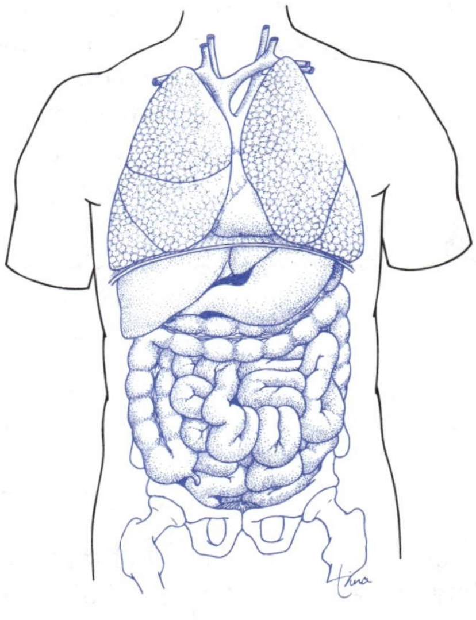

26. The nurse is interviewing an older adult client who came to the health clinic reporting frequent constipation. Which assessment findings increase the risk for constipation in the older adult client? **Select all that apply.**
1. _____ Limited mobility r/t arthritic pain
2. _____ Consumption of milk with every meal
3. _____ Consumption of coffee and soda with every meal
4. _____ Use of antacids to treat heartburn
5. _____ Use of oral iron supplements to treat anemia

TEST-TAKING TIP: Identify the words in the stem that direct attention to content.

27. The nurse is performing the skill shown in the photograph. Which actions are appropriate when performing this skill? **Select all that apply.**

1. _____ Don sterile gloves
2. _____ Cleanse the port with an alcohol swab for 15 seconds
3. _____ Use a needleless connector to collect a urine sample
4. _____ Insert a needle into the port to collect a urine sample
5. _____ Collect a sample from the drainage collection bag

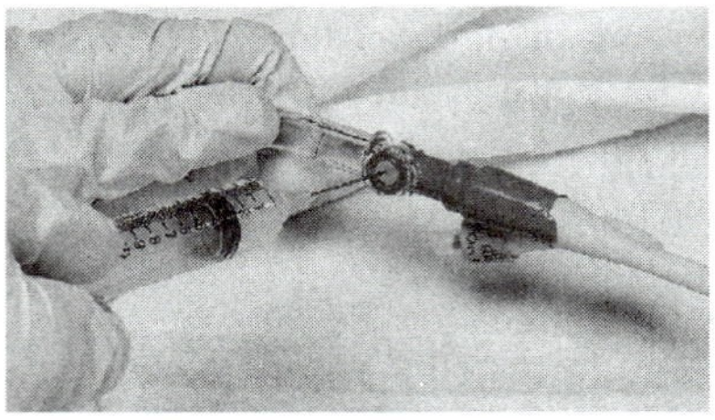

28. Which should the nurse consider when planning for the bowel elimination needs of a client? **Select all that apply.**

1. _____ Peristalsis increases after ingestion of food.
2. _____ Emotional stress initially decreases peristalsis.
3. _____ People taking opioid analgesics may experience constipation.
4. _____ Intrathoracic pressure decreases with straining during defecation.
5. _____ Daytime control of feces generally is achieved by two and a half years of age.

29. A home health nurse is interviewing a client who has been receiving physical therapy in the home because of muscular weakness of the left upper arm and left leg (hemiparesis) resulting from a brain attack (cerebrovascular accident, stroke). The nurse obtains the client's vital signs, collects data from the client, and reviews the client's diet. Which is the **primary** nursing intervention for this client?

1. Discuss with the client the importance of performing more exercise.
2. Teach the client about foods that can result in constipation.
3. Refer the client to the primary health-care provider.
4. Encourage the client to drink more fluids.

CLIENT'S CLINICAL RECORD

Vital Signs

Temperature: 97.8°F, oral
Pulse: 90 beats/min, regular rhythm
Respirations: 22 breaths/min, unlabored
Blood pressure: 142/90 mm Hg

Client Interview

Client states that physical therapy can be tiring at times but that the exercises are conscientiously carried out several times a day in addition to a half-mile walk daily. Reports feeling bloated and has to strain to have a bowel movement about twice a week. States voiding sufficient quantities of yellow urine 3 to 4 times a day.

Dietary History

Usually eats yogurt and a banana for breakfast, a cheese omelet for lunch, and meat with rice and one vegetable for dinner. Client has a chocolate candy bar or chocolate ice cream for dessert with dinner. Client states, "I eat to live. I do not live to eat." Consumes approximately 10 cups of fluid a day, mostly water.

30. A client's urinary retention catheter collection bag must be emptied at the end of a shift. The nurse washes the hands with soap and water and dons clean gloves. Place the following steps in the order in which they should be performed.
1. Drain urine in the urinary tubing into the bag.
2. Calculate the volume of urine and discard the urine into the toilet.
3. Reclamp the drainage spout just as the last of the urine exits the collection bag.
4. Unclamp the drainage spout and direct the flow of urine into the measuring device.
5. Place a calibrated container on a waterproof barrier on the floor just under the collection bag.
6. Wipe the drainage spout with an alcohol swab and replace it into the slot on the collection bag.

Answer: ____________

31. Which is a natural physiological function of the body that helps prevent infection? **Select all that apply.**
1. _____ Low pH of urine
2. _____ Increased body temperature
3. _____ Flushing action of urine flow
4. _____ High pH of gastric secretions
5. _____ Presence of sebum on the skin

TEST-TAKING TIP: Identify key words in the stem that direct attention to content.

32. A client experiencing urinary retention requires the insertion of the catheter shown in the illustration. Which is an **essential** nursing action associated with the use of this urinary catheter?

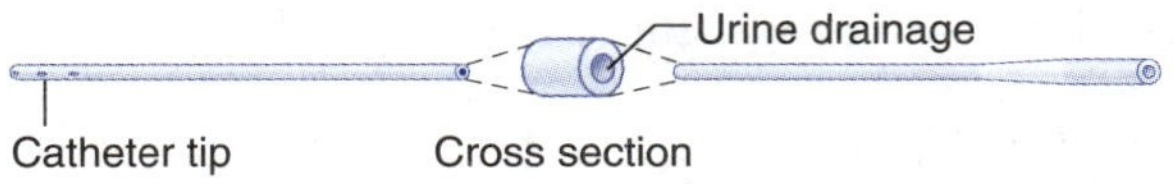

1. Use a sterile catheter kit when inserting the catheter.
2. Empty the collection bag at the end of each shift.
3. Prevent dependent loops in the collection tubing.
4. Secure the catheter to the client's thigh.

TEST-TAKING TIP: Identify the word in the stem that sets a priority. Identify the clang associations.

33. Which action should the nurse include in all bladder-retraining programs? **Select all that apply.**
1. _____ Toilet the client every 2 hours.
2. _____ Provide 3000 mL of fluids a day.
3. _____ Discuss adult incontinence underwear.
4. _____ Have the client void after eating a meal.
5. _____ Encourage the client to urinate first thing in the morning.

TEST-TAKING TIP: Identify key words in the stem that direct attention to content. Identify the option with a specific determiner.

34. A colostomy can be surgically created in a variety of places along the length of the large intestine. Which colostomy site will result in stool that is pasty in consistency?

1. 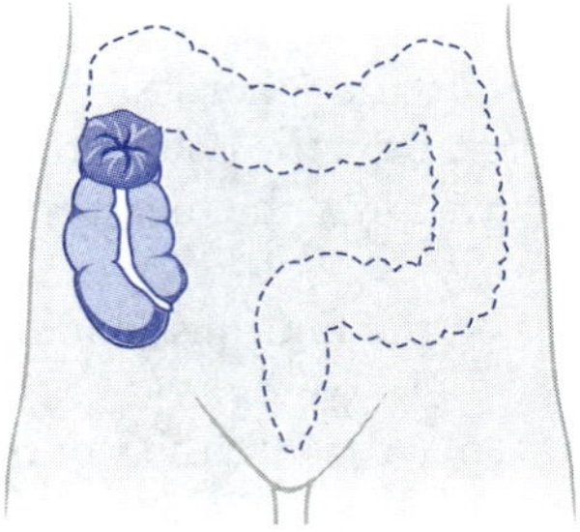

2. 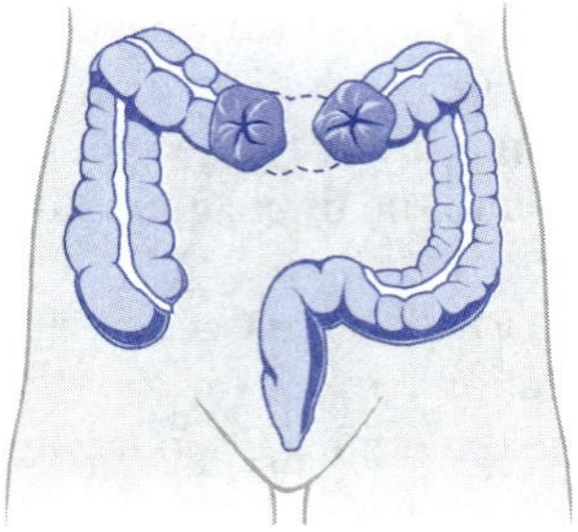

3. 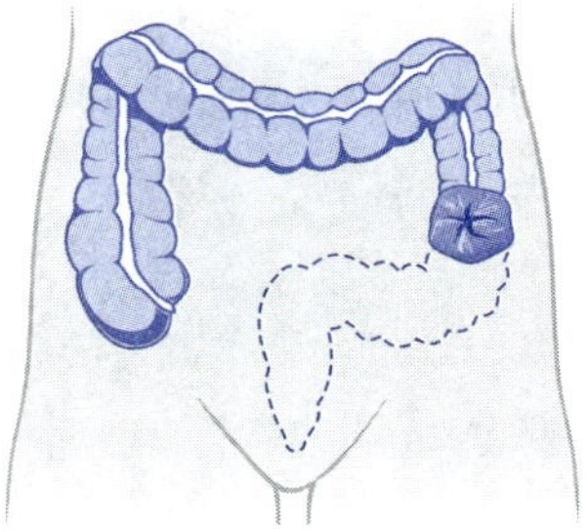

4. 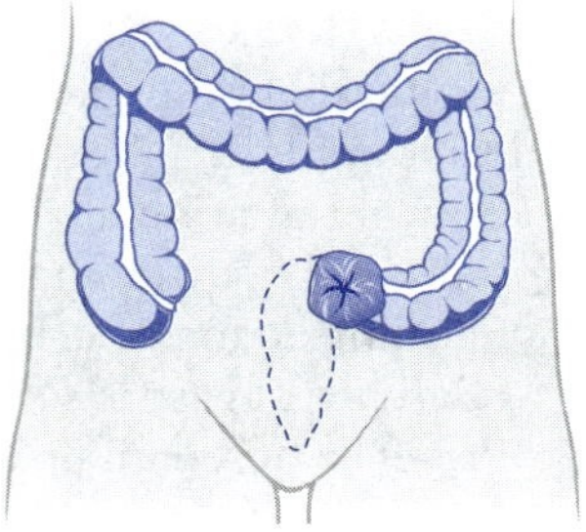

35. The nurse is caring for a client receiving continuous bladder irrigation after prostate surgery. At the completion of a 12-hour shift, the client received a total of 1000 mL of fluid via the oral route, 900 mL of fluid via the IV route, and 4050 mL of bladder irrigant. The volume of fluid emptied from the urinary collection bag totaled 5600 mL. Which was the actual urine output for the 12 hours the nurse cared for the client? **Record your answer using a whole number.**

Answer: __________ **mL**

1. **TEST-TAKING TIP: The words *common finding* in the stem direct attention to content.**
   1. Bright red stools indicate bleeding in the lower gastrointestinal tract.
   2. An infection in the gastrointestinal tract may manifest as orange or green mucoid stools.
   3. **Black (tarry) stools indicate upper gastrointestinal bleeding. Enzymes acting on the blood turn it black. In addition, iron supplements, excessive intake of red meat, and dark green vegetables can cause greenish-black stools.**
   4. Pancreatic dysfunction may manifest as pale, bulky, and foul-smelling stools.

2. **TEST-TAKING TIP: The word *bowel* is the key word in the stem that directs attention to content because surgeons performing abdominal surgery generally prefer that the bowel be free of stool. Options 1 and 3 are equally plausible because abdominal distention is often caused by intestinal gas. The word *bowel* in the stem and in option 2 is a clang association.**
   1. A Harris drip (Harris flush), not a tap-water enema, helps evacuate intestinal gas.
   2. **A tap-water enema introduces hypotonic fluid into the intestinal tract; distention and pressure against the intestinal mucosa increase peristalsis and evacuation of stool.**
   3. Reducing intestinal gas is a secondary gain because flatus and stool are evacuated along with the enema solution.
   4. A tap-water enema increases, not decreases, loss of electrolytes because it is a hypotonic solution.

3. **TEST-TAKING TIP: The words *most appropriate* set a priority in the stem. Options 1 and 3 deny the client's need to use the toilet and include the determiners *just* and *only*. Option 2 delays the client's immediate needs. Option 4 is client-centered.**
   1. Reminding a client that they recently returned from the toilet does not meet their basic physiological toileting needs. A client living with Alzheimer's disease may be unaware that they used the toilet 30 minutes prior.
   2. Inserting a Foley catheter is inappropriate. It increases the risk for urinary tract infection and does not address the client's immediate needs.
   3. Clients should be assisted to the toilet when they need to use the toilet. Although it is routine practice to offer toileting once per hour, clients may require more frequent toileting.
   4. **Assisting the client to the toilet or delegating the task to appropriate personnel who are available supports meeting the client's basic physiological needs. This is the most appropriate action.**

4. 1. **The question in option 1 relates to painful or difficult urination (dysuria). This is most often caused by bladder or urethral inflammation or trauma.**
   2. The question in option 2 may be asked when there is concern that the person is experiencing difficulty initiating urination (hesitancy) or when the passage of urine after a strong need to void occurs (urge incontinence), not when assessing for the presence of dysuria.
   3. The question in option 3 relates to stress incontinence, which is the immediate involuntary loss of urine during an increase in intraabdominal pressure, not to the presence of dysuria.
   4. The question in option 4 may be asked when there is a concern that the person is retaining urine in the bladder after urinating (residual urine), not when assessing for the presence of dysuria.

5. **TEST-TAKING TIP: The word *greatest* in the stem sets the priority.**
   1. The use of antibiotics and a diagnosis of *C. difficile* increase the risk for diarrhea, not constipation.
   2. Clients preparing to discharge are likely tolerating a full diet. Poor intake is a risk factor for constipation, and this client is not at the greatest risk for constipation in this scenario.
   3. **Older adults are at increased risk for constipation. An NPO diet order can increase the risk for constipation r/t the potential for dehydration. Opioids, the mainstay of pain management, frequently cause constipation. This client is at the highest risk.**
   4. Diarrhea, not constipation, often occurs with ulcerative colitis. The client is also

receiving IV hydration, which typically prevents constipation.

6. **TEST-TAKING TIP: The words *unable to tolerate a large volume of enema solution* are the key words in the stem that direct attention to content.**
   1. **A hypertonic enema solution uses only 120 to 180 mL of solution. Hypertonic solutions expend osmotic pressure that draws fluid out of interstitial spaces; fluid pulled into the colon and rectum distends the bowel, causing an increase in peristalsis, resulting in bowel evacuation. This type of enema usually is tolerated by clients who cannot endure a large volume of enema solution.**
   2. A normal saline enema is isotonic and requires a volume of 500 to 750 mL to be effective; the volume of fluid, not its saline content, causes an evacuation of the bowel. Five hundred to 750 mL is too large a volume of fluid for some clients to tolerate.
   3. A soapsuds enema requires a volume of 750 to 1000 mL of fluid to evacuate the bowel effectively. Seven hundred and fifty mL is too large a volume of fluid for some clients to tolerate.
   4. A tap-water enema usually requires a minimum of 750 mL of water to evacuate the bowel effectively. Seven hundred and fifty mL is too large a volume of fluid for some clients to tolerate.

7. **TEST-TAKING TIP: Options 1 and 3 are equally plausible. Options 2 and 4 are basically opposites.**
   1. The dorsal recumbent position does not use the natural curve of the rectum and sigmoid colon to facilitate instillation of enema solution.
   2. The right lateral position does not use the natural curve of the rectum and sigmoid colon to facilitate instillation of enema solution.
   3. The back-lying position does not use the natural curve of the rectum and sigmoid colon to facilitate instillation of enema solution.
   4. **The left semi-prone position permits enema solution to flow downward via gravity along the natural curve of the rectum and sigmoid colon, promoting instillation and retention of the solution.**

8. **TEST-TAKING TIP: The word *avoid* in option 4 indicates negative polarity. It is also the opposite of the other three options, which instruct the client to add something to the diet.**
   1. Dairy products increase the production of gas and should be avoided in clients with an ostomy who wish to reduce gas production.
   2. Green vegetables (including asparagus, broccoli, Brussels sprouts, cabbage, and cucumbers) increase gas and should be avoided in clients with an ostomy who wish to reduce gas production.
   3. Fish or cod liver oil increase gas and should be avoided in clients with an ostomy who wish to reduce gas production.
   4. **Carbonated beverages, including beer, increase gas and should be avoided in clients with an ostomy who wish to reduce gas production. Alcohol should also be avoided in order to reduce gas.**

9. **TEST-TAKING TIP: Options 1, 3, and 4 ignore the client's concern related to being assessed to the toilet by a male nurse or UAP.**
   1. Ignoring the comment is inappropriate. This fails to address the client's psychosocial needs. Although the client must be assisted to the toilet, they must be assisted in a way that provides dignity and respect.
   2. **Offering to find a female nurse or UAP to assist the client supports psychosocial needs while also maintaining safety when ambulating to the toilet. This is the only option that does not ignore the client's needs.**
   3. Although this statement is true, it does not address the client's concern related to embarrassment about requiring assistance with toileting from a male nurse.
   4. This action blatantly disregards the client's feelings and fails to meet their psychosocial needs related to elimination. This is inappropriate.

10. **TEST-TAKING TIP: The words *stress incontinence* in the stem direct attention to content.**
    1. Incontinence in response to a specific volume of urine in the bladder occurs in reflex, not stress, incontinence.
    2. **When intraabdominal pressure increases, the person with stress**

incontinence usually experiences urinary dribbling (i.e., a loss of less than 50 mL of urine). In some clients, once urination begins it continues until the bladder is empty.

3. Urinary tract infections often cause frequency as a result of irritation of the mucosal wall of the bladder, not stress incontinence.
4. Emotional strain may cause frequency, not stress incontinence.

11. Answer: 2, 1, 4, 5, 3

TEST-TAKING TIP: Using the If-Then technique can assist in ordering the steps via process of elimination. Procedure steps generally follow the nursing process.

1. **Option 2: Assessment is the first step in the nursing process. Obtaining baseline vital signs, auscultating bowel sounds, and assessing tissue integrity are assessment strategies.**
2. **Option 1: Positioning the client on the left side allows easier rectal tube insertion for the nurse and promotes comfort for the client. If the client is positioned on the left side, then rectal tube insertion will be easier.**
3. **Option 4: Once the client is on the left side, the tip of the rectal tube should be lubricated and inserted. If the client is on the left side and the rectal tube is lubricated, insertion will be easier for the nurse and more comfortable for the client.**
4. **Option 5: A rectal tube is typically left in place for 15 to 20 minutes and then removed.**
5. **Option 3: Performing peri-care is the last step in inserting a rectal tube. It is not required before inserting a rectal tube because the rectum is not a sterile environment.**

12. **TEST-TAKING TIP: The word *patency* is the key word in the stem that directs attention to content. Option 3 is the unique option. Options 1, 2, and 4 address the concept of characteristics of urine. The word *volume* in option 3 addresses the concept of quantity. Also, option 3 is the only option that does not begin with the letter "C."**

1. The color of urine reflects urine concentration, blood in the urine (hematuria), or a reaction to a specific drug or food, not catheter patency.
2. Clarity is an expected characteristic of urine; it does not indicate catheter patency. Cloudy urine indicates the presence of products such as red or white blood cells, bacteria, prostatic fluid, or sperm.
3. **If urine volume is minimal or nonexistent, it indicates that the catheter is obstructed, the ureters are obstructed, or the kidneys are not producing urine.**
4. Abnormal constituents of urine such as pus or blood indicate a possible pathological process, not catheter patency.

13. **TEST-TAKING TIP: The word *most* in the stem sets a priority. Option 4 is unique; options 1, 2, and 3 are related to physical concerns, whereas option 4 relates to a psychological concern.**

1. Although maintenance of skin integrity is important, it is not the most common concern of clients with a colostomy.
2. Although frequency of defecation may be a concern of some clients, it is not the most common concern of clients with a colostomy.
3. Consistency of the feces is not as major a concern as another factor. The consistency of feces varies according to the location of the stoma along the intestinal tract.
4. **The ability to control odor is a major psychological concern of people with a colostomy because the odor can be offensive if not controlled.**

14. **TEST-TAKING TIP: The words *most appropriate* in the stem set a priority. Options 2 and 4 are opposites, and options 1 and 3 are opposites.**

1. **Sticky greenish-black stools that become yellow in color 12 to 24 hours after birth are an expected finding called *meconium*. The nurse should continue to monitor and document the stools.**
2. Formula should be prepared according to package instructions. Meconium is a normal finding that requires no further intervention and this action could lead to dangerous fluid and electrolyte imbalances.
3. Meconium is a normal finding that does not require the nurse to notify the primary health-care provider.
4. Meconium is a normal finding in newborns. Asking the infant's mother about dietary patterns is not necessary in this situation.

15. **TEST-TAKING TIP: The words *culture and sensitivity* are key words in the stem that direct attention to content. The word *only* in option 3 is a specific determiner.**
   1. Two specimens are unnecessary.
   2. **A midstream urine sample contains a specimen that is relatively free of microorganisms from the urethra. After perineal care, cleansing of the urethral opening, and initiation of urination, a specimen is collected during the midportion of the stream. This technique avoids collection of urine during the initial stream, which may be contaminated with bacteria from the urethra.**
   3. Specimens collected from the first urine voided in the morning should be avoided; stagnant urine does not reflect urine that is recently produced by the urinary system.
   4. Twenty-four hours of urine is required for special tests such as the measurement of levels of adrenocortical steroids and hormones and creatinine clearance tests, not for a urine culture and sensitivity test.

16. 1. **When an intestinal muscle spasm occurs when receiving an enema, interrupting the flow of fluid allows the client to cope with discomfort during the spasm. The flow of fluid can resume once the spasm has subsided.**
   2. **Slow, deep breaths should be encouraged to prevent the client from holding the breath. Holding the breath increases intraabdominal pressure, which impedes the instillation and retention of fluid in the intestines and can result in the premature evacuation of fluid before a therapeutic effect has been achieved.**
   3. **In the left lateral position, the sigmoid colon is below the rectum and anus, facilitating the instillation of fluid.**
   4. A fluid temperature of 98.6°F is too cool and can contribute to intestinal muscle spasms and discomfort. Enema fluid should be between 105°F and 110°F because warm fluid promotes muscle relaxation and comfort.
   5. **The slow administration of enema fluid minimizes the probability of intestinal muscle spasms and premature evacuation of the fluid before a therapeutic effect has been achieved.**

17. **TEST-TAKING TIP: The words *high in fiber* are the key words that direct attention to content.**
   1. Chicken does not contain much fiber.
   2. **Most vegetables are high in fiber, which adds bulk to stool, promoting intestinal peristalsis. Generally, dark vegetables (e.g., broccoli, collard greens, Swiss chard, spinach, and beets) are high-fiber foods.**
   3. **Legumes and beans are high in fiber and are flavorful. The fiber in legumes and beans adds bulk to stool, which promotes intestinal peristalsis.**
   4. **Most fresh fruits are high in fiber. Fiber adds bulk to stool, which promotes intestinal peristalsis.**
   5. Plain yogurt is not high in fiber.
   6. **Whole-grain breads (e.g., dark rye, cracked wheat, and pumpernickel) are high in fiber. Fiber adds bulk to stool, which promotes intestinal peristalsis.**

18. 1. Applying an antiseptic ointment to the insertion site daily is unnecessary. Soap and water is adequate.
   2. **Eliminating dependent loops in the tubing prevents urine from inadvertently flowing back into the bladder; gravity allows the urine to flow from the urinary bladder to the collection bag without staying in dependent loops for prolonged periods.**
   3. **Positioning the catheter collection bag below the level of the pelvis prevents urine from flowing back into the bladder; urine flows out of the bladder by gravity.**
   4. Carrying the bag at waist level allows urine to flow back into the bladder, which can contribute to a urinary tract infection.
   5. An indwelling urinary catheter and collection bag constitute a closed system and should be changed only every 4 to 6 weeks unless crusting or sediment collects on the inside of the tubing.
   6. It is unnecessary to clamp an indwelling urinary catheter when a client is out of bed.

19. **TEST-TAKING TIP: The words *uncircumcised* and *after perineal care* are key words in the stem that direct attention to content. Options 1 and 3 are opposites.**
   1. **The foreskin should be replaced over the glans to protect the head of the penis. If the foreskin is not replaced to cover the distal portion of the penis, it can tighten around the shaft of the penis, causing local edema and pain.**

2. A condom catheter should be secured farther up the shaft of the penis, not immediately behind the glans.
3. If the foreskin is not returned over the glans, it can tighten around the shaft of the penis, causing local edema and pain.
4. **The area around the glans and the shaft of the penis must be dry to help the condom device stay in place securely.**
5. **This space prevents irritation of the tip of the penis; in addition, the 1-inch space allows urine to flow unimpeded and is not long enough to permit the condom sheath to twist.**

20. 1. This is a double-lumen urinary retention catheter. One lumen is used to inflate the balloon, and one lumen is used for urine drainage, which is connected to a collection bag.
2. This is a single-lumen (straight) urinary catheter generally used to drain the bladder of urine or to obtain a sterile urine specimen.
3. **This is a triple-lumen urinary catheter. One lumen is used to inflate the balloon, one lumen is used for the introduction of the irrigation solution and is connected to a 3000-mL bag of irrigant, and one lumen is used for drainage that eventually accumulates in a collection bag.**

21. **A urinary retention catheter is inserted into the meatus of the urethra, which leads to the urinary bladder. The urethra is directly behind the pubic symphysis and anterior to the vagina. The urinary meatus is between the clitoris and vaginal opening.**

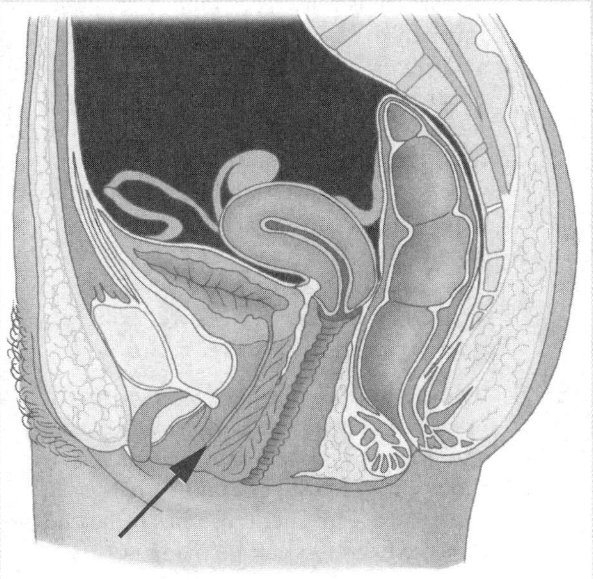

22. Answer: 250 mL/hr
Use ratio and proportion to solve for *x*.
Using Dimensional Analysis:
Find mL/hr: $\frac{250\text{ mL}}{1\text{ hour}}$
Divide to find 250 mL/hr

23. 1. Painful micturition (dysuria) generally is caused by infection, inflammation, or injury, not urinary retention.
2. Concentrated urine is caused by inadequate fluid intake and indicates dehydration, not urinary retention.
3. **Abdominal distention occurs as a result of collection of urine in the bladder. Outlet obstruction, decreased bladder tone, neurological dysfunction, opioids, and trauma can precipitate urinary retention.**
4. Functional incontinence is unrelated to retention. Functional incontinence occurs when a person who is aware of the need to void is unable to reach the toilet in time.
5. **Voiding small amounts of urine is associated with urinary retention with overflow; the bladder fills until pressure builds within it to the point that the urinary sphincters release enough urine to relieve the pressure.**

24. 1. In a 4-year-old child, nocturnal enuresis typically resolves with time. Occasional bed-wetting is normal in this age group.
2. The parent should be instructed to decrease fluid intake in the evening before bed. The child should consume adequate fluids throughout the day and then avoid fluids before bed.
3. **Covering the child's mattress with a plastic-backed pad is appropriate. This reduces the time required to clean the child's mattress and bedding and reduces odors.**
4. A thorough medical evaluation can be used to rule out underlying disease processes if nocturnal enuresis continues in a 10- or 12-year-old. Occasional nocturnal enuresis is common in a 4-year-old.
5. **Bathing the child in the morning is an appropriate education point. This reduces odor and may prevent feelings of embarrassment in the child.**

25. **Answer: Hypogastric region**
Two transverse (horizontal) planes and two sagittal planes divide the abdomen into nine areas. When a urinary bladder fills with urine, it rises upward into the

abdominal cavity (shaded). When a distended urinary bladder is assessed, palpation will reveal a round, firm mass above the symphysis pubis. Percussion will elicit a hollow, drumlike sound.

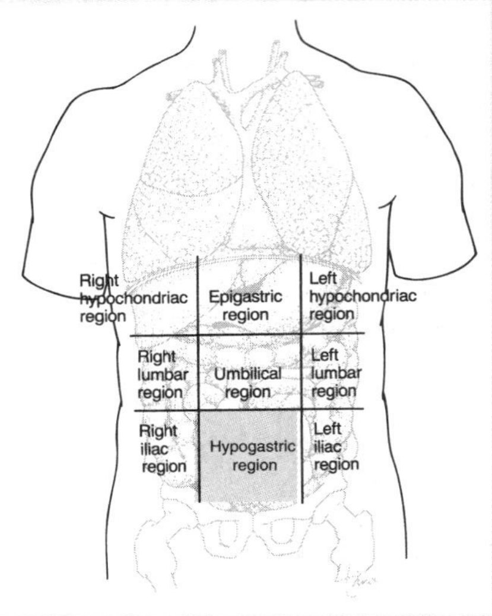

26. **TEST-TAKING TIP: The words *increased risk for constipation* are the words in the stem that direct attention to content.**
   1. **Limited mobility increases the risk for constipation in the older adult client. Increasing physical activity increases peristalsis and prevents constipation.**
   2. **Consuming dairy products such as milk can cause constipation in some clients.**
   3. Coffee and sugary beverages such as soda can increase peristalsis, causing diarrhea, in some clients.
   4. **Over-the-counter antacids used to treat heartburn can slow peristalsis and lead to constipation in the older adult client.**
   5. **Over-the-counter iron supplements used to treat anemia can slow peristalsis and lead to constipation and nausea in the older adult client.**

27. 1. Sterile gloves and sterile technique are not required when collecting a urine specimen from a urinary retention catheter. Clean gloves are appropriate.
   2. **Cleansing the port with an antiseptic swab prevents the introduction of pathogens into the closed urinary drainage system. Using an alcohol swab is appropriate and requires scrubbing for at least 15 seconds with friction.**
   3. **A needleless connector should be used to prevent puncturing the catheter tubing and introducing microorganisms into the system. Additionally, a needleless collection system reduces the risk for needle-stick injury.**
   4. The nurse in the photograph is using a needle to obtain a urine sample from the urinary catheter system. This is not best practice because it could result in needle-stick injuries or could damage the catheter tubing and introduce microorganisms into the system.
   5. A urine sample should be collected from the collection port of the urinary catheter system. A sample from the drainage collection bag may be 12 hours old and produce inaccurate results. The catheter tubing should be clamped for 15 to 20 minutes, providing a sample from the port that is current and collected from the bladder.

28. 1. **Food or fluid that enters and fills the stomach or the duodenum stimulates peristalsis; this is called the *gastrocolic reflex* or *duodenocolic reflex*.**
   2. Emotional stress initially increases peristalsis because the bowel evacuates its contents to prepare for a "fight."
   3. **Opioid analgesics depress the central nervous system, slowing peristalsis, which places a person at risk for constipation. Slowed peristalsis allows more fluid to be reabsorbed in the large intestine, resulting in hard, formed fecal material.**
   4. Straining at defecation increases, not decreases, intrathoracic pressure. Forcible exhalation against a closed glottis (Valsalva maneuver) increases intrathoracic pressure, which impedes venous return. When the breath is released, blood is propelled through the heart, causing tachycardia and increased blood pressure; a reflex bradycardia immediately follows. With an increase in intrathoracic pressure, immediate tachycardia and bradycardia occur in succession; clients with heart problems can experience a cardiac arrest.
   5. **At two and a half years of age, the child has mature muscles and nerves and can typically gain daytime bowel control after a program of toilet training.**

29. 1. The client does not have to perform more exercises. The client is physically active and does physical therapy exercises several times a day, as well as taking a half-mile walk daily. The client also has indicated that the exercises can be tiring at times.

2. **The client is experiencing constipation, a human response the nurse is legally permitted to treat. Constipation is infrequent fecal elimination (less than three stools weekly) or the passage of hard, dry feces. The client is consuming foods that are low in fiber (e.g., yogurt, eggs, cheese, and rice) and high in fat (dairy products, chocolate, and meat). Low-fiber foods leave little residue after they are digested.**

   High-fiber foods leave residue after they are digested, which promotes the formation of feces as well as peristalsis. Foods high in fat take longer to pass through the gastrointestinal system, allowing more fluid to be reabsorbed before being eliminated. Unripe bananas can cause constipation because they contain approximately 80% starch and a small amount of pectinase. Ripe bananas do not cause constipation because they contain approximately 5% starch and a large amount of pectinase, which breaks down the pectin between the cells in bananas and makes them easier to digest. The nurse must explore what type of bananas the client is consuming.
3. Referring the client to the primary health-care provider is not necessary. The nurse has the legal responsibility and expertise to address this client's problem. The nurse is abdicating nursing responsibilities to another health-care professional.
4. Increasing fluid intake is not necessary. Two and a half liters of fluid a day is an adequate fluid intake to maintain metabolic functions and prevent constipation.

30. Answer: 1, 5, 4, 3, 6, 2

1. **Draining urine from the urinary tubing into the bag ensures that all the urine excreted within a specified time frame is included in the amount of urinary output.**
5. **Placing a clean, waterproof barrier between the calibrated container and the floor prevents contamination of the calibrated container. Placing the calibrated container under the urine collection bag allows the urine to flow into it without contaminating the drainage spout.**
4. **Unclamping the drainage spout allows urine to flow out of the collection bag and into the container by gravity.**
3. **Reclamping the drainage spout just as the last amount of urine exits the system prevents microorganisms from entering the system. A urinary retention catheter system is a closed, sterile system.**
6. **Wiping the drainage spout with an alcohol swab reduces the amount of bacteria present, limiting the risk of a urinary infection.**
2. **Calculating the volume of urinary output is an essential part of the client's output when intake and output is ordered by the health-care provider. Clients with a urinary retention catheter generally are on intake and output. Discarding urine into a toilet eliminates exposure of the client's urine to others.**

31. TEST-TAKING TIP: The words *physiological* and *prevent infection* are key words in the stem that direct attention to content.

1. **Freshly voided urine is slightly acidic; this medium is unfavorable to microorganisms.**
2. An increased temperature may help to limit an existing infection, but it does not prevent an infection. An increased temperature results from released toxins in the presence of infection.
3. **Microorganisms congregate at the urinary meatus because it is warm, moist, and dark; when urine flows down the urethra and out of the urinary meatus, the force of the urine carries away microorganisms, which minimizes ascending infections.**
4. Gastric secretions are acidic and have a low pH.
5. **The sebaceous glands in the skin secrete sebum (oil) onto the skin surface. Sebum lubricates the skin, preventing drying and cracking.**

32. TEST-TAKING TIP: The word *essential* in the stem sets a priority. The word *catheter* in the stem and in options 1 and 4 are clang associations. Examine options 1 and 4 carefully.

1. **Using sterile technique when inserting a straight catheter reduces the risk of introducing a pathogen into the bladder.**
2. This type of urinary catheter (straight catheter) is not attached to a collection bag. The straight catheter in the illustration is left in the urinary bladder just long

enough to empty the bladder of urine and is then immediately removed.

3. No urine collection tubing is used with this type of urinary catheter (straight catheter). The urine usually is collected in the container associated with the catheterization kit.
4. A straight urinary catheter does not remain in the bladder once the bladder has been emptied of urine. A double-lumen catheter used with an indwelling urinary catheter and collection set should be secured to the client to prevent tension on the catheter that has been left in place. It should be attached to the thigh area for women and the abdomen for men.

33. **TEST-TAKING TIP: The words *all bladder-retraining programs* are key words in the stem that direct attention to content. The word *every* in option 1 is a specific determiner.**

1. Toileting is not automatically implemented every 2 hours but is based on the individual needs of the client.
2. The volume of scheduled fluid intake is based on the individual needs of the client.
3. Incontinence pads generally are not encouraged when a bladder-retraining program is implemented.
4. Toileting a client should be done before a meal. Toileting after a meal is done to promote a bowel movement by taking advantage of the gastrocolic reflex.
5. **Toileting first thing in the morning is done for all clients on a bladder-retraining program; it empties the urinary bladder in the morning before other activities of daily living. When one moves from lying down to a vertical position, urine moves toward the trigone and urinary meatus. The increased pressure of urine in this area stimulates the desire to void.**

34.
1. This site is the ascending colon; it contains the most liquid stool because it is at the beginning of the large intestine, where little fluid has been reabsorbed.
2. **This site is the transverse colon with a double-barreled colostomy. The stool produced will be soft and pasty because just a little fluid has been reabsorbed. As fecal material progresses through the large intestine, 80% of the fluid that enters the bowel is eventually reabsorbed.**
3. This site is the descending colon, where stool is soft but formed. More fluid has been reabsorbed than in the transverse colon, but less fluid has been reabsorbed than in the sigmoid colon.
4. This site is the sigmoid colon. The stool produced is formed and firm because this is the final small segment of the large intestine. The sigmoid colon is the intestinal section just before the rectum, anal canal, and anus.

35. **Answer: 1550 mL**

The nurse should deduct the volume of bladder irrigant from the total output in the urinary collection bag (5600 – 4050 = 1550 mL) to arrive at the client's total urine output for 12 hours. The oral and intravenous intake is unrelated to calculating the actual urine output.

MEETING CLIENTS' OXYGEN NEEDS

This section includes questions related to assessments and interventions associated with expected and abnormal respiratory and circulatory functions. Questions focus on topics such as aspiration, emergency care for clients with respiratory difficulties, techniques and devices that assess or increase respiratory or circulatory function, and assessments and interventions associated with the administration of oxygen.

QUESTIONS

1. The client recently diagnosed with COPD is being discharged with oxygen via nasal cannula. The client states, "I know I'm not supposed to, but I cannot wait to smoke a cigarette on my back porch." Which of the following is a priority action?
   1. Lubricate the nares with water-soluble jelly
   2. Explain oxygen-related safety concepts to the client
   3. Adjust the flow rate before applying the prongs
   4. Ensure that electrical devices have three-pronged plugs

   TEST-TAKING TIP: Identify the word in the stem that sets a priority.

2. A client with a history of chronic respiratory disease begins to have difficulty breathing. For which **most** serious responses should the nurse assess the client?
   1. Orthostatic hypotension when rising and the need to sit in the orthopneic position
   2. Wheezing sounds on inspiration and the need to sit in the orthopneic position
   3. Mucus tinged with frank red streaks and wheezing sounds on inspiration
   4. Chest pain and mucus tinged with frank red streaks

   TEST-TAKING TIP: Identify the word in the stem that sets a priority. Identify duplicate facts among options.

3. The nurse is caring for several pediatric clients and their families. The nurse recognizes that infants, toddlers, and preschool-age children are at increased risk for respiratory compromise for what reasons? **Select all that apply.**
   1. Infants born after 36 weeks have underdeveloped surfactant systems.
   2. Infants have a small airway diameter.
   3. Toddlers are frequently exposed to lower respiratory infections at day care.
   4. Infants and toddlers have relatively large lymph organs in their throats.
   5. A growing number of young people use electronic nicotine delivery systems.

   TEST-TAKING TIP: Identify key words in the stem that direct attention to content.

4. While eating, a male client clutches his upper chest with his hands, makes choking sounds, and has a frightened facial expression. Which should the nurse do **first?**
   1. Start artificial respirations
   2. Perform abdominal thrusts
   3. Slap the client on the back
   4. Assess the client's ability to breathe

   TEST-TAKING TIP: Identify the word in the stem that sets a priority. Identify the unique option.

5. The nurse is monitoring a client with a respiratory problem for the presence of cyanosis. Which are the **most** appropriate sites to assess?
   1. Around the mouth and fingernail beds
   2. Lower extremities and around the mouth
   3. Fingernail beds and conjunctiva of the eyes
   4. Conjunctiva of the eyes and lower extremities

   TEST-TAKING TIP: Identify the word in the stem that sets a priority. Identify duplicate facts among options.

6. The nurse is providing oropharyngeal suctioning with a Yankauer (tonsil-tip) device for a client with dysphagia who is in the low Fowler position. During the procedure, the client begins to gag and vomit. Which should the nurse do?
   1. Raise the head of the bed higher
   2. Turn the client onto a lateral position
   3. Give the client oxygen via nasal cannula
   4. Continue the procedure to clear the mouth of debris

7. The nurse is caring for an 86-year-old client on postoperative day 1 after a complex abdominal surgery. The nurse recognizes that which of the following physiological changes occur in the older adult that increase the risk for respiratory infection? **Select all that apply.**
   1. Recoil ability increases in the lungs
   2. Costal cartilage calcification
   3. Decreased diaphragm strength
   4. Increased response to oxygen demand
   5. Less effective cough reflex

   TEST-TAKING TIP: Identify opposites in options.

8. The nurse is caring for an 8-year-old client newly diagnosed with asthma. Which of the following statements about asthma is true?
   1. Asthma is an allergic reaction occurring in the small airways of the lungs.
   2. Asthma is uncommon, but life-threatening in children.
   3. Asthma is an allergic reaction effectively treated with antihistamines.
   4. Asthma affects only children.

   TEST-TAKING TIP: Identify the word in the stem that sets a priority. Identify key words in the stem that direct attention to content. Identify the clang association.

9. The nurse identifies that a client has excessive sputum. Which intervention is effective for maintaining a patent airway in this client?
   1. Active coughing
   2. Incentive spirometry
   3. Nebulizer treatments
   4. Abdominal breathing

10. The nurse is caring for a client who is experiencing respiratory difficulty. Which **most** accurately measures the adequacy of tissue oxygenation and requires monitoring by the nurse?
    1. Hematocrit values
    2. Hemoglobin levels
    3. Arterial blood gases
    4. Pulmonary function tests

    TEST-TAKING TIP: Identify the word in the stem that sets a priority. Identify the key words in the stem that direct attention to content.

11. The nurse identifies that a client with an infection has tachypnea. Which should the nurse consider is the reason for this response?
    1. Increase in the metabolic rate
    2. Need to retain carbon dioxide
    3. Decrease in carbon dioxide levels
    4. Attempt to compensate for respiratory alkalosis

12. A client comes to the emergency department in respiratory distress, and the nurse identifies the presence of wheezing breath sounds. Which does the nurse determine is the cause of these sounds?
    1. Fluid in the lung
    2. Sitting in the orthopneic position
    3. Air moving through a narrowed airway
    4. Pleural surfaces that rub against each other

13. The nurse is caring for a client in the emergency department diagnosed with diabetic ketoacidosis. The nurse identifies which pattern of breathing associated with this emergency condition?
   1. Recurring pattern of quick, shallow respirations alternating with irregular periods of apnea
   2. Repeating pattern of increasing rate and depth of respirations alternating with apnea
   3. Labored respirations, with breathlessness, that are possibly painful
   4. High rate and depth of respirations that are regular

   TEST-TAKING TIP: Identify opposites in options.

14. The nurse is caring for a client with a medical diagnosis of anemia. Which physiological activity is altered as a result of the pathophysiology of anemia?
   1. Perfusion of oxygen
   2. Diffusion of oxygen
   3. Exchange of oxygen
   4. Transport of oxygen

15. The nurse is caring for a client in her 38th week of pregnancy. The client states, "I'm young and healthy, why am I so short of breath?" What is the nurse's most accurate response?
   1. "Metabolism decreases in the last half of pregnancy."
   2. "The diaphragm can't move downward."
   3. "Respiratory infections are common in pregnancy and can cause shortness of breath."
   4. "Oxygen demand decreases in the last half of pregnancy."

   TEST-TAKING TIP: Identify the key word in the stem that directs attention to content.

16. The nurse is caring for a client who presents to the emergency room with a dry cough. The client was prescribed an ACE inhibitor for newly diagnosed hypertension approximately 1 month ago. The nurse anticipates which of the following orders?
   1. STAT sputum sample
   2. Discontinue the ACE inhibitor
   3. 500 mg amoxicillin PO three times daily
   4. 250 mg tetracycline PO four times daily

   TEST-TAKING TIP: Identify equally plausible options.

17. The nurse collects a sputum sample and documents that the sample appeared "pink and frothy." The nurse understands that the sputum of this appearance is related to which state?
   1. Viral infection
   2. Bacterial infection
   3. Lung cancer
   4. Pulmonary edema

18. A client has chronic impaired peripheral arterial circulation. For which response should the nurse assess the client? **Select all that apply.**
   1. _____ Sores on the legs that do not heal
   2. _____ Diminished pulse in feet or legs
   3. _____ Brittle, slow-growing toenails
   4. _____ Lack of hair below the knees
   5. _____ Continuous leg discomfort
   6. _____ Cool lower extremities

   TEST-TAKING TIP: Identify the key words in the stem that direct attention to content.

19. A client who is hospitalized has difficulty swallowing. Which should the nurse do to help prevent this client from aspirating? **Select all that apply.**
1. _____ Ensure a small amount of food is included with each mouthful
2. _____ Encourage that fluids be mixed with food in the mouth
3. _____ Allow time between spoonfuls for chewing
4. _____ Avoid conversation during meals
5. _____ Cut up meat into small pieces

TEST-TAKING TIP: Identify the unique option.

20. A child diagnosed with otitis media is prescribed amoxicillin 500 mg every 8 hours PO. The amoxicillin is supplied in 250 mg/5 mL. How many mL should be administered every 8 hours? **Record your answer using a whole number.**

Answer: ___________ mL

21. The nurse is educating a client who has impaired circulation to the lower extremities. Which action should the nurse include in the teaching program about how to care for the feet? **Select all that apply.**
1. _____ Wear sturdy, well-fitting, closed-toe shoes.
2. _____ Apply moisturizing lotion between the toes after bathing.
3. _____ Use a mirror to check the under-surfaces of the feet daily.
4. _____ Use warm socks rather than a heating pad when the feet are cold.
5. _____ Report breaks in the skin of the feet to the primary health-care provider.

TEST-TAKING TIP: Identify the key words in the stem that direct attention to content. Identify clang associations.

22. The nurse is auscultating a client's breath sounds. Place an X over the site where the nurse should place the stethoscope when assessing breath sounds in the right middle lobe via the lateral approach.

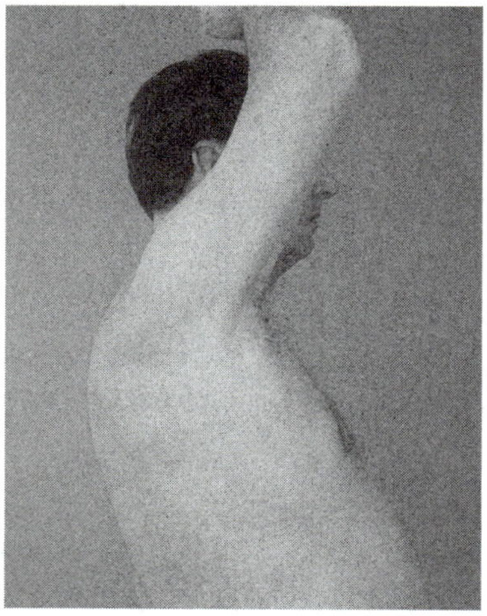

23. A client ambulating in the hall reports having sudden chest pain. Which should the nurse do? **Select all that apply.**
1. _____ Obtain vital signs
2. _____ Perform a pain assessment
3. _____ Walk the client back to bed slowly
4. _____ Return the client to bed via a wheelchair
5. _____ Have the client stand still until the discomfort subsides

TEST-TAKING TIP: Identify the key words in the stem that direct attention to content. Identify the option with a clang association.

24. The nurse is performing a physical assessment and notes a nail plate angle greater than 180°, as shown in the illustration. The nurse understands that this finding is associated with which of the following? **Select all that apply.**

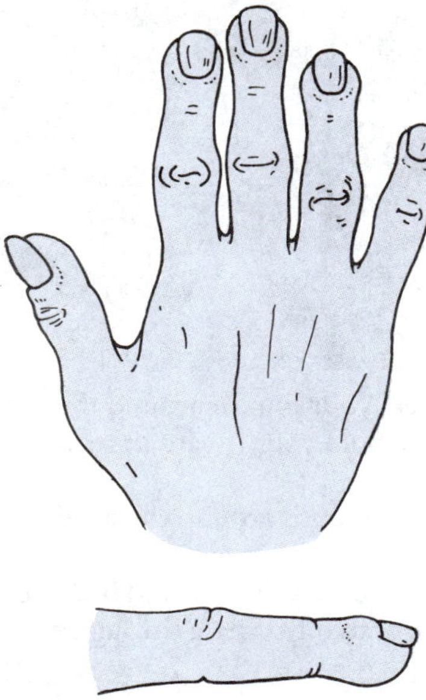

1. _____ Oxygen administration
2. _____ Chronic tobacco use
3. _____ Chronic impaired gas exchange
4. _____ Well-controlled asthma
5. _____ Acute respiratory distress syndrome

TEST-TAKING TIP: Identify opposites in options.

25. The nurse is preparing to discharge a 12-year-old child diagnosed with asthma on this admission. Place the steps in the correct order for using a peak flow meter at home.

1. Forcefully exhale.
2. Adjust medication according to the highest reading and the treatment plan.
3. Take a deep breath.
4. Repeat three times.
5. Place the mouthpiece between the teeth and close the lips around it.

Answer: ____________

26. A client has dysphagia. Which should the nurse do to prevent aspiration after meals? **Select all that apply.**

1. _____ Keep the head of the bed elevated 45° for 45 to 60 minutes
2. _____ Position the client in the low Fowler position
3. _____ Administer mouth care when necessary
4. _____ Inspect the mouth for pocketed food
5. _____ Remove fluids from the bedside

TEST-TAKING TIP: Identify key words in the stem that direct attention to content. Identify options that are opposites. Identify the unique option.

27. The nurse is responsible for monitoring clients for aspiration. Which of the following clients are at increased risk for aspiration? **Select all that apply.**

1. _____ The client with a Glasgow Coma Scale score of 6
2. _____ The client with a Glasgow Coma Scale score of 15
3. _____ The client unable to clear secretions independently
4. _____ The client with NPO orders awaiting a swallow study
5. _____ The adolescent client with no comorbidities attending rehab for a fractured femur

28. Which instruction should the nurse give a client who is using the device in the illustration?

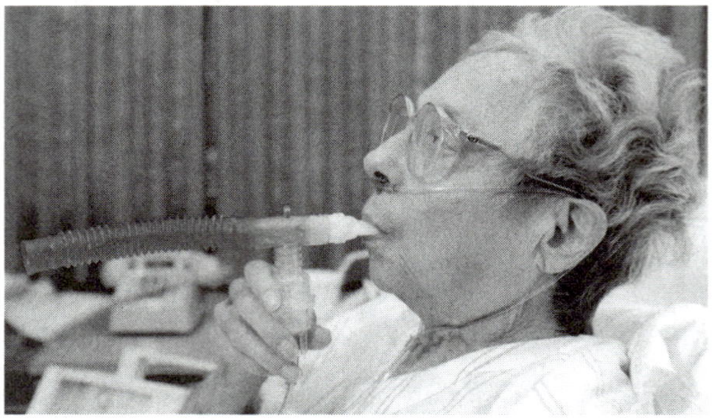

1. Breathe out normally, seal your mouth around the mouthpiece, breathe in slowly and as deeply as possible, hold your breath at least 3 seconds, and remove the mouthpiece and exhale.
2. Hold the device, seal your mouth around the mouthpiece, and breathe in and out slowly and deeply.
3. Seal your mouth around the mouthpiece and breathe in and out normally.
4. Take a deep breath and forcefully exhale through the mouthpiece.

29. The nurse assesses the respiratory pattern of four clients. Each option represents a 30-second interval. Which client's respiratory pattern reflects bradypnea?

1. 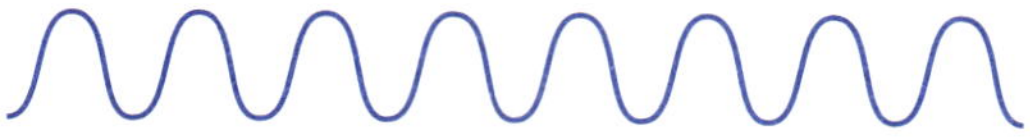
2. 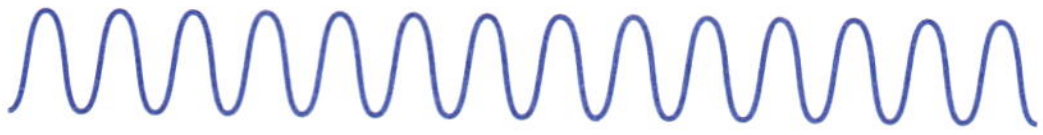
3. 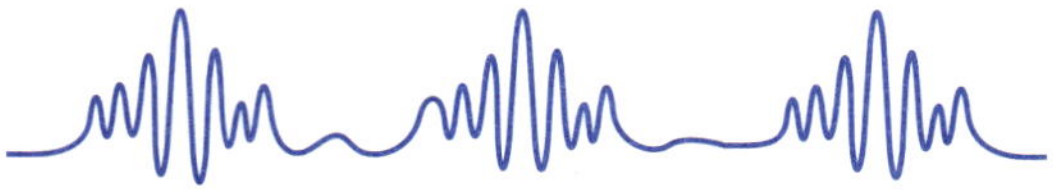
4. 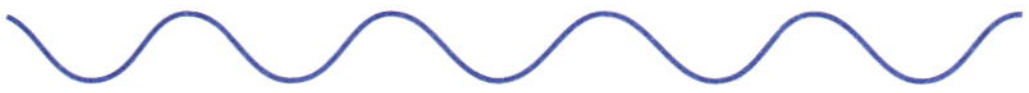

30. The nurse has just documented in the client's clinical record. When repositioning the client at 0930, the client reports sudden, severe substernal chest pain and becomes diaphoretic and anxious. Pulse is now weak, rapid, and noted at 110 BPM. Respirations are shallow, labored, and noted at 22 per minute. What is the nurse's **priority** action?
1. Call the respiratory therapist to obtain a pulse oximetry reading
2. Initiate the rapid response team and elevate the head of the bed.
3. Notify the primary care provider and start oxygen via nasal cannula
4. Take the client's blood pressure and start an IV line with 0.9% sodium chloride

CLIENT'S CLINICAL RECORD

Nurse's Progress Note 0900

Client 4 days postoperative for a right total hip replacement. Alert, oriented times 3. Reports dull ache in operative site on a level 2 that increases to a level 4 with movement. Right lower extremity peripheral pulses are present and strong. 2 sec capillary refill BLE. Suture line dry, edges approximated with no signs of inflammation or dehiscence. Abduction maintained. Decreased bowel sounds noted in the upper right quadrant. Voiding sufficient quantity. No adventitious breath sounds. Client reports a slight ache in right calf. No swelling or heat observed at site. Encouraged client to remain in bed with entire right extremity supported on 1 pillow; primary health-care provider's office notified and awaiting a response.

Vital Signs 0900

Blood pressure: 140/75 mm Hg
Pulse: 84 beats/min, regular rhythm
Respirations: 18 breaths/min

TEST-TAKING TIP: Identify the word in the stem that sets a priority.

31. The nurse teaches a client how to self-administer a corticosteroid via a metered-dose inhaler with an extender. Which behavior indicates that the client understands the teaching? **Select all that apply.**
1. _____ Assumes a sitting position for the procedure
2. _____ Rinses the mouth with water after the treatment
3. _____ Waits at least 1 minute before taking the next puff
4. _____ Shakes the canister vigorously several times before using the device
5. _____ Positions the mouthpiece over the tongue with the teeth and lips tight around the mouthpiece while inhaling

TEST-TAKING TIP: Identify the key words in the stem that direct attention to content.

32. Oseltamivir (Tamiflu®) 45 mg twice a day for 5 days is prescribed for a child with influenza. The medication is supplied in an oral suspension of 6 mg/mL. How much oral suspension should the nurse administer for each dose? **Record your answer using one decimal place.**

Answer: __________ mL

33. Place an X on the site that the nurse **most** commonly assesses for the presence of a pulse when administering cardiopulmonary resuscitation to an adult.

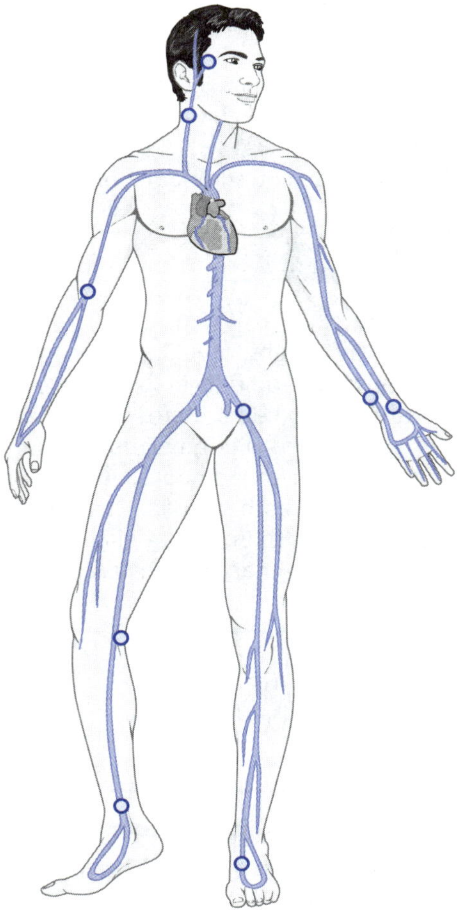

TEST-TAKING TIP: Identify the word in the stem that sets a priority.

34. Which nursing intervention increases both circulation and respiration in a client? **Select all that apply.**

1. _____ Encourage the use of a spirometer.
2. _____ Reposition the client every 2 hours.
3. _____ Rub the bony prominences with lotion.
4. _____ Assist the client with ambulating in the hall.
5. _____ Teach the client to cough after breathing deeply every 4 hours.

TEST-TAKING TIP: Identify the key words in the stem that direct attention to content.

35. The nurse is caring for a client who is receiving a continuous nasogastric tube feeding via a volume-control pump. Which should the nurse do to prevent aspiration when assisting this client with hygiene and changing the linens? **Select all that apply.**

1. _____ Lower the height of the bag containing the formula
2. _____ Place the bed flat and change the sheets quickly
3. _____ Slow the rate of flow on the infusion pump
4. _____ Obtain additional assistance
5. _____ Shut off the infusion pump

TEST-TAKING TIP: Identify key words in the stem that direct attention to content. Identify equally plausible options. Identify the option with clang associations. Identify options that are opposites.

MEETING CLIENTS' OXYGEN NEEDS ANSWERS AND RATIONALES

1. **TEST-TAKING TIP: The word *first* in the stem sets a priority.**
   1. Lubricating the nares with water-soluble jelly is not the priority. Nares can be moisturized with water-based lubricants if needed. Vaseline should be avoided.
   2. **Safety is a priority. This client should understand the dangers related to the use of continuous oxygen therapy and cigarette smoking. The nurse should also offer cessation counseling.**
   3. Although adjusting the oxygen level before applying the nasal prongs is important, it is not the priority.
   4. Using three-pronged plugs whenever possible is a safety strategy. However, explaining oxygen-related safety concepts to the client is of greater importance in this scenario.

2. **TEST-TAKING TIP: The word *most* in the stem sets a priority. Five client responses are presented in different combinations for you to choose the most serious one in this situation. If you are able to identify one response that is most serious and it appears in two options, you can narrow the choice to these two options. If you can identify one response that is least significant and it appears in two options, you can eliminate these two distractors from consideration.**
   1. Orthostatic hypotension when rising and the need to sit in the orthopneic position are common clinical findings in individuals with chronic respiratory disease and are not as serious as another option. Rising slowly permits the circulation to adjust to the change in position, thereby minimizing orthostatic hypotension. Elevating the head helps breathing by lowering the abdominal organs via gravity, which allows the diaphragm to contract more efficiently on inspiration.
   2. Wheezing sounds on inspiration and the need to sit in the orthopneic position are common responses associated with respiratory disease and are not as serious as another option. Raising the head of the bed helps breathing by lowering the abdominal organs by gravity, which allows the diaphragm to contract more efficiently on inspiration. Wheezing on inspiration is a response to an increase in airway resistance.
   3. Although mucus tinged with frank red streaks and wheezing are common responses to respiratory disease, this combination of responses is not as serious as another combination of responses among the options.
   4. **Although mucus tinged with frank red streaks can be a response to chronic respiratory disease, chest pain is not. Chest pain may indicate a pneumothorax. When these clinical manifestations occur together, they should be addressed immediately by a rapid response team or the primary health-care provider.**

3. **TEST-TAKING TIP: The words *infants, toddlers, and preschool-age children* direct attention to content.**
   1. Infants born before 35 weeks, premature infants, have underdeveloped surfactant systems. This statement is false.
   2. **Infants and toddlers have a small airway diameter. This physiological feature of these age groups predisposes them to choking on small objects. Additionally, less airway inflammation is required to compromise the airway.**
   3. Infants and toddlers are frequently exposed to upper respiratory infections, not lower respiratory infections, at preschool and day care.
   4. **Infants and toddlers have relatively large tonsils and adenoids, lymph organs, in their throats. This predisposes them to tonsillitis and requires less airway inflammation to compromise the airway.**
   5. Although this statement is true, it applies to people as young as middle school and not infants, toddlers, and preschoolers.

4. **TEST-TAKING TIP: The word *first* in the stem sets a priority. Option 4 is unique because it is the only option that is an assessment. Options 1, 2, and 3 are all actions.**
   1. Action before assessment is inappropriate. The client is not in respiratory arrest; food is lodged in the respiratory passages.
   2. Action before assessment is inappropriate. Abdominal thrusts may be done after it is determined that the client cannot breathe because of a totally obstructed airway. The American Heart Association recommends that abdominal thrusts be done to attempt to clear the airway of foreign matter.
   3. Action before assessment is inappropriate. Slapping the client on the back five times alternating with five abdominal thrusts is recommended by the American Red Cross

to clean the airway of foreign matter. Some resources state that slapping the client on the back may cause the aspirated object to lodge deeper in the respiratory passages.

4. **Assessment is the priority because each situation requires a different intervention. If the client is able to breathe, a "wait and watch" stance is appropriate. If the client cannot breathe, then the guidelines to clear the airway recommended by either the American Heart Association or the American Red Cross should be implemented.**

5. **TEST-TAKING TIP: The word *most* in the stem sets a priority. Four different sites are presented as preferred sites to assess for the presence of cyanosis. If you are able to identify one site that is the least desirable to use for the assessment of cyanosis, you can eliminate two distractors and narrow the choice to two options. If you are able to identify one site that is desirable to use for the assessment of cyanosis, you can narrow the choice to two options.**
   1. **Nail beds, lips, and mucous membranes of the mouth are the primary sites to assess for signs of oxygen deprivation. The mucous membranes of the mouth are highly vascular, and the presence of an excessive concentration of deoxyhemoglobin in the blood is observable.**
   2. Although the lips and mucous membranes of the mouth are primary sites to assess for early signs of oxygen deprivation, the lower legs are not the first sites to assess for systemic oxygen deprivation.
   3. Although the nail beds are a primary site to assess for signs of oxygen deprivation, pallor of the conjunctiva of the eyes, not cyanosis, reflects reduced oxyhemoglobin.
   4. Pallor of the conjunctiva of the eyes, not cyanosis, reflects reduced oxyhemoglobin. The lower legs are not the first sites to assess for systemic oxygen deprivation.

6. 1. Raising the head of the bed should be done when the client is finished vomiting. Raising the head of the bed will facilitate respirations by allowing the abdominal contents to drop by gravity, thereby not exerting pressure against the diaphragm.
   2. **Turning the client to a side-lying position will permit the vomitus to exit the mouth by gravity. This will prevent the vomitus from flowing to the back of the oropharynx, where it can enter the respiratory tract when the client inhales (aspiration).**
   3. Oxygen may or may not be given when the client is done vomiting. The use of oxygen will depend on the client's respiratory status.
   4. It is unrealistic and traumatic to continue suctioning the oral cavity of a client who is gagging and vomiting. The vomitus can still enter the respiratory tract when the client inhales (aspiration).

7. **TEST-TAKING TIP: Each option is related to either increased function or decreased function.**
   1. As the body ages, elasticity in the alveoli is lost and the ability of the lungs to recoil decreases. Oximetry measures the degree to which hemoglobin is saturated with oxygen; it provides some indication of the efficiency of lung ventilation.
   2. **The costal cartilage calcifies with age and results in decreased ability to expand with the movements of breathing. This results in decreased ability to move air.**
   3. **The diaphragm is an important muscle involved in moving air in and out of the lungs. As the body ages, the diaphragm loses strength. This results in a decreased ability to move air effectively.**
   4. As the body ages, the ability to respond to increased oxygen demand decreases.
   5. **The cough reflex becomes less effective as the body ages. This phenomenon, combined with drier mucus and decreased cilia in the airways, results in less efficient clearing of the airways.**

8. **TEST-TAKING TIP: The word *most* in the stem sets a priority. The words *dramatic increase* are key words in the stem that direct attention to content. The word *individual* in the stem and in option 2 is a clang association.**
   1. **Asthma is an allergic reaction to triggers such as tobacco smoke, dust mites, or air pollution. These environmental triggers cause airway constriction and lead to difficulty breathing.**
   2. Asthma is the most common serious chronic disease of childhood. It can lead to life-threatening airway constriction and should be managed promptly.
   3. Asthma is an allergic reaction. However, because histamines are not a major factor of the response, antihistamines are not effective at treating asthma.
   4. Asthma is a chronic disease. Although most commonly diagnosed in childhood, it requires daily management across the life span. Additionally, it can be diagnosed in adulthood.

9. **1. A cough forcefully expels air from the lungs and is an effective self-protective reflex to clear the trachea and bronchi of secretions.**
   2. An incentive spirometer is a device used to encourage voluntary deep breathing, not to clear an airway; it is used to prevent or treat atelectasis.
   3. A nebulizer treatment does not clear an airway; it adds moisture or medication to inspired air to alter the tracheobronchial mucosa. After the respiratory passages have been dilated or mucolytic agents have reduced the viscosity of secretions, the client can cough more productively.
   4. Abdominal breathing does not clear the air passages. It helps to decrease air trapping and reduce the work of breathing.

10. **TEST-TAKING TIP: The word *most* in the stem sets a priority. The words *accurately* and *tissue oxygenation* are key words in the stem that direct attention to content.**
   1. Although hematocrit is the percentage of red blood cell mass in whole blood, it is not an accurate test for adequacy of tissue oxygenation; a low hematocrit value may indicate possible water intoxication, and an increased hematocrit value may indicate dehydration.
   2. Although hemoglobin is a protein molecule in red blood cells that carries oxygen, its measurement is not an accurate test for adequacy of tissue oxygenation; a decreased hemoglobin value is evidence of iron-deficiency anemia or bleeding.
   3. Arterial blood gases include the levels of oxygen, carbon dioxide, bicarbonate, and pH. Blood gases determine the adequacy of alveolar gas exchange and the ability of the lungs and kidneys to maintain an acid-base balance of body fluids.
   4. Pulmonary function tests measure lung volume and capacity; although these tests provide valuable information, they do not provide specific data about tissue oxygenation.

11. **1. Because of the energy required to "fight" an infection, the basal metabolic rate increases, resulting in increased respiratory rate (tachypnea).**
   2. The body has a need to exhale, not retain, carbon dioxide.
   3. Tachypnea occurs in the presence of increased levels of carbon dioxide and carbonic acid, not decreased carbon dioxide levels.
   4. The client with an infection is more likely to be experiencing metabolic acidosis; tachypnea that progresses to hyperventilation causes respiratory alkalosis.

12. 1. Sounds caused by fluid in the alveoli of the lung are called *crackles* or *rales*, and sounds caused by fluid or resistance in the bronchi of the lung are called *rhonchi* or *gurgles*.
   2. Sitting in the orthopneic position is not the cause of adventitious breath sounds (abnormal breath sounds).
   3. *Wheezes* occur as air passes through airways narrowed by secretions, edema, or tumors; these high-pitched squeaky musical sounds are best heard on expiration and usually are not changed by coughing.
   4. A *pleural friction rub* is a superficial grating sound heard particularly at the height of inspiration that is not relieved by coughing; it is caused by the rubbing together of inflamed pleural surfaces.

13. **TEST-TAKING TIP: Options 1 and 4 are opposites. In option 1, respirations are shallow and irregular. In option 4, respirations have a high depth and are regular.**
   1. A recurring pattern of quick, shallow respirations alternating with irregular periods of apnea is characteristic of Biot's respiration. This pattern is seen with damage to the pons, such as in stroke or trauma.
   2. A repeating pattern of increasing rate and depth of respirations alternating with apnea is characteristic of Cheyne-Stokes respiration. This pattern is seen when the respiratory center of the brain is damaged due to stroke, encephalitis, tumors, or increased intracranial pressure. It is also associated with heart failure and chronic pulmonary edema.
   3. Dyspnea is a general term for the subjective feeling of difficulty breathing. Dyspnea can be painful and is associated with many conditions that impair gas exchange.
   4. A high rate and depth of respirations is known as Kussmaul respirations. It is the body's effort to correct severe metabolic acidosis, particularly diabetic ketoacidosis (DKA), by blowing off excess carbon dioxide.

14. 1. Perfusion relates to the extent of inflow and outflow of air between the alveoli and

pulmonary capillaries or the extent of blood flow to the pulmonary capillary bed; perfusion is not related to red blood cell levels.
2. Diffusion occurs at the alveolar capillary beds and is not related to anemia.
3. Exchange of oxygen occurs in the capillary beds of the alveoli via the process of diffusion; this is unrelated to anemia.
4. **The hemoglobin portion of red blood cells transports oxygen from the alveolar capillaries in the lungs to distant tissue sites.**

15. **TEST-TAKING TIP: The word *pregnancy* is the key word in the stem that directs attention to content.**
1. This statement is false. Metabolism increases in the last half of pregnancy, resulting in an increased oxygen demand.
2. **This statement is correct. In a client with an uncomplicated pregnancy, the uterus limits the diaphragm's ability to move downward during lung expansion. This results in the feeling of shortness of breath.**
3. Although respiratory infections can cause shortness of breath, this statement does not make sense in this scenario. The client described themselves as healthy and respiratory infections are independent of pregnancy.
4. This statement is false. Metabolism increases in the last half of pregnancy, resulting in an increased oxygen demand.

16. **TEST-TAKING TIP: Options 3 and 4 are extremely similar and can be eliminated.**
1. Collecting a sputum sample in a client with a dry cough would be challenging. This is not a likely order for this client.
2. **ACE inhibitors are known to cause a dry, nagging cough. This is a side effect that frequently limits adherence. For this client, an Angiotensin Receptor Blocker (ARB) may be more appropriate because ARBs treat hypertension without the dry, nagging cough.**
3. Antibiotics are reserved for bacterial infections. This order would not be appropriate without first identifying a bacterial infection.
4. Antibiotics are reserved for bacterial infections. This order would not be appropriate without first identifying a bacterial infection.

17. 1. White or clear sputum is associated with a viral infection, although this must be confirmed with laboratory testing.
2. Green or yellow sputum is associated with bacterial infection, although this must be confirmed with laboratory testing.
3. Hemoptysis, or blood in the sputum, is sometimes associated with lung cancer.
4. **Pink and frothy sputum is associated with severe pulmonary edema. It is a result of fluid in the alveoli.**

18. **TEST-TAKING TIP: The words *impaired peripheral arterial circulation* are the key words in the stem that direct attention to content.**
1. **A decrease in oxygen and nutrients to the area due to impaired arterial circulation results in sores that do not heal.**
2. **A buildup of fatty deposits reduces blood flow through the arteries of the lower extremities, causing the pulses of the legs to be weak.**
3. **A decrease in oxygen and nutrients to the lower extremities causes toenails to be brittle, yellow, and slow growing.**
4. **A decrease in oxygen and nutrients to the lower part of the legs due to impaired arterial circulation results in a lack of hair. The lack of hair progresses from the toes to the knees over time.**
5. Leg discomfort related to impaired peripheral arterial perfusion usually is intermittent, not continuous. Mild activity increases leg discomfort, which is relieved by rest (intermittent claudication).
6. **The skin on the legs feels cool when there is a decrease in the amount of circulating blood volume to the lower legs and feet.**

19. **TEST-TAKING TIP: Option 4 is unique. It is the only option that identifies something that should be avoided; the other options are stated from a positive perspective.**
1. **The act of chewing (mastication) is facilitated by taking smaller portions of food in the mouth. The risk for aspiration increases when the mouth is overwhelmed by a large volume of food at one time.**
2. Ingesting fluids before swallowing can flush food into the breathing passages rather than down the esophagus.
3. **Well-chewed food is broken down and mixed with saliva, forming a bolus; a bolus of food that is well chewed is easier to swallow, causing less risk for aspiration.**
4. **Talking while eating can increase the risk for aspiration. People should not**

talk with food in their mouths; people need to inhale before talking, and this action may cause aspiration of food when food is in the mouth.

5. Meat that is cut into small pieces may be easier to chew than larger portions; the client still must take the time to chew the food adequately before attempting to swallow.

20. Answer: 10 mL

Have: $\frac{5\ \text{mL}}{250\ \text{mg}}$

Desired: $\frac{500\ \text{mg}}{X\ \text{mL}}$

Solve for X = (500 ÷250) x 5 = 10 mL

21. **TEST-TAKING TIP:** The words *impaired circulation* and *lower extremities* are key words in the stem that direct attention to content. The word *feet* in the stem and in options 3, 4, and 5 is a clang association.

1. People with impaired circulation to the feet should always wear sturdy, well-fitting, closed-toe shoes to protect the feet from injury.
2. Applying moisturizing lotion to the feet keeps skin supple. However, moisturizing lotion should not be applied between the toes because doing so supports fungal and bacterial growth. Also, it can macerate the skin.
3. Checking the feet daily using a mirror to monitor all surfaces is an excellent way to identify problems early.
4. Warm socks and blankets should be used when the feet are cold because heating pads and hot water bottles may cause burns. Often, people with impaired circulation to the feet also have reduced sensation, which compromises their ability to identify injury to the feet.
5. Reporting a break in the skin or injury to the feet to a primary health-care provider ensures that the client receives appropriate medical intervention with topical or systemic treatment to prevent infection and/or to facilitate healing.

22. The right lung has three lobes: the right upper lobe (RUL), right middle lobe (RML), and right lower lobe (RLL). Using the lateral approach, the RML is auscultated above the eighth rib in front of the anterior axillary line.

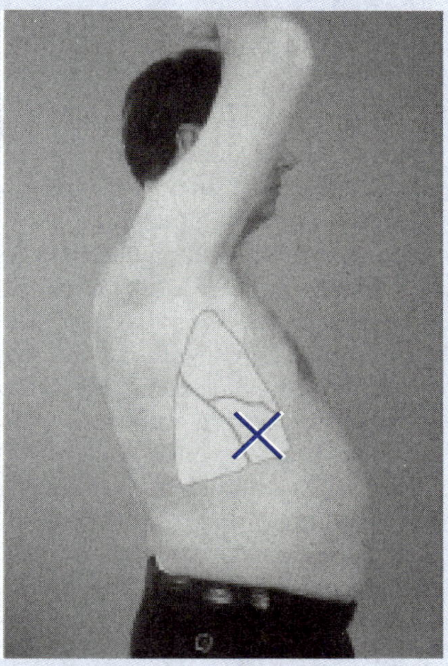

23. **TEST-TAKING TIP:** The words *sudden chest pain* are the key words in the stem that direct attention to content. The word *pain* in the stem and in option 2 is a clang association.

1. The client's vital signs should be taken and compared with baseline data. Alterations in vital signs may reflect a cardiopulmonary event (e.g., angina, myocardial infarction, pulmonary embolism).
2. A detailed pain assessment (e.g., description, intensity, location, precipitating activity) will help the primary health-care provider to establish a diagnosis.
3. Walking should be avoided; activity increases the demand on the heart and will increase pain.
4. Reducing activity and increasing bed rest will decrease oxygen demand on the heart; this in turn will limit the pain. After the activity has been interrupted, the nurse should obtain the vital signs and conduct a thorough pain assessment.
5. Standing still will continue to place a demand on the heart and should be avoided. The pain may take a long time to subside.

24. **TEST-TAKING TIP:** Acute and chronic are opposites that appear in this solution set. Clubbing is related to the chronic impairment of oxygen exchange.

1. The administration of oxygen promotes oxygen available for exchange. This is

not associated with clubbing. Clubbing is caused by chronically low oxygen levels in the peripheral circulation.

2. **Chronic tobacco use impairs oxygen exchange and can lead to clubbing of the fingertips. Chronic tobacco use is a major cause of COPD, a condition where clubbing is often observed.**
3. **Clubbing is the result of chronically low oxygen levels in the peripheral circulation. This state is often due to impaired gas exchange. COPD is a condition where clubbing is often observed.**
4. Asthma is a common and severe chronic lung condition that begins in childhood. In well-controlled asthma, however, oxygen exchange is optimized. Clubbing is not associated with well-controlled asthma.
5. Clubbing is associated with chronic impaired gas exchange. Acute respiratory distress syndrome is just that, acute. It is not associated with clubbing.

25. Answer: 3, 5, 1, 4, 2

3. **The client should first be instructed to move the marker to the lowest setting of the peak flow meter and then take a full deep breath in.**
5. **The client should then hold the breath while placing the teeth around the mouthpiece and closing the lips tightly around it. The client should not block the mouthpiece with their tongue.**
1. **The client should then forcefully exhale into the mouthpiece of the peak flow meter and record the height of the marker.**
4. **The client should repeat this process three times in order to identify the highest reading.**
2. **Once the highest of three readings is identified, the client should use this reading and adjust medication according to their individualized treatment plan.**

26. **TEST-TAKING TIP: The words *dysphagia* and *after meals* are key words in the stem that direct attention to content. Options 1 and 2 are opposites. One or the other is the correct answer. Option 1 is unique because it is the only option with numbers. Examine option 1 carefully.**

1. **Keeping the head of the bed elevated (45° or higher) after meals for 45 to 60 minutes promotes retention of food in the stomach rather than regurgitation, which increases the risk for aspiration.**
2. A low Fowler position (15°) can promote regurgitation and aspiration of food.
3. Frequent mouth care provides comfort, but it does not reduce the risk of aspiration.
4. **Clients who have difficulty swallowing unknowingly can have food trapped in the buccal cavity, which can eventually be aspirated.**
5. **Fluids can be aspirated by a client who has difficulty swallowing; fluid intake should be supervised.**

27.

1. **Clients with decreased level of consciousness are at risk for aspiration. The Glasgow Coma Scale measures level of consciousness from 3 to 15. The higher the score, the higher the level of consciousness. A score of 6 represents a decreased level of consciousness and increased risk for aspiration.**
2. Clients with decreased level of consciousness are at increased risk for aspiration. A Glasgow Coma Scale score of 15 represents the highest level of consciousness possible. This client is not at increased risk for aspiration.
3. **Clients with diminished gag or cough reflex or difficulty swallowing are at increased risk for aspiration. These could be factors causing this client to be unable to clear secretions independently. This client is at increased risk for aspiration.**
4. **Clients with difficulty swallowing are at increased risk for aspiration. The client with NPO orders awaiting a swallow study may have impaired swallow and should be treated as increased risk for aspiration until assessment is complete.**
5. This client has no comorbidities that would indicate increased risk for aspiration. Attending rehab is an indicator that this client is mobile and not at increased risk for aspiration.

28.

1. These are the instructions for using an incentive spirometer. An incentive spirometer requires that a person take a deep breath and expand the lungs to help prevent deflated alveoli (atelectasis).
2. **These are the instructions for using a nebulizer, which is the device in the photograph. A nebulizer is a**

medication delivery system that produces an aerosol spray, which is inhaled via a mouthpiece. Breathing deeply and slowly facilitates contact of the medication with the respiratory tract mucosa.

3. These are instructions for assessing tidal volume. Tidal volume is the volume of air inhaled and exhaled with each normal breath, which is approximately 500 mL.
4. These are the instructions for using a peak expiratory flow meter (PEFM), which measures the peak expiratory flow rate (PEFR). A PEFR is the volume of air that can be forcefully exhaled after taking in a deep breath.

29. 1. This pattern shows a regular pattern of respirations and 16 breaths per minute. The expected respiratory rate is 12 to 20 breaths per minute. *Eupnea* is the term for a normal respiratory pattern.
2. This pattern represents tachypnea, a regular but accelerated pattern of breathing. Tachypnea is defined as a rate exceeding 20 breaths per minute. This pattern represents 28 breaths per minute.
3. This pattern represents Cheyne-Stokes respirations, a pattern of increasing depth and frequency of respirations.
4. **This pattern represents bradypnea, a regular but decreased rate of respiration. This pattern represents 10 breaths per minute.**

30. TEST-TAKING TIP: The word *first* in the stem sets a priority.

1. Obtaining a pulse oximetry reading is within the nurse's scope of practice and does not require a respiratory therapist. This is not the priority action, as it delays care.
2. **These signs are consistent with a pulmonary embolism. The rapid response team should be notified to assess and restore oxygenation as soon as possible. Elevating the head of the bed promotes oxygenation in a client who is experiencing dyspnea.**
3. Notifying the primary care provider and initiating oxygen therapy are appropriate. However, activating the rapid response team identifies and resolves the problem faster than notifying the primary care provider, who may not be immediately available.
4. Although these actions are important, the actions in another option should be implemented first. The nurse needs a primary health-care provider's prescription to initiate an IV infusion.

31. TEST-TAKING TIP: The words *metered-dose inhaler* and *extender* are key words in the stem that direct attention to content.

1. **The client should be in an upright (standing, sitting, or high Fowler) position to promote lung expansion when inhaling.**
2. **Rinsing the mouth removes any remaining medication. This prevents irritation to the oral mucosa and tongue as well as oral fungal infections.**
3. **Waiting between puffs of the inhaler allows time for the medication from the first puff to be absorbed.**
4. **Shaking the canister vigorously several times before using the device mixes the medication sufficiently, resulting in an adequate dose.**
5. **When an extender (spacer) is used with a metered-dose inhaler, the mouthpiece of the extender should be placed in the mouth over the tongue with the teeth and lips tightly around the mouthpiece. This ensures that the tongue does not occlude the end of the extender. Tightly positioning the teeth and lips around the extender mouthpiece ensures that the dose is not diluted with air from outside the mouth.**

32. Answer: 7.5 mL

Solve the problem using ratio and proportion.

$$\frac{\text{Desire}}{\text{Have}} \quad \frac{45 \text{ mg}}{6 \text{ mg}} = \frac{x \text{ mL}}{1 \text{ mL}}$$

$$6x = 45$$

$$x = 45 \div 6$$

$$x = 7.5 \text{ mL}$$

33. TEST-TAKING TIP: The word *most* in the stem sets a priority.

The carotid artery should be assessed during cardiopulmonary resuscitation because when a person is in cardiac arrest, circulation to the extremities is reduced in an attempt to perfuse core organs. Therefore, a carotid artery may have a pulse while the pulses at other sites are weak or absent.

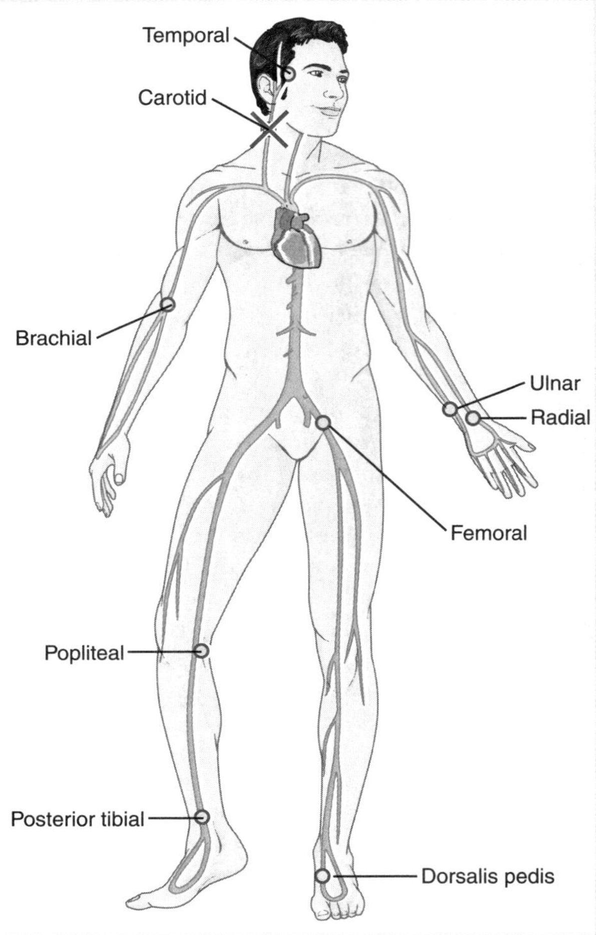

34. **TEST-TAKING TIP: The words *both circulation and respiration* are the key words in the stem that direct attention to content. The interventions chosen must increase both circulation and respiration.**
   1. The use of a spirometer helps to prevent only respiratory complications.
   2. **Repositioning the client every 2 hours helps prevent fluid from collecting in the lung fields, which can contribute to infection and interfere with respiration. Repositioning the client also relieves pressure and increases activity, thereby promoting circulation.**
   3. Rubbing bony prominences with lotion increases only local circulation.
   4. **Ambulation requires the upright position, which relieves pressure against body tissues. The activity of walking increases cardiac output, which increases circulation. Also, the activity of walking increases oxygen demands on the body, which increases the depth and rate of respirations.**
   5. Coughing and deep breathing help to prevent only respiratory complications. Also, coughing and deep breathing should be performed hourly when awake.

35. **TEST-TAKING TIP: The words *nasogastric tube feeding* and *prevent aspiration* are key words in the stem that direct attention to content. Options 3 and 5 are opposites.**
   1. Lowering the height of the bag containing the feeding formula will have no effect on the rate of flow of the formula when it is regulated by an infusion pump.
   2. The head of the bed should remain elevated during the bath and linen change. The bed can be made from the top of the bed to the foot of the bed rather than from side to side. Elevation of the head of the bed keeps the feeding contents in the client's stomach by gravity. A bed in the flat position places the client at risk for gastric reflux and aspiration. Quickly turning the client from side to side to change the linen may unnecessarily jostle the client, which can precipitate gastric reflux and aspiration.
   3. Slowing the flow rate of the feeding still introduces formula, which may promote aspiration.
   4. Seeking additional assistance does not reduce the risk of aspiration.
   5. **Shutting off the feeding reduces the risk of aspiration by temporarily halting the volume of feeding being administered.**

MEETING THE NEEDS OF PERIOPERATIVE CLIENTS AND CLIENTS WITH WOUNDS

This section includes questions related to meeting the needs of clients before, during, and after surgery (perioperative period). The questions focus on physical assessment and on prevention and care related to common complications associated with the perioperative period, such as hemorrhage, wound dehiscence, atelectasis, infection, and thrombophlebitis. The principles of perioperative teaching, meeting clients' emotional needs, sterile technique, and types of dressings and wounds are also tested. In addition, assessment and care of postoperative tubes and wound drainage systems are addressed.

QUESTIONS

1. When a client is brought to the care unit, the nurse is told that the client lost 2 units of blood during surgery. Which responses are significant to this information and should be assessed by the nurse?
1. Rapid, deep breathing and increased blood pressure
2. Rapid, deep breathing and decreased blood pressure
3. Slow, shallow breathing and increased blood pressure
4. Slow, shallow breathing and decreased blood pressure

TEST-TAKING TIP: Identify duplicate facts among options. Identify opposites in options.

2. The nurse is caring for a client on postoperative day 4 after a below-the-knee amputation. The nurse notes opaque, yellow drainage from the wound site and an elevated white blood cell count. What is the nurse's most appropriate next action?
1. Irrigate the wound and replace the sterile dressing
2. Assess the client's pain level, including phantom limb pain
3. Notify the primary health-care provider
4. Monitor for warmth and redness at the incision site

TEST-TAKING TIP: Identify the word in the stem that sets a priority.

3. The nurse is admitting a client who is scheduled for a colon resection in the morning. While reconciling the client's medication list, the nurse notes the client is taking apixaban, ibuprofen, and aspirin. Which assessment question reduces the risk of surgical complications?
1. "Could you describe why you are taking each of these medications?"
2. "When did you last take each of these medications?"
3. "When did you start taking each of these medications?"
4. "Did you know that these medications increase the risk of bleeding during surgery?"

TEST-TAKING TIP: Identify client-centered options.

4. A surgical client is transferred from the postanesthesia care unit to a medical-surgical unit, and the nurse reviews the surgeon's prescriptions. Which vitamin that is commonly prescribed postoperatively should the nurse be alert for?
1. Vitamin C
2. Vitamin A
3. Vitamin K
4. Vitamin B

5. The nurse on a surgical unit routinely assesses clients' incisions as part of postoperative care associated with nontraumatic and noncontaminated incisions. When should the nurse be alert for clinical signs of a wound infection?
1. Between 24 and 48 hours after surgery
2. Between 5 and 10 days after surgery
3. Within the first 24 hours after surgery
4. Later than 12 days after surgery

TEST-TAKING TIP: Identify key words in the stem that direct attention to content.

6. Unlike a T-tube or indwelling urinary catheter, which intervention is unique to a Hemovac® or Jackson-Pratt® drain?
   1. Assessing characteristics of the effluent
   2. Maintaining patency of the conduit
   3. Ensuring negative pressure
   4. Measuring output

   TEST-TAKING TIP: Identify the key words in the stem that direct attention to content.

7. An enema is ordered for a client scheduled for bowel surgery. Which potential event associated with surgery is the enema **primarily** designed to prevent?
   1. Intraoperative peristalsis
   2. Postoperative constipation
   3. Contamination of the operative field
   4. Fecal incontinence during the procedure

   TEST-TAKING TIP: Identify the word in the stem that sets a priority.

8. The nurse is admitting a preoperative client and notes that the client has smoked two packs of cigarettes a day for 15 years. The nurse notes that this is not documented. What are the nurse's two best actions?
   1. Document the client's history and notify the surgeon.
   2. Document the client's history and provide smoking cessation counseling.
   3. Document the client's history and facilitate a referral for smoking cessation counseling.
   4. Document the client's history and request an order for a nicotine patch.

   TEST-TAKING TIP: Identify options that deny client feelings, concerns, or needs. Identify the unique option. Identify words in the stem that set a priority.

9. After a client has a procedure that uses the femoral artery as an access, a pressure dressing is applied at the catheter insertion site. Which is the **primary** purpose of this pressure dressing?
   1. Prevents pain
   2. Limits infection
   3. Decreases drainage
   4. Promotes hemostasis

   TEST-TAKING TIP: Identify the word in the stem that sets a priority. Identify the unique option.

10. The nurse is caring for a client reporting 5/10 pain when returning to the nursing unit after a knee replacement surgery. The nurse notes the following orders on the client's chart: NPO and 1000 mg IV acetaminophen Q6 hours PRN for pain. The nurse recognizes that the client's top two concerns are most likely what?
    1. Pain and eating
    2. Pain and bathing
    3. Pain and discharge planning
    4. Pain and seeing family members

    TEST-TAKING TIP: Identify the word in the stem that sets a priority. Use Maslow's hierarchy of needs to establish the priority.

11. The nurse is caring for a client who just had thoracic surgery. Which is the **most** specific assessment related to this type of surgery?
    1. Blood pressure
    2. Urinary output
    3. Intensity of pain
    4. Rate and depth of respirations

    TEST-TAKING TIP: Identify the word in the stem that sets a priority. Identify key words in the stem that direct attention to content. Identify the unique option.

12. The nurse is caring for a client with a nasogastric tube attached to low continuous suction. Which should the nurse do to prevent dislodgement of the nasogastric tube?
    1. Pin it to the client's pillow
    2. Attach it to the client's gown
    3. Secure the tube to the client's nose
    4. Instruct the client not to touch the tube

    TEST-TAKING TIP: Identify equally plausible options. Identify clang associations.

13. The nurse is caring for a client who repeatedly asks, "Why is this happening to me?" The pattern repeats more frequently as the client's scheduled wrist repair surgery approaches. The nurse prioritizes which nursing diagnosis for this client?
    1. Knowledge Deficit
    2. Airway Clearance Impairment
    3. Ineffective Coping
    4. Disturbed Sleep Pattern

    TEST-TAKING TIP: Identify the word in the stem that sets a priority.

14. A client has a portable wound drainage system after resection of a tumor in the neck. When should the nurse empty the portable wound drainage collection chamber?
    1. After it is full
    2. Every 2 hours
    3. Every 4 hours
    4. When it is half full

15. A postoperative client has a history of heart disease. Which nursing assessment is **most** significant when monitoring this client?
    1. Pain at the site of the incision
    2. Alterations in fluid balance
    3. Irregular pulse rhythm
    4. Dependent edema

    TEST-TAKING TIP: Identify the word in the stem that sets a priority. Identify equally plausible options. Identify the obscure clang association.

16. The nurse is assessing a postoperative client who has just been extubated. Which client response indicates mild postoperative laryngospasm after extubation?
    1. Wheezing
    2. Crackles
    3. Gurgles
    4. Rales

    TEST-TAKING TIP: Identify key words in the stem that direct attention to content. Identify equally plausible options.

17. A client has an order for a wound to be packed with a wet-to-damp gauze dressing. Which should the nurse explain to the client is the **primary** reason for this type of dressing?
    1. "It minimizes the loss of protein."
    2. "It facilitates the healing process."
    3. "It increases the resistance to infection."
    4. "It prevents the entry of microorganisms."

    TEST-TAKING TIP: Identify the word in the stem that sets a priority.

18. The nurse is caring for a postoperative client who had abdominal surgery. Which should the nurse do to help prevent postoperative wound dehiscence? **Select all that apply.**
1. _____ Keep the area clean and dry
2. _____ Change the dressing every 8 hours
3. _____ Medicate the client for pain around the clock
4. _____ Teach the client how to avoid the Valsalva maneuver
5. _____ Encourage the client to support the incision during activity

TEST-TAKING TIP: Identify the key words in the stem that direct attention to content. Identify the obscure clang association.

19. The nurse is caring for a client who had abdominal surgery. Which routine intervention helps prevent atelectasis during the postoperative period? **Select all that apply.**
1. _____ Use of an incentive spirometer
2. _____ Humidification of oxygen
3. _____ Diaphragmatic breathing
4. _____ Progressive activity
5. _____ Postural drainage

TEST-TAKING TIP: Identify the key words in the stem that direct attention to content.

20. The nurse is caring for a client with a nasogastric tube attached to suction. Which is an **essential** nursing action in relation to the nasogastric tube? **Select all that apply.**
1. _____ Use sterile technique when instilling fluid into the system.
2. _____ Record the intake and output at the end of each shift.
3. _____ Maintain suction at the ordered level.
4. _____ Check for tube patency every hour.
5. _____ Provide oral care every 2 hours.

TEST-TAKING TIP: Identify the word in the stem that sets a priority. Identify the clang association.

21. Which intervention is related to the prevention of postoperative thrombophlebitis? **Select all that apply.**
1. _____ Walking regularly
2. _____ Increasing fluid intake
3. _____ Performing feet and leg exercises
4. _____ Applying antiembolism stockings
5. _____ Wearing a sequential compression device

TEST-TAKING TIP: Identify key words in the stem that direct attention to content.

22. Which of the following actions maintain the appropriate strategies to prevent hospital-acquired infections in the perioperative period? **Select all that apply.**
1. _____ Alcohol-based hand rub after caring for the client in contact precautions
2. _____ Chlorhexidine gluconate to access an implanted port the same day it was placed
3. _____ Alcohol-based hand rub before discharge education on an orthopedic nursing unit
4. _____ Discarding sterile gloves found open in the supply room
5. _____ Consider the outer 1-inch border of the sterile field to be sterile

23. The nurse is applying the dressing depicted in the illustration. Place the following steps in the order in which they should be implemented.
1. Peel paper backing from the dressing.
2. Place your hand on the dressing for approximately 10 seconds.
3. Document the date, time, and your initials on the edge of the dressing.
4. Place the dressing over the wound and gently use a hand to smooth it toward the edges.

Answer: ____________

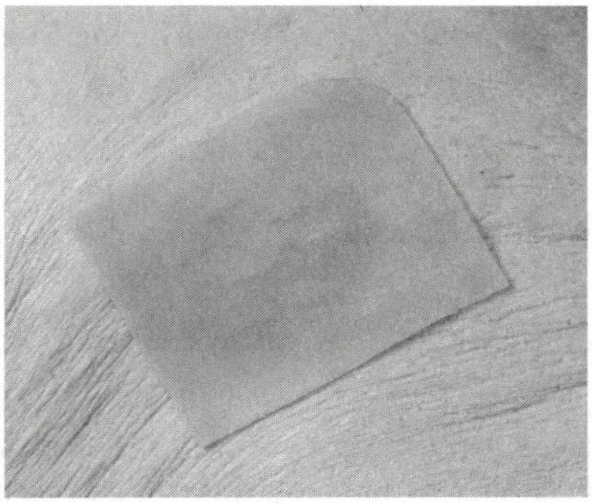

24. A client who received spinal anesthesia is transferred to the postanesthesia care unit. Which assessment of the client during the postoperative period is related to spinal anesthesia? **Select all that apply.**
1. _____ Peripheral circulation
2. _____ Level of consciousness
3. _____ Orientation to time and place
4. _____ Sensation in the legs and toes
5. _____ Ability to move the lower extremities

TEST-TAKING TIP: Identify the key words in the stem that direct attention to content.

25. A postoperative client voids for the first time after surgery. The nurse measures the amount of urine in a graduate as indicated in the illustration. How many milliliters should the nurse document that the client voided? Record your answer using a whole number.

Answer: ____________ **mL**

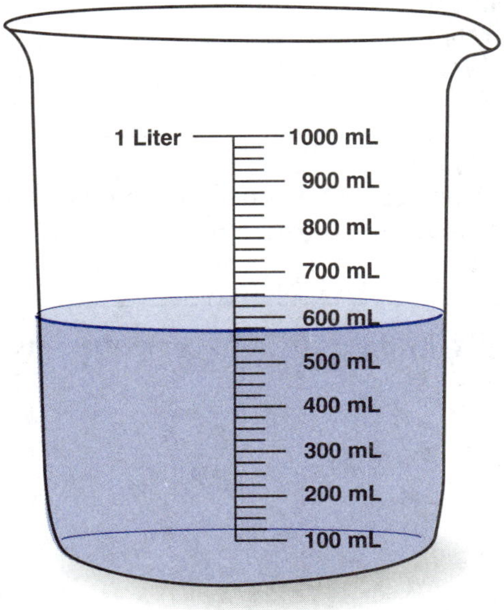

26. Which factor places an older adult at **greater** risk during surgery than a younger person? **Select all that apply.**
1. _____ Increased glomerular filtration rate
2. _____ Increased rigidity of arterial walls
3. _____ Increased basal metabolic rate
4. _____ Decreased hepatic function
5. _____ Decreased cardiac reserve

TEST-TAKING TIP: Identify the word in the stem that sets a priority. Identify key words in the stem that direct attention to content.

27. The nurse is caring for clients with a variety of wounds. Which type of wound heals by primary intention? **Select all that apply.**
1. _____ Pressure ulcer
2. _____ Excoriation
3. _____ Deep burn
4. _____ Paper cut
5. _____ Abrasion

TEST-TAKING TIP: Identify the key words in the stem that direct attention to content.

28. The nurse compares a client's current status with the client's previous information. The nurse bases this analysis on common protocols established for the postanesthesia care unit. Before notifying the surgeon, the nurse should **first:**
1. reinforce the dressing.
2. increase the flow rate of the IV infusion.
3. raise the oxygen flow rate to 12 L/minute.
4. elevate the head of the bed to a high Fowler position.

CLIENT'S CLINICAL RECORD

Admitting Note

0800: Client accepted from circulating nurse and anesthesiologist after having a 2-cm noncancerous tumor removed from right side of neck. Oral airway in place. Oxygen face tent set at 10 L/min. Dressing dry and intact. IV of 1000 mL of 0.9% sodium chloride at 125 mL/hr in progress, with 400 mL left in the bag. IV insertion site dry and intact; no signs of infiltration or inflammation.

Vital Signs

Blood pressure: 140/75 mm Hg
Pulse: 78 beats/min, regular rhythm
Respirations: 22 breaths/min
Oxygen saturation: 97%

Nurse's Progress Note

0900: Airway in place. Client still unresponsive. Moderate amount of blood identified on linen under client's neck. Blood pressure, 100/60 mm Hg; pulse, 90 beats/min; respirations, 24 breaths/min, unlabored.

TEST-TAKING TIP: Identify the word in the stem that sets a priority.

29. The nurse is caring for four clients with abdominal wounds. Identify the wound that should cause the **most** concern.

1. 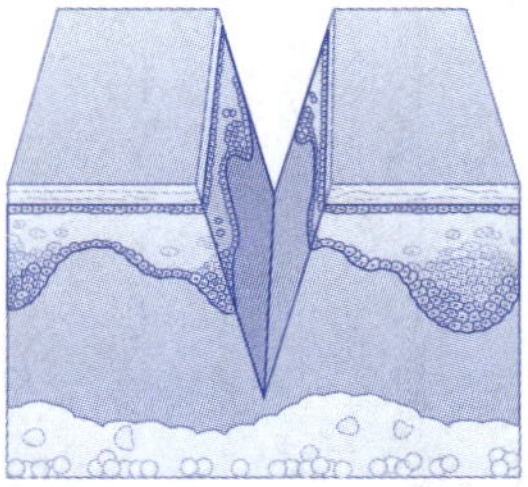

2. 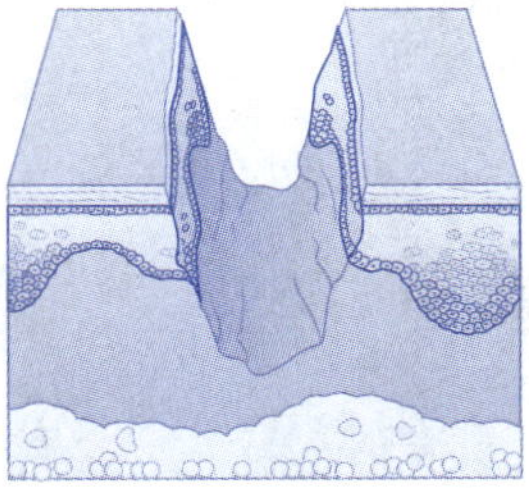

3. 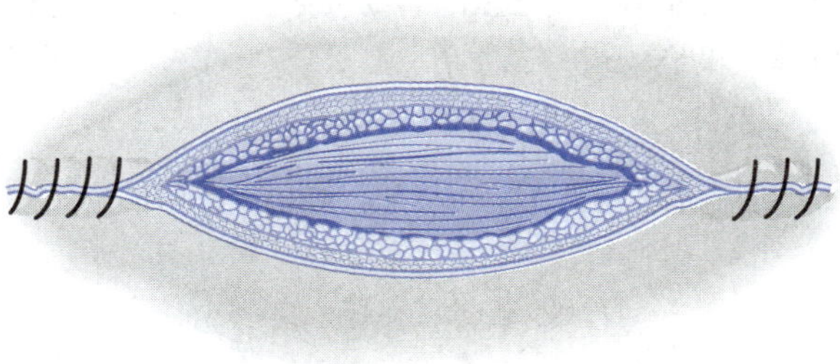

4. 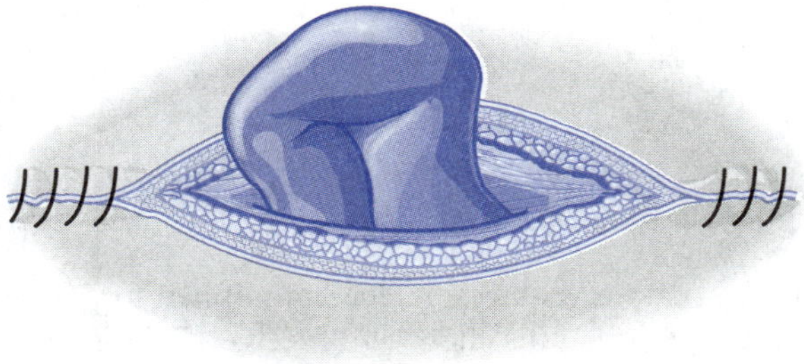

30. The nurse is caring for a client scheduled for abdominal surgery the following morning. Which statements prompt the nurse to provide additional education? **Select all that apply.**

1. _____ "I am worried about having a bowel movement when I come out of surgery."
2. _____ "It will hurt less if I apply pressure against the incision when coughing."
3. _____ "I have been practicing the foot and leg exercises for after surgery."
4. _____ "I want to stay in the postanesthesia care unit as long as possible."
5. _____ "It is important for me to lie still while I am on bed rest."

TEST-TAKING TIP: Identify words in the stem that direct attention to content. Identify the clang association.

31. The nurse is caring for a client with the type of wound dressing depicted in the illustration. Which type of wound should the nurse generally expect to see under this dressing?
  1. Wound with a Hemovac drain
  2. Wound with excessive secretions
  3. Wound with negative pressure therapy
  4. Wound with approximated wound edges

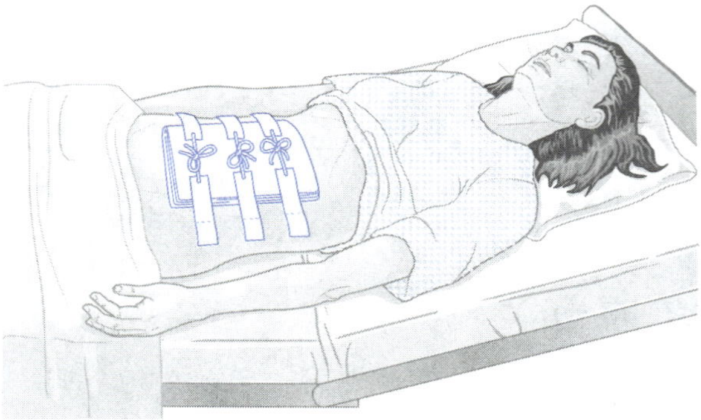

32. The nurse is assessing a client's wound postoperatively. Place an X on the section of this wound that causes the **most** concern.

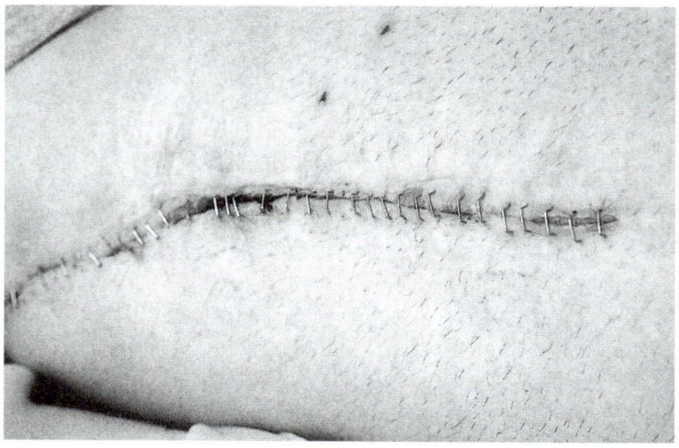

33. An 8-year-old client weighing 23 pounds requires IV acetaminophen for pain management in the postoperative period. This client will receive 12.5 mg/kg every 4 hours. IV acetaminophen is supplied in 10 mg/mL. How many mg will this child receive every 4 hours? **Record your answer using a whole number.**

Answer: ____________ mg

34. The device in the photograph is ordered for a client after surgery. The client asks the nurse, "Why do I have to wear these things?" Which information should the nurse include in the response to the client's question? **Select all that apply.**
 1. _____ Keeps the lower extremities warm
 2. _____ Helps prevent deep vein thrombosis
 3. _____ Accelerates the rate of wound healing
 4. _____ Promotes circulation of blood back to the heart
 5. _____ Eliminates the need for leg and foot exercises after surgery

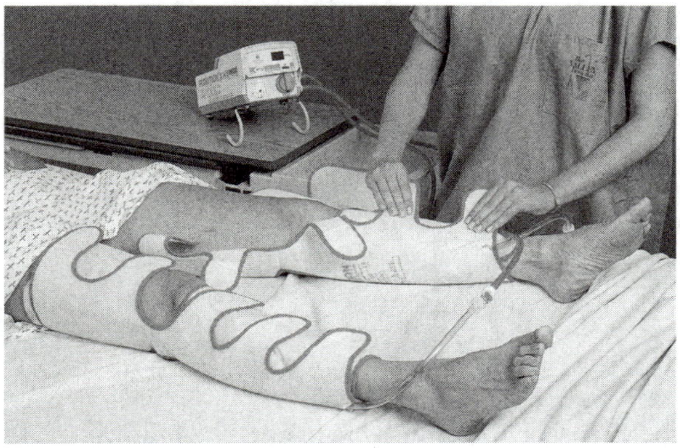

35. The nurse is caring for a client with the wound therapy portrayed in the illustration. Which action should be implemented by the nurse? **Select all that apply.**
 1. _____ Apply a skin protectant around wound edges.
 2. _____ Cut the dressing to the approximate size of the wound.
 3. _____ Pack the deep crevices of the wound with the dressing.
 4. _____ Irrigate the wound as prescribed, moving from dirty to clean areas.
 5. _____ Place the transparent occlusive film covering 2 inches beyond the edges of the wound.

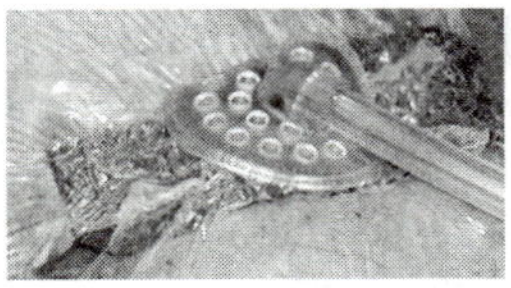

CLINICAL JUDGMENT CASE STUDY

The nurse is caring for a client who is scheduled to undergo a laparoscopic partial colectomy of the transverse colon the following morning. The nurse verifies that the informed consent form has been signed by the client and is documented in the client's chart. The client explains to the nurse that they are "going to have a small surgery, there are no risks and the surgeon is only going to take a couple lymph nodes to make sure that the lump the doctor saw on the x-rays won't move."

36. **Recognize cues—What matters most?** What is the nurse's **most** important action?
 1. Contact the surgeon to reobtain informed consent
 2. Complete preoperative orders on time to prevent delays in surgery
 3. Demonstrate colostomy care to prepare for postoperative care
 4. Explain the rationale for removing lymph nodes

37. **Analyze cues—What could it mean?** The following day, the client returns to the medical-surgical floor after recovering in the postanesthesia care unit (PACU). The nurse notes a 9-cm incision and a stoma in the left upper abdominal quadrant that is beefy red in color. What do these assessment findings indicate?
1. The client will have less scarring and their bowel function will return earlier.
2. The client will have a shorter hospital stay and is at a lower risk for complications.
3. The client underwent an open colectomy and the colon could not be sutured back together.
4. The client experienced complications during the intraoperative period and the stoma was created to decrease length of stay.

38. **Prioritize hypotheses—Where do I start?** The nurse notes the client's vital signs.

Temperature	98.9°F (37.2°C)
Pulse	82
BP	128/82
Respirations	18/min

1. The nurse assesses the client's incision and documents the following: "9-cm surgical incision noted at abdominal midline. Edges well-approximated and 10 staples present. Scant red blood noted on dressing. No edema or redness noted." The nurse understands that preventing infection is a priority for this client. Based on this assessment and the client's surgery type, the nurse classifies this incision as which of the following?
2. Clean wound
3. Clean-contaminated wound
4. Contaminated wound
5. Infected wound

39. **Generate solutions—What can I do?** The client is now postoperative day 4. Place an X in the box indicating whether each assessment finding is expected or requires intervention.

Finding	Expected	Requires Intervention
Client reports feeling a "pop" at the wound site		
Absence of bowel sounds and abdominal pain		
Moderate amount of "toothpaste" consistency stool		
Cramping in the left calf during ambulation		

40. **Take action—What will I do?** The client reports pain 8/10 that prevents the client from sleeping at night and interferes with their appetite. Which of the following are appropriate nursing interventions to manage this client's postoperative pain? **Select all that apply.**
1. Ask the primary health-care provider to order around-the-clock NSAIDs in addition to opioids.
2. Use binders or splint the incision.
3. Promote adequate oral hydration.
4. Reassess pain every 12 hours.
5. Avoid progressive muscle relaxation or guided imagery.

41. **Evaluate outcomes—Did it help?** The nurse is providing discharge education to this client. The nurse knows that the client understands the information when the client makes which of the following statements?
1. "Severe abdominal pain will happen and I don't need to bother the doctor about it."
2. "I should call the doctor if I have a fever."
3. "I need to rest as much as possible in my recliner."
4. "If the pain becomes severe, it is okay to take extra pain pills."

MEETING THE NEEDS OF PERIOPERATIVE CLIENTS AND CLIENTS WITH WOUNDS ANSWERS AND RATIONALES

1. **TEST-TAKING TIP: The question is testing your knowledge about the type of breathing and type of blood pressure associated with hypovolemia secondary to blood loss. If you know just one of these clinical indicators related to hypovolemia, you can reduce your final selection to two options. Options 1 and 4 are opposites, and options 2 and 3 are opposites. Although there are two sets of opposites in this item, it is easier and more productive to focus instead on the duplicate facts to help eliminate distractors.**
   1. Although rapid, deep breathing is associated with hypovolemia, blood pressure decreases, not increases.
   2. **With a decrease in circulating red blood cells, respiration increases in rate and depth to meet oxygen needs. With a reduction in blood volume, there is a decrease in blood pressure.**
   3. With hypovolemia, breathing is rapid and deep, not slow and shallow, and blood pressure decreases, not increases.
   4. Although blood pressure decreases with hypovolemia, respirations are rapid and deep, not slow and shallow.

2. **TEST-TAKING TIP: The words *most appropriate* and *next* in the stem set the priority.**
   1. Purulent drainage and an elevated WBC count are signs of an infection. This is not the most appropriate next action.
   2. Assessing pain is an important aspect of postsurgical care for a client who has had an amputation. Clients who have had an amputation often experience phantom limb pain. However, this is not the most appropriate next action.
   3. **Purulent drainage from a surgical wound and an elevated white blood cell count indicate infection. Notifying the primary health-care provider is the most appropriate next action, as this client requires further assessment and management to prevent negative outcomes.**
   4. Purulent drainage and an elevated white blood cell count indicate infection. Monitoring for warmth and redness identify additional signs of infection. However, this action does not address the infection that is already identifiable based on the other findings. The most appropriate next action is to notify the primary health-care provider.

3. **TEST-TAKING TIP: Option 4 is not a client-centered option and can be ruled out. Think about what apixaban, ibuprofen, and aspirin have in common.**
   1. Although a client should understand why they are taking each of their medications, this question does not lower the risk of surgical complications.
   2. **Apixaban, ibuprofen, and aspirin all carry the risk of bleeding. Generally, these medications are held for a defined period of time before a major surgery, such as a colon resection. This assessment question is important and can reduce the risk of the surgical complication of bleeding by identifying if the client understood and adhered to preoperative instructions.**
   3. This assessment question does not reduce the risk of surgical complications. The nurse should identify whether or not the client followed preoperative instructions, which are designed to prevent complications, such as the risk for bleeding.
   4. This question is not client-centered. It may contribute to anxiety that a client is already experiencing in the perioperative period and does not address the issue of apixaban, ibuprofen, and aspirin increasing the risk for bleeding.

4. 1. **Vitamin C (ascorbic acid) is essential for collagen formation, the single most important protein in connective tissue. The recommended daily dose is 60 mg; however, a postoperative client may need up to 1000 mg of vitamin C for tissue repair, necessitating supplementation.**
   2. Although vitamin A is associated with epithelial tissue, it is not usually prescribed individually but rather as part of a multivitamin.
   3. Although vitamin K promotes blood clotting by increasing the synthesis of prothrombin by the liver, it is not usually prescribed unless the client has liver disease or a bleeding tendency.
   4. Although the B-complex vitamins are related to protein synthesis and cross-linking of collagen fibers, they are not usually prescribed individually but rather as part of a multivitamin.

5. **TEST-TAKING TIP: The words *wound infection* in the stem direct attention to content.**

1. One to 2 days is too short a time for an infectious process to develop from a surgical incision; a contaminated traumatic wound may precipitate an infection this early.
2. **Microorganisms in a surgical incision can precipitate an infection, which generally manifests in 5 to 10 days after surgery; erythema, pain, edema, chills, fever, and purulent drainage indicate infection.**
3. Within 24 hours after surgery is too short a time for an infectious process to develop from a surgical incision; a contaminated traumatic wound may precipitate an infection this early.
4. An infectious process generally manifests before 12 days.

6. **TEST-TAKING TIP: The words *intervention is unique to a Hemovac® or Jackson-Pratt®* are key words in the stem that direct attention to content.**
   1. All drainage must be assessed for quantity, color, consistency, and odor.
   2. All conduits (e.g., tubes, catheters) must be patent for drainage to occur.
   3. **Portable wound drainage systems work by continuous low negative pressure as long as the suction bladder is less than half full; T-tubes and indwelling urinary catheters work via gravity.**
   4. The volume of fluid over specific time periods must be measured for all drainages.

7. **TEST-TAKING TIP: The word *primarily* in the stem sets a priority.**
   1. Although an enema may reduce bowel peristalsis intraoperatively (during surgery) because the bowel will be empty of stool, it is not the purpose of an enema before bowel surgery.
   2. Postoperative constipation is prevented by activity and adequate fluid intake.
   3. **If feces are present in the bowel when the intestine is incised, the excrement spills into the abdominal cavity, causing contamination and increasing the risk of peritonitis.**
   4. Although an enema prevents fecal incontinence during surgery, it is not the purpose of thorough bowel preparation for intestinal surgery.

8. **TEST-TAKING TIP: Options 2, 3, and 4 deny client feelings, concerns, or needs. Options 2, 3, and 4 involve interacting with the client. Option 1 is unique because it involves communicating information to the surgeon. The word *best* in the stem sets a priority.**
   1. **This important finding should be documented and the surgeon should be informed of this information because it may influence the type of anesthesia administered and the perioperative medical regimen.**
   2. This finding should be documented. Smoking cessation counseling is important, but this is not the best action because it does not address the client's immediate perioperative needs. Additionally, the client must consent to smoking cessation counseling. Counseling is more effective if the client is ready to quit.
   3. This finding should be documented and a referral to an expert for smoking cessation counseling may be appropriate. However, this action does not address the client's immediate perioperative needs. The client must consent to smoking cessation counseling. Counseling is more effective if the client is ready to quit.
   4. This finding should be documented. There are many pharmacological strategies to support clients who use tobacco during a hospital admission. These options must first be discussed with the client in order to involve them in their care. This is not the best action because it does not address the client's immediate needs during the perioperative period.

9. **TEST-TAKING TIP: The word *primary* in the stem sets a priority. Option 4 is unique because it is from a positive perspective, expressed by the word *promotes*. Options 1, 2, and 3 are from a negative perspective, expressed by the words *prevents*, *limits*, and *decreases*.**
   1. Although a pressure dressing may help prevent the accumulation of interstitial fluid, thereby limiting pain, it does not prevent pain; also, this is not the primary purpose of a pressure dressing.
   2. Surgical asepsis, not a pressure dressing, limits infection.
   3. Dressings usually do not decrease drainage; they absorb drainage.
   4. **Pressure causes the constriction of peripheral blood vessels, which prevents bleeding; it also eliminates dead space in underlying tissue so that healing can progress.**

10. **TEST-TAKING TIP: The word *most* in the stem sets a priority. Meeting nutritional**

needs is a physiological need, a first-level need according to Maslow's hierarchy of needs theory.

1. **After concerns about pain, eating is the most common concern for many postoperative clients. According to Maslow, it has the highest priority of the options presented. The nurse must investigate why the client has NPO orders, advocate for appropriate diet orders, or educate the client accordingly.**
2. Although knowing when one can shower may be important to some clients, it is not the most basic common concern of the majority of clients. Showering refers to microbiological safety, which is a second-level need according to Maslow.
3. Although wanting to know when one can go home may be important to some clients, it is not the most basic common concern of the majority of clients. Going home refers to love and belonging, which is a third-level need according to Maslow.
4. Although having visitors may be important to some clients, it is not the most basic common concern of the majority of clients. Having visitors is related to love and belonging needs, which are third-level needs according to Maslow.

11. **TEST-TAKING TIP: The word *most* in the stem sets a priority. The words *thoracic* and *specific* are key words in the stem that direct attention to content. Option 4 is unique because it is the only option with two assessments.**

1. Monitoring blood pressure is important after any surgery but is not specific to thoracic surgery.
2. Monitoring fluid intake and urinary output is important after all types of surgery; it is not unique to thoracic surgery.
3. Monitoring the characteristics of pain is required after all types of surgery but is not specific to thoracic surgery.
4. **Thoracic surgery involves entering the thoracic cavity; respiratory function becomes a priority.**

12. **TEST-TAKING TIP: Options 1 and 2 are equally plausible. The word *tube* in the stem and in options 3 and 4 is a clang association.**

1. Pinning the tubing to the client's bed linen is unsafe; tension on the tube will increase with client movement, which may result in displacement of the tube.
2. Attaching the tubing to the gown is unsafe. Client movement will increase tension on the tubing and may result in displacement of the tube.
3. **Attaching a nasogastric tube to the client's nose via tape or a tube fixation device anchors the tube and helps prevent dislodgement.**
4. Although the client should be instructed not to touch the tube, this is not the most effective way to prevent dislodgement of the tube because clients tend to touch foreign objects that irritate the body.

13. **TEST-TAKING TIP: The word *prioritizes* in the stem sets a priority. Avoid reading into the question. Use only the information provided.**

1. Although the client may have a knowledge deficit related to the rationale for their surgery, this nursing diagnosis is not the priority.
2. This scenario does not provide any information on an underlying condition that may increase this client's risk for airway clearance impairment. This is not the priority nursing diagnosis.
3. **The client is increasingly questioning why they must undergo the surgery. This pattern of behavior may be related to anxiety that can interfere with coping. The nurse should prioritize this nursing diagnosis because it is having the greatest effect on the client at this time.**
4. This scenario does not provide any information on factors that may influence sleep. This nursing diagnosis is not the priority.

14.

1. Waiting until after the device is full is undesirable because of the reduced effectiveness of the system's negative pressure.
2. This may be unnecessary because the device may not have filled to the level where it should be emptied. Opening the device increases the risk of infection and should be done only when necessary.
3. This may be unnecessary because the device may not have filled to the level where it should be emptied. Opening the device increases the risk of infection and should be done only when necessary.
4. **The force of the vacuum within the system reduces as the collection chamber fills. Therefore, the collection chamber should be emptied when it is half full to ensure the effectiveness of suction.**

15. **TEST-TAKING TIP: The word *most* in the stem sets a priority. Options 2 and 4 are equally plausible; they both relate to problems with fluid balance. The words *heart* in the stem and *pulse* in option 3 are obscure clang associations. Left ventricular contraction of the heart precipitates the pulse.**
    1. Pain at the incisional site is common in postoperative clients and is not specific to a postoperative client with a history of heart disease.
    2. Although changes in fluid balance are important assessments, an alteration in fluid balance is not immediately life threatening.
    3. **An irregular pulse rhythm may indicate a life-threatening dysrhythmia.**
    4. Although assessment of dependent edema is important, it is not as critical as another assessment.

16. **TEST-TAKING TIP: The words *mild* and *laryngeal spasm* are key words in the stem that direct attention to content. Options 2 and 4 are equally plausible. Rales and crackles describe the same adventitious lung sound heard on auscultation caused by air passing through secretions.**
    1. **Wheezing, which consists of high-pitched whistling sounds, is caused by air moving through a narrowed or partially obstructed airway. Mild laryngeal spasm narrows the airway.**
    2. Crackles, also known as rales, are sounds caused by air passing through respiratory passages containing excessive secretions.
    3. Gurgles, formerly known as rhonchi, are sounds caused by air moving through tenacious mucus.
    4. Rales, more commonly known as crackles, are sounds caused by air passing through respiratory passages containing excessive secretions.

17. **TEST-TAKING TIP: The word *primary* in the stem sets a priority.**
    1. Wet-to-damp packing of a wound is not done to minimize the loss of protein from a wound. Protein loss occurs until the wound heals.
    2. **Packing a wound with wet-to-damp dressings allows epidermal cells to migrate more rapidly across the bed of the wound surface than dry dressings, thereby facilitating wound healing.**
    3. Although packing a wound with wet-to-damp dressings will wick exudate up and away from the base of the wound and therefore help to increase resistance to a wound infection, this is not the primary reason for its use.
    4. This is not the primary purpose of a wet-to-damp gauze dressing. Dry sterile dressings are used to prevent the entry of microorganisms into a wound.

18. **TEST-TAKING TIP: The words *prevent* and *dehiscence* are the key words in the stem that direct attention to content. The word *wound* in the stem and the word *incision* in option 5 are obscure clang associations.**
    1. Keeping the wound clean and dry should prevent infection, not wound dehiscence.
    2. Changing the wound dressing every 8 hours should prevent infection, not wound dehiscence.
    3. Pain medication promotes comfort; it does not limit the occurrence of dehiscence.
    4. **Attempted exhalation against a closed glottis (Valsalva maneuver) is unconsciously performed when attempting elimination, moving around in bed, or rising from a sitting to a standing position. The Valsalva maneuver increases intraabdominal pressure, which exerts tension behind the sutured incision that can result in separation of the wound edges (dehiscence).**
    5. **Pressure against the incision supports the integrity of the approximation of the edges of the wound.**

19. **TEST-TAKING TIP: The words *prevent atelectasis* are the key words in the stem that direct attention to content.**
    1. **Atelectasis occurs when the alveoli are deflated, resulting in reduced or absent gas exchange. An incentive spirometer provides a visual cue that promotes a progressive increase in the volume of inspired breath. Also, the device promotes the maintenance of a deep breath at the height of inhalation, which helps to expand alveoli.**
    2. Humidification of oxygen keeps the mucous membranes of the respiratory tract moist; it does not prevent atelectasis.
    3. **Diaphragmatic breathing expands the alveoli, which prevents atelectasis. Also, it precipitates coughing, which prevents the accumulation and stagnation of secretions.**
    4. **Although progressive activity does not directly affect the lungs, it does promote cardiopulmonary and circulatory functioning in general.**

Activity requires muscle contraction, which increases the need for oxygen. When there is an increased need for oxygen at the cellular level, the heart rate increases and the depth and rate of respirations increase. Also, activity mobilizes respiratory secretions where they can be expectorated.

5. Postural drainage promotes the flow of mucus out of segments of the lung; it is not done routinely after surgery to prevent atelectasis.

20. **TEST-TAKING TIP: The word *essential* in the stem sets a priority. The word *suction* in the stem and in option 3 is a clang association.**

1. Medical, not surgical, asepsis is necessary. The stomach is not considered a sterile space.
2. **The intake and output must be recorded at routine intervals per hospital policy, such as at the end of each shift and every 24 hours.**
3. **The level of suctioning is part of the order for nasogastric decompression. Low suction pressure is between 80 and 100 mm Hg, and high suction pressure is between 100 and 120 mm Hg. Suctioning must be maintained continuously with a Salem sump to prevent reflux of gastric secretions into the vent lumen, which will obstruct its functioning and may result in mucosal damage. A single-lumen tube requires low intermittent suction, which helps to prevent the tube from adhering to the stomach mucosa.**
4. **Functioning of the tube must be maintained; therefore, its patency should be checked every hour. Gastric contents will accumulate in the stomach when a nasogastric tube is not functioning; this can result in nausea and vomiting.**
5. **Oral hygiene should be provided every 2 hours and more frequently if necessary. The mouth becomes dry because there is no food or fluid to stimulate salivary gland secretion, and the tube in the nose may interfere with breathing, precipitating mouth breathing.**

21. **TEST-TAKING TIP: The words *prevention* and *thrombophlebitis* are key words in the stem that direct attention to content.**

1. **Ambulating increases circulation in the lower extremities, which helps to prevent thrombus formation.**
2. **Increasing fluid intake promotes hemodilution, which helps limit thrombus formation.**
3. **Flexing and extending the feet requires muscle contraction. Muscle contraction requires oxygen; thus, circulation increases to bring more blood cells and therefore oxygen to the area. When muscles contract and relax, they rhythmically compress the capillary beds, promoting venous return.**
4. **Antiembolism stockings promote venous return, which helps to prevent thrombus formation.**
5. **A sequential compression device helps to prevent venous pooling in the lower extremities by promoting venous return to the heart; this helps to prevent thrombus formation.**

22. **TEST-TAKING TIP: The word *sterile* in the stem directs attention to content. Option 1 contains the word *always*, which is a specific determiner. The word *sterile* in the stem and in option 5 is a clang association.**

1. Clients in contact precautions are being managed for infections such as *C. diff.* When caring for clients in contact precautions, the nurse should wash hands using soap and water, not an alcohol-based hand rub.
2. **Chlorhexidine gluconate is the most appropriate cleansing agent when accessing an implanted port. Implanted ports can be safely accessed the same day they are surgically placed. The nurse should be aware that, when accessing an implanted port the same day it is placed, they are managing both a central line and surgical site.**
3. **Alcohol-based hand rub is appropriate before discharge education is conducted on an orthopedic nursing unit. This activity requires minimal physical contact.**
4. **Any time that the sterility of a supply item is questionable, the product should be discarded to prevent the contamination of a sterile field. An example of questionable sterility is finding a pair of sterile gloves with open packaging in the supply room.**
5. The outer 1-inch border of a sterile field is considered contaminated. All sterile

equipment must remain inside this border to be considered sterile.

23. Answer: 3, 1, 4, 2
   3. **Documenting important information on this hydrocolloid dressing before it is applied prevents unnecessary pressure over the wound compared with documenting the information on the dressing after it is applied. Pressure against a dressing after it has been applied may be uncomfortable or painful for the client. Documenting important information on the outside of the dressing ensures that others know the date and time the dressing was applied and the identity of the nurse applying the dressing.**
   1. **Removing the paper exposes the adhesive backing of this hydrocolloid dressing before the dressing is applied.**
   4. **Placing this hydrocolloid dressing gently on the wound and smoothing it toward the edges ensures that the dressing is against the wound and the edges adhere to the skin surrounding the wound. Working gently avoids undue pressure against the wound.**
   2. **Placing a hand on this hydrocolloid dressing for approximately 10 seconds uses body heat to mold the dressing to the skin. This action improves adherence of the dressing to the client's skin.**

24. **TEST-TAKING TIP: The words *spinal anesthesia* are the key words in the stem that direct attention to content.**
   1. Spinal anesthesia does not alter peripheral circulation.
   2. General anesthesia, not spinal anesthesia, acts on the cerebral centers to produce loss of consciousness.
   3. General anesthesia, not spinal anesthesia, acts on the cerebral centers and alters orientation to time, place, and person.
   4. **Spinal anesthesia causes loss of sensation in the toes, perineum, legs, and abdomen. When sensations in the legs and toes return, the client is considered to have recovered from the effects of the spinal anesthetic.**
   5. **Spinal anesthesia causes loss of motion in the lower extremities. When mobility of the legs and toes returns, the client is considered to have recovered from the effects of the spinal anesthetic.**

25. Answer: 575 mL
   Each line represents 25 mL of urine.

26. **TEST-TAKING TIP: The word *greater* in the stem sets a priority. The words *older adult* are key words in the stem that direct attention to content.**
   1. Older adults have a decreased, not increased, glomerular filtration rate.
   2. **Older adults have increased rigidity of the arterial walls because of changes in the mechanical and structural properties of arterial walls. There is fragmentation of elastic tissue, changes in structural proteins, and increased collagen in vascular walls; stiffness of vascular smooth muscle cells; and presence of atherosclerotic plaques and calcifications.**
   3. Older adults have a decreased, not increased, basal metabolic rate.
   4. **The size of the liver, blood flow in the liver, and enzyme production by the liver decrease; the half-life of anesthetic agents and medications increases, which may result in toxicity.**
   5. **As one ages, cardiac output and the strength of cardiac contractions decrease and the heart rate takes longer to return to the resting rate. Sudden physical or emotional stresses may result in cardiac dysrhythmias and heart failure.**

27. **TEST-TAKING TIP: The words *primary intention* are the key words in the stem that direct attention to content.**
   1. A pressure ulcer heals by secondary intention. A pressure ulcer does not have close approximated edges. It usually appears as a circular wound.
   2. An excoriation is an abrasion, a loss of superficial skin layers caused by trauma, friction, chemicals, or digestive enzymes. An excoriation heals by secondary intention.
   3. A burn has wound edges that are not approximated, and the wound usually is wide and open. A burn heals by secondary intention.
   4. **A paper cut is a slice or sliver-like wound with very close approximated edges. It heals by primary intention. Primary intention is a healing process that consists of defensive, reconstructive, and maturative healing stages. It involves a clean wound that has closely approximated edges.**

5. An abrasion, like an excoriation, is the loss of superficial skin layers caused by trauma, friction, chemicals, and digestive enzymes. An abrasion heals by secondary intention.

28. TEST-TAKING TIP: The word *first* is the word in the stem that sets a priority.

1. Reinforcing the dressing should be done eventually, but it is not the priority.
2. **When a postoperative client in the postanesthesia care unit demonstrates signs of hemorrhage, protocols generally permit the nurse to increase the flow rate of an IV infusion until the surgeon can be notified. The decrease in blood pressure, increases in pulse and respiratory rates, and blood on the linen under the client's neck support the conclusion that the client is hemorrhaging.**
3. This intervention does not address the client's immediate need. The suggested flow rate for a face tent is 8 to 10 L/min.
4. Elevating the head of the bed higher than the semi-Fowler position is too high for an unresponsive client. A high Fowler position may be assumed after recovery from anesthesia.

29. 1. This is the least serious of the wounds presented. This wound appears to be clean, with edges that can be approximated with sutures. This wound will heal by primary intention.

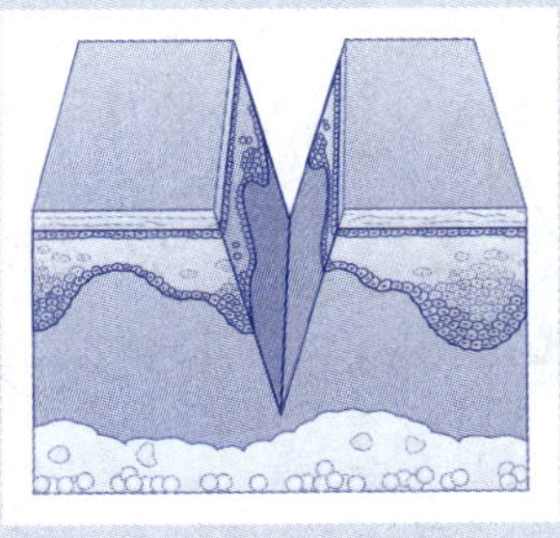

2. This wound is less serious than two other wounds presented. This wound has irregular wound edges that will heal by secondary intention.

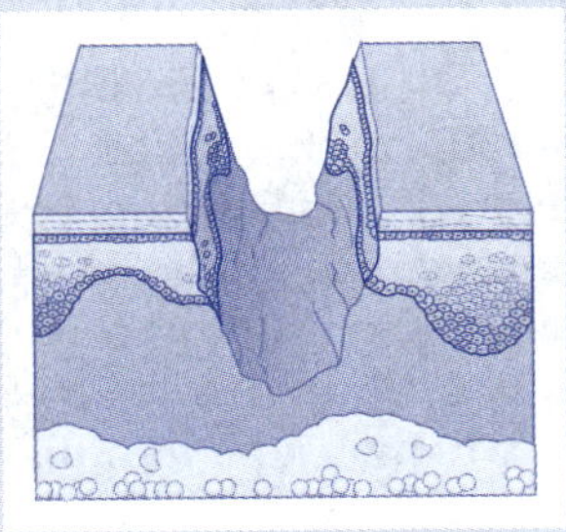

3. This wound has wound edges that have separated, and the muscle layer is visible (dehiscence). Although this is a serious complication of wound healing, it is not as serious as another wound presented in the question. Dehiscence occurs in approximately 0.3% to 3% of clients with abdominal surgery, with studies documenting mortality rates of 14% to 30%. Dehiscence generally occurs between the fifth and twelfth day postoperatively.

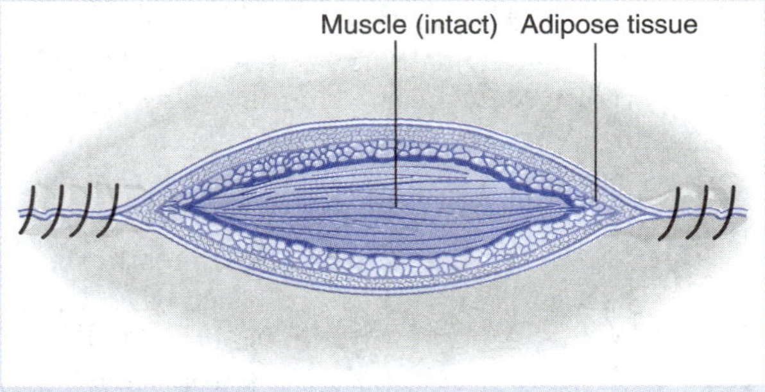

4. **This illustration exhibits evisceration, which is a life-threatening condition. Evisceration occurs when abdominal contents protrude through separated wound edges, precipitating necrosis of the intestines or overwhelming sepsis. Evisceration occurs in approximately 1% to 2% of clients with abdominal surgery, with the largest number appearing between the seventh and tenth day postoperatively. Evisceration has a mortality rate of 30% to 37%.**

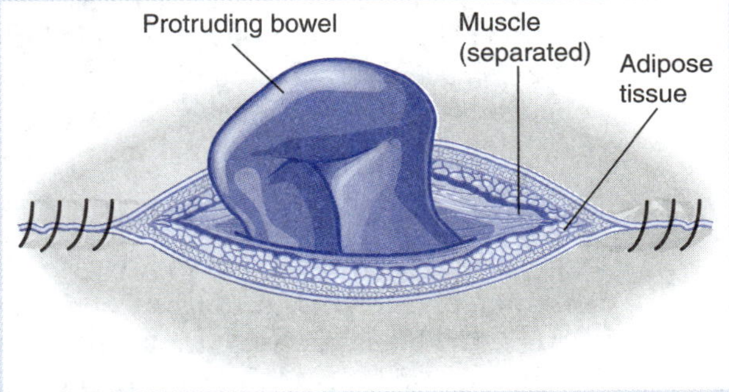

30. TEST-TAKING TIP: The words *prompt* and *additional education* direct attention to content. The nurse must recognize when client statements do not make sense, clarify meaning, and provide additional information to support client understanding.

1. **It takes a minimum of 2 to 3 days for peristalsis to return after abdominal surgery because of the effects of**

anesthesia and manipulation of the abdominal organs, particularly the intestines. The nurse should give this information to the client and discuss strategies to reduce pain with bowel movements after an abdominal surgery.

2. When performing any activity that increases intraabdominal pressure, applying pressure against an incision is an acceptable practice to minimize incisional pain and help prevent dehiscence. This client has accurate expectations of the postoperative period.
3. Foot and leg exercises should be performed after abdominal surgery to increase venous return to the heart. These exercises will help prevent deep vein thrombosis. This client is preparing appropriately for the postoperative period.
4. **Clients are kept in the postanesthesia care unit until they are reactive and stable, not as long as possible. This client may require reassurance that they will receive good care beyond the postanesthesia care unit.**
5. **Remaining immobile after surgery is not recommended because it promotes cardiopulmonary, vascular, and gastrointestinal complications. Many types of exercises can be performed when on bed rest. This client should receive additional information about preventing complications after surgery.**

31. 1. The illustrated dressing generally is not necessary for a wound with a Hemovac drain. In addition, a drainage tube exiting the dressing and terminating in a Hemovac collection container would be visible when examining the client's abdominal area; however, none is present.

2. **An open wound with excessive (i.e., large, profuse, abundant, copious) amounts of secretions requires frequent changing. This minimizes drainage coming into contact with intact tissue, avoiding maceration of the skin. The Montgomery straps dressing in the illustration does not require the constant removal and reapplication of tape when frequent dressing changes are necessary. The nurse unties the straps, removes the soiled dressing, cleanses the wound, applies a sterile dressing, and reties the straps to hold the dressing in place.**
3. This is not an illustration of a wound with negative pressure therapy. A wound with negative pressure therapy has a transparent dressing with a tube leading from the center of the dressing to a machine that maintains negative pressure and collects drainage.
4. A wound with approximated wound edges does not need the dressing in the illustration. A wound with approximated wound edges generally has only small amounts of serosanguineous drainage, requiring a dry sterile dressing for 1 to 2 days.

32. The section indicated by the X marks the wound edges that are separating. A partial or complete parting of the outer layers of a wound (dehiscence) occurs in approximately 3% of clients with abdominal surgery. The critical time when dehiscence commonly occurs is between the fifth and twelfth postoperative days. Sutures or staples that are too close together or too far apart or that have been removed prematurely can contribute to dehiscence. In addition, edema or infection at the incisional site and obesity may contribute to dehiscence.

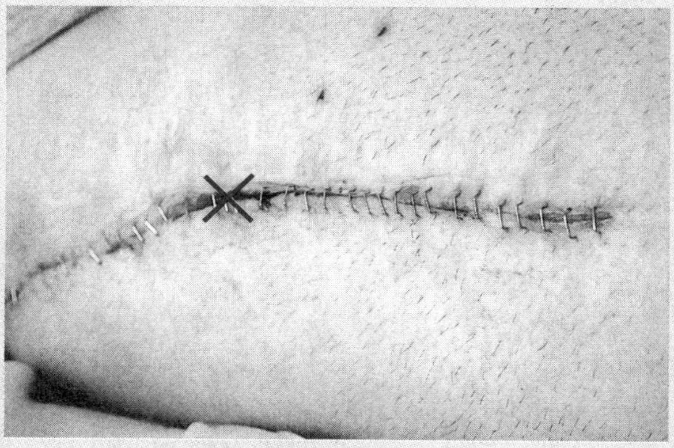

33. Answer: 125 mg
First, convert pounds to kilograms by dividing.
22 pounds ÷ 2.2 kilograms = 10 kg
Then, multiply.
12.5 mg/kg
12.5 mg × 10 kg = 125 mg

34. 1. Keeping the lower extremities warm is not the purpose of this device.

2. **Sequential compression devices help prevent venous pooling by facilitating venous return to the heart. Venous stasis contributes to deep vein thrombosis, which can be minimized with the**

use of sequential compression devices and foot and leg exercises.

3. This device does not accelerate the rate of wound healing.
4. **Sequential compression devices inflate and deflate chambers in the device, moving from distal to proximal, promoting venous blood return to the heart. This action helps prevent venous stasis, which is associated with the development of deep vein thrombosis.**
5. The use of this device does not eliminate the need to implement foot and leg exercises after surgery. Both interventions should be employed to reduce the risk of deep vein thrombosis associated with postoperative recovery.

35.
1. **This is a photograph of negative pressure wound therapy. Applying a skin protectant around wound edges helps reduce the risk of skin breakdown.**
2. **This is a photograph of negative pressure wound therapy. Cutting the dressing to the approximate size of the wound prepares the equipment for the dressing change. The dressing should be small enough to not touch the skin but large enough to fill the wound.**
3. The dressing should be gently placed into the wound cavity with this wound therapy system. Packing the dressing into deep crevices or overfilling the wound is contraindicated because it compresses tissue, which may impair circulation.
4. This photograph does not illustrate wound irrigation. In addition, when irrigating a wound, the nurse should always move from the clean end to the dirty end of the wound because doing so reduces the risk of contaminating the clean end of the wound.
5. **The transparent occlusive film covering should be applied so that it extends 1 to 2 inches beyond the wound edges. It should be compressed gently to ensure that the edges of the transparent occlusive film covering adhere to the skin.**

CLINICAL JUDGMENT CASE STUDY ANSWERS AND RATIONALES

36.
1. **This client does not understand the nature of the surgery that they are scheduled for. There are multiple risks involved with abdominal surgery, including bleeding, blood clots, and infection. The client's signature and documentation in the chart is only part of informed consent. The client must understand the procedure.**
2. Although completing preoperative orders on time is important, it is not the nurse's most important action in this scenario. Preoperative orders may include nothing by mouth (NPO) diet orders, prophylactic antibiotics, and holding certain medications.
3. This client may or may not have a colostomy postoperatively. Although educating this client about colostomy care is an important nursing intervention that should be discussed preoperatively, it is not the most important action in this scenario.
4. Although it is important for the patient to understand the rationale for removing lymph nodes, it is not the most important action in this scenario. A partial colectomy is performed to remove a tumor found in the colon. Multiple lymph nodes are also removed to determine the stage or grade of a cancerous tumor. Staging and grading of a cancerous tumor are used to determine the most appropriate treatment strategy.

37.
1. When a laparoscopic colectomy is performed, less scarring, earlier return of colon function, fewer expected complications, and a shorter hospital stay are expected. A 9-cm incision indicates that the laparoscopic colectomy that was planned was converted to an open colectomy.
2. When a laparoscopic colectomy is performed, less scarring, earlier return of colon function, fewer expected complications, and a shorter hospital stay are expected. A 9-cm incision indicates that the laparoscopic colectomy that was planned was converted to an open colectomy.
3. **A 9-cm incision indicates that the laparoscopic colectomy that was planned was converted to an open colectomy. Possible causes for this change in plan include the presence of adhesions from prior surgery, bleeding, a client who is overweight, or a tumor that is large.**
4. There are instances when a laparoscopic colectomy must be converted to an

open colectomy in the context of an operation that occurs without complications. A 9-cm incision indicates that the laparoscopic colectomy was converted to an open colectomy, and this may increase the client's length of stay. The creation of a stoma would likely increase the length of stay, rather than decrease it, and decisions to create a stoma are made based on colon function, not to reduce length of stay.

38. 1. Clean wounds are not infected, have minimal inflammation, and have little risk of infection. Examples include surgeries of the eye, joint replacements, breast biopsies, and tonsillectomies. Surgical incisions of the gastrointestinal tract, such as a colectomy, are considered clean-contaminated wounds.

2. **Clean-contaminated wounds are not infected but are at an increased risk for developing an infection. Surgical incisions that enter the gastrointestinal, respiratory, or genitourinary tract are considered clean-contaminated wounds due to the increased risk of infection.**

3. Contaminated wounds are not infected but carry a high risk for developing an infection. Examples include surgeries to repair trauma, such as compound fractures.

4. Infected wounds have evidence of infection, such as purulent drainage, necrotic tissue, or elevated bacterial counts. This client's wound is not showing signs of infection.

39.

Finding	Expected	Requires Intervention
Client reports feeling a "pop" at the wound site		X
Absence of bowel sounds and abdominal pain		X
Moderate amount of "toothpaste" consistency stool	X	
Cramping in the left calf during ambulation		X

40. Correct Answer: 1, 2, 3

1. **Administering around-the-clock NSAIDs in addition to opioids is an effective strategy for managing post-operative pain. It is recommended to use analgesics from different drug classes. This strategy has the potential to reduce the necessary dose of opioids required for pain relief. Reducing the dose reduces the associated adverse effects.**
2. **Binders or splinting the incision, as with a pillow while in bed, are nursing interventions that can help manage pain in clients who have undergone abdominal surgery.**
3. **Adequate hydration is an intervention to avoid constipation and straining. Stool softeners may also be ordered for the same reason. Straining to defecate can contribute to pain. Constipation, nausea, and fatigue are experiences that can increase the client's perception of pain, and managing them is a strategy to manage postoperative pain.**
4. Pain should be reassessed more frequently than every 12 hours. Pain should be assessed before and after each activity and each pharmacological and nonpharmacological intervention. Pain should be treated as the fifth vital sign and the plan of care should be adjusted to manage pain.
5. Complementary therapies such as progressive muscle relaxation, guided imagery, visualization, meditation, yoga, aroma therapy, and many others are useful in managing pain. They are evidence-based pain management strategies and generally considered safe.

41. Correct Answer: 2

1. Severe abdominal pain could indicate a postoperative complication. Although mild pain is expected, it should be managed. The care team must be notified if pain continues, increases, or occurs with abdominal distention or signs of infection so that the cause of the pain can be identified and appropriately managed.
2. **Fever is a systemic sign of infection and should be reported as soon as possible. Other signs of infection include swelling, redness, or purulent drainage from the incision.**

3. The client should walk frequently and practice deep breathing to prevent pneumonia and blood clots. Rest is also important to healing, but the client must also understand the importance of these strategies.
4. Pain medication should be taken as prescribed. If the prescribed regimen is not adequately managing the client's pain, communication must occur between the client and the care team and the pain medication regimen must be adjusted accordingly. Taking extra pain medications, especially narcotics, can lead to dangerous adverse effects.

MEETING THE NEEDS OF CLIENTS IN THE COMMUNITY SETTING

This section encompasses questions related to caring for an individual, a family, a subgroup, or the population within a community. The questions include topics such as health-care delivery settings (e.g., nursing homes, day-care centers, assisted-living residences, occupational settings, and private homes), the focus of nursing actions (e.g., prevention of illness, health promotion, maintenance of safe environments, protection and restoration of health), and specific nursing activities (e.g., screening, health education). The questions also focus on levels of health-care services (e.g., primary, secondary, and tertiary health-care delivery), levels of disease prevention (e.g., primary, secondary, and tertiary levels of prevention), and community-focused examples related to nursing intervention (e.g., developmental stresses, common health problems, crisis intervention, and the needs of individuals in the community according to Maslow's hierarchy of needs).

QUESTIONS

1. The nurse is assessing and making recommendations to modify the home environment to promote energy conservation in a client diagnosed with stage 3 heart failure. This nursing activity demonstrates which of the following types of intervention?
1. Primary
2. Secondary
3. Tertiary
4. Quaternary

TEST-TAKING TIP: Identify words in the stem that direct attention to content.

2. The nurse is caring for a population of students in an elementary school. Which of the following school nurse activities represents a primary intervention strategy?
1. Vision and hearing screening
2. Scoliosis screening
3. Ensuring immunizations are current
4. Manage asthma and diabetes during school hours

TEST-TAKING TIP: Identify the clang association.

3. The nurse is driving to a client's home to conduct an initial assessment. During the drive, the nurse observes large and well-kept homes, "high-end" grocery stores, and several sprawling green golf courses. Which of the following are appropriate considerations when approaching this client's home? **Select all that apply.**
1. Cleaning and preparing meals is always part of home health services
2. Nicer neighborhoods require less environmental awareness
3. Home health often includes supporting family caregivers
4. Home health visits are extremely structured
5. Nurses are guests in client homes

TEST-TAKING TIP: Identify specific determiners in options.

4. Which of the following individuals is eligible for home health services under Medicare?
1. 24-year-old requiring continuous monitoring for suicidal ideation
2. 24-year-old requiring special equipment while recovering from a car accident
3. 69-year-old requesting assistance with groceries and meal preparation
4. 69-year-old requesting diabetes education who is homebound

TEST-TAKING TIP: Identify the clang associations.

5. A person is exposed to an individual diagnosed with severe acute respiratory syndrome (SARS). Which method should the nurse expect to be implemented to control the spread of infection?
   1. Isolation
   2. Quarantine
   3. Segregation
   4. Surveillance

6. Which statement reflects the concept of prevalence?
   1. "On Monday morning, the school nurse determined that six children had measles."
   2. "During the last 5 years, 1% of the population of the United States had tuberculosis."
   3. "Last year, of the people at risk for developing breast cancer, 9% actually developed the disease."
   4. "On the first day of June this year, 10% of the population of Middletown had cardiovascular disease."

7. Which of the following nursing actions are aligned with the National Patient Safety Goals defined by the Joint Commission? **Select all that apply.**
   1. The nurse memorizes a client's full name and date of birth and no longer asks.
   2. The nurse prints a current medication list for the client.
   3. The nurse double-checks that metformin and metronidazole are correctly placed in the client's pill box.
   4. The nurse educates the client on the side effects of aspirin.
   5. The nurse double-checks that they are at the right address before administering medications during a home visit.

8. The nurse is caring for an older adult in the community. Which of the following instructions is appropriate regarding medication disposal?
   1. OTC medications can be used safely after their expiration date.
   2. Save leftover prescription medications in case you need them again.
   3. Recap insulin syringes and dispose of them in the trash.
   4. Place insulin syringes in a plastic jar and return them to the pharmacy.

9. Which categories of health-care delivery are associated mainly with community-based nursing?
   1. Primary and tertiary
   2. Secondary and primary
   3. Tertiary and rehabilitation
   4. Rehabilitation and secondary

   TEST-TAKING TIP: Identify the word in the stem that sets a priority. Identify duplicate facts among options.

10. The nurse is planning care for a rural community. The nurse understands that rural communities tend to have fewer resources than urban or suburban communities. The nurse is aware that this community may include what type of population?
    1. Healthy
    2. Vulnerable
    3. Cultural
    4. Unhealthy

    TEST-TAKING TIP: Identify opposites in the options.

11. Which population trend will continue to have the greatest impact on health-care funding and the nursing shortage into the future?
    1. Downward trend in the number of people living in poverty
    2. Upward trend in the number of multiple birth deliveries
    3. Upward trend in the number of adults over age 65 living with chronic disease
    4. Downward trend in the number of people immigrating

    TEST-TAKING TIP: Identify words in the stem that draw attention to content. Identify the option that is the most specific.

12. The concept of community coalition is accurately associated with:
    1. wellness programs.
    2. growing diversity.
    3. shared purpose.
    4. home care.

    TEST-TAKING TIP: Identify the key word in the stem that directs attention to content.

13. People living in which community have the **most** difficulty ensuring their health-care needs are met?
    1. Metropolitan areas
    2. Suburban areas
    3. Urban areas
    4. Rural areas

    TEST-TAKING TIP: Identify the key word in the stem that sets a priority.

14. Which action by the nurse in the occupational setting reflects the lowest-level need according to Maslow?
    1. Identifying hazards in the environment
    2. Assessing the health status of employees
    3. Initiating a prescribed immunization program
    4. Promoting the social adjustment of employees

    TEST-TAKING TIP: Identify key words in the stem that direct attention to content.

15. Which of the following nurses is taking on the role of advocate in the community health setting?
    1. The nurse educating a group of high school students on STI prevention strategies
    2. The nurse attending a local city council meeting to discuss the opioid epidemic
    3. The nurse facilitating a referral for lung cancer screening
    4. The nurse surveying clients about barriers to health care in a community

16. The nurse is sharing information with aging female adults at a community center. Information from which program addresses the leading cause of death in aging female adults?
    1. The American Heart Association's Go Red for Women initiative
    2. The World Health Organization resources for cervical cancer screening
    3. The Department of Veterans Affairs' Veterans Crisis Line
    4. The National Health Service Act FAST campaign

    TEST-TAKING TIP: Identify the word in the stem that sets a priority. Identify equally plausible options.

17. An older adult who needs help with dressing and bathing and who takes prescription medication twice a day is to be discharged from the hospital. Which facility appropriately meets this individual's needs?
    1. Group home
    2. Nursing home
    3. Day-care center
    4. Assisted-living facility

18. A visiting nurse is caring for a bedbound client with a pressure ulcer. Which nursing intervention associated with providing pressure ulcer care in the home often differs from pressure ulcer care provided in the acute-care setting? **Select all that apply.**
   1. _____ Measuring a wound weekly rather than daily
   2. _____ Employing medical asepsis rather than sterile technique
   3. _____ Changing dressings once a day rather than three times a day
   4. _____ Irrigating the wound with tap water rather than normal saline
   5. _____ Using a bulb syringe rather than a piston syringe when irrigating the wound

   TEST-TAKING TIP: Identify the key words in the stem that direct attention to content.

19. Which nursing activity in the community addresses the **most** basic needs according to Maslow's hierarchy of needs? **Select all that apply.**
   1. _____ Arranging for Meals on Wheels
   2. _____ Exploring the meaning of one's life
   3. _____ Teaching a family member to remove throw rugs
   4. _____ Obtaining low-income energy assistance for a family
   5. _____ Supervising a client performing a colostomy irrigation
   6. _____ Presenting a program at the senior center regarding strategies to improve sleep

   TEST-TAKING TIP: Identify the word in the stem that sets a priority. Identify key words in the stem that direct attention to content.

20. A home health-care nurse has had several visits with an older adult who previously had type 2 diabetes and is now insulin dependent. The client has a prescription for a mixture of NPH and regular insulin in the morning. The client also has a prescription for self-monitoring of blood glucose level before each meal and at bedtime with insulin coverage. The nurse has been educating the client about blood glucose monitoring and injections of insulin. In the most recent home visit, the nurse determines that the client has appropriate knowledge about type 2 diabetes, insulin, and how to perform self-monitoring of blood glucose and insulin injections safely, but occasionally forgets to perform glucose monitoring before lunch. The client's blood glucose levels have been within acceptable limits. Occasionally, the client requires insulin coverage before a meal, which is effective. The home health-care nurse uses the Omaha Problem Rating Scale for Outcomes to document the client's knowledge, behavior, and status. What is the client's total score? **Record your answer using a whole number.**

   Answer: __________

Omaha Problem Rating Scale for Outcomes

Concepts	1	2	3	4	5
KNOWLEDGE: Ability of the client to remember and interpret information	No knowledge	Minimal knowledge	Basic knowledge	Adequate knowledge	Superior knowledge
BEHAVIOR: Observable responses, actions, or activities of the client fitting the occasion or purpose	Not appropriate behavior	Rarely appropriate behavior	Inconsistently appropriate behavior	Usually appropriate behavior	Consistently appropriate behavior
STATUS: Condition of the client in relation to objective and subjective defining characteristics	Extreme signs and symptoms	Severe signs and symptoms	Moderate signs and symptoms	Minimal signs and symptoms	No signs and symptoms

21. "Upstream thinking" is a conceptual approach used in public health efforts. Which action implemented by a community health nurse demonstrates upstream thinking? **Select all that apply.**
1. _____ Encouraging parents who live in old buildings to test for lead-based paint
2. _____ Urging parents to ensure that their children's vaccinations are up to date
3. _____ Facilitating support groups for people who are giving up smoking
4. _____ Conducting a nutrition class on the MyPlate food guide
5. _____ Urging clients to enroll in a physical fitness program

22. Which should the nurse do **first** on the basis of information identified during the home visit?
1. Administer insulin coverage as prescribed
2. Implement the dressing change as per the order
3. Immediately call 911 for an ambulance to transport the client to the hospital
4. Ask the supervisor to notify the primary health-care provider about the client's status

POSTANESTHESIA CLINICAL RECORD

Client History

A 65-year-old adult lives alone and has type 1 diabetes and a stage II pressure ulcer on the lateral malleolus of the right extremity. The primary health-care provider ordered a 1500-calorie diabetic diet, twice-a-day insulin doses, and insulin coverage ac and hs. The primary health-care provider also ordered daily dressing changes for the pressure ulcer and evaluation of the client's ability to implement self-monitoring of blood glucose and self-administration of insulin.

Vital Signs During Home Visit

Blood pressure: 100/65 mm Hg
Pulse: 110 beats/min, thready
Respirations: 24 breaths/min

Nursing Assessment

Client answered the door using a walker but walked slowly and reported feeling weak and fatigued. The client expressed experiencing an increase in urination, blurred vision, and nausea. The client also stated, "I don't remember what my last blood glucose was or when I had insulin last." Vital signs were taken, and the blood glucose level was 350 mg/dL. There was no dressing on the wound.

TEST-TAKING TIP: Identify the word in the stem that sets a priority.

23. The nurse is caring for a 17-year-old adolescent client in the community. Which of the following nurse activities are most appropriate for this client? **Select all that apply.**
1. _____ Education about safe tattoo/body piercing
2. _____ Discussion about wearing seat belts
3. _____ Information about suicide and depression warning signs
4. _____ Repeat scoliosis screening
5. _____ Review childhood immunization schedule

TEST-TAKING TIP: Identify the word in the stem that sets a priority. Identify the key word in the stem that directs attention to content.

24. Which recent trend in health-care delivery has influenced how health-care services are provided in the United States? **Select all that apply.**
1. _____ Urgent care centers that are caring for clients with minor acute illnesses
2. _____ Agencies experiencing an increase in the numbers of volunteers
3. _____ Extended-care facilities providing a variety of new therapies
4. _____ Older adult day-care centers providing support for wellness
5. _____ Hospitalized clients being discharged before full recovery

25. The nurse is visiting a grandparent in a skilled nursing facility when they notice papers in their grandparent's roommate's trash can catch fire. Place the following actions in the correct order.
1. Pull the fire extinguisher from the hallway
2. Move the grandparent and their roommate away from the fire
3. Pull the fire alarm and alert staff
4. Extinguish the fire
5. Pull the pin from the fire extinguisher and aim at the fire

Answer: ___________

CLINICAL JUDGMENT CASE STUDY

26. Recognize cues—What matters most? The nurse is preparing materials for a community health screening clinic for a population of people who speak English as a second language. Before leaving the office, the nurse notices that the provider version of the health education materials was printed instead of the client version. This mistake affects which important concept?
1. Cultural competency
2. Health literacy
3. Overcoming language barriers
4. Access to care

27. Analyze cues—What could it mean? At the community health screening clinic, the nurse is caring for a 65-year-old client whose clothing smells of cigarette smoke. The nurse calculates the client's BMI of 29 and the client states that they seldom take metformin and atorvastatin. The nurse recognizes that this client is at the greatest risk for which of the following?
1. Cardiovascular disease
2. Bladder cancer
3. Diabetes mellitus
4. Lung cancer

28. Prioritize hypotheses—Where do I start? While exploring medication adherence, the client states "those pills are expensive." The nurse prioritizes which of the following interventions?
1. Offer support with smoking cessation
2. Offers support with prescription drug coverage
3. Offer support with weight loss
4. Offer support with nutrition counseling

29. Generate solutions—What can I do? The nurse understands that which of the following strategies can support this client in adherence to the prescribed medications? **Select all that apply.**
1. Request generic prescriptions
2. Referral to a Licensed Social Worker
3. Request more refills on each prescription
4. Refer the client to another health-care provider for a second opinion
5. Advocate for better prescription coverage

30. **Take action—What will I do?** While describing available resources, the client asks "What good are these pills? Everybody says they are good." What is the nurse's best response?
   1. "They help you quit smoking."
   2. "They help you become a healthier weight."
   3. "They help lower the risk of heart disease."
   4. "They help lower the risk for cancer."

31. **Evaluate outcomes—Did it help?** After discussing the client's risk factors for cardiovascular disease using motivational interviewing techniques, the nurse knows that the client has a better understanding when the client makes which of the following statements?
   1. "Only my spouse smokes cigarettes."
   2. "I will walk to the store and buy frozen vegetables."
   3. "I will stop taking the pills when I feel well."
   4. "I can't control a heart attack."

MEETING THE NEEDS OF CLIENTS IN THE COMMUNITY SETTING ANSWERS AND RATIONALES

1. **TEST-TAKING TIP: The words *energy conservation* and *diagnosed* draw attention to content indicating a level of intervention.**
   1. Primary interventions prevent disease from occurring in the first place. Examples include applying sunscreen, avoiding the use of tobacco, and educating individuals without diseases about how to prevent disease.
   2. Secondary interventions minimize the impact of a disease by identifying it and treating it early. Examples include mammograms, scoliosis screening, and identifying risk for sexually transmitted diseases.
   3. **Tertiary interventions work to slow disease progression or to improve client function. Examples include symptom management and modifying the home environment. In this scenario, the nurse is making recommendations for home environment modifications that support the client in conserving energy and maintaining function.**
   4. Quaternary interventions are related to the appropriate use of resources. For example, clients between the ages of 45 and 75 are screened for colon cancer because research has shown that this age group benefits the most from this resource. Screening clients over age 76 for colon cancer offers less benefit and is not a recommended use of resources.

2. **TEST-TAKING TIP: Options 1 and 2 are both related to screening and can be ruled out as answers.**
   1. Screening is an example of secondary intervention. Secondary intervention minimizes the impact of disease by identifying and treating it early.
   2. Screening is an example of secondary intervention. Secondary intervention minimizes the impact of disease by identifying and treating it early.
   3. **Immunizations are an example of a primary intervention. Immunizations improve the immune response to diseases before a person is exposed to the disease.**
   4. Asthma and diabetes are chronic conditions that a school nurse frequently manages. This is an example of tertiary intervention. Tertiary intervention slows disease progression and improves client functionality. The school nurse plays an important role in ensuring that pediatric clients living with these conditions are able to fully participate in education-related activities with minimal absences.

3. **TEST-TAKING TIP: The words *always* in option 1 and *extremely* in option 4 are specific determiners.**
   1. Cleaning and preparing meals are services that may be included in home health-care services. However, they are not considered skilled services and may not be appropriate under some health programs.
   2. Personal safety of the nurse is of greater concern when making home visits. The nurse must be aware of the surrounding environment and alert to possible risks, regardless of the appearance of the community.
   3. **Caregivers are frequently overburdened and may require support from the nurse during a home visit. Caregivers may also wish to observe care and determine whether or not they are willing to allow the nurse into the home.**
   4. The nurse is responsible for ensuring necessary supplies are available. The nurse functions independently without other team members immediately available for assistance during a home visit. The client's home may be chaotic and the nurse must be flexible and able to modify their plan because the home environment is much less controlled than the hospital environment.
   5. **The nurse must consider themselves a guest in the client's home. The client and their household members decide whether or not to let the nurse into the home. The nurse must ask permission to enter and work to establish a positive working relationship.**

4. **TEST-TAKING TIP: The word *homebound* in option 4 is a clang association for home health services in the stem.**
   1. Medicare is a program for clients over age 65 requiring intermittent health-care services. This client is 24 and requires continuous health-care services.
   2. Medicare is a program for clients over age 65 requiring skilled care including supportive devices. This client requires supportive

devices, but is 24 and not eligible for Medicare.

3. Medicare does not cover services that are not skilled care. Grocery shopping and meal preparation are not skilled services. Medicare covers services based on skilled care. Unless this client establishes a need for skilled care, they are not eligible for additional services such as assistance with bathing or dressing.
4. **Medicare is a program for clients over age 65 who require skilled care and who are homebound. Clients with a condition that restricts their ability to leave the home or require special assistance to leave the home are considered homebound. Diabetes education is considered skilled care.**

5\. 1. Isolation is used to separate an infected person during the time the disease is communicable. The person in the question has been exposed to the SARS pathogen but is not yet infected.
2. **Quarantine is used to prevent further transmission of the disease in case the person has become infected as a result of exposure to the SARS pathogen. The exposed person is kept separate for the duration of the longest incubation period known for the disease.**
3. Segregation is used to separate a group of infected individuals to control the spread of a disease. In the early 1900s, sanatoriums were established to separate infected individuals with tuberculosis from the general population.
4. Surveillance is associated with either monitoring individuals or investigating the disease within a population. Personal surveillance is supervision without limitations on movement. Disease surveillance is the continuing investigation of an incidence and spread of disease relevant to effective control.

6\. 1. This statement represents a simple count of the number of people with a disease.
2. Calculating the prevalence rate over a period of time is called a period prevalence rate. It is calculated with the following formula:

$$\text{Period prevalence rate} = \frac{\text{Number of persons with a characteristic during period of time}}{\text{Total number in the population}}$$

3. This reflects an incidence rate. It is calculated with the following formula:

$$\text{Incidence} = \frac{\text{Number of persons developing a disease}}{\text{Total number at risk per unit of time}}$$

4. **Prevalence refers to all people with a health condition existing in a given population at a given point in time. It is calculated with the following formula:**

$$\text{Prevalence rate} = \frac{\text{Number of persons with a characteristic on a particular day}}{\text{Total number in the population}}$$

7\. **TEST-TAKING TIP: Full name and date of birth are the most commonly used patient identifiers.**

1. The nurse may memorize a client's full name and date of birth after providing care to the same client on a regular basis. However, the nurse must continue to positively identify the client using two patient identifiers with every encounter.
2. **Clients should keep a current and accurate medication list and be instructed to take it to all medical appointments. This promotes safety with medication prescriptions. The nurse can support patient safety by providing a current medication list any time that the list changes or if the client does not have one.**
3. **This action supports patient safety when look-alike or sound-alike medications are prescribed.**
4. **One of the National Patient Safety Goals is to educate clients about anticoagulants. A side effect of aspirin is increased risk for bleeding. This action is aligned with the National Patient Safety Goals defined by The Joint Commission.**
5. The National Patient Safety Goals outlined by The Joint Commission require that clients are positively identified using two identifiers. An address may be used as one, but a second is required. Full name and date of birth are the most common identifiers used.

8\. **TEST-TAKING TIP: The principles of medication disposal are comparable in the acute-care and community health-care settings.**

1. OTC medications should be properly disposed of after their expiration date.

The chemical makeup of the drug may change after the expiration date. Some communities have OTC take-back programs. A local pharmacy may have further disposal instructions.

2. Prescription medications should be properly disposed of. Prescription antibiotics should be taken as prescribed until the prescription is complete. Keeping prescription medications such as narcotics has been shown to contribute to the opioid epidemic.
3. Recapping insulin syringes and placing them in the trash increases the risk for needle-stick injuries. This should not be recommended.
4. **Insulin syringes should not be recapped. They should be placed in a sharps container or a plastic jar if a sharps container is not available. They can then be safely returned to a pharmacy or other community facility for proper disposal.**

9. **TEST-TAKING TIP: The word *mainly* in the stem sets a priority. Four concepts of health-care delivery are being associated with community-based nursing: primary, secondary, tertiary, and rehabilitation. If you know one concept (either primary or tertiary) that is associated with health-care delivery in the community setting, two options can be deleted from consideration. If you know one concept (either secondary or rehabilitation) that is not related to health-care delivery in the community setting, two options can be deleted from consideration.**

1. **Primary care is associated with health promotion, screening, education, and protection. Although tertiary care is associated with specialized diagnostic and therapeutic care that is generally delivered in the acute-care setting, it also includes specialized services such as rehabilitation and hospice services, which are most often delivered in community settings.**
2. Although primary health-care activities generally take place in the community setting, secondary health-care activities take place in the acute-care setting and generally not in the community setting.
3. Although tertiary care is associated with specialized services such as rehabilitation, rehabilitation is not a category of health-care delivery. Rehabilitation is a specialized service provided in acute-care and community settings. Activities that help people maintain or restore function after an illness are in the tertiary prevention, not primary prevention, category.
4. Rehabilitation is not considered a category of health care but rather a type of service provided in acute care and community settings. Secondary health care is associated with hospital-based service (e.g., critical, emergency, and acute care).

10. **TEST-TAKING TIP: Options 1 and 4 are opposites.**

1. The nurse must first assess a community in order to determine its health status. This cannot be determined with the information given.
2. **A population at increased risk for health disparities and adverse outcomes due to particular characteristics is considered a vulnerable population. Rural communities tend to have fewer health-care resources than suburban or urban communities due to their geographical location.**
3. Although rural communities may belong to a particular culture and culture deeply affects the approach to health care, this is not the best answer.
4. The nurse must first assess the community in order to determine its health status. This cannot be determined with the information given.

11. **TEST-TAKING TIP: The words *will continue* draw attention to content. This indicates that the answer is a current issue.**

1. This statement is inaccurate. The number of people living in poverty is trending upward, not downward.
2. Although the number of multiple birth deliveries is trending upward, this is not the best option as another option has a greater impact on health-care funding and the nursing shortage.
3. **The number of adults over age 65 is expected to reach 77 million by 2035 and 94 million by 2060. As strategies to manage chronic disease improve, the demand for health care in this growing population will increase. This has significant effects on available funding for health-care services and the nursing shortage.**
4. The number of people immigrating to new countries is not trending downward. This option does not have the greatest impact on health-care funding and the nursing shortage.

12. **TEST-TAKING TIP: The word *coalition* is the key word in the stem because it is related**

to words such as *partnership*, *alliance*, and *unification*. The definition of the word *coalition* should lead you to the word *shared* in option 3.

1. A "wellness program" and a "community coalition" are two different concepts. A wellness program is a health promotion program that focuses on the reduction of risks and the development of positive health habits.
2. Growing diversity speaks to increasing differences in culture and ethnicity in the population. People of different cultures maintain cultural values, traditions, and beliefs that contribute to the texture and complexity of a community. Although a group of people from one cultural or ethnic group may share a common purpose, this concept is different from a community coalition.
3. **Synonyms for the word *coalition* include *alliance*, *unification*, and *combination*. A community coalition is the unification of individuals and groups to address issues related to a shared purpose.**
4. "Home care" and "community coalition" are two different concepts. Home care is associated with providing services for a client in the individual's place of residence.

13. TEST-TAKING TIP: The word *most* in the stem sets a priority.

1. A metropolitan area is a major city with smaller surrounding communities. Cities in the United States have a high concentration of health-care organizations, health professionals, and specialty medical services that provide opportunities for access to health care.
2. A suburban area is a residential district on the outskirts of a city. Cities in the United States have a high concentration of health-care organizations, health professionals, and specialty medical services that provide opportunities for access to health care. Because of the close proximity of a suburb to a city, residents usually have opportunities to access the health care available in the city.
3. An urban area is a city or town with the characteristics of a city. Urban areas in the United States have a high concentration of health-care organizations, professionals, and specialty services, which provide opportunities for access to health care.
4. **Rural areas usually are geographically remote areas with few health-care providers. Health-care organizations may be hundreds of miles away, and specialty medical services may be thousands of miles away. In addition, rural areas tend to have a health-care culture that values self-sufficiency, and many people are self-employed and do not have health insurance.**

14. TEST-TAKING TIP: The words *lowest-level need* and *Maslow* are key words in the stem that direct attention to content.

1. Identifying hazards in the environment is a health promotion activity that supports the safety of employees. Safety and security are second-level needs according to Maslow's hierarchy of needs.
2. **Assessing the health of an employee includes identifying the physical status of the individual, which addresses first-level needs necessary for survival, such as air, food, water, shelter, rest, sleep, and activity.**
3. An immunization program is a specific health protection activity that helps to keep a person safe from a specific disease. Safety and security are second-level needs according to Maslow's hierarchy of needs.
4. Promoting social adaptation addresses people's love and belonging needs. The need to feel loved and the need to attain a place within a group are third-level (love and belonging) needs according to Maslow's hierarchy of needs.

15.

1. The nurse assumes the role of educator when sharing evidence-based information to high school students on the topic of STI prevention.
2. **The nurse attending a city council meeting to discuss the opioid epidemic at the local level is playing the role of advocate in the community health setting. Nurses are among the most respected professions and bring valuable information and perspectives to such discussions.**
3. The nurse plays the role of case manager when facilitating referrals for preventive screenings such as lung cancer.
4. The nurse assumes the role of collaborator when gathering information from clients via surveys. This is a strategy to better understand a problem and to take appropriate steps toward solving the problem.

16. **TEST-TAKING TIP: The words *female adults* draw attention to content.**

1. **The leading cause of death in older adults and females is heart disease. The American Heart Association's Go Red for Women initiative strives to raise awareness about heart disease in women.**
2. Cancer is the second leading cause of death in older adults. Cervical cancer screening is recommended until age 65.
3. The Veterans Crisis Line is a suicide hotline. Suicide is not a leading cause of death in older adults.
4. The Act FAST campaign is a campaign to encourage the early recognition and prompt treatment of a stroke. Stroke is the fifth leading cause of death in older adults.

17.

1. Group homes are for specific populations, such as people who are developmentally disabled, have a mental illness, or are recovering from alcohol or drug misuse.
2. A nursing home provides skilled nursing care, which this client does not need.
3. This client needs more care than can be provided in a day-care center. This person needs assistance with dressing and bathing, which occur before arrival at a day-care center.
4. **Assisted-living facilities help clients with activities of daily living (such as dressing, bathing, grooming, and toileting), prepare meals, and dispense medications as prescribed.**

18. **TEST-TAKING TIP: The words *differs from* are the key words in the stem that direct attention to content.**

1. Pressure ulcers should be measured at least weekly whether the client is in the hospital or in the home. It may be done more frequently depending on the needs of the individual.
2. **Medical aseptic technique often is used when changing a wound dressing in the home. People in a home environment usually are farther along in recovery and less susceptible to infection than people in a hospital and have built up resistance to the "familiar microorganisms." Sterile technique is used when a hospitalized person requires a wound dressing change to prevent the occurrence of a hospital-acquired infection. The risk of infection for a hospitalized person is increased at several stages of the chain of infection.**
3. The frequency of changing the dressing on a wound is individualized depending on the client's needs. The setting is irrelevant.
4. Tap water is not used to irrigate an open wound whether the procedure is done in a hospital or a home. Sterile solutions are used for wound irrigations.
5. Both bulb and piston syringes can be used in either a home or an acute-care setting.

19. **TEST-TAKING TIP: The word *most* in the stem sets a priority. The words *basic* and *Maslow's hierarchy of needs* are key words in the stem that direct attention to content.**

1. **Meals on Wheels delivers meals daily to those at home who need assistance with preparing nutritious meals. Adequate nutrition (food) is essential for survival and is a first-level (physiological) need according to Maslow's hierarchy of needs.**
2. Exploring the meaning of one's life relates to self-actualization, which is the highest level in Maslow's hierarchy of needs.
3. Removing throw rugs protects a person from falls. According to Maslow's hierarchy of needs, safety and security needs become significant after basic physiological needs are met.
4. **Being warm is a basic physiological need according to Maslow's hierarchy of needs. Helping an income-eligible household to acquire assistance in offsetting the rising cost of home energy will help meet the family's need to be warm.**
5. **Performing a colostomy irrigation is a skill related to the basic need for fecal elimination. Meeting elimination needs is a basic physiological need identified by Maslow.**
6. **Sleep is a basic physiological need. Presenting a program regarding strategies to improve sleep is an intervention that addresses a basic physiological need according to Maslow's hierarchy of needs.**

20. Answer: 11
Knowledge: The client received a score of 4 for having adequate knowledge about type 2 diabetes, self-monitoring of blood glucose, and injection of insulin. *Behavior:* The client received a score of 3 because the client is inconsistent in monitoring blood glucose levels before lunch. *Status:* The client received a score of 4 because the

client exhibited minimal signs and symptoms associated with the condition of type 2 diabetes. The client's total score is 11.

21. 1. **Identifying the presence of lead paint and then having the lead paint removed is an example of "upstream thinking." Upstream thinking challenges providers to look "upstream" to identify the etiology of disease and intervene to prevent illness rather than to provide care "downstream," when the person is in the "river of illness."**
2. **A vaccine contains attenuated or killed microorganisms or antigen proteins derived from them to prevent an infectious disease. Preventing disease is associated with upstream thinking.**
3. **Cigarette smoke is a known carcinogen. By eliminating smoking, a person reduces the risk of developing oral cancer and lung cancer. Eliminating smoking is an example of upstream thinking.**
4. **Research demonstrates that following the MyPlate food guide can help prevent obesity, type 2 diabetes, and heart disease and decrease the risk of developing hypertension, kidney stones, bone loss, and some forms of cancer. Upstream thinking challenges providers to look "upstream" to identify the etiology of disease and intervene to prevent illness.**
5. **Urging clients to enroll in a physical fitness program is an example of upstream thinking. Regular physical activity has reduced the morbidity and mortality of various chronic illnesses such as coronary heart disease, type 2 diabetes, colon cancer, and hypertension.**

22. **TEST-TAKING TIP: The word *first* in the stem sets a priority.**
1. **Administering insulin coverage as prescribed is the first thing the nurse should do according to the information presented in the scenario. The blood glucose level is too high, and the client must have insulin immediately.**
2. Of the options presented, implementing the dressing change as ordered is the last action the nurse should implement. At this time, the wound is not as serious as the concern associated with another option.
3. Another action is the priority. Immediately calling 911 for an ambulance to transport the client to the hospital is the second action the nurse should implement because the client demonstrates an inability to manage self-care and is unsafe at home. The client's vital signs support the conclusion that the client is most likely dehydrated and needs medical intervention beyond the administration of insulin.
4. Once actions are implemented to ensure that the client's immediate metabolic needs are met, the primary health-care provider should be notified.

23. **TEST-TAKING TIP: The word *adolescent* is the key word in the stem that directs attention to content.**
1. **Adolescents may be interested in tattoos and body piercings. If an adolescent chooses to get a tattoo or body piercing, education should be provided about preventing the transmission of bloodborne diseases.**
2. **The rate of morbidity and mortality due to motor vehicle accidents is relatively high among adolescents. A discussion about wearing seat belts, not texting and driving, and not driving while using drugs or alcohol is a strategy to promote safety among adolescents.**
3. **Adolescents are at increased risk for depression and suicide. Providing information about warning signs is a strategy to promote safety in this population.**
4. Scoliosis screening is routinely performed around 12 years old or sixth grade. Repeating a screening is not necessary at age 17 unless the client has not previously been screened.
5. Reviewing childhood immunizations is not routinely performed with a 17-year-old client. According to the CDC's recommended immunization schedule, the majority of vaccines are received during the school-age years. This is not the most appropriate activity for this client based on the information provided.

24. 1. **Urgent-care centers, also known as *acute-care centers,* provide medical care for clients with minor acute illnesses. These centers have decreased the number of clients seen in primary health-care practitioners' offices and the emergency department of hospitals.**
2. The number of volunteers generally has remained the same because of two factors: more women are working to help support their families and do not have the time to volunteer and people are retiring earlier and engaging in volunteer work.

3. **Extended-care facilities traditionally provided nursing care for clients who required long-term "custodial" care. Many extended-care facilities now can care for clients who require therapies such as hemodialysis and mechanical ventilation.**
4. Older adult day-care centers have always supported wellness and do not represent a new trend in health-care delivery.
5. **Diagnostic related groups (DRGs), pretreatment diagnosis reimbursement categories, were designed to decrease the average length of a hospital stay, reducing costs. As a result, clients are being discharged before they are fully recovered and while still in need of medical and nursing support services. These services are being provided in a variety of extended-care facilities, such as nursing homes and rehabilitation centers, as well as in the home. This trend has dramatically changed the way health-care services are provided to all but those who are acutely ill.**

25. **Answer: 2, 3, 1, 5, 4**

2. **Generally, the acronym used to manage a fire in a situation like this is RACE. The first step is to remove or rescue anyone in the immediate area of the fire. In this case, the first action is to remove the grandparent and their roommate from danger.**
3. **The second step of RACE is to alarm or alert others to the fire.**
1. **The third and fourth steps of RACE are to confine and to extinguish or evacuate. In this case, the fire is very small and can easily be extinguished with a fire extinguisher.**
5. **When using a fire extinguisher, the acronym PASS is often used. The first two steps of PASS are to "Pull the pin" and "Aim at the base" of the fire.**
4. **The third and fourth steps when using the PASS acronym to use a fire extinguisher are to "Squeeze the handle" and "Sweep back and forth" until the fire is extinguished.**

CLINICAL JUDGMENT CASE STUDY ANSWERS AND RATIONALES

26. 1. Cultural competency is an awareness of cultural factors that influence communication. This situation deals with printed materials. Therefore, health literacy is the most appropriate answer.

2. **Health literacy refers to a person's ability to find, read, and understand health-related information. It is generally accepted that printed written materials should be at a fifth-grade reading level. The provider version of health education materials is likely higher than a fifth-grade reading level and may be difficult for clients to understand.**
3. Overcoming language barriers is accomplished by offering services in the client's first language. Education materials may be printed in a client's first language. Even when printed in the client's first language, health literacy must be considered.
4. Access to care is the ability of a client to access health services. Access to care can be affected by geographical location, socioeconomic status, and language barriers. When dealing with printed materials, health literacy is the most appropriate answer.

27. 1. **First- and second-hand tobacco smoke, a BMI indicating the client is overweight, metformin indicating the client is living with diabetes, and atorvastatin indicating the client is living with hyperlipidemia point to risk factors for cardiovascular disease.**

2. Although smoking cigarettes does increase the risk for bladder cancer, the nurse should not assume that clothes that smell like tobacco smoke mean the client uses tobacco products. This requires further assessment.
3. The nurse can infer that a client prescribed metformin has already been diagnosed with type 2 diabetes mellitus. Clients diagnosed with diabetes are no longer categorized as at risk for diabetes. They are at risk for complications related to diabetes, and these complications should be managed by promoting things such as drug adherence.
4. Although smoking cigarettes increases the risk for lung cancer, the nurse should not assume that clothes that smell like tobacco smoke mean the client uses tobacco products. This requires further assessment.

28. 1. Clothes that smell like tobacco smoke do not necessarily mean that the client uses tobacco. Clients who are tobacco users must be ready to quit before smoking cessation support is successful. This is not the priority for this client.

2. **The client has defined a barrier to adhering to prescribed medications. The nurse must recognize the role of diabetes management in reducing the client's risk for cardiovascular disease. The nurse must prioritize eliminating barriers to adhering to prescription drugs.**
3. Although weight loss will positively influence outcomes for this client, it is not the priority. The client has defined a barrier to prescription drug adherence that must be addressed. Weight loss is typically a long process and just one component of managing cardiovascular disease risk.
4. Although appropriate nutrition will positively influence outcomes for this client, it is not the priority. The client has defined a barrier to prescription drug adherence that must be addressed. Changing diet and nutrition is typically a long process and just one component of managing cardiovascular disease risk.

29. 1. **Generic prescriptions are often more affordable than name-brand prescriptions.**
2. **A Licensed Social Worker is skilled in finding resources for clients requiring financial assistance for things such as prescription drug coverage. This is an important and effective strategy.**
3. Increasing the number of refills on a prescription does not affect the cost of the prescription.
4. Referral to another physician is not necessary. The client can be better served by using resources such as generic prescriptions, communicating with their pharmacy, and working with a Licensed Social Worker to identify financial resources.
5. **The nurse can practice advocacy for better prescription drug coverage at the local, state, and national levels. The nurse can also advocate for this client by requesting generic prescriptions and facilitating a referral to a Licensed Social Worker for financial assistance.**

30. 1. Although smoking is a risk factor for cardiovascular disease, metformin and atorvastatin are medications to manage diabetes and high blood cholesterol, respectively.
2. Although weight reduction lowers the risk for cardiovascular disease, metformin and atorvastatin are medications to manage diabetes and high blood cholesterol, respectively.
3. **Risk factors for cardiovascular disease include tobacco smoke, diabetes, high blood cholesterol, hypertension, and obesity. Metformin is a prescription medication used to manage type 2 diabetes. Atorvastatin is a prescriptive medication used to manage high blood cholesterol. Therefore, these medications help lower risk factors for cardiovascular disease.**
4. Metformin and atorvastatin are used to manage diabetes and high blood cholesterol, respectively. Although cardiovascular disease and lung cancer share the risk factor of smoking, this answer is incorrect.

31. 1. This statement clarifies that the client is exposed to second-hand smoke. It does not demonstrate understanding of risk factors.
2. **This statement demonstrates that the client is taking action to lower risk factors related to cardiovascular disease. Walking is a safe and effective exercise that can help with weight loss. Frozen vegetables are an affordable way to consume more nutritious foods.**
3. Metformin and atorvastatin are evidence-based strategies for managing diabetes and lowering blood cholesterol. These interventions lower the risk for cardiovascular disease. Often, clients with diabetes and high blood cholesterol do not have acute symptoms. Stopping these medications when the client feels well is not appropriate.
4. This statement indicates a lack of understanding about how to lower risk factors for cardiovascular disease. This client can be supported in reducing exposure to tobacco smoke, adhering to prescription medications that manage diabetes and lower blood cholesterol, and weight loss and diet management to reduce the risk for cardiovascular disease.

ADMINISTRATION OF MEDICATIONS

This section includes questions related to the principles associated with the administration of medications via the oral, parenteral (IV, intramuscular, intradermal, and subcutaneous injections), topical, ear, eye, vaginal, and rectal routes. The questions focus on allergies, untoward effects, toxic effects, developmental considerations associated with medications, the Z-track method, peak and trough levels of medications, pain assessment before administering medication for pain, and computation of dosage.

QUESTIONS

1. The nurse has safely opened an ampule of promethazine and drawn the medication into a syringe. Before injecting the medication into a diluent, what is the critical step in protecting client safety?
   1. Crack the ampule using gauze.
   2. Change the needle.
   3. Dispose of the ampule in the sharps container.
   4. Dispose of the needle used to instill the medication into the diluent.

   TEST-TAKING TIP: Identify the key word in the stem that directs attention to content. Identify the unique option.

2. The nurse must administer a 2-mL intramuscular injection to an adult client who is in severe pain and lying in the supine position. Which muscle is the safest for the nurse to use to administer an intramuscular injection to this client?
   1. Deltoid
   2. Dorsogluteal
   3. Ventrogluteal
   4. Vastus lateralis

   TEST-TAKING TIP: Identify the word in the stem that sets a priority. Identify the key word in the stem that directs attention to content. Identify equally plausible options.

3. The nurse is injecting preprandial insulin aspart into a client with a BMI of 18. What is the appropriate angle for this injection?
   1. 90 degrees
   2. 45 degrees
   3. 20 degrees
   4. 10 degrees

   TEST-TAKING TIP: Identify key words in the stem that direct attention to content.

4. The nurse is administering oral medications to a child. Which is the **most** important factor concerning a child that the nurse must consider?
   1. Age
   2. Weight
   3. Level of anxiety
   4. Developmental level

   TEST-TAKING TIP: Identify the word in the stem that sets a priority. Identify the key word in the stem that directs attention to content.

5. A client is receiving IV piggyback (IVPB) medication every 4 hours. Because the medication has a narrow therapeutic window, a peak blood level is prescribed. The nurse should plan to obtain a blood specimen for this test:
   1. 3 hours after administering a dose.
   2. 1 hour before administering a dose.
   3. halfway between two scheduled doses.
   4. 1 hour after administering a dose.

   TEST-TAKING TIP: Identify the key word in the stem that directs attention to content. Identify opposites in options. Identify equally plausible options.

6. In addition to inhibiting microbial growth, an antibiotic also may depress bone marrow. In which category is the depression of bone marrow classified?
   1. Overdose
   2. Side effect
   3. Habituation
   4. Idiosyncratic effect

7. Which route of administration is used only for its local therapeutic effect?
   1. Eye
   2. Skin
   3. Nose
   4. Rectum

   TEST-TAKING TIP: Identify key words in the stem that direct attention to content.

8. The nurse plans to inject a medication via an existing IV line. Which should the nurse do **first?**
   1. Select the port closest to the needle entry site
   2. Pinch the tubing above the port being used
   3. Clean the injection port with an antiseptic
   4. Determine the patency of the IV line

   TEST-TAKING TIP: Identify the word in the stem that sets a priority. Identify the clang association.

9. The nurse is filling a syringe with medication from a multiple-dose vial. Which should the nurse do?
   1. Keep the needle above the level of the liquid and maintain sterile technique
   2. Keep the needle below the level of the liquid and record the date and time on the vial when opened
   3. Keep the needle below the level of the liquid and change the needle after withdrawing the solution
   4. Keep the needle above the level of the liquid and inject air at 1.5 times the volume of the prescribed dose

   TEST-TAKING TIP: Identify duplicate facts among options. Identify the clang association.

10. The nurse is preparing to administer an extended-release tablet. Which of the following considerations for this tablet is correct?
    1. This tablet has immediate effect
    2. This tablet is not susceptible to the first-pass effect
    3. This tablet should not be crushed
    4. This tablet should be taken every 4 hours

    TEST-TAKING TIP: Identify the key word in the stem that directs attention to content.

11. The nurse is caring for a 4-year-old child who has a prescription for IV fluids. The nurse is unable to obtain an IV volume control device and decides to administer the IV via gravity until a volume control device can be acquired. The nurse selects the **most** appropriate IV administration set with a drop factor. Which is the drop factor of the IV administration set?
    1. 10
    2. 15
    3. 20
    4. 60

    TEST-TAKING TIP: Identify key words in the stem that direct attention to content. Identify the word in the stem that sets a priority.

12. The nurse is preparing to administer IV vancomycin to a client who is allergic to penicillin and has been diagnosed with a MRSA infection. The nurse recognizes that vancomycin is a vesicant drug and identifies which of the following vascular access devices as most appropriate for the administration of this drug?
    1. 22 gauge IV in the left forearm
    2. 18 gauge IV in the right antecubital space
    3. Midline catheter
    4. Peripherally inserted central catheter

    TEST-TAKING TIP: Identify words in the stem that draw attention to content. Identify the unique option.

13. The nurse is administering a drug via the Z-track injection method. Which action is unique to this procedure?
    1. A "Z" is formed when dividing a buttock into several quadrants.
    2. The injection sites are rotated along a "Z" pattern on the abdomen.
    3. An air lock is established behind the bolus of medication in Z-track injections.
    4. The skin is pulled laterally throughout Z-track injections and is released after needle withdrawal.

    TEST-TAKING TIP: Identify key words in the stem that direct attention to content. Identify options with a clang association.

14. Peak and trough levels are prescribed to monitor the plasma profile of an antibiotic. When the trough level of a drug is being measured, when should the nurse plan for a blood specimen to be drawn?
    1. First thing in the morning
    2. Halfway between scheduled doses
    3. A half hour before a scheduled dose
    4. A half hour after drug administration

    TEST-TAKING TIP: Identify the key word in the stem that directs attention to content. Identify opposites in options.

15. The nurse is administering a medication in the form of a troche. The nurse should place the medication in the client's:
    1. rectal vault.
    2. buccal cavity.
    3. vaginal vault.
    4. auditory canal.

16. The nurse is educating a client prescribed a nicotine patch. Which of the following instructions are incorrect?
    1. Change the patch every 24 hours.
    2. Replace the patch in the same place every day.
    3. Apply the patch to clean, dry skin.
    4. Fold the patch in half before disposal.

    TEST-TAKING TIP: Identify opposites in options. Identify the option with a specific determiner.

17. Which route is considered the **most** desirable when administering medications?
    1. Via injection
    2. Intravenous
    3. By mouth
    4. Topical

    TEST-TAKING TIP: Identify the word in the stem that sets a priority.

18. The nurse is preparing to administer an influenza immunization to an infant. The nurse considers which of the following pertaining to the correct route of administration?
1. Choose a syringe with a retractable needle
2. Choose an age-appropriate IM site
3. Administer the age-appropriate dose
4. Document the route of administration

TEST-TAKING TIP: Identify the word in the stem that sets a priority.

19. Medication that must be administered via an intramuscular injection is prescribed for an infant. Which muscle should the nurse use to administer the injection?
1. Deltoid
2. Dorsogluteal
3. Ventrogluteal
4. Rectus femoris

TEST-TAKING TIP: Identify the unique option.

20. Which route of delivery for medication should be used cautiously by the nurse if the client is an older adult who is cachectic?
1. Intradermal
2. Intravenous
3. Subcutaneous
4. Intramuscular

TEST-TAKING TIP: Identify the key word in the stem that directs attention to content. Identify the word in the stem that indicates negative polarity. Identify the unique option.

21. The nurse is preparing to instill a vaginal cream. Which client position facilitates the instillation of a vaginal cream? **Select all that apply.**

1. _____ Dorsal recumbent position
2. _____ Low Fowler position
3. _____ Left-lateral position
4. _____ Orthopneic position
5. _____ Supine position

22. A client is admitted to the hospital with a diagnosis of congestive heart failure and pulmonary edema. Furosemide (Lasix®) 30 mg IM STAT is prescribed for the client. The available furosemide is 10 mg/mL. Calculate how many mL of furosemide the nurse should administer.

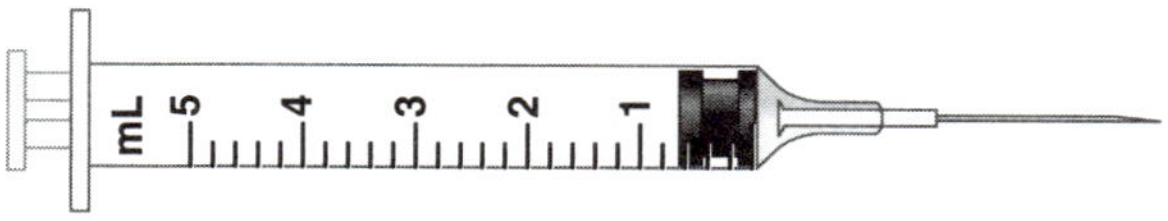

23. The client's most current blood pressure reading is 182/102. The nurse has obtained an order for an antihypertensive agent. Place the following steps in the correct order.
1. Verify the prescription.
2. Perform thorough hand hygiene.
3. Obtain the client's blood pressure.
4. Document outcomes.
5. Identify the client using two identifiers

Answer: ____________

24. Ear drops are prescribed for an adult client. Which should the nurse do when instilling ear drops into the client's ear? **Select all that apply.**
1. _____ Press a cotton ball gently into the ear canal
2. _____ Pull the pinna of the ear upward and backward
3. _____ Tug the pinna of the ear downward and backward
4. _____ Direct the flow of fluid down the center of the ear canal
5. _____ Hold a dropper approximately 2 inches above the ear canal

TEST-TAKING TIP: Identify the key word in the stem that directs attention to content. Identify opposites in options.

25. The nurse is caring for a 28-year-old female recently diagnosed with hypertension and prescribed an ACE inhibitor. Which of the following assessment questions promote safety should the client become pregnant? **Select all that apply.**
1. _____ "Have you ever had an anaphylactic reaction?"
2. _____ "Are you considering becoming pregnant?"
3. _____ "Have you ever been treated for a drug addiction?"
4. _____ "Do you have any allergies?"
5. _____ "What form of birth control do you use?"

26. Place an X where the nurse should look along a primary administration set to determine whether an IV solution, infusing by gravity, is running at the rate prescribed.

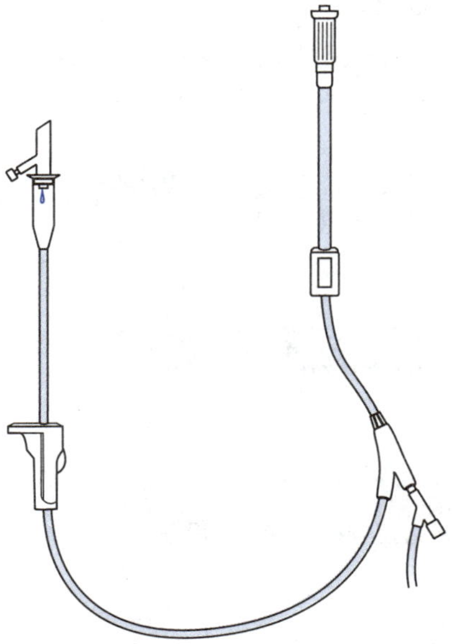

27. The nurse is checking medication prescriptions written by a primary health-care provider to ensure that the prescriptions meet the standards identified by The Joint Commission. Identify the prescription that the nurse should clarify with the provider. **Select all that apply.**
1. _____ Morphine sulfate 2 mg IV every 2 hours PRN for severe incisional pain
2. _____ Gentamicin ophthalmic solution 2 gtts AU qid
3. _____ Regular insulin 5 units Sub-Q STAT
4. _____ Docusate sodium 100 mg PO qd
5. _____ Alprazolam 0.5 mg PO tid

TEST-TAKING TIP: Identify the words in the stem that indicate negative polarity.

28. Which statement indicates to the nurse that the client with an eye infection understands teaching regarding the self-administration of eye drops? **Select all that apply.**
1. _____ "I can wipe away excess medication on my eyelid."
2. _____ "I should gaze upward while instilling the eye drops."
3. _____ "I should close my eyes gently after the medicine is in my eye."
4. _____ "I should place one drop of the medication inside my lower eyelid."
5. _____ "I can easily transmit the infection from one eye to the other if I do not use precautions."

TEST-TAKING TIP: Identify the clang associations.

29. The nurse is administering a liquid medication to a toddler who is in tears. Which of the following strategies promote medication adherence for this client? **Select all that apply.**
1. _____ Mix the medication in the toddler's favorite juice
2. _____ Consult the parent
3. _____ Offer a popsicle before medication administration
4. _____ Ask the parent to lie the child back in their lap
5. _____ Administer the medication at the same time every day

30. The nurse receives an order to administer 1.5 milligrams of an oral medication. This medication is supplied in 500 micrograms per tablet. How many tablets should the nurse administer? **Record your answer using a whole number.**

Answer: ____________ **tablets**

31. A client has a prescription for regular insulin 20 units subcutaneously STAT. Which syringe should the nurse use to administer this medication?

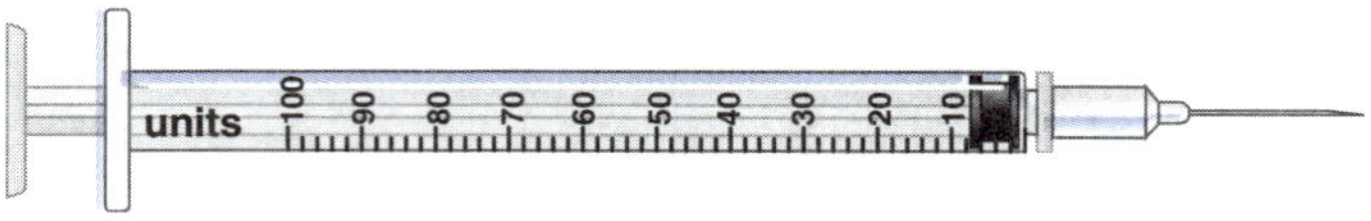

1.

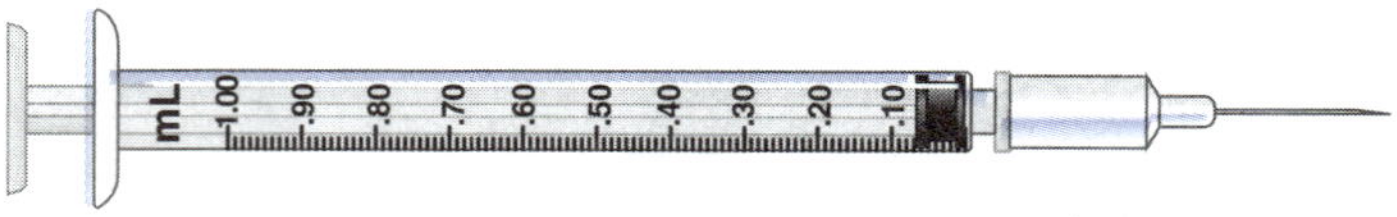

2.

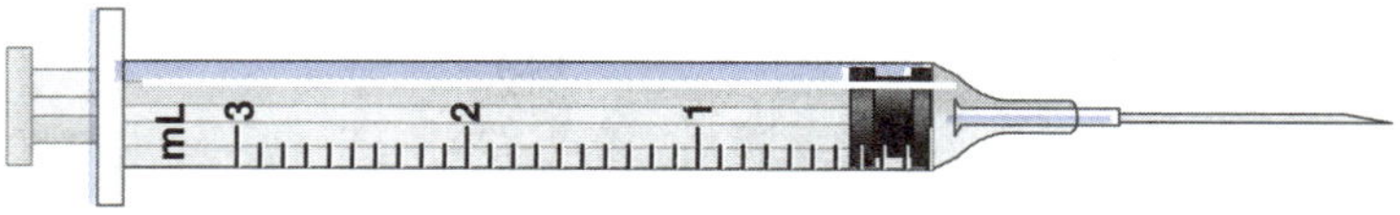

3.

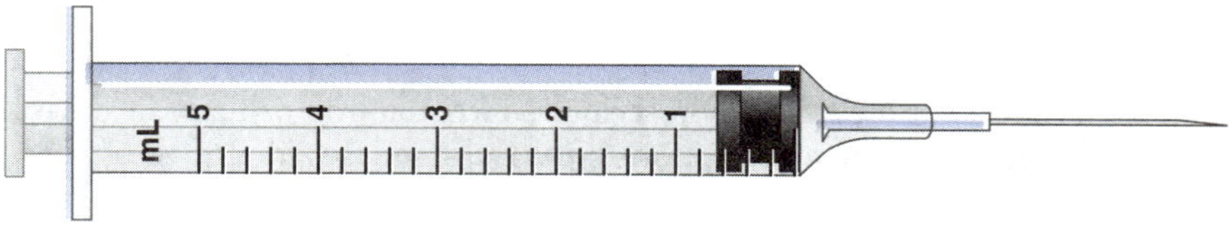

4.

32. The nurse is administering medications to a group of older adults. For which response specifically related to aging should the nurse assess these clients? **Select all that apply.**
1. _____ Toxicity
2. _____ Side effects
3. _____ Drug interactions
4. _____ Allergic reactions
5. _____ Teratogenic effects

TEST-TAKING TIP: Identify key words in the stem that direct attention to content.

33. The nurse is evaluating a mother's ability to administer nose drops to her child. Which action indicates that the mother is administering the nose drops correctly? **Select all that apply.**

1. _____ Encouraging sniffing the medication into the lungs
2. _____ Tilting the head backward while instilling the medication
3. _____ Instructing the child to blow the nose gently before instillation
4. _____ Positioning the dropper outside the nostril without touching the nose
5. _____ Discarding excess fluid in the dropper after administering the medication and then putting the dropper back into the bottle

TEST-TAKING TIP: Identify key words in the stem that direct attention to content. Identify the clang associations.

34. The nurse must administer a prescribed medication via the rectal route. Place the following steps in the order in which they should be implemented.

1. Position the client in the semi-prone position.
2. Use water-soluble jelly to lubricate the suppository.
3. Instruct the client to remain in a side-lying position for at least 10 minutes.
4. Determine if there are any contraindications to the insertion of a suppository.
5. Insert the suppository 1 to 3 inches past the internal sphincter using an index finger.

Answer: ___________

35. The nurse encounters the situation pictured in the illustration. What is the nurse's priority action?

1. Document the time the secondary infusion completed.
2. Verify the rate of the primary infusion.
3. Clamp and discard the secondary infusion set.
4. Replace the primary fluids with a new bag.

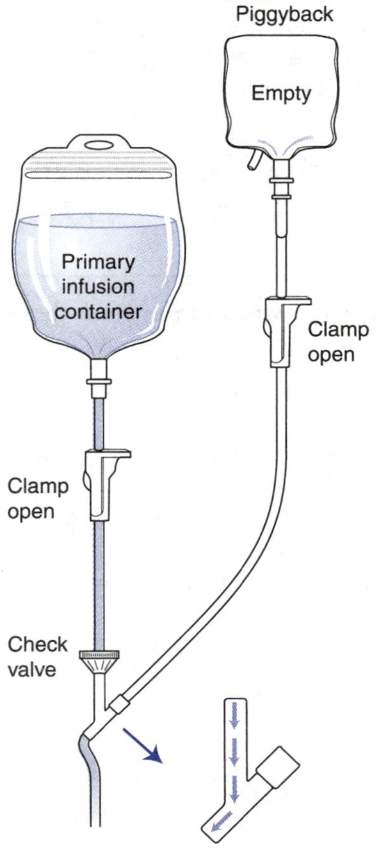

TEST-TAKING TIP: Identify the word in the stem that sets a priority.

36. The nurse is preparing to administer four daily prescription medications in pill form, plus a potassium tablet, to an 82-year-old client living with Alzheimer's disease with a history of swallowing difficulty. Which of the following actions are appropriate? **Select all that apply.**

1. _____ Administer all of the pills in one cup
2. _____ Allow additional time for medication administration
3. _____ Confirm that each pill has been swallowed
4. _____ Avoid confusing the client with verbal instructions
5. _____ Offer sips of water to assess swallow before administering medications

37. The nurse is caring for a client with cancer who is experiencing pain at 7 p.m. (1900 hours). The nurse assesses the client and reviews the client's prescribed medications and the medication administration record. Which nursing intervention is **most** appropriate for this client?

1. Notify the primary health-care provider about the client's status.
2. Wait 1 hour to give the prescribed hydromorphone 4 mg.
3. Administer the prescribed acetaminophen 650 mg.
4. Reassess the client in half an hour.

CLIENT'S HOME CARE CLINICAL RECORD

Primary Health-Care Provider's Prescriptions

Acetaminophen 325 mg PO every 6 hours for mild pain
Acetaminophen 650 mg PO every 4 hours for moderate pain
Hydromorphone 4 mg PO every 4 hours for severe pain

Medication Administration Record

0200: Acetaminophen 325 mg PO for mild abdominal pain (3 on 0 to 10 scale)
0800: Acetaminophen 650 mg PO for moderate abdominal pain (7 on 0 to 10 scale)
1200: Hydromorphone 4 mg PO for severe abdominal pain (8 on 0 to 10 scale)
1600: Hydromorphone 4 mg PO for severe abdominal pain (8 on 0 to 10 scale)

Client Assessment

Client reporting sharp abdominal pain of 9 on a scale of 0 to 10. Vital signs are pulse, 68 beats/min, regular rhythm; respirations, 10 breaths/min, shallow, unlabored; BP, 106/72 mm Hg.

TEST-TAKING TIP: Identify the word in the stem that sets a priority.

38. A client has a prescription for albuterol 90 mcg/spray, two puffs via a metered-dose inhaler every 12 hours. Place the following steps in the order in which they should be implemented by the nurse.

1. Instruct the client to breathe in slowly and deeply while activating the canister.
2. Tell the client to seal the lips around the mouthpiece of the spacer.
3. Remove the cap on the metered-dose inhaler and shake it well.
4. Ask the client to rinse the mouth with water and spit it out.
5. Direct the client to exhale fully through the mouth.

Answer: ___________

39. Which part of a syringe must remain sterile when drawing up medication from a vial and administering an injection? **Select all that apply.**
1. _____ Flange
2. _____ Plunger
3. _____ Needle hub
4. _____ Needle shaft
5. _____ Outside barrel

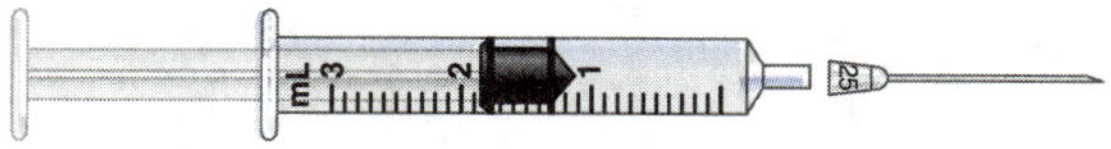

40. The nurse teaches a parent to administer an ophthalmic antibiotic to a child diagnosed with pinkeye. Which statement by the parent indicates that the teaching was understood? **Select all that apply.**
1. _____ "I will apply gentle pressure to the inner corner of the eye after giving the medication."
2. _____ "I will wipe my eye, moving from the inner corner of the eye outward."
3. _____ "My child should blink several times after instilling the medication."
4. _____ "I should hold the eyedropper about a half inch above my eye."
5. _____ "I will put the antibiotic in a pocket in the lower lid of my eye."

CLINICAL JUDGMENT CASE STUDY

The nurse is caring for a male client with a history of substance use disorder admitted for management of sickle cell crisis. The nurse notes a Hgb count of 9 g/dL and the following vital signs:

Temperature	98.9°F (37.2°C)
Pulse	88
BP	148/82
Respirations	20/min, shallow
Oxygen	96% on RA
Pain	8 out of 10

41. **Recognize cues—What matters most?** The nurse understands that which of the following should be prioritized when caring for this patient?
1. Manage pain
2. Avoid using controlled substances
3. Treating anemia
4. Supporting oxygenation

42. **Analyze cues—What could it mean?** The nurse completes a 5-minute head-to-toe assessment and notes an ashen gray appearance of the client's skin and increased respiratory rate when the client ambulates. The client states "Why am I so tired?" What is the nurse's **best** response?
1. "Fatigue is common when a person is admitted to the hospital."
2. "Pain is the number one cause of fatigue."
3. "A low red blood cell count can cause fatigue."
4. "Difficulty breathing can cause a person to feel tired."

43. **Prioritize hypotheses—Where do I start?** The nurse reviews the WHO Analgesic Ladder and prescribed medications for this client. Mark an X to indicate whether the order is appropriate or inappropriate.

	Appropriate	Inappropriate
1000 mg PO acetaminophen QID		
PRN 2 mg IV morphine, every 2 hours		
2 L O_2 via NC		
Hold SQ LMWH QAM		
IV NS 200 mL/hr, continuous		

44. **Generate solutions—What can I do?** The nurse is preparing to administer morphine and buprenorphine to this client for pain management. The nurse is unfamiliar with buprenorphine. What is the nurse's most appropriate action?
1. Look up the drug in a current drug guide.
2. Look up the drug on an Internet search engine.
3. Ask a colleague about the medication.
4. Notify the physician that the nurse is unfamiliar with this medication.

45. **Take action—What will I do?** The nurse understands that nonpharmacological interventions can improve the efficacy of pharmacological interventions for pain. Which of the following interventions can the nurse implement to support pain relief in this client? **Select all that apply.**
1. Keep the room as cool as possible.
2. Offer appropriate distractions.
3. Offer warm packs.
4. Turn on the lights and open blinds.
5. Minimize noise.

46. **Evaluate outcomes—Did it help?** The nurse conducts a follow-up phone call 2 days after discharge. The client was sent home with fentanyl patches. Which of the following indicate that the client requires further education?
1. "The skin under the patch looks normal."
2. "I always wear the patch in the same spot."
3. "I wear the patch on my arm because I can't reach my shoulder."
4. "I change the patch every 3 days after I shower."

TEST-TAKING TIP: Identify specific determiners in the solution.

ADMINISTRATION OF MEDICATIONS ANSWERS AND RATIONALES

1. **TEST-TAKING TIP: The word *ampule* is the key word in the stem that directs attention to content. Option 2 is unique because it directly affects client safety. The other three options protect both nurse and client safety.**
   1. The nurse has already opened the ampule safely. Ampules can be opened safely using an ampule opener or, when an ampule opener is not available, protecting the fingers with gauze and opening the ampule away from the nurse's body.
   2. **Ampules are made of glass that must be broken before removing the medication. The medication must be removed with a filter needle and the filter needle must be replaced before transferring the medication from an ampule to a diluent. This step prevents introducing any particles caught by the filter needle into the diluent.**
   3. Although disposing of the ampule in a sharps container is appropriate, changing the needle is a critical step to protect the client from exposure to unsafe particles in the diluent when the promethazine is administered.
   4. The needle used to instill medication into the diluent should be properly disposed of to protect patient safety. However, the critical step in this process is changing the needle to prevent the client from being exposed to unsafe particles in the diluent when the promethazine is administered.

2. **TEST-TAKING TIP: The word *safest* is the word in the stem that sets a priority and is the key word in the stem that directs attention to content. Options 2 and 3 are equally plausible because they both require repositioning the client.**
   1. The deltoid is not well developed in many adults and children. The radial and ulnar nerves and brachial artery lie in the upper arm along the humerus. The deltoid should not be used for intramuscular injections unless other sites are unavailable.
   2. To access the dorsogluteal site, the client must be repositioned, which may increase pain. Historically, the dorsogluteal was the preferred site for an intramuscular injection; however, there is a risk of hitting the sciatic nerve, blood vessels, or greater trochanter. Piercing the sciatic nerve can cause partial or permanent paralysis of the leg.
   3. To access the ventrogluteal site, the client must be repositioned, which may increase pain. The ventrogluteal is the preferred site after the vastus lateralis; it is safe to use in cachectic clients and children older than 18 months.
   4. **The vastus lateralis is the preferred site for this client because this muscle has no major nerves and blood vessels nearby and absorbs drugs rapidly. In addition, using this muscle does not require the client, who is in pain, to be moved and repositioned.**

3. **TEST-TAKING TIP: The words *insulin* and *½-inch long needle* are key words in the stem that direct attention to content.**
   1. This client is considered underweight based on their BMI. Injecting insulin, a subcutaneous injection, at a 90-degree angle carries the risk of inappropriate route of administration.
   2. **Subcutaneous injections are generally administered at a 45-degree angle in order to place the medication into the connective tissue under the dermis. The abdomen and tissue on the back of the upper arm are common sites of subcutaneous injections.**
   3. Administering a subcutaneous injection at 20-degree angle risks administering the medication via the inappropriate route. Inserting an IV is done at an angle less than 25 degrees.
   4. A 10-degree angle is appropriate for an intradermal route of administration, not a subcutaneous injection such as insulin.

4. **TEST-TAKING TIP: The word *most* in the stem sets a priority. The word *child* is the key word in the stem that directs attention to content.**
   1. Age is not reliable for calculating a pediatric dose of medication.
   2. **Children's body sizes are different, necessitating calculation of drug dosage by weight. Weight is an objective and accurate way to calculate appropriate medication dosages for children.**
   3. Level of anxiety does not influence calculation of dosage of medication for a child.
   4. Developmental level does not influence calculation of dosage of medication for a child.

5. **TEST-TAKING TIP: The word *peak* is the key word in the stem that directs attention to content. Options 2 and 4 are opposites. Options 1 and 2 are equally plausible because they both refer to obtaining a blood specimen 1 hour before administering the next dose. The drug is to be given every 4 hours. Three hours after a dose (option 1) is the same as 1 hour before the next dose (option 2).**
   1. A blood test taken 3 hours after administration of a dose that is given every 4 hours will not provide an accurate peak blood level. A blood level 3 to 3.5 hours after administration of a drug given every 4 hours provides information about a trough level.
   2. A blood specimen taken 1 hour before administration of a dose will not provide an accurate peak blood level. A blood level at 30 to 60 minutes before the next dose measures the trough level.
   3. A blood level specimen taken halfway between two scheduled doses will not provide an accurate result when testing for a peak blood level for a drug administered every 4 hours.
   4. **Most medications administered every 4 hours have a peak concentration about 1 hour after administration.**

6. 1. An overdose occurs when a person receives a dose larger than the usual recommended dose; this rarely is planned and usually is an accident or error.
   2. **A side effect is a secondary effect. Side effects can be harmless or can cause injury; if injurious, the drug is discontinued.**
   3. Habituation is an acquired tolerance from continued exposure to a substance.
   4. An idiosyncratic effect is an unexpected effect; it can be an overreaction, an underreaction, or an unusual reaction.

7. **TEST-TAKING TIP: The words *only* and *local* are key words in the stem that direct attention to content.**
   1. **Medications are instilled into the eye only for local effect; part of the procedure for instillation of eye drops is to apply gentle pressure to the nasolacrimal duct for 10 to 15 seconds to prevent absorption of the medication into the systemic circulation.**
   2. Medications can be administered via the skin for either local or systemic effect.
   3. Medication can be administered via the nose for either local or systemic effect.
   4. Medication can be administered via the rectum for either local or systemic effect; medications can be absorbed through the rich vascular bed in the mucous membranes.

8. **TEST-TAKING TIP: The word *first* in the stem sets a priority. The words *IV line* in the stem and in option 4 are clang associations.**
   1. Although selecting the port closest to the catheter insertion site is part of the procedure, it is not what the nurse should do first.
   2. Although pinching the tubing above the port being used is part of the procedure, it is not what the nurse should do first.
   3. Although cleaning the injection port is part of the procedure, it is not what the nurse should do first.
   4. **For medication to enter a vein, the IV line must be unobstructed; therefore, the nurse should determine the patency of the IV line. The nurse also must ensure that the medication is administered into a vein, not into subcutaneous tissue.**

9. **TEST-TAKING TIP: Options 1 and 4 contain a duplicate fact, and options 2 and 3 contain a duplicate fact. If you know whether a needle should be kept above or below the level of fluid in a vial, you can reduce your final selection to two options. The word *vial* in the stem and in option 2 is a clang association.**
   1. Although sterile technique should be maintained, the bevel of the needle should be kept below the level of the fluid to prevent the syringe from filling with air.
   2. **The bevel of the needle must be kept below the level of the fluid to prevent air from entering the syringe. Once opened, medications should be marked with the date and time of opening because there is generally a recommended period of viability before they should be discarded. A second dose from a multiple-dose vial must be obtained only by the nurse who obtained and documented the first dose.**
   3. Although the bevel of the needle should be kept below the level of the fluid, changing the needle is unnecessary. The needle must be changed only when the solution is caustic to tissues.
   4. The bevel of the needle should be kept below the level of the fluid when withdrawing medication, or the syringe will fill with air. The amount of air injected into the vial before withdrawing the medication should equal the amount of solution to be withdrawn; extra air will result in excessive pressure within the closed space of the vial.

10. **TEST-TAKING TIP: The word *extended-release* is the key word in the stem that directs attention to content.**

1. An extended-release tablet is designed to provide the desired effect over an extended period of time. Medications taken orally, as a tablet indicates, do not have immediate effect.
2. The first-pass effect is related to medications metabolized by the liver resulting in a decreased bioavailability of the medications. Medications administered via the oral route, as a tablet indicates, are susceptible to this effect.
3. **Extended-release tablets are typically coated with a substance that is dissolved slowly in the stomach. Crushing an extended-release tablet interferes with this feature.**
4. Extended-release tablets are designed for 12- or 24-hour dosing. Administering an extended-release tablet every 4 hours is inappropriate.

11. **TEST-TAKING TIP: The words *child* and *drop factor* are key words in the stem that direct attention to content. The word *most* in the stem sets a priority.**

1. IV tubing with a drop factor of 10 represents 10 drops per 1 mL and is considered a macrodrip. It is difficult to regulate the rate of an IV with 10 drops per mL to children.
2. IV tubing with a drop factor of 15 represents 15 drops per 1 mL and is considered a macrodrip. It is difficult to regulate the rate of an IV with 15 drops per mL to children.
3. IV tubing with a drop factor of 20 represents 20 drops per 1 mL and is considered a macrodrip. It is difficult to regulate the rate of an IV with 20 drops per mL to children.
4. **IV tubing with a drop factor of 60 represents 60 drops per 1 mL and is considered a microdrip. It is easier to regulate the rate of an IV with 60 drops per mL than it is to regulate tubing that requires fewer drops to deliver 1 mL, especially to children. Children usually receive fewer milliliters per hour than adults.**

12. **TEST-TAKING TIP: The word *vesicant* draws attention to content in the stem. Option 4 is a central line and options 1, 2, and 3 are peripheral lines.**

1. A 22-gauge IV in the forearm is not the best option for administering a vesicant drug.
2. An 18-gauge IV in the antecubital space is a better option than a 22-gauge IV in the forearm because it is a larger-bore needle in a larger vein. However, it is not the best option from the choices given for administering a vesicant drug.
3. A midline catheter is a better option than an IV in the forearm or antecubital space. However, it is not the best option from the choices given for administering a vesicant drug. A midline is still a type of peripheral line.
4. **A peripherally inserted central catheter (PICC) is the best option for administering a vesicant drug. It is a central line, meaning that the medication is instilled into central circulation and quickly diluted in the bloodstream. Vancomycin in this situation will likely be required over an extended period of time, and administering a vesicant via a central line lowers the risk of tissue damage.**

13. **TEST-TAKING TIP: The words *Z-track* and *unique* are key words in the stem that direct attention to content. The word *injection* in the stem and the words *injection(s)* in options 3 and 4 are clang associations.**

1. A buttock is not divided by a "Z." When a buttock (dorsogluteal) is used for intramuscular injections, the usual bony landmarks must be used to identify the correct insertion site. The dorsogluteal site is no longer recommended because of its proximity to the sciatic nerve.
2. A "Z" pattern is not used for medications administered via the Z-track technique. An intramuscular site, preferably the dorsogluteal, is used for Z-track medication administration, not the abdomen, which is used for subcutaneous injections.
3. The air-lock technique also can be done with intramuscular injections. When air is injected behind the medication, the air clears the needle of medication. This technique is controversial and is being researched for evidence-based practice. This generally is not used with Z-track injections.
4. **The "Z" in the Z-track method refers to pulling the skin to the side before and during an intramuscular injection. This technique alters the position of skin layers so that once the needle**

is removed and the skin released, the injected fluid is kept within the muscle tissues and does not rise in the needle tract, which can irritate subcutaneous tissues. Pulling the skin to the side causes the needle tract to take the shape of the letter Z.

14. **TEST-TAKING TIP: The word *trough* is the key word in the stem that directs attention to content. Options 3 and 4 are opposites.**
    1. The peak and trough of a blood plasma level depend on the time the last dose was administered.
    2. Halfway between scheduled doses is not the time period when a drug is at its lowest concentration in the blood.
    3. **"Trough level" refers to the level when a drug is at its lowest concentration in the blood in response to biotransformation; this usually occurs during the period just before the next scheduled dose.**
    4. Many variables affect the time when a drug reaches its peak plasma level within an individual; however, a half hour after the administration of an antibiotic, one can safely plot the antibiotic plasma level on the rising side of the curve of its plasma level profile, not within the trough.

15.
    1. A suppository is designed for administering medication into the rectum.
    2. **A troche (lozenge) is placed in the space between the upper or lower molar teeth and the gums (buccal cavity) so that it can release medication as it dissolves.**
    3. A suppository, solution, or cream can be delivered to the vaginal vault by a vaginal applicator.
    4. Medication in a suspension can be administered via a dropper into the auditory canal.

16. **TEST-TAKING TIP: The word *incorrect* draws attention to content.**
    1. This statement is correct. The patch should be changed every 24 hours.
    2. **This statement is incorrect. The patch should be placed in a different location each day to prevent irritation of the skin.**
    3. This statement is correct. The patch should be applied to clean, dry skin, and areas covered in hair should be avoided. Skin that is oily, soiled, hairy, or wet interferes with absorption.
    4. This statement is correct. The patch should be folded in half with the sticky sides connected to each other before disposal. This prevents inadvertent exposure to the nicotine in the patch.

17. **TEST-TAKING TIP: The word *most* in the stem sets a priority.**
    1. Administering a medication via an injection is not the most desirable route because a needle enters the skin and the medication is absorbed more rapidly than many other routes.
    2. The IV route is not the most desirable route for medication administration. The IV route carries the highest risk because a needle enters the skin and the medication is delivered directly into the bloodstream.
    3. **Using the oral route is the safest way to administer medication because it is convenient, it does not require piercing the skin, it usually does not cause physical or emotional stress, and the medication is absorbed slowly.**
    4. Because absorption is affected by a variety of factors, such as the extent of the capillary network and condition of the skin, the topical route is not the most accurate and therefore not the most desirable method of medication administration.

18. **TEST-TAKING TIP: The words *infant* and *route* in the stem draw attention to content.**
    1. Although the nurse should choose a syringe with a retractable needle to prevent needle-stick injuries, this action does not pertain to the correct route of administration.
    2. **An influenza immunization is administered via the IM route. An important component of ensuring the medication is administered via the correct route is choosing an age-appropriate IM injection site. The anterolateral thigh is the preferred IM injection site in infants under 12 months.**
    3. Although the age-appropriate dose is important, this pertains to the correct dose, not the correct route.
    4. Although the route of administration, including the age-appropriate site, must be documented, this pertains to the right documentation of medication administration and not the right route.

19. **TEST-TAKING TIP: Option 4 is unique because it is the only option with two words.**

1. The deltoid muscle is contraindicated for intramuscular injections in infants and children. This site has a small amount of muscle mass, and it lies close to the radial nerve and brachial artery.
2. The dorsogluteal muscle is contraindicated for an intramuscular injection in children younger than 18 months because the muscle mass is inadequate to allow a safe injection. Also, the sciatic nerve and gluteal artery lie close to the site.
3. An infant should not receive an intramuscular injection into the ventrogluteal muscle; the muscle is not well developed until the child begins to walk.
4. **The rectus femoris muscle, which belongs to the quadriceps muscle group, is the site of choice for intramuscular injections in infants. It is the largest and most well-developed muscle in infants, is easy to locate, and is away from major blood vessels and nerves.**

20. **TEST-TAKING TIP: The word *cachectic* is the key word in the stem that directs attention to content. The word *cautiously* in the stem indicates negative polarity. The question is asking which administration route is associated with an undesirable increase in drug absorption, which may be unsafe when administering a medication to a client who has insufficient subcutaneous tissue. Option 3 is unique because the first word begins with "S," not with the prefix *Intra-*.**
    1. An intradermal injection is administered by inserting the needle of a syringe through the epidermis into the dermis, where the fluid is injected. This is a safe procedure in an older adult who is cachectic.
    2. IV medications can be administered safely to cachectic older adults.
    3. **Older adults and cachectic individuals have a decrease in subcutaneous tissue. When a subcutaneous injection is administered to a client with insufficient subcutaneous tissue, the medication usually is absorbed faster; this may be unsafe.**
    4. Although muscle mass may be smaller in older adults and cachectic individuals, an intramuscular injection can be administered safely by using a 1-inch rather than a 1.5-inch needle.

21. 1. **The dorsal recumbent position (supine position with the hips and knees flexed) exposes and allows easy access to the vaginal orifice. Lying in this position for 10 minutes after administration of the vaginal cream prevents its drainage from the vaginal canal.**
    2. The low Fowler position does not expose the vaginal orifice.
    3. **A left- or right-lateral position exposes and allows easy access to the vaginal orifice. Maintaining this position for 10 minutes after insertion of the vaginal cream prevents its drainage from the vaginal canal.**
    4. The orthopneic position does not expose the vaginal orifice.
    5. The supine position does not expose the vaginal orifice.

22. **Answer: 3 mL**
    Solve the problem using ratio and proportion.

$$\frac{\text{Desire}}{\text{Have}} \quad \frac{30\text{ mg}}{10\text{ mg}} = \frac{x\text{ mL}}{1\text{ mL}}$$

$$10x = 30$$

$$x = 30 \div 10$$

$$x = 3\text{ mL}$$

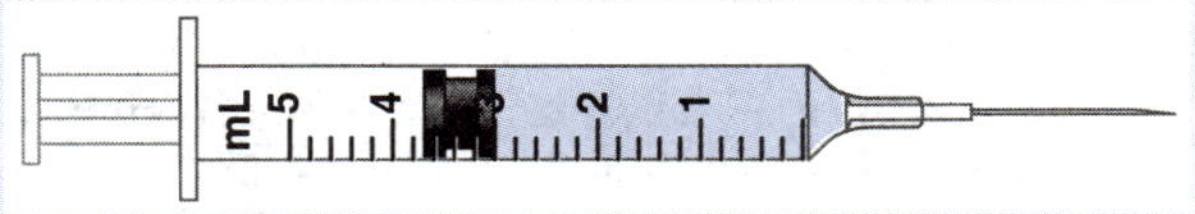

23. **Answer: 1, 2, 5, 3, 4**
    1. **Administering medication is a dependent function of the nurse. The nurse must verify the primary health-care provider's original prescription.**
    2. **Verifying the prescription requires the nurse to touch a computer or a clinical record, both of which are considered contaminated objects. Hand hygiene reduces the number of microorganisms on the nurse's hands before touching a unit dose package that will be given to a client.**
    5. **The client must be positively identified using two identifiers before medication administration. This ensures that the correct client receives the correct medication.**
    3. **An antihypertensive agent is administered to decrease blood pressure. To determine whether or not the intervention was effective, the nurse must obtain a second reading**

at the appropriate interval after administration.

4. **The nurse must document all care provided, including the medication administered and related outcomes. In this case, the second blood pressure reading is the most obvious outcome of administering an antihypertensive agent.**

5. **ACE inhibitors are teratogenic, meaning they can harm a developing fetus. Clients prescribed ACE inhibitors must be made aware of this risk, and counseling about the utility of birth control must be provided to all clients who are sexually active.**

24. **TEST-TAKING TIP: The word *adult* is the key word in the stem that directs attention to content. Options 2 and 3 are opposites.**
   1. A cotton ball may be placed in the outermost part of the ear; it should not be pressed into the ear canal.
   2. **Pulling the pinna of the ear upward and backward straightens the ear canal of an adult. This action facilitates the distribution of the medication into the external ear canal.**
   3. The pinna of the ear should be pulled downward and backward to straighten the ear canal of a child younger than 3 years, not an adult.
   4. This action may injure the eardrum. The flow of fluid should be directed against the wall of the ear canal to prevent fluid from falling against the eardrum, which can cause trauma.
   5. The force exerted by a drop falling from a height of 2 inches can injure the eardrum. The dropper should be held ½ inch (1 cm) above the ear canal, and the drop should fall against the wall of the canal and then flow toward the eardrum.

25. 1. This question is an appropriate assessment question, but it is not specific to safety during pregnancy.
   2. **This question appropriately assesses client-specific factors related to the administration of teratogenic drugs. ACE inhibitors are teratogenic, meaning they can harm a developing fetus. If a client is considering becoming pregnant, additional counseling related to the management of hypertension during pregnancy must be provided to promote safety.**
   3. This question is unrelated to a teratogenic drug. Drug addiction refers to an uncontrollable craving for a chemical substance because of physical or psychological dependence.
   4. This question is unrelated to a teratogenic. Allergies are unpredictable hypersensitive reactions to allergens such as drugs.

26. **The nurse should count the drops per minute falling in the drip chamber to determine whether the IV solution is running at the rate prescribed. The administration set indicates the number of drops per 1 mL (drop factor). The following formula can be used to determine the prescribed rate, and then the product of that formula can be compared with the actual rate being delivered to the client. A discrepancy between these rates indicates an inaccurate flow rate.**

$$\textbf{Drop Rate} = \frac{\textbf{Total mL prescribed} \times \textbf{the drop factor}}{\textbf{Total time in minutes}}$$

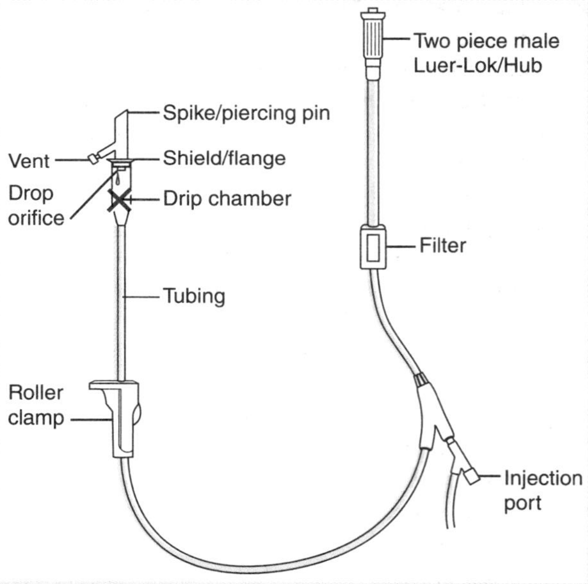

27. **TEST-TAKING TIP: The words *clarify with the provider* are the words in the stem that indicate negative polarity. The question is testing if you know when a prescription does not meet the standards identified by The Joint Commission.**
   1. This is a correctly written prescription. It contains the medication spelled out (morphine sulfate). It contains the dose (2 mg), the route (IV), the frequency (every 2 hours), and a parameter for administration (for severe incisional pain).

2. **There is an error in this prescription. *AU* indicates both ears, and gentamicin ophthalmic solution is a medication administered to the eyes. Although the abbreviation *AU* has not been disallowed by The Joint Commission, many agencies require AU to be written out (i.e., both ears).**
3. This is a correctly written prescription. It contains the medication spelled out (regular insulin). It contains the dose (5 units), and the term *units* is spelled out. It contains the route (Sub-Q) and frequency (STAT, now). The Joint Commission has not disallowed the use of Sub-Q, SQ, or SC. However, many agencies require that these abbreviations be avoided and the word *subcutaneously* be spelled out.
4. **The abbreviation *qd* for *daily* is disallowed by The Joint Commission. The prescription should state *daily*, meaning *every day*. When *qd* is written, it may be misinterpreted as *qid*, which is four times a day and thus four times the dose.**
5. **The dosage for alprazolam (Xanax®) should contain a "0" before the decimal point (0.5). This is done so that the decimal point is not overlooked. If 5 mg is given instead of 0.5 mg, the client will receive 10 times the prescribed dose. This must be clarified with the prescribing provider.**

28. TEST-TAKING TIP: The words *drops* in the stem and option 2 and *drop* in option 4 are clang associations.

1. **Excess medication is unneeded and can be wiped away; also, doing this promotes comfort.**
2. **Gazing upward moves the cornea upward and away from the conjunctival sac, where medication should be instilled.**
3. **Eyes should be closed gently to disperse medication and not force it out of the eye. Closing the eyes tightly will force medication out of the eye, reducing the dose of the medication being delivered.**
4. **The conjunctival sac, the correct location to instill eye drops, is inside the lower eyelid.**
5. **Eye infections can be easily transmitted from one eye to the other; however, it must be stressed that if aseptic principles are followed, cross-infection can be minimized.**

29. 1. Medications, especially medications with a bad taste, should not be mixed with milk or juice that the child enjoys because this can create an aversion to these beverages.
2. **Asking a parent what strategies have been successful is appropriate. A parent is a trusted adult who can be of great help when administering medications to toddlers.**
3. **Offering a cold popsicle before administering a medication can support establishing trust with this client. Additionally, it can numb the taste buds and reduce the unpleasant taste of some medications.**
4. The parent may hold the child while the nurse administers a medication, but the child should be sitting up. This prevents aspiration of the liquid.
5. **Administering the medication at the same time every day is appropriate. This action establishes routine and limits unpleasant surprises.**

30. Answer: 3 tablets

Use dimensional analysis, starting with what is needed:

$$\frac{1.5 \text{ mg}}{1} \times \frac{1000 \text{ mcg}}{1 \text{ mg}} \times \frac{1 \text{ tablet}}{500 \text{ mcg}}$$

Multiply what is above the line: 1.5 × 1000 = 1500

Then divide by what is below the line: 1 × 1 × 500 = 500

1500 ÷ 500 = 3 tablets

31. 1. **This is an insulin syringe marked in units. It has a small-gauge (27- to 29-gauge) needle. Insulin syringes usually are 5⁄16-inch, ½-inch, or ⅝-inch long. This syringe is used to administer insulin via the subcutaneous route.**
2. This syringe is inappropriate for administering insulin via the subcutaneous route. This is a 1-mL tuberculin syringe marked in 0.01-mL increments. It has a small-gauge (26- to 27-gauge) needle that is ¼-inch long. This syringe is used to administer a tuberculin (TB) skin test (tuberculin purified protein derivative [PPD]) via the intradermal route.
3. This is the appropriate syringe for administering medications via the intramuscular route. It has a 21-gauge needle that is ½-inch long to penetrate tissue to the level of a muscle.
4. This is the appropriate syringe to use when preparing medications with a

volume of 5 mL or less that is being reconstituted or added to a larger volume of solution. Although this 5-mL syringe is marked in whole milliliters, has a 20- to 21-gauge needle, has a 1.5-inch length needle, and can be used to administer an intramuscular injection, a 3-mL volume syringe with an appropriate needle gauge and length is used more often for intramuscular injections.

32. **TEST-TAKING TIP: The words *specifically* and *older adults* are key words in the stem that direct attention to content.**
    1. **Biotransformation of drugs is less efficient in older adults than in clients of younger developmental ages; when drugs are not fully metabolized, degraded, or excreted, toxic levels can accumulate.**
    2. Harmless or injurious side effects (secondary effects) are common to people of all ages, not just older adults.
    3. **Drug interactions are common in people of all ages, but more so in older adults. Older adults tend to have chronic health problems that require a multiplicity of medications. Also, older adults may take over-the-counter medications to address problems that occur with aging, such as insomnia and constipation.**
    4. Allergic reactions are common to people of all ages, not just older adults.
    5. *Teratogenic* refers to agents that cause physical defects in a developing fetus. This is a concern in women of childbearing age.

33. **TEST-TAKING TIP: The words *administering nose drops correctly* are key words in the stem that direct attention to content. The word *child* in the stem and in option 3 is a clang association. The word *nose* in the stem and in option 3 is a clang association.**
    1. Sniffing the medication is contraindicated because sniffing pulls the medication to the oropharynx, where it will be swallowed rather than inhaled into the upper respiratory tract. Nose drops should be directed toward the midline of the superior concha of the ethmoid bone as the client breathes through the mouth.
    2. **Tilting the head backward allows the instilled drops to flow well back into the nostril.**
    3. **Blowing the nose clears the nose of mucus and debris before the medication is administered. This ensures that more surface area of the mucous membrane comes into contact with the medication.**
    4. The dropper should be placed approximately a third of an inch inside the nostril to ensure that the entire drop enters the nostril. The dropper should not touch the mucous membranes of the nostril to prevent contamination of the dropper and avoid precipitating a sneeze.
    5. **Discarding excess fluid in the dropper after administering the medication and then returning the dropper to the bottle reduces the risk of contaminating the fluid in the bottle.**

34. **Answer: 4, 1, 2, 5, 3**
    4. **Assessing for any contraindications protects the client from complications, such as stimulation of vagal nerves in the rectal area, which is inappropriate when a client has a cardiac problem, or from trauma if a client is already experiencing rectal bleeding.**
    1. **Placing the client in the semi-prone position provides access to and visualization of the client's perianal area. The left semi-prone position is preferred because the suppository will follow the natural curve of the rectum and sigmoid colon.**
    2. **Lubricating the suppository reduces friction, which eases its insertion and limits trauma to the anal and rectal mucosa.**
    5. **Inserting the suppository 1 to 3 inches past the internal sphincter facilitates the retention of the suppository.**
    3. **Remaining in the side-lying position facilitates retention and absorption of the medication.**

35. **TEST-TAKING TIP: The word *priority* sets the priority in the stem.**
    1. Although the nurse should document the time the secondary infusion completed, this does not take priority over ensuring the primary infusion is running at the prescribed rate.
    2. **Ensuring that the primary infusion is running at the prescribed rate is the priority. The flow rate of the secondary infusion is often faster than that of the primary infusion. Once the secondary infusion is complete, the primary infusion will continue to flow at the rate**

set for the secondary infusion, which is often faster than the rate prescribed for the primary infusion.

3. Although the nurse should clamp, remove, and discard the empty secondary infusion bag and set, this is not the priority.
4. This action is not necessary. Generally, a new primary solution bag is hung when the current primary bag is empty.

36. 1. Administering all of the pills in one cup at the same time is inappropriate. This does not promote safety in a client with a history of difficulty swallowing. The pills should be administered one at a time.

2. This is appropriate. Clients with difficulty swallowing should not be rushed to swallow oral medications. The nurse should allow additional time to promote safety in this client.

3. The nurse must administer one pill at a time and ensure that each pill has been swallowed before offering the next pill. This promotes safety and ensures the correct dose is administered.

4. The client living with Alzheimer's disease must still receive appropriate instructions. Rather than avoiding verbal instructions, the nurse should choose simple sentences and repeat them as frequently as necessary.

5. This is appropriate. A client with a history of swallowing difficulty should be assessed before attempting to administer medications that require the client to swallow. This can be accomplished by offering sips of water or by facilitating a referral to speech therapy, if appropriate.

37. **TEST-TAKING TIP:** The word *most* in the stem sets a priority.

1. Notifying the primary health-care provider of the client's status is the appropriate intervention. The client's pain has become progressively more intense over the course of the day, and the medication protocol must be examined and possibly revised to adequately relieve this client's pain. Opioids depress the central nervous system, resulting in depressed respirations, heart rate, and blood pressure. The rapid response team should be notified when the client's respirations, heart rate, and blood pressure are very depressed or the client is excessively sedated.

2. Waiting 1 hour to administer hydromorphone is an inappropriate intervention. The client will unnecessarily be in severe pain for 1 hour. Also, the client's pain has become progressively more intense over the course of the day. The client's respirations are depressed and may become further depressed if hydromorphone is administered.
3. Administering acetaminophen 650 mg is an inappropriate intervention. The client is experiencing severe, not moderate, pain.
4. Reassessing the client in 30 minutes is inappropriate. The client will continue to be in severe pain during this time.

38. Answer: 3, 5, 2, 1, 4

3. Shaking the canister of albuterol (Ventolin® HFA) ensures that the ingredients in the medication are well mixed.

5. Exhaling through the mouth efficiently clears air from the lungs. The goal of an inhaler is to have medication reach deep into the lungs. When a person efficiently exhales, a large lung surface is available to come into contact with the subsequent inhaled medication.

2. Sealing the lips around the mouthpiece prevents medication from escaping from around the mouth and mouthpiece and allows delivery of an accurate dose.

1. Inhaling slowly allows for prolonged contact of the medication with the lining of the respiratory tract. Breathing in deeply delivers medication deep into the lungs.

4. Medication in a metered-dose inhaler may cause irritation of the oral mucosa or a fungal infection of the oral cavity. A swish and spit with water after the procedure reduces exposure of the oral mucosa to the medication, reducing the risk of irritation to or a fungal infection of the oral cavity.

39.

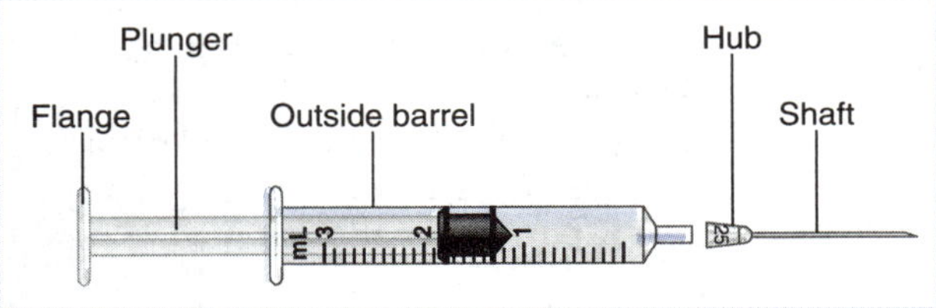

1. The flange does not have to be kept sterile. It is pulled back with the hands when drawing up air or medication and is depressed when injecting air into a vial or when administering medication to the client.

2. The plunger must remain sterile because it comes into contact with the sterile inside of the barrel when it is depressed as air is injected into the medication vial. Then, the plunger is withdrawn, pulling sterile medicated solution into the sterile inside of the barrel.

3. The needle hub must remain sterile because it may come into contact with the break in the skin caused by insertion of the needle into the client's body.

4. When the shaft of a needle is sterile, it will not insert pathogens into the client's body when the skin is pierced.

5. The outside of the barrel does not come into contact with sterile medication solution and therefore does not have to be sterile.

40. 1. Applying gentle pressure with a finger on the inner corner of the eye over the tear duct for 30 seconds after instillation of eye drops prevents medication from entering the nose and eventually the bloodstream. If the medication travels to the bloodstream, it can cause unwanted systemic side effects.

2. The eye should be wiped moving from the inner to the outer canthus; this promotes comfort, prevents trauma, and moves excess medication away from the nasolacrimal duct, minimizing systemic absorption and infection. The client should also use a new towel to wipe the child's second eye to avoid spreading the infection from one eye to the other.

3. It is unnecessary to blink the eyes after eye medication has been instilled. Keeping the eyes closed for a full 2 minutes allows time for the medication to completely penetrate the surface of the eye.

4. It is desirable to hold the dropper a half inch above the conjunctival sac. Holding it higher may injure the eye because of the force exerted by the drop; holding it lower increases the risk of contaminating the dropper or injuring the eye.

5. Instilling the eye drops in a pocket in the lower lid of the eye is appropriate because it permits medication to remain in the eye and promotes its even distribution.

CLINICAL JUDGMENT CASE STUDY ANSWERS AND RATIONALES

41. 1. Managing pain is the priority when caring for this client. Sickle cell crisis is a painful experience and the client's other vital signs are relatively stable.

2. Although a history of substance use disorder requires additional considerations, managing pain is still a priority. Pain management, especially severe pain as in this client's case, often requires the use of controlled substances. Controlled substances can be used safely for this client.

3. Treating anemia is an important component of sickle cell crisis management. However, a Hgb count of 9 g/dL is stable and pain management is the priority when caring for this client.

4. The client's oxygen saturation and respiratory rate are stable. Pain management is the priority for this client.

42. 1. Although fatigue is common due to interrupted sleep while admitted to the hospital, the most likely cause of this client's fatigue, pallor, and increased respiratory rate with ambulation is the low red blood cell count associated with sickle cell crisis and evidenced by a low Hgb count.

2. Pain can contribute to fatigue, but it is not necessarily the cause of this client's fatigue.

3. The most likely cause of this client's fatigue, pallor, and increased respiratory rate with ambulation is anemia caused by sickle cell crisis. Anemia is the reduction of red blood cells. Red blood cells are responsible for carrying oxygen to tissues. This is the nurse's most appropriate response in this scenario.

4. Although difficulty breathing can result in increased energy expenditure to maintain oxygenation and result in fatigue, this is not the best response. Anemia is the most likely cause of this client's fatigue.

43.

	Appropriate	Inappropriate
1000 mg PO acetaminophen QID		X
PRN 2 mg IV morphine, every 2 hours	X	
2 L O2 via NC	X	
Hold SQ LMWH QAM		X
IV NS 200 mL/hr, continuous	X	

44. 1. **If ever in doubt about a medication, the most appropriate action is to look up the drug in a reputable source. A current drug guide is a reputable source and a drug guide is often built into the electronic medication administration record.**
2. An Internet search engine is not the most reputable source for looking up medications. Search engines may provide outdated information or information from Web sites that are not evidence based.
3. Asking a colleague for information is a common practice. Unfortunately, this is not the best resource for the most accurate and up-to-date information.
4. Notifying the physician that the nurse is unfamiliar with a medication is inappropriate. It is fully within the scope of nursing practice to administer this medication. The appropriate action is to fill the knowledge gap of the nurse by looking up the medication.

45. 1. The room should be kept at a temperature that is comfortable to the client. This may be to cool or to warm the room.
2. **Distraction can be a powerful nonpharmacological intervention to reduce pain. The nurse should choose distractions appropriately. For example, the use of humor can be effective, but it is very easy to use humor inappropriately.**
3. **Offering warm or cool packs is appropriate. These strategies are nonpharmacological, within the scope of nursing practice, and effective ways to decrease pain.**
4. Generally, dimming lights can help to reduce pain. This is an example of creating a calming environment to promote comfort.
5. **Minimizing noise is an effective strategy for promoting comfort and helping to reduce pain. Clients can be offered ear plugs or to keep the door to the room closed. Nurses can avoid conversations in hallways and advocate for quiet hours.**

46. **TEST-TAKING TIP: The word *always* in option 2 is a specific determiner.**
1. This statement indicates that the client is assessing the skin under the patch. This is appropriate and does not require further intervention.
2. **It is best practice to choose a new site each time a fentanyl patch is replaced. This prevents skin damage and promotes adequate absorption of the medication in the patch. A client who wears the patch in the same spot requires additional teaching.**
3. Like the shoulder, the arm is an appropriate place to wear a fentanyl patch. This is an example of a client appropriately adapting to this administration route.
4. A fentanyl patch should be replaced every 72 hours, or every 3 days. It should be applied to clean, intact skin. This is an appropriate statement that does not require further teaching.

PHARMACOLOGY

This section encompasses questions related to how drugs physiologically and biochemically affect the body (pharmacodynamics) and how drugs are absorbed, distributed, metabolized, and eliminated from the body (pharmacokinetics). The questions include topics such as the therapeutic and side effects of classifications of drugs, medication toxicity, peak and trough values, factors affecting drug action, common assessments before and after drug administration, use of the nursing process in drug therapy, and the role of the nurse in client education and adherence to a medication regimen.

QUESTIONS

1. A client is receiving a medication that has a narrow therapeutic window. The medication is administered every 6 hours at 12 a.m., 6 a.m., 12 p.m., and 6 p.m. There is a prescription for the nurse to assess the peak plasma level of the medication. At what time should the nurse obtain a blood specimen for this test?
   1. 0500 hr (5 a.m.)
   2. 0800 hr (8 a.m.)
   3. 1200 hr (12 p.m.)
   4. 1900 hr (7 p.m.)

   TEST-TAKING TIP: Identify the words in the stem that direct attention to content.

2. The nurse is preparing to administer furosemide to a 62-year-old client with a history of hypertension and congestive heart failure. The nurse reviews the client's basic metabolic panel and identifies which of the following as the most concerning?
   1. Sodium: 136 mEq/L
   2. Potassium: 3.3 mEq/L
   3. Cholesterol: 180 mg/dL
   4. Blood urea nitrogen: 20 mg/dL

3. Which classification of drugs does the nurse anticipate is **most** likely to be prescribed when a client has difficulty sleeping?
   1. Benzodiazepines
   2. Barbiturates
   3. Analgesics
   4. Opioids

   TEST-TAKING TIP: Identify the word in the stem that sets a priority. Identify equally plausible options.

4. The nurse is teaching a client about tricyclic antidepressants. Which potential side effect should the nurse include?
   1. Polyuria
   2. Diarrhea
   3. Severe hypertension
   4. Orthostatic hypotension

   TEST-TAKING TIP: Identify the key words in the stem that direct attention to content. Identify the options that are opposites.

5. Which classification of medications is at risk for a drug interaction with digoxin?
   1. Glucocorticoids
   2. Sulfonamides
   3. Antibiotics
   4. Antacids

   TEST-TAKING TIP: Identify equally plausible options.

6. Which client response indicates a therapeutic outcome after receiving a cathartic?
   1. Has a bowel movement
   2. Describes pain relief
   3. Falls asleep
   4. Voids urine

7. A primary health-care provider prescribes montelukast 10 mg PO daily for a client with asthma. The nurse should teach this client to:
   1. take the medication before lunch.
   2. report behavioral changes immediately.
   3. discontinue taking the drug when symptoms subside.
   4. understand that this drug is used to treat an acute respiratory episode.

8. The nurse is caring for a group of clients receiving drugs in the following classifications. Which classification of drug may precipitate a superinfection?
   1. Diuretic
   2. Antibiotic
   3. Antiemetic
   4. Thrombolytic

9. An antibiotic to be administered via IV piggyback (IVPB) every 12 hours is prescribed for a client. When the drug is administered at 2:00 p.m., at which time should the nurse schedule a blood sample to be drawn to determine a trough level?
   1. 1:30 a.m.
   2. 2:30 a.m.
   3. 3:00 p.m.
   4. 8:00 p.m.

   TEST-TAKING TIP: Identify opposites in options.

10. The nurse is evaluating a client's response to an antitussive. Which clinical finding when **decreased** indicates that the antitussive was effective?
    1. Fever
    2. Mucus viscosity
    3. Nasal congestion
    4. Frequency of coughing

11. When giving a health history, a client states, "I take one package of Metamucil® every day no matter what." Which drug effect should the nurse expect to occur?
    1. Tolerance
    2. Synergistic
    3. Habituation
    4. Idiosyncratic

12. A client is receiving an antibiotic that has a 4 to 10 mcg/mL therapeutic range, an optimum peak value of 8 to 10 mcg/mL, and a minimum trough level of 0.5 mcg/mL. Which value requires the nurse to notify the primary health-care provider?
    1. Peak value of 5 mcg/mL
    2. Peak value of 9 mcg/mL
    3. Trough value of 0.7 mcg/mL
    4. Trough value of 0.3 mcg/mL

    TEST-TAKING TIP: Identify the words in the stem that indicate negative polarity.

13. Codeine for pain is prescribed for a client of Asian descent. Which element of pharmacokinetics does the nurse understand is critical when assessing this client's response to the medication?
    1. Excretion
    2. Absorption
    3. Distribution
    4. Biotransformation

14. The therapeutic blood level range for an antibiotic is 4 to 10 mcg/mL. Which should the nurse conclude when the laboratory test indicates a peak level of 12 mcg/mL?
1. The drug dose is safe.
2. The drug dose is subtherapeutic.
3. The client is at risk for drug accumulation.
4. The client's next dose of the drug should be given over a longer period of time.

TEST-TAKING TIP: Identify opposites in options. Identify the unique option.

15. The nurse is caring for a client who experienced an excess fluid volume exhibited by lower extremity edema, increased blood pressure, dyspnea, and distended neck veins. Furosemide is prescribed. The nurse is monitoring the client's daily potassium level. On which day should the nurse inform the primary health-care provider of the client's potassium level and seek a prescription for potassium supplementation?
1. Day 1—Serum potassium: 5.5 mEq/L
2. Day 2—Serum potassium: 4.2 mEq/L
3. Day 3—Serum potassium: 3.6 mEq/L
4. Day 4—Serum potassium: 2.8 mEq/L

16. The nurse is completing a medication reconciliation and identifies that which of the following medication combinations puts the client at the highest risk for bleeding?
1. Rivaroxaban and enoxaparin
2. Omeprazole and metoprolol
3. Amoxicillin and metformin
4. Oxycodone and acetaminophen

TEST-TAKING TIP: Identify words in the stem that draw attention to content.

17. A client is receiving digoxin 0.25 mg every day. The nurse should provide further teaching when the client states:
1. "I should not take antacids with this medication."
2. "I will not take the digoxin if my pulse is less than 60."
3. "I should call the doctor if I have nausea, vomiting, or weakness."
4. "If I forget to take my digoxin, I should take 2 pills the next day."

TEST-TAKING TIP: Identify the words in the stem that indicate negative polarity.

18. The client taking Percocet® to manage 7 out of 10 pain states, "The other nurse said that this pill is two drugs in one and that makes it safer. How can that be?" What is the nurse's best response?
1. "Using both drugs completely eliminates pain."
2. "One drug reduces the dose of the other drug needed to manage pain."
3. "It is not safer than any other pain medication."
4. "The two drugs work the same way to manage pain."

TEST-TAKING TIP: Identify clang associations.

19. The nurse is collecting a health history from a client who will be receiving IV heparin sodium therapy. Which statement by the client requires further exploration by the nurse?
1. "I may be pregnant."
2. "I eat a lot of green, leafy vegetables."
3. "I always experience heavy menstrual periods."
4. "I stopped taking my daily aspirin tablet several days ago."

TEST-TAKING TIP: Identify the words in the stem that indicate negative polarity.

20. A 20-year-old client attending college full time was recently prescribed bupropion to manage depression and attention-deficit/hyperactivity disorder (ADHD). The client asks how long the drug takes before they "start to feel better." What is the nurse's best response?
1. "The drug begins to work within two to five hours."
2. "You'll feel better in a couple days."
3. "About two weeks after taking the medication, you should notice its effects."
4. "It takes over two months for this drug to work."

TEST-TAKING TIP: Identify key words in the stem that direct attention to content.

21. The nurse is caring for a client who is receiving chemotherapy for cancer. The client has a nose bleed and reports that brushing the teeth causes the gums to bleed for several minutes. The nurse reviews the client's laboratory results. Which laboratory result should cause the **most** concern?
1. White blood cell count—5000 cells/mcL
2. Platelets—80,000 cells/mcL
3. Hemoglobin—10 g/dL
4. Hematocrit—37%

TEST-TAKING TIP: Identify the word in the stem that sets a priority.

22. A client is receiving a neuroleptic antipsychotic medication. For which extrapyramidal reaction should the nurse assess the client? **Select all that apply.**
1. _____ Protrusion of the tongue
2. _____ Spasm of neck muscles
3. _____ Motor agitation
4. _____ Muscle rigidity
5. _____ Shuffling gait

TEST-TAKING TIP: Identify the key words in the stem that direct attention to content.

23. The nurse administers an expectorant to a client. Which result indicates that the client is experiencing a therapeutic response to the medication? **Select all that apply.**
1. _____ Reduced fever
2. _____ Productive cough
3. _____ Relieved nasal congestion
4. _____ Dilation of respiratory airways
5. _____ Decrease in itchy, watery eyes

TEST-TAKING TIP: Identify the key words in the stem that direct attention to content.

24. The nurse is administering heparin to a client daily for a week. For which undesirable clinical response to heparin that indicates the need to discontinue the heparin therapy should the nurse assess the client? **Select all that apply.**
1. _____ Activated partial thromboplastin time of 70 sec
2. _____ International normalized ratio of 2.5
3. _____ Platelet count of 5000 cells/mcL
4. _____ Hematuria
5. _____ Gastritis

TEST-TAKING TIP: Identify the word in the stem that indicates negative polarity.

25. A client is receiving prednisone, a glucocorticoid. For which response should the nurse monitor the client's electrolytes? **Select all that apply.**

1. _____ Hypokalemia
2. _____ Hypocalcemia
3. _____ Hyperkalemia
4. _____ Hyponatremia
5. _____ Hypercalcemia
6. _____ Hypernatremia

TEST-TAKING TIP: Identify opposites in options.

26. Which medication increases bulk to stimulate intestinal peristalsis? **Select all that apply.**

1. _____ Methylcellulose
2. _____ Polycarbophil
3. _____ Bisacodyl
4. _____ Psyllium
5. _____ Senna

TEST-TAKING TIP: Identify the key words in the stem that direct attention to content.

27. The nurse is preparing to administer analgesic medication to a client with severe pain. Which route of administration, represented in the illustration, is most appropriate for this client?

1. Intravenous
2. Oral
3. Sublingual
4. Rectal

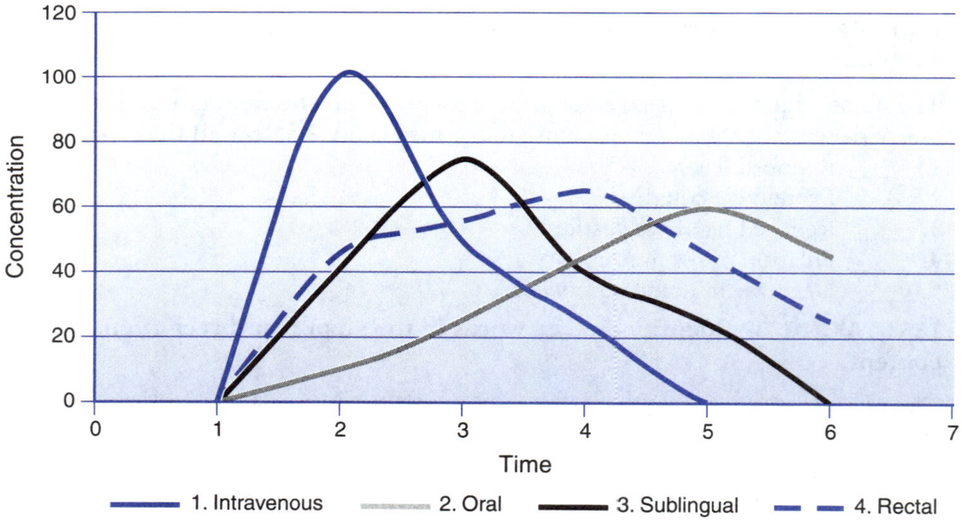

28. The client has been referred to a cardiac rehabilitation program after a coronary artery bypass graft. Which medications play a role in improving mortality for this client? **Select all that apply.**

1. _____ Bupropion
2. _____ Oxycodone
3. _____ Ondansetron
4. _____ Acetaminophen
5. _____ Atorvastatin
6. _____ Metformin

TEST-TAKING TIP: Identify the key word in the stem that directs attention to content.

29. Clorazepate (Tranxene®) 7.5 mg PO twice a day was prescribed for a client. This sedative/hypnotic was prescribed for its skeletal muscle relaxant effect. The medication is supplied as 3.75 mg per tablet. How many tablets should the nurse administer? **Record your answer using a whole number.**

Answer: ___________ tablets

30. The nurse has been administering a diuretic to a client. Which clinical finding should the nurse assess to reflect a therapeutic response to the diuretic? **Select all that apply.**
1. _____ Decreased weight
2. _____ Improved heart function
3. _____ Increased urinary output
4. _____ Decreased blood pressure
5. _____ Decreased white blood cell count

TEST-TAKING TIP: Identify the words in the stem that direct attention to content.

31. The nurse identifies that it is most appropriate to advocate for the continued use of a patent peripheral IV based on what information in this client's medical record?
1. Elevated heart rate
2. Clopidogrel (Plavix) 75 mg once daily
3. Elevated blood pressure
4. Open wound

CLIENT'S CLINICAL RECORD

Client diagnosed with lower extremity arterial disease with 1-cm ulcer on the distal end of the right large toe. Client has a history of coronary artery disease and hypothyroidism. Client reports intermittent joint pain on a level 5. Daily wound irrigation with NS and wet-to-moist dressings to right large toe as well as education regarding drug therapy prescribed by the primary health-care provider.

Vital Signs

Blood pressure: 138/86 mm Hg
Pulse: 100 beats/min, regular
Respirations: 22 breaths/min, unlabored
Temperature: 98.9°F

Current Medications

Levothyroxine (Synthroid) 125 mcg, PO, once daily
Clopidogrel (Plavix) 75 mg once daily
Ibuprofen (Motrin IB) 2 caplets every 6 hours for joint discomfort
Cleanse wound on right large toe with NS and apply wet-to-moist dressing daily

32. The nurse is administering an antineoplastic drug that is neurotoxic. For which side effect should the nurse assess this client? **Select all that apply.**
1. _____ Diarrhea
2. _____ Renal failure
3. _____ Paralytic ileus
4. _____ Electrolyte imbalances
5. _____ Peripheral neuropathies
6. _____ Decreased red blood cell count

TEST-TAKING TIP: Identify the key word in the stem that directs attention to content. Identify the clang association.

33. The nurse is caring for a client with a history of falls and who is receiving multiple medications. Which classification of medication may increase this client's risk for falls? **Select all that apply.**
1. _____ Antibiotic
2. _____ Antiemetic
3. _____ Antihistamine
4. _____ Antidepressant
5. _____ Antihypertensive
6. _____ Antidysrhythmic

TEST-TAKING TIP: Identify the key word in the stem that directs attention to content.

34. The nurse is caring for several clients who are receiving an antipsychotic medication as well as another medication. The nurse plans to assess these clients for signs of drug interactions. Which classification of drugs can the action of antipsychotic medication potentiate? **Select all that apply.**
1. _____ Amphetamines
2. _____ Anticoagulants
3. _____ Opioid analgesics
4. _____ Antihypertensives
5. _____ Oral hypoglycemic agents

35. A client has a prescription for the administration of NPH insulin. The nurse must understand the pharmacokinetics of this medication to assess the client's response to it, especially when the client is at risk for developing hypoglycemia. Which time action profile reflects the onset, peak, and duration pharmacokinetics of NPH insulin?

CLIENT'S HOME CARE CLINICAL RECORD

1.	ONSET: 1 to 1.5 hr	PEAK: No peak action	DURATION: 20 to 24 hr
2.	ONSET: 1.5 to 4 hr	PEAK: 4 to 12 hr	DURATION: 18 to 24 hr
3.	ONSET: 30 to 60 min	PEAK: 2 to 5 hr	DURATION: 5 to 8 hr
4.	ONSET: 10 to 20 min	PEAK: 1 to 3 hr	DURATION: 3 to 5 hr

36. A client who has a history of sensitivity reactions to new drugs is being cared for in a primary health-care provider's office. A new medication is prescribed. The office nurse administers the first dose from a sample pack of the drug provided by a pharmaceutical representative. List the nurse's actions in order of priority.
1. Give the client the drug according to the prescription.
2. Ask the client if this drug was ever received in the past.
3. Instruct the client to remain in the waiting room for at least 30 minutes.
4. Ask the client if this drug has ever caused a sensitivity reaction in the past.
5. Instruct the client to notify the primary health-care provider immediately if any sensitivity reactions occur.

Answer: ___________

37. A primary health-care provider prescribes the diuretic hydrochlorothiazide (HCTZ) for a client with hypertension. What should the nurse teach the client to do while taking this medication? **Select all that apply.**

1. _____ Avoid drinking orange juice
2. _____ Limit salt intake to 4 grams daily
3. _____ Take it in the evening before going to sleep
4. _____ Monitor for signs of hypernatremia such as thirst, dry mouth, and confusion
5. _____ Report muscle weakness, cramps, nausea, vomiting, diarrhea, dizziness, or irregular heartbeats if they occur

38. The nurse is caring for a client receiving hydrocodone/acetaminophen for back pain. For which effect should the nurse monitor the client? **Select all that apply.**

1. _____ Nausea
2. _____ Diplopia
3. _____ Euphoria
4. _____ Drowsiness
5. _____ Hypotension

39. A client with panic disorder has been taking alprazolam (Xanax®) 0.5 mg by mouth three times a day. After a week of therapy, the prescription is increased to 1 mg by mouth three times a day. The client has leftover alprazolam tablets 0.25 mg. How many tablets should the nurse instruct the client to take for each dose? **Record your answer using a whole number.**

Answer: ____________ **tablets**

40. Which physiological change in the older adult should the nurse consider as contributing to prolonged drug half-life? **Select all that apply.**

1. _____ Decreased liver function
2. _____ Reduced subcutaneous tissue
3. _____ Reduced glomerular filtration rate
4. _____ Decreased hydrochloric acid production
5. _____ Decreased gastrointestinal absorptive surface

TEST-TAKING TIP: Identify key words in the stem that direct attention to content.

1. **TEST-TAKING TIP: The words *peak plasma level* are the words in the stem that direct attention to content.**
   1. Five a.m. (0500 hr) is an appropriate time to obtain a blood specimen to test the lowest, not highest, plasma concentration of the medication for this client. Trough levels are assessed via a blood specimen obtained 30 to 60 minutes before the next dose.
   2. Eight a.m. (0800 hr) is an inappropriate time to assess either a peak or trough level of the medication for this client. It is approximately halfway between two doses.
   3. Twelve p.m. (1200 hr) is an inappropriate time to assess either a peak or trough level of the medication for this client.
   4. **Seven p.m. (1900 hr) is an appropriate time to obtain a blood specimen to assess the peak level of the medication for this client. Blood specimens for assessing the peak level of the medication should be obtained 30 to 60 minutes after a dose is administered. Additional acceptable times to obtain a blood specimen to measure a peak plasma concentration of the medication in this client are 0100 hr (1 a.m.), 0700 hr (7 a.m.), and 1300 hr (1 p.m.).**

2.
   1. The reference range for sodium is 135 to 145 mEq/L. Furosemide (Lasix®) blocks renal absorption of sodium, which can cause a low serum sodium level (hyponatremia). A sodium level of 136 mEq/L is within the reference range, but should be monitored. Values less than 120 and higher than 160 mEq/L are critical findings.
   2. **The reference range for potassium is 3.5 to 5.0 mEq/L. Furosemide (Lasix®) can cause a loss of potassium, resulting in hypokalemia. A potassium level of 3.3 is considered hypokalemia. Hypokalemia may precipitate a cardiac dysrhythmia that can be life threatening. Values less than 2.5 mEq/L and higher than 6.5 mEq/L are critical findings.**
   3. The desired cholesterol level is less than 200 mg/dL. Although clients with heart disease often have elevated cholesterol levels, this client does not, and cholesterol is not significantly affected by furosemide.
   4. The reference range of blood urea nitrogen (BUN) is 8 to 21 mg/dL. Congestive heart failure can cause an elevated BUN level, but that is not the case for this client. A BUN level greater than 100 mg/dL is a critical finding.

3. **TEST-TAKING TIP: The word *most* in the stem sets a priority. Options 3 and 4 are equally plausible because they are both categories of drugs that relieve pain.**
   1. **Benzodiazepines, such as temazepam (Restoril®) and zolpidem (Ambien®), are a group of nonbarbiturate sedative-hypnotics. They influence the neurons in the central nervous system that suppress responsiveness to stimuli, thereby decreasing levels of arousal.**
   2. Barbiturates, such as pentobarbital sodium (Nembutal® sodium), have many side effects and have been replaced by benzodiazepines as the drugs of choice to induce sleep.
   3. Analgesics are administered primarily to reduce pain, not to induce sleep.
   4. Opioids are administered primarily to reduce pain, not to induce sleep.

4. **TEST-TAKING TIP: The key words in the stem that draw attention to content are *tricyclic antidepressants* and *side effect*. Options 3 and 4 are opposites.**
   1. Urinary retention, not polyuria, is a side effect of tricyclic antidepressants.
   2. Constipation, not diarrhea, is a common side effect of tricyclic antidepressants that usually can be managed with stool softeners and a high-fiber diet.
   3. Hypertension is not a side effect of tricyclic antidepressants.
   4. **Orthostatic hypotension is a common side effect of tricyclic antidepressants; the client should be instructed to rise slowly from a sitting to a standing position.**

5. **TEST-TAKING TIP: Options 2 and 3 are equally plausible. Sulfa drugs are antibiotics.**
   1. **Prednisone, a glucocorticoid with mineralocorticoid activity, can precipitate hypokalemia. Hypokalemia increases the sensitivity of the myocardium to digitalis. Hypokalemia can precipitate digitalis toxicity, even when digoxin serum levels are in the therapeutic range of 0.5 to 2.0 ng/mL.**
   2. Sulfonamides do not interact with digoxin.
   3. Antibiotics do not interact with digoxin.
   4. Antacids do not interact with digoxin.

6.
   1. **Cathartics, also called *laxatives*, induce defecation.**
   2. Analgesics relieve pain. Also, some cathartics may cause slight abdominal discomfort due to increased intestinal peristalsis.

3. Sedatives and hypnotics promote sleep.
4. Diuretics increase urinary output.

7. 1. Montelukast (Singulair®) should be taken in the evening, not before lunch. Most people with asthma experience worsening symptoms at night. When montelukast (Singulair®) is taken at night, its peak action (3 to 4 hours after ingestion) will be optimal when asthma symptoms generally peak.

2. Agitation, aggression, depression, irritability, hallucinations, and thoughts of hurting oneself are serious adverse reactions to montelukast (Singulair®) that should be reported immediately to the primary health-care provider. Montelukast (Singulair®) may need to be discontinued if these responses occur.

3. Montelukast (Singulair®) is used for the maintenance treatment of asthma and should not be discontinued when symptoms subside without consulting the primary health-care provider.
4. Montelukast (Singulair®) is not used to treat an acute asthma attack; it is used to prevent and treat chronic asthma and seasonal allergic rhinitis and to prevent exercise-induced bronchoconstriction.

8. 1. Diuretics increase the formation and excretion of urine. They can cause dehydration and electrolyte imbalance; they do not precipitate a superinfection.

2. Prolonged or inappropriate use of antibiotics can stimulate bacterial growth as normal flora of the gastrointestinal tract and skin are destroyed. Infections that occur while a client is receiving antimicrobial therapy are called *superinfections*.

3. Antiemetics are used to prevent nausea and vomiting. They may cause side effects such as headache, dizziness, fatigue, and diarrhea, not superinfections.
4. Thrombolytics dissolve thrombi or emboli; they also prolong coagulation processes, which may increase the risk of bleeding. Thrombolytics do not precipitate superinfections.

9. TEST-TAKING TIP: Options 1 and 2 are opposites. Option 1 is 30 minutes before the drug is administered, and option 2 is 30 minutes after the drug is administered.

1. The blood level of an antibiotic is at its lowest level just before the next scheduled dose.

2. After the drug is administered, the blood level of the drug increases. A value taken 30 minutes after the drug is administered does not reflect the lowest serum level, which is the purpose of identifying a trough level.
3. This is too soon for a trough level. This time is appropriate for a peak level.
4. This is too soon for a trough level. This time is halfway between two doses.

10. 1. Antipyretics reduce a fever; antitussives do not.
2. Mucolytics reduce mucus viscosity; antitussives do not.
3. Nasal decongestants reduce nasal congestion; antitussives do not.

4. Antitussives reduce the frequency and intensity of a cough. They act on the central or peripheral nervous system or on the local mucosa.

11. 1. Tolerance occurs when an individual requires increases in the dosage of a drug to maintain its therapeutic effect.
2. A synergistic effect occurs when the effect of two medications given together is greater than the effect of the medications when given individually.

3. Drug habituation occurs when an individual develops a mild form of psychological dependence and relies on the use of a substance such as psyllium (Metamucil).

4. An idiosyncratic effect occurs when a person's response to a drug is an underresponse, an overresponse, or a different response from that which is expected.

12. TEST-TAKING TIP: *Notify the primary health-care provider* are words that reflect negative polarity. The question is asking which blood level result is unacceptable.

1. Although this is below the optimal peak value of 8 to 10 mcg/mL, it is within the therapeutic window of 4 to 10 mcg/mL, which is acceptable.
2. This falls within the optimal peak value range of 8 to 10 mcg/mL, which is acceptable.
3. A value of 0.7 mcg/mL is higher than 0.5 mcg/mL, which is the minimum trough value necessary for a dose to be effective.

4. The primary health-care provider should be notified because the dose of the antibiotic should be increased. A value of 0.3 mcg/mL is below

0.5 mcg/mL, which is the lowest trough value of the antibiotic necessary to inhibit bacterial growth.

13. 1. Another element of pharmacokinetics is of more concern than elimination of an opioid from the body (excretion) by a person of Asian descent.
2. Another element of pharmacokinetics is of more concern than the process of movement of a medication into the bloodstream (absorption) by a person of Asian descent.
3. Another element of pharmacokinetics is of more concern than transport of a medication from the site of absorption to the site of medication action (distribution) by a person of Asian descent.
4. **Genes can cause liver metabolism to be slower in individuals of Asian descent. Because conversion of a medication to a less active form (biotransformation) in preparation for excretion from the body occurs in the liver, toxic levels of a medication may occur when liver metabolism is slowed in a client of Asian descent. Nurses must assess clients of Asian descent for drug toxicity when they receive an opioid that includes clinical manifestations such as decreased respiratory rate and depth, drowsiness, sedation, confusion, and hypotension. A person of Asian descent may require a lower dose of an opioid to achieve a therapeutic effect.**

14. **TEST-TAKING TIP: Options 2 and 3 are opposites. Option 3 is unique. It is the only option that does not include the word *dose*.**
1. The drug dose is not safe. A peak level of 12 mcg/mL indicates that the drug dose is too high and should be reduced by the primary health-care provider. The optimum peak value should be between 8 and 10 mcg/mL.
2. The drug level will be less than 4 mcg/mL if the dose is subtherapeutic.
3. **A value of 12 mcg/mL is 2 mcg/mL more than is necessary to be effective and will contribute to drug accumulation and toxicity if it continues for 3 to 5 days.**
4. The dose should be adjusted by the primary health-care provider and not just given at a slower rate.

15. 1. The client's serum potassium level of 5.5 mEq/L is higher than the expected range of 3.5 to 5.0 mEq/L; therefore, supplemental potassium is unnecessary and inappropriate.
2. The client's serum potassium level of 4.2 mEq/L is within the expected range of 3.5 to 5.0 mEq/L; therefore, supplemental potassium is unnecessary and inappropriate.
3. **Although the client's serum potassium level of 3.6 mEq/L is within the expected range of 3.5 to 5.0 mEq/L, the level has progressively decreased over the last 72 hours. Furosemide (Lasix®), a loop diuretic, decreases sodium and chloride reabsorption in the ascending loop of Henle and distal renal tubule. This in turn inhibits potassium reabsorption mechanisms. If the client continues to receive furosemide without potassium supplementation, the potassium level will continue to decrease, placing the client at risk for a cardiac dysrhythmia and other signs and symptoms associated with a low serum potassium level (hypokalemia).**
4. When a client is receiving furosemide, potassium supplementation should begin when the client's serum potassium level is in the low expected range, not when it decreases below the expected range. A low potassium level (hypokalemia) can result in cardiac dysrhythmias, muscle weakness, fatigue, nausea and vomiting, decreased gastric motility, decreased reflexes, and abdominal distention, which can be avoided with prophylactic potassium supplementation.

16. **TEST-TAKING TIP: The word *bleeding* draws attention to content.**
1. **Rivaroxaban is a factor Xa inhibitor with a black box warning related to bleeding. Enoxaparin is a low-molecular-weight heparin (LMWH) with a black box warning related to bleeding.**
2. Omeprazole is a proton pump inhibitor and metoprolol is a beta blocker. Both drugs may cause bleeding, but not to the degree of rivaroxaban and enoxaparin in option 1.
3. Amoxicillin is a penicillin antibiotic and metformin is a biguanide. Both drugs may cause bleeding, but not to the degree of rivaroxaban and enoxaparin in option 1.
4. Oxycodone is an opiate and acetaminophen is a nonsteroidal antiinflammatory

drug (NSAID). They are often given in combination as an analgesic. NSAIDs can cause bleeding, but not to the same degree of rivaroxaban and enoxaparin in option 1.

17. **TEST-TAKING TIP: The words *provide further teaching* in the stem indicate negative polarity.**
    1. Antacids can interfere with the absorption of digoxin and should not be taken at the same time.
    2. Digoxin slows the heart rate and strengthens cardiac contractions. If the apical pulse is below a predetermined parameter set by the primary health-care provider (usually below 60 beats per minute), the dose should be withheld.
    3. Nausea, vomiting, and weakness are signs of toxicity. The client needs a test to determine the serum blood level of digoxin.
    4. **This action is unsafe and may lead to toxicity. If a dose is missed, it should be taken within 12 hours of the scheduled dose.**

18. **TEST-TAKING TIP: The word *pain* in the stem and options 1 and 2 are clang associations.**
    1. This statement is false. Percocet® is a combination of oxycodone and acetaminophen. Although it can effectively reduce pain, it does not completely eliminate pain in all clients.
    2. **Percocet® is a combination of oxycodone and acetaminophen. The addition of acetaminophen, which acts on pain by a different mechanism, reduces the dose of oxycodone needed to manage pain in some clients. This reduces the required dose of opiate and therefore reduces the risk for dangerous adverse effects and improves safety.**
    3. This statement is inappropriate. It negates the statements of the other nurse and compromises the client's trust in the health-care team. Additionally, using oxycodone and acetaminophen in combination is considered safer than using high doses of an opiate to manage pain.
    4. This statement is false. Oxycodone is an opiate that blocks receptors and therefore the transmission of pain signals. Acetaminophen is an NSAID whose exact mechanism of action is unknown. Acetaminophen possibly inhibits COX pathways to reduce pain.

19. **TEST-TAKING TIP: The words *requires further exploration* in the stem indicate negative polarity. The question is asking which situation is unsafe when a person is receiving IV heparin.**
    1. Heparin does not cross the placental barrier and has no effects on the fetus or newborn.
    2. Eating a lot of green, leafy vegetables can contribute to the ineffectiveness of warfarin sodium (Coumadin®), not heparin sodium.
    3. **Heavy menstrual periods are a contraindication for the use of heparin because of an increased risk of prolonged bleeding during menstruation.**
    4. Although aspirin can prolong bleeding time when given with heparin, several days is sufficient time to be aspirin free for safe administration of heparin.

20. **TEST-TAKING TIP: The words *how long* and *feel better* are key words in the stem that direct attention to content.**
    1. Bupropion is an antidepressant that is also used for smoking cessation and ADHD management. The serum concentration peaks 2 to 5 hours after administration, but this is too fast for the client to notice therapeutic effects.
    2. Two days is too short a time to experience a therapeutic response to bupropion.
    3. **Most clients experience a therapeutic effect after 2 weeks of regular bupropion administration. All clients should be monitored for suicidal ideation when starting a new antidepressant because suicidal ideation may increase during this time.**
    4. The client should be monitored during the first few months after a new antidepressant is prescribed. However, bupropion is expected to have therapeutic effects before 2 months.

21. **TEST-TAKING TIP: The word *most* in the stem sets a priority.**
    1. The white blood cell (WBC) count of 5000 cells/mcL is within the expected range of 4500 to 10,500 cells/mcL and is not as much of a concern as another option. Chemotherapy can cause bone marrow depression, resulting in a decreased WBC count (leukopenia, neutropenia). The WBC count should be monitored because a low count can place this client at risk for infection.

2. **The low platelet count is the laboratory result of most concern. The client's platelet count of 80,000 cells/mcL is a seriously low count and should be reported immediately to the primary health-care provider. An expected range for a platelet count is 150,000 to 450,000 per microliter of blood. An adequate platelet count is essential for blood clotting. A low count predisposes a client to hemorrhage, which is a life-threatening situation.**
3. Although a hemoglobin level of 10 g/dL is below the expected range of 12.6 to 17.4 g/dL, it is not low enough to indicate the need for a blood transfusion. A blood transfusion generally is necessary when the hemoglobin level is 8.5 g/dL or less. A hemoglobin level of less than 6 g/dL is a critical finding.
4. The client's hematocrit of 37% is within the expected range of 36% to 52% and is not a concern. A hematocrit level indicates the volume of solutes in the blood. If a person hemorrhages, the hematocrit level will decrease. A hematocrit level less than 18% is a critical finding.

22. **TEST-TAKING TIP: The words *extrapyramidal reaction* are the key words in the stem that direct attention to content.**
1. **Extrapyramidal side effects such as tardive dyskinesia can result from use of neuroleptic antipsychotic medications. This condition is characterized by involuntary movements of the tongue and face, such as rolling or protrusion of the tongue, lip smacking, teeth grinding, chewing motions, and tics.**
2. **Spasm of neck muscles (torticollis) is an acute dystonic reaction that occurs because of lack of modulation of muscle contraction, causing excessive contraction and muscle spasms.**
3. **Motor agitation (akathisia) may occur with neuroleptic antipsychotic medications. Akathisia occurs in response to dopamine blockage or depletion in the basal ganglia.**
4. **Extrapyramidal side effects such as Parkinsonism-like responses can occur with neuroleptic antipsychotic medications. These responses include muscle rigidity, mask-like face, tremors, drooling, and stooped posture.**
5. **Extrapyramidal side effects such as Parkinsonism-like responses can occur with neuroleptic antipsychotic medications. These responses include shuffling gait (cogwheel gait), mask-like face, tremors, drooling, and stooped posture.**

23. **TEST-TAKING TIP: The words *expectorant* and *therapeutic response* are the key words in the stem that direct attention to content.**
1. An antipyretic, not an expectorant, reduces a fever.
2. **Expectorants lubricate the irritated lining of the respiratory tract, which helps to mobilize secretions toward the trachea and oral cavity; this promotes a productive cough. A productive cough is a cough that results in the elimination of mucus from the oral cavity.**
3. A nasal decongestant, not an expectorant, relieves nasal edema and congestion.
4. A bronchodilator, not an expectorant, dilates the airways of the respiratory tract.
5. Antihistamines, not expectorants, block the release of histamine, which occurs when the body is exposed to allergens. Itchy, watery eyes; sneezing; coughing; and nasal discharge are additional signs of exposure to allergens.

24. **TEST-TAKING TIP: The word *undesirable* in the stem indicates negative polarity.**
1. This value is within the therapeutic range for an activated partial thromboplastin time (aPTT), which is between 60 and 85 seconds.
2. An international normalized ratio (INR) value is obtained to assess the effectiveness of warfarin sodium (Coumadin®) therapy, not heparin therapy.
3. **Heparin-induced thrombocytopenia (HIT) of 5000 cells/mcL necessitates discontinuing heparin. HIT can lead to increased resistance to heparin therapy and may progress to the development of venous and arterial thrombosis.**
4. **Blood in the urine (hematuria), bleeding gums, nosebleeds, and black tarry stools are serious side effects of heparin therapy that require the termination of therapy.**
5. Heparin is administered parenterally, not by mouth, and does not cause gastritis. Gastritis may be a contraindication for heparin therapy.

25. **TEST-TAKING TIP: Options 1 and 3 are opposites. Options 2 and 5 are opposites.**

Options 4 and 6 are opposites. Examine opposites carefully because they cannot both be correct answers.

1. **Prednisone, a glucocorticoid, has significant water- and sodium-retaining (mineralocorticoid) activities. As sodium is retained, potassium is depleted, resulting in hypokalemia.**
2. **Prednisone interferes with the absorption of calcium; as a result, the client may experience hypocalcemia.**
3. Prednisone does not cause hyperkalemia.
4. Prednisone does not cause hyponatremia.
5. Prednisone does not cause hypercalcemia.
6. **Prednisone, a glucocorticoid, has significant water- and sodium-retaining (mineralocorticoid) activities. As sodium is retained, the client may develop hypernatremia.**

26. **TEST-TAKING TIP: The words *increase bulk* are the key words in the stem that direct attention to content.**

1. **Methylcellulose (Citrucel®) increases bulk in the intestine to stimulate peristalsis.**
2. **Polycarbophil (FiberCon®) forms a viscous gel that holds water, which increases the size of stool, thereby stimulating peristalsis.**
3. Bisacodyl (Dulcolax®) is a stimulant laxative that irritates the intestinal mucosa, increasing intestinal motility.
4. **Psyllium (Metamucil®) forms a viscous gel that holds water, which increases the size of stool, thereby stimulating peristalsis.**
5. Senna (Senokot®) is a stimulant laxative that irritates the intestinal mucosa, increasing intestinal motility.

27.

1. **The intravenous route produces the fastest pharmacological response because the medication is administered directly into the intravascular compartment and bypasses absorption. This is the most appropriate route for a client in severe pain because they benefit from immediate action of an analgesic.**
2. The oral route is the slowest route because the medication must reach the small intestine and then be absorbed before effects are seen. Absorption is influenced by many factors, such as the amount of food in the stomach, physical activity, and comorbidities. The client in severe pain requires a more immediate effect.
3. The sublingual route is faster than the oral route because absorption in the sublingual tissue bypasses the first-pass effect. However, it is not the most appropriate route for this client because the intravenous route is faster.
4. The rectal route is faster than the oral route, but slower than the sublingual route. The first-pass effect is reduced by approximately 50% via the rectal route. However, a client in severe pain requires more immediate pain relief, which is provided by the intravenous route.

28. **TEST-TAKING TIP: The word *palliative* is the key word in the stem that directs attention to content.**

1. **Bupropion (Zyban®) is an antidepressant used in smoking cessation. Smoking is a major modifiable risk factor for cardiac disease. Cardiac rehabilitation programs focus on aggressive management of cardiac risk factors.**
2. Oxycodone (OxyContin®), an opioid analgesic, relieves the symptoms of a disease. It does not play a large role in improving mortality.
3. Ondansetron (Zofran®), an antiemetic, is used to prevent or treat nausea and vomiting. It does not play a large role in improving mortality in clients with cardiac disease.
4. Acetaminophen (Tylenol®), a pain reliever and fever reducer, relieves clinical symptoms. It does not play a large role in improving mortality in clients with cardiac disease.
5. **Atorvastatin (Lipitor®) is used to lower cholesterol. Hyperlipidemia is a major modifiable risk factor in clients with cardiac disease.**
6. Metformin (Glucophage®) is the first-line drug for managing type 2 diabetes. Diabetes is a major modifiable risk factor for clients with cardiovascular disease.

29. **Answer: 2 tablets**

Solve the problem using a formula for ratio and proportion.

$$\frac{\text{Desire}}{\text{Have}} \quad \frac{7.5 \text{ mg}}{3.75 \text{ mg}} = \frac{x \text{ tablets}}{1 \text{ tablet}}$$

$$3.75x = 7.5$$

$$x = 7.5 \div 3.75$$

$$x = 2 \text{ tablets}$$

30. **TEST-TAKING TIP: The words *diuretic* and *therapeutic response* are key words in the stem that direct attention to content.**

1. **A diuretic enhances the selective excretion of water and various electrolytes. One liter of fluid is equal to 2.2 pounds. A rapid decrease in weight indicates fluid loss.**
2. **A person with heart failure may receive a prescription for a diuretic. A weak heart pumps less blood through the kidneys and causes water retention, resulting in edema of the ankles, legs, and abdomen.**
3. **A diuretic enhances the selective excretion of water and various electrolytes by affecting renal mechanisms for tubular secretion and reabsorption, thereby increasing urinary output.**
4. **Blood pressure level will decrease as excess fluid is excreted from the body because there is less fluid in the intravascular compartment.**
5. Diuretics are not antibiotics and therefore will not destroy microorganisms, resulting in a decrease in the white blood cell count.

31. **TEST-TAKING TIP: Think of why it would be important to avoid starting an IV.**

1. **This client is at risk for infection due to the open wound. The elevated heart rate should be communicated to the primary health-care provider. However, this is not the most appropriate reason to advocate for continued use of a patent IV in this situation.**
2. Ibuprofen (Motrin® IB) can cause an increased risk of bleeding when the client is concurrently taking clopidogrel (Plavix®). IV sticks should be minimized in order to reduce the risk of bleeding in this client. Although the primary health-care provider should be notified of the client's high blood pressure result, it is not the priority of the options presented.
3. An elevated blood pressure should be identified, monitored, and managed. However, this is not the most appropriate reason to advocate for the continued use of a patent IV in this situation.
4. This client is at risk for infection due to the presence of an open wound. This wound should be appropriately managed. However, this is not the most appropriate reason to advocate for the continued use of a patent IV in this situation.

32. **TEST-TAKING TIP: The word *neurotoxic* is the key word in the stem that directs attention to content. The word *neurotoxic* in the stem and the word *neuropathies* in option 5 are closely related and are obscure clang associations. Consider option 5 carefully. In this question, it is one of the correct answers.**

1. **The cause of diarrhea with antineoplastic drugs is unclear. There is believed to be complex overlapping pathophysiology related to inflammation, secretory dysfunction, and gastrointestinal dysmotility and innervation.**
2. Renal failure is related to the urinary, not the neurological, system.
3. **Decreased innervation of the bowel causes a decrease or absence of intestinal peristalsis (paralytic ileus), resulting in constipation or obstipation.**
4. Electrolyte imbalances are not related to the neurological system.
5. **A peripheral neuropathy occurs in almost every client, particularly depression of the Achilles tendon reflex.**
6. Red blood cells are part of the hematopoietic, not the neurological, system.

33. **TEST-TAKING TIP: The word *falls* is the key word in the stem that directs attention to content.**

1. Postural hypotension is not a common side effect of antibiotics.
2. Postural hypotension is not a common side effect of antiemetics.
3. Postural hypotension is not a common side effect of antihistamines.
4. **Essentially all antidepressants have been correlated with an increase in falls because of their sedative and orthostatic hypotension properties.**
5. **Most antihypertensives contribute to postural hypotension because of actions such as peripheral vasodilation, decreased peripheral resistance, decreased heart rate, and decreased cardiac contraction.**
6. **Antidysrhythmics affect the conduction system of the heart. Common side effects are decreased blood pressure (hypotension) and decreased heart rate (bradycardia), both of which may predispose a person to falls.**

34. 1. Antipsychotics decrease, not potentiate, the effectiveness of amphetamines.

2. Antipsychotics decrease, not potentiate, the effectiveness of anticoagulants.
3. Antipsychotics potentiate the effects of other central nervous system depressants, such as opioid analgesics.
4. Antipsychotics potentiate the effects of antihypertensives, increasing the risk of hypotension.
5. Antipsychotics decrease, not potentiate, the effectiveness of oral hypoglycemic agents.

35. 1. This time action profile reflects the pharmacokinetics of glargine (Lantus®), a long-acting insulin.
2. This time action profile reflects the pharmacokinetics of NPH insulin, an intermediate-acting insulin.
3. This time action profile reflects the pharmacokinetics of regular insulin, a short-acting insulin.
4. This time action profile reflects the pharmacokinetics of aspart (NovoLog®) insulin, a rapid-acting insulin.

36. Answer: 2, 4, 1, 3, 5
2. The first step involves identifying whether the client has ever received the drug in the past.
4. The second step is to determine whether the client has ever had a sensitivity reaction to the drug.
1. Once a prior sensitivity reaction to the drug has been eliminated, the medication can be administered.
3. Once the drug is administered, the client should be monitored for at least 30 minutes to ensure that an immediate anaphylactic reaction does not occur.
5. After 30 minutes without a sensitivity reaction, the client can be sent home with instructions to notify the primary health-care provider immediately if a sensitivity reaction occurs.

37. 1. Thiazide diuretics reduce potassium concentration in the blood via various mechanisms. Orange juice contains potassium and is often recommended for clients to ingest to avoid thiazide diuretic–induced hypokalemia.
2. A 4-g sodium diet provides an excessive amount of sodium. A 2-g sodium diet limits the retention of fluid, which should lower blood pressure. Excessive salt intake contributes to fluid retention, which in turn increases blood pressure.
3. Clients should take hydrochlorothiazide (HCTZ) in the morning to avoid nocturia and interruption of sleep.
4. Hyponatremia, not hypernatremia, is associated with thiazide diuretic therapy. Hyponatremia occurs when the serum level of sodium falls below the normal range of 135 to 145 mEq/L. The signs and symptoms of hyponatremia include nausea and vomiting; headache; confusion; lethargy; fatigue; loss of appetite; restlessness; irritability; and muscle weakness, spasms, or cramps and can lead to decreased consciousness and coma.
5. These clinical manifestations indicate that the client may have electrolyte imbalances. A thiazide diuretic inhibits sodium reabsorption in the distal tubule of the kidney, thereby increasing the excretion of sodium and water. It also promotes the excretion of potassium, chloride, magnesium, and bicarbonate, resulting in electrolyte imbalances.

38. 1. Hydrocodone/acetaminophen (Vicodin®) is an opioid/nonopioid analgesic combination. The acetaminophen in Vicodin® may weaken the ability of the stomach lining to resist stomach acid, thus contributing to nontherapeutic gastrointestinal responses such as nausea.
2. Diplopia (double vision) is not an expected response to Vicodin®.
3. Vicodin® contains hydrocodone and acetaminophen, which comprise an opioid/nonopioid analgesic combination. The hydrocodone in Vicodin® is a central nervous system depressant that can cause an exaggerated sense of well-being in the physical and mental realm.
4. Vicodin® contains hydrocodone and acetaminophen, which comprise an opioid/nonopioid analgesic combination. The hydrocodone in Vicodin® is a central nervous system depressant that causes drowsiness.
5. Vicodin® contains hydrocodone and acetaminophen, which comprise an opioid/nonopioid analgesic combination. The hydrocodone in Vicodin® is a central nervous system depressant, which relaxes the neurovascular system and contributes to hypotension.

39. Answer:
Solve the problem using a formula for ratio and proportion.

$$\frac{\text{Desire}}{\text{Have}} \quad \frac{1 \text{ mg}}{0.25 \text{ mg}} = \frac{x \text{ tablets}}{1 \text{ tablet}}$$

$$0.25x = 1$$

$$x = 1 \div 0.25$$

$$x = 4 \text{ tablets}$$

40. TEST-TAKING TIP: The words *older adult* are key words in the stem that direct attention to content.

1. **The hepatic microsomal enzyme system causes biotransformation of drugs within the body. Aging decreases the effectiveness of this system.**
2. Reduced subcutaneous tissue is unrelated to drug accumulation.
3. **A reduced glomerular filtration rate contributes to reduced excretion of a drug, thereby prolonging the drug half-life.**
4. Drugs that rely on gastric acid for absorption are less effective when there is reduced hydrochloric acid production in older adults; this decreases, not increases, the risk of a prolonged half-life of a drug.
5. A diminished absorptive surface reduces the absorption of drugs, thereby decreasing, not increasing, the risk of a prolonged half-life of a drug.

12 Comprehensive Final Book Examination

This test is provided to give you an opportunity to practice your test-taking skills. It is designed to measure your knowledge of nursing content and motivate you to continue with your efforts to succeed in testing situations.

When self-administering this 100-question practice test, simulate a testing environment by sitting at a table and selecting a time when you will not be disturbed. Set aside 2 hours for the test. This will allow approximately 1 minute per question, with 20 minutes for review. If you spend less than 1 minute on a question, you can use this time for the questions you find more difficult or add it to the time you have reserved for your review at the end of the test. Use the full 2 hours to complete this practice test. If your school allots more or less time than 1 minute per question, adjust your time accordingly. If your examinations are not timed, use all the time you need to complete the test.

Answer every question. If you do not know the answer to a question, attempt to eliminate as many options as you can by using test-taking skills, and then make an educated guess. If you are preparing for a computer-administered test that does not permit you to return to previous questions, answer each question before moving on to the next question. Do not go back to answer or change the answer to a previous question.

After you complete this practice test, compare your answers with the answers and rationales provided at the end of the chapter. Evaluate your performance by following the directions in Chapter 10, "Analyze Your Test Performance." This will help you diagnose information-processing errors and identify knowledge deficits; suggestions for corrective actions are also provided. Do not be tempted to avoid this important step in taking a practice test. In addition, see whether you were able to identify the test-taking techniques presented at the end of the rationales for each question. The ability to use test-taking techniques to eliminate distractors and focus on potential correct answers should improve your success when taking a nursing examination. It is through this self-analysis that you can eventually maximize your strengths and address your educational needs in preparation for your next test.

QUESTIONS

1. A debilitated client is admitted to the hospital with the diagnoses of heart failure and osteoporosis. Which should the nurse do to help prevent injury to this client who has bone demineralization? **Select all that apply.**
   1. _____ Apply emollients to the skin every day
   2. _____ Encourage walking in the hall once daily
   3. _____ Have the client drink several liters of fluid daily
   4. _____ Support joints when changing the client's position
   5. _____ Teach the client to wear well-fitting, flat, rubber-soled shoes

2. A primary health-care provider prescribes 1 mg hydromorphone to be delivered via IV push as needed to a client with severe acute pain. Hydromorphone is supplied in 2-mg/mL vials. How much medication should the nurse draw up into the syringe shown in the picture?

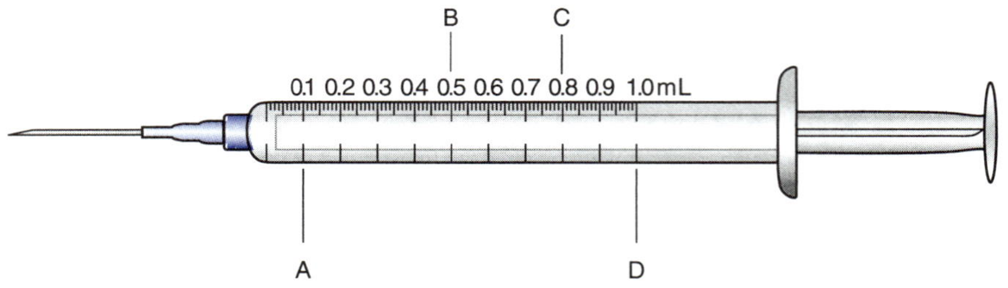

1. A
2. B
3. C
4. D

3. A client was diagnosed with multiple sclerosis (MS) 10 years ago. The client's MS is well controlled with ocrelizumab. The client is tearful and states, "I'm so worried about missing my kids' futures." The nurse recognizes that this is an example of which of the following psychological responses to stress?
   1. Anxiety
   2. Fear
   3. Depression
   4. Anger

4. The nurse is routinely monitoring a client's blood pressure. Which should the nurse do **first** when an assessment reveals an **increase** in the client's blood pressure?
   1. Notify the primary health-care provider immediately
   2. Report the change to the nurse in charge
   3. Document the observed change
   4. Obtain the other vital signs

5. The client tells the nurse about problems with constipation. Which should the nurse teach the client to avoid eating?
   1. Cheese and broccoli
   2. Yogurt and cheese
   3. Broccoli and peas
   4. Peas and yogurt

6. A client who is comatose begins to vomit while lying in bed. In which position should the nurse **immediately** place the client?
   1. Dorsal recumbent
   2. High Fowler
   3. Supine
   4. Lateral

7. The spouse of a client who died a month ago continues to experience intense emotions and reports they are less painful than the previous week. The nurse recognizes this as which type of grief?
   1. Uncomplicated
   2. Chronic
   3. Masked
   4. Anticipatory

8. A nurse is assessing a client who is having difficulty sleeping. Which client response supports the nurse's conclusion that an adequate night's sleep was attained? **Select all that apply.**
1. _____ Awakens only once during the night
2. _____ Has the ability to remember dreams
3. _____ Walks in the hall after breakfast
4. _____ Expresses renewed strength
5. _____ Sleeps 6 hours each night

9. Which of the following actions demonstrate critical thinking skills among nurses? **Select all that apply.**
1. _____ The novice nurse who accepts information from the preceptor that differs from what they learned in school.
2. _____ The experienced nurse who inflates the catheter balloon to check patency before inserting a Foley catheter.
3. _____ The experienced nurse who calls the primary health-care provider to seek clarification on conflicting orders.
4. _____ The novice nurse who calls the primary health-care provider to seek clarification on conflicting orders.
5. _____ The novice nurse who spends more time reviewing the client's medication list before administering medications.
6. _____ The experienced nurse who pauses before assessing a client with chronic pain to reflect on personal bias.

10. A client is admitted to the postanesthesia care unit after abdominal surgery. The client's vital signs are blood pressure, 150/90 mm Hg; pulse, 88 beats per minute and bounding; and respirations, 24 breaths per minute with some crackles. Which response does the nurse conclude that the client is experiencing?
1. Hypoglycemia
2. Hyponatremia
3. Hyperkalemia
4. Hypervolemia

11. A client has left-sided hemiplegia as the result of a brain attack (cerebrovascular accident). While being dressed, the client states in a disgusted tone of voice, "I feel like a 2-year-old. I can't even get dressed by myself." Which is the nurse's **best** response?
1. "It's hard to feel dependent on others."
2. "Most people who have had a stroke feel this way."
3. "It must be terrible not being able to move your arm."
4. "You are feeling down today, but things will get better."

12. A newly admitted client reports not having had a good bowel movement in 10 days. Which question should the nurse ask the client to identify a possible fecal impaction? **Select all that apply.**
1. _____ "Do you find yourself straining to have a bowel movement?"
2. _____ "How long has it been since you had a formed stool?"
3. _____ "Have you had small amounts of liquid stool?"
4. _____ "Do you notice a bad odor to your breath?"
5. _____ "Have you been eating food with fiber?"
6. _____ "Are you having any vomiting?"

13. A client is receiving droplet precautions. Which is an effective way to reduce the transmission of microorganisms to or from this client? **Select all that apply.**
1. _____ Placing a surgical mask on the client during transport outside the room
2. _____ Wearing a respirator mask when entering the room
3. _____ Having the client wash the hands after eating
4. _____ Wearing gloves when removing a food tray
5. _____ Using disposable dishes and utensils

14. The nurse is caring for a client who is actively dying. Their spouse states, "Please, please God let them stay a little longer." This statement represents which stage of grief according to Kübler-Ross?
1. Denial
2. Anger
3. Bargaining
4. Depression

15. The nurse is caring for five clients in a medical-surgical nursing unit. Which of the following clients most likely require contact precautions? **Select all that apply.**
1. The client awaiting blood culture results for suspected MRSA infection
2. The client with a fever 2 days postoperative after a hip replacement
3. The client with a history of acute lymphocytic leukemia in childhood
4. The client due for a metronidazole IVPB infusion to manage severe diarrhea
5. The client on antiretroviral therapy for an HIV infection with an undetectable viral load

16. The nurse is caring for a client diagnosed with COVID-19. This client is placed under droplet precautions to prevent the spread of this virus. The client's family member asks why the nurses need to wash their hands after removing their PPE. The nurse's response is based on which principle?
1. Hand washing is a priority to protect nurses from infection.
2. Nurses are in the habit of always washing their hands.
3. COVID-19 is spread by direct person-to-person contact only.
4. Droplet precautions are used in addition to standard precautions.

17. A bedbound older adult has a stage I pressure ulcer in the sacral area. In which position should the nurse place the client to relieve pressure and promote circulation to the sacral area? **Select all that apply.**
1. _____ Dorsal recumbent
2. _____ Semi-Fowler
3. _____ Lateral
4. _____ Supine
5. _____ Semi-prone

18. The nurse is triaging a client in the emergency department who reports headache, nausea, vomiting, and abdominal pain. The client reports that they have taken the following over-the-counter medications to manage their symptoms in the last 24 hours:
- Nyquil® (650 mg acetaminophen, 20 mg dextromethorphan, 12.5 mg doxylamine succinate) × 2 doses
- Dayquil® (325 mg acetaminophen, 10 mg dextromethorphan, 200 mg guaifenesin, 5 mg phenylephrine) × 4 doses
- Excedrin® (500 mg acetaminophen, 500 mg aspirin, 130 mg caffeine) × 2 doses

What is the total amount of acetaminophen that this client ingested in the past 24 hours?

Record your answer using a whole number.

Answer: _______________ **mg**

19. The linen under the buttocks of a client who has an indwelling urinary retention (Foley) is found wet with urine. The nurse determines that the catheter is patent and immediately places a waterproof pad under the client's buttocks. Which should the nurse do **next?**
1. Provide perineal care
2. Insert a larger-size catheter
3. Change all the linen on the bed
4. Remove the indwelling urinary catheter

20. The nurse is reviewing the nurse's note from the previous shift in the electronic health record of a client. Which information from this note indicates that personal bias influenced this nurse's pain assessment?
1. Client reports 8/10 pain in lower back.
2. PRN IV morphine administered, per order.
3. Client reports moderate improvement in pain 15 minutes after IV morphine administered.
4. Client overusing call bell to report pain.

21. The nurse enters a client's room and observes the client depicted in the photograph. What should the nurse do **first?**
1. Put shoes on the client's feet and position them on the floor
2. Position pillows under the client's arms and behind the back
3. Drape a sheet under the client on the wheelchair and another over the client's legs
4. Ensure that the wheels of the wheelchair are locked and that a call bell is within the client's reach

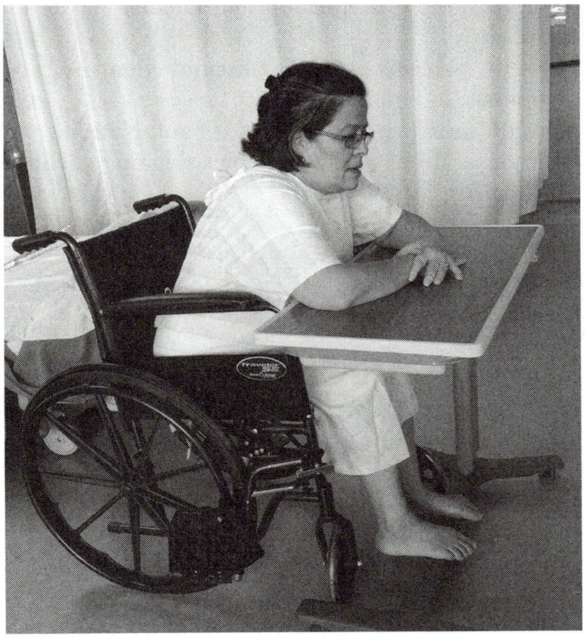

22. The nurse is caring for a client who is in a coma because of a traumatic brain injury. Which should the nurse do when providing oral hygiene for this client? **Select all that apply.**
1. _____ Place a padded tongue blade between the client's teeth before starting oral care
2. _____ Use glycerin and lemon swabs to cleanse the client's mouth
3. _____ Keep a suction device at the bedside during the procedure
4. _____ Apply petroleum jelly to the client's tongue and lips
5. _____ Position the client in the dorsal recumbent position
6. _____ Explain to the client what will be done

23. The nurse is operating a booth at an annual health fair offered for adults over the age of 65. When talking to members of this community, the nurse recognizes that which of the following clients is experiencing a physiological change that is not a normal part of aging?
1. "It takes longer, but I'm still getting dressed and looking sharp every day."
2. "If I don't carry hard candies and peppermints, my mouth is dry."
3. "I have always loved to read, and now I need snazzy reading glasses to do it!"
4. "My daughter has to help me button my blouses because I can't feel them with my fingertips."

24. A pediatric client is receiving valproic acid to treat seizures. The therapeutic range for this medication is 50 to 100 mcg/mL. What can the nurse conclude if the client's current serum drug level is 125 mcg/mL?

1. The drug dose is appropriate.
2. The drug dose is subtherapeutic.
3. The client's next dose should be given over a longer period of time.
4. The drug dose should be adjusted.

25. A 1000-mL daily fluid restriction is prescribed for a client with kidney failure. Which should the nurse do? **Select all that apply.**

1. _____ Provide fluids that the client likes
2. _____ Eliminate liquids between mealtimes
3. _____ Indicate the need for clear liquids in the client's plan of care
4. _____ Divide the fluids by three and give the resulting amount every 8 hours
5. _____ Give proportionally more fluids during the daytime hours than during the night

26. The nurse receives a bedside shift report on four clients. Which finding requires **immediate** intervention?

1. Rattling sounds in the pharynx of an unconscious client
2. Expectorating copious amounts of mucus
3. Anxiety related to the anticipation of pain with ambulation
4. Twelve unlabored respirations per minute by a sleeping client

27. Which action by a nurse **supports** a client's right to privacy? **Select all that apply.**

1. _____ Leaving a crying client alone
2. _____ Addressing a client by the last name
3. _____ Closing the door when interviewing the client
4. _____ Positioning a bath blanket over the client during a bath
5. _____ Pulling a curtain closed when changing a sterile dressing

28. Identify the range of motion being performed in the following illustration.

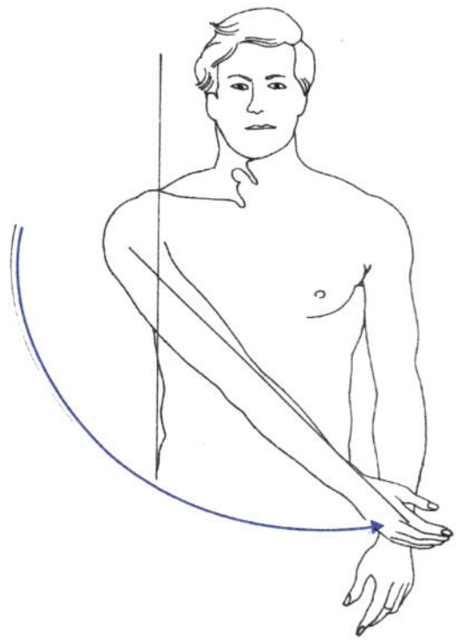

1. Flexion
2. Inversion
3. Adduction
4. Circumduction

29. Which should the nurse do when washing the genitals of an uncircumcised client? **Select all that apply.**

1. _____ Wash the head of the penis with a circular motion from the meatus outward
2. _____ Retract the foreskin before washing the head of the penis
3. _____ Wash down the shaft of the penis toward the meatus
4. _____ Use a rubbing motion to remove debris effectively
5. _____ Employ a light touch throughout the procedure

30. An older adult who received 4 weeks of rehabilitation after a brain attack (cerebrovascular accident, stroke) and has mild left-sided hemiparesis is preparing for discharge to a daughter's home. Which recommendation concerning safety in the home should the nurse discuss with the client and daughter? **Select all that apply.**
1. _____ Mount safety bars around the toilet.
2. _____ Position a shower chair in the shower.
3. _____ Install a higher toilet seat in the bathroom.
4. _____ Limit scatter rugs to those with a rubber backing.
5. _____ Use a walker without wheels for support when ambulating.

31. Which piece of information documented in the clinical record of an adult client should the nurse consider problematic?
1. Temperature: 99.2°F
2. Potassium: 3.0 mEq/L
3. Pulse: 62 beats per minute
4. Ibuprofen 200 mg, PO, every 4 hours for joint pain

CLIENT'S CLINICAL RECORD

Laboratory Results
Calcium: 5.4 mEq/L
Sodium: 137 mEq/L
Potassium: 3.0 mEq/L

Physical Assessment
Temperature (oral): 99.2°F
Pulse: 62 beats per minute
Respirations: 20 breaths per minute
Blood pressure: 110/76 mm Hg

Medication Reconciliation Form
Ibuprofen 200 mg, PO, every 4 hours for joint pain
Digoxin 0.125 mg, PO, daily

32. The nurse administers an antiemetic to a client. A **decrease** in which client response indicates to the nurse that the client is experiencing a therapeutic response?
1. Nausea and anxiety
2. Vomiting and nausea
3. Coughing and anxiety
4. Vomiting and coughing

33. Daily weights are prescribed for the purpose of evaluating a client's fluid loss or gain. When should the client be weighed by the nurse?
1. Twice a day
2. One hour before meals
3. At the same time each day
4. Before urination in the morning

34. The nurse identifies reactive hyperemia over a client's bony prominence. Which is the cause of this response?
1. Applying a warm soak
2. Using the effleurage technique when doing a back rub
3. Pulling the client up in bed without using a pull sheet
4. Turning a client who was in one position for several hours

35. The nurse is assessing a variety of clients with respiratory problems. Which client response should cause the **most** concern?
  1. Inspiratory stridor
  2. Pleural friction rub
  3. Expiratory wheezing
  4. Nonproductive cough

36. After working diligently for 4 years, a nursing student completes a BSN from an accredited nursing program. This student nurse refers to which entity that authorizes licensure in the United States?
  1. Nurse Licensure Compact
  2. Nurse Practice Acts
  3. Accreditation Commission for Education in Nursing
  4. American Nurses Association

37. The primary nurse is responsible for a group of clients. Which client should the nurse attend to before the others?
  1. A client who is waiting to be escorted to the lobby after being discharged
  2. A client admitted for hypertension who wants pain medication for a headache
  3. A client who got dizzy when the nursing assistant was transferring the client from a wheelchair to the bed
  4. A client who is anxious to have an IV line removed after being informed by the primary health-care provider that it can be discontinued

38. The nurse is caring for a client who is diagnosed with hypernatremia caused by excessive watery diarrhea. For which additional clinical indicator should the nurse assess the client? **Select all that apply.**
  1. _____ Muscle twitches
  2. _____ Tachycardia
  3. _____ Confusion
  4. _____ Agitation
  5. _____ Thirst

39. Which action is associated with the correct administration of medication delivered by the Z-track method? **Select all that apply.**
  1. _____ Using a special syringe designed for Z-track injections
  2. _____ Pulling laterally and downward on the skin before inserting the needle
  3. _____ Giving the injection in the muscle on the anterior lateral aspect of the thigh
  4. _____ Waiting 5 to 10 seconds after instilling the solution before removing the needle
  5. _____ Inserting the needle in a separate spot for each dose on a Z-shaped grid on the abdomen

40. The nurse is caring for a client with a hearing deficit. Which is the **most** significant intervention to ensure that the client heard what the nurse said?
  1. Speaking clearly
  2. Facing the client
  3. Obtaining feedback
  4. Raising the volume of speech

41. How much fluid should the nurse use when preparing a soapsuds enema to effectively stimulate the bowel of an adult?
  1. 250 mL
  2. 500 mL
  3. 700 mL
  4. 900 mL

42. A nursing assistant informs the nurse that a client's pulse seems irregular. Which should the nurse do **first** to reassess this client's pulse?
1. Take it for a full minute
2. Use two different sites
3. Employ a Doppler probe
4. Obtain it at the carotid artery

43. The nurse is recording fluid intake for a postoperative client. The client has consumed one 4-ounce container of Italian ice, half of an 8-ounce container of flavored gelatin, and 150 mL of ginger ale. How many milliliters of fluid should the nurse document on the intake section of the client's Intake and Output Sheet? **Record your answer using a whole number.**

Answer: ________________ **mL**

44. The nurse is teaching oral care to a client with a history of gingivitis and dental plaque. Which should the nurse teach the client to do to prevent dental plaque?
1. Rinse the mouth with diluted hydrogen peroxide.
2. Have the teeth cleaned by a licensed hygienist once a year.
3. Brush the biting surface of the teeth using a forward and backward motion.
4. Vibrate the toothbrush holding it at an angle where the teeth meet the gums.

45. The nurse reviews a client's admission note, laboratory findings, and vital signs. The nurse's assessment should focus on which of the following systems?
1. Hematological
2. Cardiac
3. Gastrointestinal
4. Respiratory

CLIENT'S CLINICAL RECORD

Admission Note

A female client was admitted to the hospital directly after reporting severe stabbing abdominal pain during a primary health-care visit. The client has a history of diverticulosis and rates the pain 8 out of 10. The client received pain medication at the primary health-care provider's office 60 minutes before admission.

VITAL SIGNS

Blood pressure: 145/90 mm Hg
Pulse: 110 beats/min, regular rhythm
Respirations: 24 breaths/min; rapid, unlabored
Temperature: 100.6°F

LABORATORY FINDINGS

Hb: 10 g/dL
Hct: 36%
WBC: 16,000 cells/mcL

46. Which action associated with restraint use can the nurse delegate to a nursing assistant? **Select all that apply.**
1. _____ Determination of a client's need for a restraint
2. _____ Evaluation of a client's response to restraint use
3. _____ Selection of the appropriate type of restraint to meet a client's needs
4. _____ Supervision of the client for a short period of time after the restraints are removed
5. _____ Performance of range-of-motion exercises to a client's joints when restraints are off

47. The nurse is caring for an adult female client who experiences incontinence at approximately 0100 every night. Which of the following are appropriate interventions to manage incontinence in this client? **Select all that apply.**
1. Ask, "Have you noticed a strong urge to void?"
2. Offer toileting at approximately 0030
3. Request an order to insert a Foley catheter
4. Teach the client exercises to strengthen pelvic floor muscles
5. Avoid using a bedside commode to encourage ambulation

48. The nurse is implementing tracheal suctioning for an adult. Which should the nurse do? **Select all that apply.**
1. _____ Suction the trachea before the oropharyngeal area
2. _____ Rotate the catheter while inserting it into the trachea
3. _____ Apply intermittent suction during removal of the catheter
4. _____ Use wall suction with a pressure setting below 90 mm Hg
5. _____ Lubricate the catheter with sterile normal saline before its insertion

49. A boy with hypospadias is born to a couple who practice a religion that celebrates ritual circumcision. When the parents are told about the baby's birth anomaly, the mother begins to cry and the father asks whether the child will be able to be circumcised in 8 days. The nurse understands that the foreskin is used in the reconstruction of the penis. Which of the following statements should the nurse **support?**
1. Circumcision is not appropriate for this infant at this time.
2. Even without a circumcision, the baby can be raised in the religious faith of the parents.
3. The parents must decide which is more important, surgical reconstruction or the religious circumcision ceremony.
4. It may be possible for the ritual circumciser to remove just a little of the foreskin without jeopardizing future reconstruction.

50. A client has dysphagia because of a stroke (brain attack). Which should the nurse do when feeding this client? **Select all that apply.**
1. _____ Insert food on the strong side of the client's mouth
2. _____ Provide small amounts of food with each forkful
3. _____ Offer fluids to assist with swallowing
4. _____ Allow adequate time between bites
5. _____ Place in a high Fowler position

51. Medicated eye drops are prescribed for a client. Place the following steps in the order in which they should be implemented after donning clean gloves.
1. Apply gentle pressure over the inner canthus.
2. Release the lower lid and instruct the client to close the eyes gently.
3. Tilt the client's head slightly back and toward the eye being medicated.
4. Clean the eyelid and lashes with sterile normal saline–soaked cotton balls from the inner to the outer canthus.
5. Place a finger just below the lower eyelashes and exert gentle downward pressure over the bony prominence of the cheek.
6. Hold the dropper close to the eye without touching the eye, and administer the prescribed number of drops so they fall into the conjunctival sac.

Answer: _______________

52. The nurse is preparing to discharge a client who has been diagnosed with hypertension. The client states that they would like to lose weight and eat healthier and asks for a diet recommendation. Which of the following diets is most appropriate for this client?
1. Ketogenic
2. Atkins
3. DASH
4. Vegan

53. An intradermal injection is prescribed for a client to assess for the presence of an allergy. Which nursing action is related to an intradermal injection? **Select all that apply.**
1. _____ Use a 1-mL syringe
2. _____ Select a 26-gauge needle
3. _____ Choose a 1-inch needle length
4. _____ Aspirate the syringe after needle insertion
5. _____ Stretch the skin over the site before insertion of the solution

54. The nurse is driving home from the hospital after a 12-hour shift. The nurse witnesses a roll-over vehicle crash and pulls their car over to help. The nurse knows which of the following protects them in this situation?
1. Mandatory Reporting
2. Good Samaritan Laws
3. Nurse Practice Acts
4. Nursing Code of Ethics

55. A client who was in an automobile collision is at risk for internal hemorrhage. For which sign should the nurse monitor this client? **Select all that apply.**
1. _____ Increasing abdominal girth
2. _____ Decreased respiratory rate
3. _____ Thready pulse
4. _____ Hypotension
5. _____ Warm skin
6. _____ Bradypnea

56. The nurse is transferring a client from the bed to a chair and sits the client on the side of the bed for several minutes. Which is the **primary** rationale for this action?
1. Provides the heart rate time to return to the expected range
2. Enables the body to adapt to a drop in blood pressure
3. Permits the client to take several deep breaths
4. Allows the client to regain energy expended

57. Sublingual nitroglycerin is prescribed for a client with the diagnosis of angina pectoris (chest pain related to transient cardiac ischemia). Which should the nurse teach the client about this medication?
1. "Take only 1 dose of nitroglycerin. If the pain continues, get immediate help."
2. "Double the dose of nitroglycerin 5 minutes after the first dose if there is no pain relief."
3. "Take 1 dose of nitroglycerin every 3 minutes as often as necessary until the pain is relieved."
4. "Repeat the dose of nitroglycerin every 5 minutes for 3 doses. If pain is unrelieved, immediately call 911."

58. The nurse is auscultating respirations in a client preparing to discharge after an emergency department visit for an ankle sprain. The nurse notes gurgling sounds until the client coughs. What term should the nurse use to document this finding?
1. Rhonchi
2. Wheezes
3. Crackles
4. Stridor

59. According to Jean Watson, the client with terminal illness with both a high level of functioning and coping can be described as which of the following?
1. Grieving
2. Uncertain
3. Healthy
4. Denying

60. A nurse is withdrawing liquid medication from an ampule. Place the following steps in the order in which they should be implemented.
1. Use a filtered needle.
2. Draw up the desired volume of solution.
3. Shake the ampule with a rapid snap of the wrist.
4. Place an ampule opener over the neck of the ampule.
5. Snap the head of the ampule away from the caregiver.
6. Replace the filtered needle with an appropriate needle.

Answer: ________________

61. The nurse is caring for five clients with hypertension. The nurse knows that beta blockers are not appropriate for which of the following clients? **Select all that apply.**
1. _____ 61-year-old male with poorly controlled type 2 diabetes
2. _____ 62-year-old female with family history of hypertension
3. _____ 36-year-old female with a positive pregnancy test
4. _____ 37-year-old female with bradycardia
5. _____ 52-year-old male with a history of myocardial infarction

62. A medication that is to be administered via the buccal route is prescribed for a client. Which illustration reflects the medication being administered via the buccal route?

1. 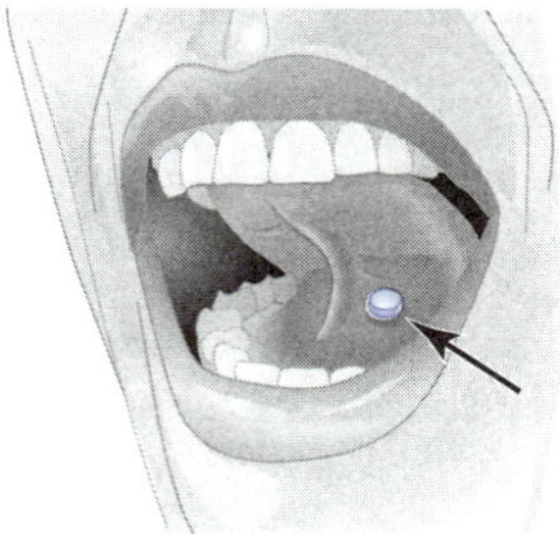

2. 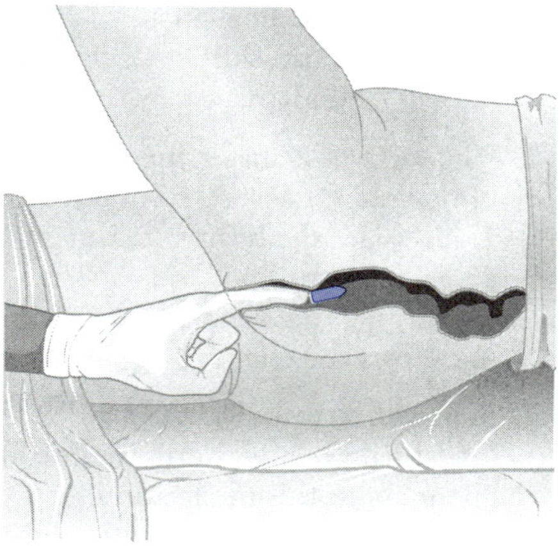

3. 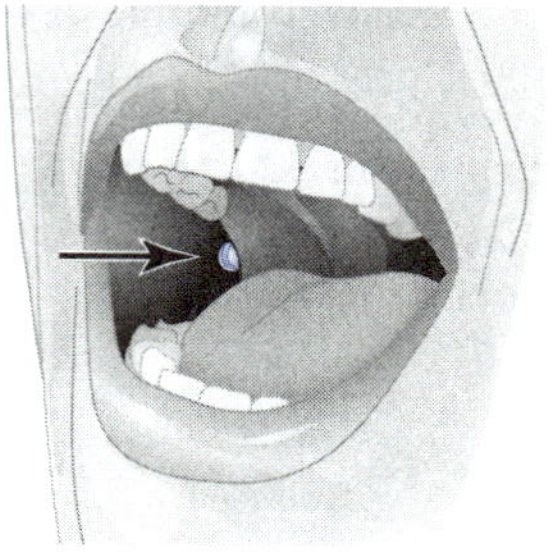

4. 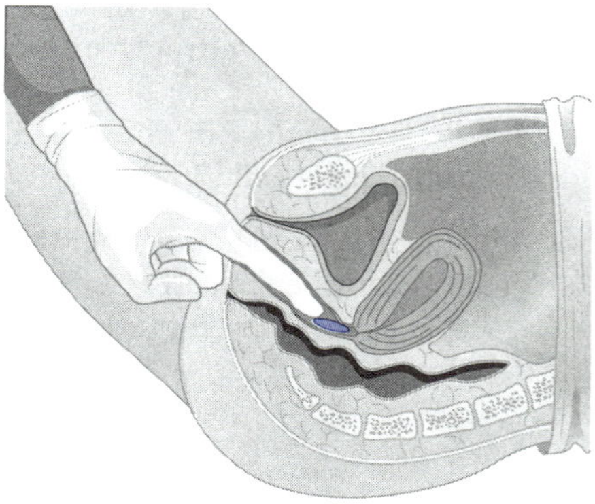

63. The nurse recognizes that which of the following clients is at increased risk for constipation? **Select all that apply.**
1. _____ An 84-year-old client who eats a low-fiber diet
2. _____ A 54-year-old client who eats a high-fiber diet
3. _____ A 60-year-old client who consumes 3.5 liters of fluids daily
4. _____ A 62-year-old client with NPO orders
5. _____ A 24-year-old client who jogs every morning
6. _____ A 29-year-old client taking opioids to treat pain related to a fractured femur

64. A nurse identifies an excoriated perineal area in a client with diarrhea. Which step of the nursing process has the nurse performed?
1. Analysis
2. Evaluation
3. Assessment
4. Implementation

65. Which must the nurse do first when providing culturally competent care?
1. Learn more about cultural beliefs related to health and illness
2. Provide ethnocentric care
3. Recognize personal beliefs and attitudes
4. Focus on similarities between cultures

66. The nurse is caring for a client admitted to the hospital after a stroke. The nurse explains to the UAP that oral hygiene is important to prevent which of the following in this client?
1. Subsequent stroke
2. Aspiration
3. Blood clots
4. Falls

67. The nurse is planning care to relieve a client's pain. Which nursing intervention is based on the gate control theory of pain relief? **Select all that apply.**
1. _____ Promoting rest
2. _____ Encouraging activity
3. _____ Providing a back rub
4. _____ Playing relaxing music
5. _____ Administering a narcotic

68. The nurse is teaching a preoperative client about active leg exercises. The client asks the nurse why these exercises are necessary. Which **primary** reason for these exercises should the nurse include in a response to the client's question?
1. Promote venous return
2. Prevent muscle atrophy
3. Limit joint contractures
4. Increase muscle strength

69. A client with a large pressure ulcer is being cared for in the home by a spouse. To promote wound healing, the nurse teaches the spouse about foods high in vitamin C. Which food selected by the spouse indicates that the teaching has been understood? **Select all that apply.**
1. _____ Brussels sprouts
2. _____ Yellow peppers
3. _____ Fresh broccoli
4. _____ Tomato juice
5. _____ Orange juice

70. Rosuvastatin (Crestor®) 10 mg PO once daily is prescribed for a client. Which should the nurse teach the client in relation to this lipid-lowering drug? **Select all that apply.**
1. _____ Follow a low-cholesterol diet.
2. _____ Avoid drinking grapefruit juice.
3. _____ Ingest this medication with food.
4. _____ Take this medication in the evening.
5. _____ Call the clinic if you experience muscle weakness.

71. The nurse is assessing a client's urinary status. Which clinical manifestation indicates urinary retention? **Select all that apply.**
   1. _____ Absence of urine
   2. _____ Wet undergarments
   3. _____ Distended suprapubic area
   4. _____ Burning sensation when voiding
   5. _____ Sudden, overwhelming urge to void

72. The nurse is caring for five clients in a medical-surgical nursing unit. The nurse classifies which of the following orders as fluid replacement? **Select all that apply.**
   1. _____ 0.9% Normal Saline at KVO
   2. _____ PO fluids 30 mL/kg/day
   3. _____ 0.45% NaCl to improve renal function
   4. _____ 5% dextrose in NaCl + potassium in the client with diarrhea
   5. _____ 0.9% Normal Saline bolus to manage hypotension

73. The nurse is repositioning an unconscious client. The client's spouse asks why so much care is taken to smooth the wrinkles in the bed sheets. What is the nurse's best explanation?
   1. "It's just a habit."
   2. "The air mattress isn't as effective when the sheets are wrinkled."
   3. "Smooth sheets are less likely to cause skin breakdown."
   4. "Smoothing wrinkles makes it easier to use the sheet to reposition the client."

74. The nurse is assessing a client for an emotional response to stress. For which response should the nurse monitor the client? **Select all that apply.**
   1. _____ Headache
   2. _____ Irritability
   3. _____ Heartburn
   4. _____ Depression
   5. _____ Hypertension

75. The nurse is teaching a client to perform a breast self-examination. The nurse understands that there are three patterns for breast examination. Which pattern should the nurse teach the client because it is considered **most** effective?

1. 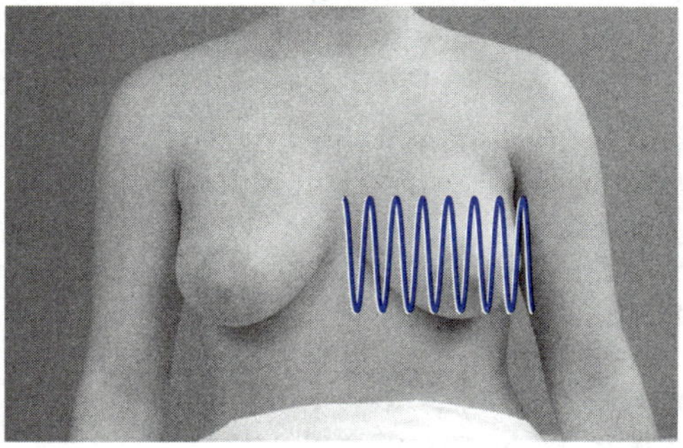

2. 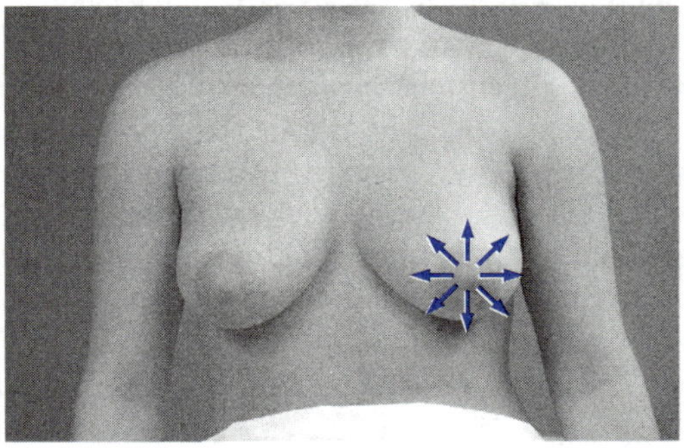

3. 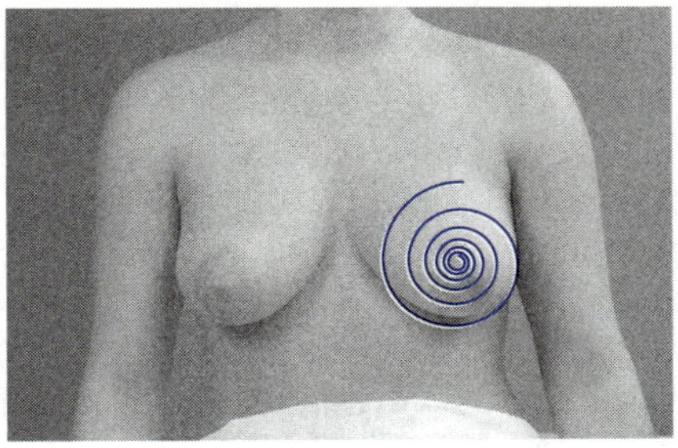

76. Which statement indicates that a client understands the teaching about diaphragmatic breathing? **Select all that apply.**

1. _____ "I should feel my abdomen rise on inspiration."
2. _____ "I should take a slow, deep breath through my nose."
3. _____ "I should raise my shoulders and chest when I inhale."
4. _____ "I should hold my breath for several seconds at the height of inspiration."
5. _____ "I should use my hands to put pressure against the abdomen when I inhale."

77. An obese client who has a history of heart failure is prescribed metoprolol (Lopressor®) 50 mg PO twice a day. Which should the nurse teach the client regarding self-administration of this antihypertensive? **Select all that apply.**

1. _____ Weigh yourself twice a week.
2. _____ Check your pulse before taking the medication.
3. _____ Stop taking the medication when you feel better.
4. _____ Take the medication at the same times every day.
5. _____ Move from a sitting to a standing position slowly.
6. _____ Monitor your blood pressure before taking each dose of the medication.

78. The nurse is caring for the client reporting nausea and stating, "I think I'm going to puke." Which of the following is an appropriate intervention to reduce nausea?
1. Apply pleasant-smelling perfume before caring for the client
2. Limit fluid intake to reduce volume of stomach contents
3. Encourage larger meals to replace lost nutrients
4. Keep an emesis basin nearby so the client can easily access it

79. The nurse must obtain a urine specimen from an indwelling urinary catheter. The nurse identifies the client, explains the procedure, and clamps the drainage tubing below the port 20 minutes before performing the procedure. The nurse then washes the hands and collects the necessary equipment. Place the following steps in the order in which they should be performed.
1. Remove the clamp and allow urine to drain.
2. Provide for client privacy and expose the port.
3. Don gloves and wipe the port with an alcohol swab.
4. Remove the syringe and wipe the port with an alcohol swab.
5. Insert the syringe and aspirate a minimum of five mL of urine.
6. Transfer urine into a sterile specimen cup and discard the syringe and gloves into appropriate containers.

Answer: ______________

80. The nurse is administering heparin via the intravenous (IV) route to a client with a deep vein thrombosis. Which is **most** important for the nurse to have readily available on the unit when a client is receiving IV heparin?
1. Potassium chloride
2. Protamine sulfate
3. Prothrombin
4. Plasma

81. Which nursing action interferes with the chain of infection at the level of transmission? **Select all that apply.**
1. _____ Covering the nose when sneezing
2. _____ Placing used linen into a linen hamper
3. _____ Repositioning a client every 2 hours
4. _____ Limiting talking when performing a sterile procedure
5. _____ Applying a sterile dressing over a contaminated wound

82. The nurse is supervising the activities of a nursing assistant. Which action observed by the nurse reflects inappropriate body mechanics on the part of the nursing assistant? **Select all that apply.**
1. _____ Standing on a client's weak side when assisting with ambulation
2. _____ Raising the head of the bed before moving a client up in bed
3. _____ Flexing the knees when lifting an object from the floor
4. _____ Placing the feet apart when transferring a client
5. _____ Bending from the waist when making a bed

83. Which action by a client should the nurse report to the primary health-care provider, because the client may need a restraint?
1. Climbing off the end of the bed at night
2. Pulling out an intravenous catheter
3. Wandering into other rooms
4. Picking at lint on bed linens

84. The nurse is caring for a client who is on intake and output. During the 11 to 7 shift, the client voids a total of 700 mL of dark yellow urine and vomits 200 mL of greenish-yellow fluid at 0300 hr and 150 mL of greenish-yellow fluid at 0600 hr. Place an X where the nurse should record the total amount the client vomited during the 11 to 7 shift.

Intake and Output

INTAKE	11-7	7-3	3-11	24 HR	11-
Oral/Tube					
Blood/Plasma					
I.V.					
Other					
Other					
TOTAL					
OUTPUT	**11-7**	**7-3**	**3-11**	**24 HR**	**11-**
Liquid Stool					
Urine					
G.I. Suction					
Emesis					
Bowel Movement					
Other					
TOTAL					
INITIALS					

85. The nurse is planning care for an older adult living with dementia. The frequency of falls for clients like this one increases during which time?
1. At night
2. Before meals
3. Immediately postoperative
4. During visiting hours

86. The nurse instills two medicated drops into a client's ear as prescribed. Place an X over the site the nurse should compress to help disperse the medication throughout the external auditory canal.

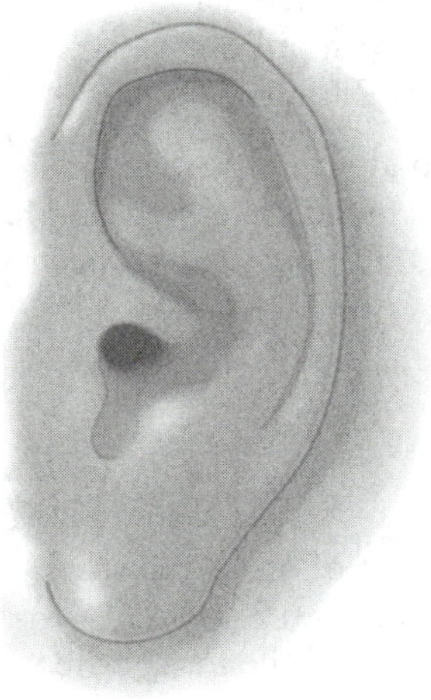

87. The client consumes a total of 2000 calories in a 24-hour period. The client consumed 60 grams of fat, 182 grams of protein, and 183 grams of carbohydrates. What percentage of calories came from fat? **Record your answer using a whole number.**

Answer: ________________%

88. The nurse just received a bedside shift report on four clients. Place the four clients in order from highest to lowest priority.
1. A 25-year-old alert male who returned from the postanesthesia care unit 2 hours ago after knee surgery and is receiving continuous passive range-of-motion exercises with the physical therapist at the bedside
2. A 60-year-old female with a new temporary colostomy who arranged for her spouse to attend a teaching session about how to care for the colostomy
3. A 75-year-old female client with a history of dementia admitted following a fall and rubbing their right hip
4. A 65-year-old male client admitted following an assault and requesting pain medication to relieve epigastric pain after a meal

Answer: ______________

89. Which action **supports** a principle of surgical asepsis? **Select all that apply.**
1. _____ Recapping a syringe after withdrawing medication from a vial
2. _____ Holding sterile gloved hands below the waist during a sterile procedure
3. _____ Holding a wet sterile gauze with sterile forceps while the handle is higher than the tip
4. _____ Failing to wipe the rubber port with alcohol the first time a multiple-dose vial is accessed
5. _____ Pouring normal saline on gauze that is lying in its opened sterile paper wrapper while on an overbed table

90. Which should the nurse assess to evaluate peripheral circulation in the lower extremities of a client? **Select all that apply.**
1. _____ Pedal pulses
2. _____ Blood pressure
3. _____ Extent of hair on the feet
4. _____ Speed of capillary refill in the toes
5. _____ Presence of discomfort in the legs when walking

91. A client who had a brain attack (stroke, cerebrovascular accident) has hemiparesis. Which should the nurse do to **best** prevent this client from developing contractures?
1. Teach the client to perform range-of-motion exercises
2. Transfer the client to a chair 2 times a day
3. Support the client's joints with pillows
4. Reposition the client every 2 hours

92. The nurse is caring for a female client who was diagnosed with a urinary tract infection. The client reports feeling nauseous and has an episode of emesis. The nurse notes a temperature of 102.1°F. The nurse suspects that these symptoms are due to which of the following?
1. *E. coli* infection
2. Kidney infection
3. Gastrointestinal infection
4. Respiratory infection

93. A confused client is incontinent of urine and stool. Which should the nurse do to **best** prevent skin breakdown in this client?
1. Instruct the client to always call the nurse when soiled
2. Check for soiling frequently and wash if necessary
3. Place sheepskin on the bed and apply a diaper
4. Reposition the client frequently

94. A client has a prescription for an opioid every 4 hours prn for pain after abdominal surgery. Which client outcome indicates that the medication is effective?
1. Is able to cough with a tolerable level of discomfort
2. Is able to maintain the semi-Fowler position
3. Requests another tablet in 3 hours
4. Has a decrease in the respiratory rate

95. A school-age child is to be hospitalized for several weeks. Which should the nurse encourage the parents to do to enhance achievement of the developmental task associated with this age group?
1. Have siblings visit several times a week
2. Bring a favorite stuffed animal from home
3. Plan for schoolwork to be brought to the hospital
4. Arrange for the television to be turned on in the room

96. The nurse is caring for a client who has a history of urge incontinence. Which should the nurse do to **best** provide for the elimination needs of this client?
1. Toilet the client every 4 hours
2. Toilet the client as soon as requested
3. Encourage the client to stay near the bathroom
4. Ask the client to limit fluid intake after 6:00 in the evening

97. The nurse is evaluating a client's use of a liquid metered-dose inhaler. Which behavior indicates that the client is using the inhaler appropriately? **Select all that apply.**
1. _____ Holding the breath at the height of inhalation when using the inhaler
2. _____ Shaking the container before pressing down on the inhaler
3. _____ Rinsing the mouth with tap water after using the inhaler
4. _____ Inhaling quickly when pressing down on the inhaler
5. _____ Tilting the head back when using the inhaler

98. Where should the nurse stand when helping a blind client to walk?
1. In front of the client while the client uses the corridor handrail
2. Next to the client while the client holds the nurse's arm
3. In front of the client while providing verbal directions
4. Next to the client while holding the client's elbow

99. A nurse is caring for a client with a nasogastric tube. Which should the nurse do to assess for correct placement of the tube?
1. Auscultate the lungs
2. Place the end of the tube in water
3. Instill a small amount of normal saline
4. Aspirate stomach contents through the tube

100. A client has metastatic lung cancer, and the primary health-care provider discusses the diagnosis and prognosis in detail with the client. After a severe episode of coughing and shortness of breath later in the day, the client says to the nurse, "This is just a cold. I'll be fine once I get over it." Which is the appropriate response by the nurse?
1. "Tell me more about your illness."
2. "It's really not a cold; it's lung cancer."
3. "I understand that you had some bad news this morning."
4. "Remember what you were told about your condition earlier today."

COMPREHENSIVE FINAL BOOK EXAMINATION ANSWERS AND RATIONALES

1\. 1. Emollients hold moisture in the skin, making it supple; they do not prevent bone injury.
2. Weight bearing helps limit bone demineralization, but it will not prevent bone injury.
3. An intake of 2500 mL of fluid daily flushes the kidneys and limits calculi formation, which can occur because of the high level of calcium salts in the urine as a result of demineralization. It does not prevent bone injury.
4. **Bone demineralization (osteoporosis) causes the bones to become weak, brittle, and fragile. Supporting joints when turning or moving limits the stress that may cause a fracture.**
5. **Falls are the leading cause of bone fractures in older adults. Inadequate footwear can contribute to a fall that can cause a bone fracture. Wearing well-fitting, flat, rubber-soled shoes provides support and stability. Also, sneakers are fine as long as they do not have a thick tread that can cause a person to trip and fall.**

TEST-TAKING TIP: The word *demineralization* is the key word in the stem that directs attention to content.

2\. 1. This would be the equivalent of 0.2 mg hydromorphone and result in the administration of an incorrect dose. Additionally, this dose would likely not achieve adequate pain relief in this client.
2. **This is correct. The syringe shown is a 1-mL syringe. The nurse should first calculate the dose: 1 mg is half of 2 mg/mL; therefore, the nurse should administer 0.5 mL of hydromorphone.**
3. This would be the equivalent of 1.6 mg and result in the administration of an incorrect dose.
4. This would be the equivalent of 2 mg hydromorphone and result in the administration of an incorrect dose.

3\. 1. **The client who expresses worry is often experiencing some level of anxiety. Anxiety is a response to the anticipation of danger.**
2. Fear and anxiety produce similar responses. Unlike anxiety, fear is related to a current event rather than a future event. Fear is a cognitive response to a physical or psychological event whereas anxiety is an emotional response to a nonphysical threat.
3. Depression may occur in response to stressors. The client experiencing depression may be tearful. However, anxiety is the more appropriate option in this situation because the client is expressing worry about a future event.
4. Anger is a strong and uncomfortable feeling of displeasure. Based on the information provided, this client is not demonstrating anger.

4\. 1. Notifying the primary health-care provider may be done later; it is not the priority at this time.
2. Reporting the change to the nurse in charge may be done later; it is not the priority at this time.
3. Documenting the observed change may be done later; it is not the priority at this time.
4. **Because of the interrelationships among the circulatory system, the respiratory system, and the basal metabolic rate, all the vital signs should be obtained for an accurate assessment.**

TEST-TAKING TIP: The word *first* in the stem sets a priority. The word *increase* in the stem directs attention to content. Option 1 contains the specific determiner *immediately*. Option 4 is unique. It is the only option that indicates additional assessment. Options 1, 2, and 3 all refer to communicating the event in some way.

5\. 1. Although cheese can contribute to constipation, broccoli facilitates defecation.
2. **Dairy products are low in roughage and lack bulk; they produce too little waste to stimulate the defecation reflex. Low-residue foods move more slowly through the intestinal tract, permitting increased fluid uptake from stool, resulting in hard-formed stools and constipation.**
3. Both broccoli and peas provide bulk that increases peristalsis, which facilitates defecation.
4. Although yogurt contributes to constipation, peas provide bulk (undigested residue), which facilitates fecal elimination.

TEST-TAKING TIP: The word *avoid* in the stem indicates negative polarity. The question is asking what foods should

the client not eat because they can contribute to constipation. The options in this question contain duplicate facts. Four nutrients are presented: cheese, broccoli, yogurt, and peas. If you know that broccoli contains fiber that helps to increase peristalsis, you can eliminate options 1 and 3. If you know that peas contain fiber that helps to increase peristalsis, you can eliminate options 3 and 4. In either event, you have increased your chances of choosing the correct answer to 50%. If you know that cheese is low in roughage, resulting in hard-formed stools and constipation, you can focus on options 1 and 2. If you know that yogurt is low in roughage, you can focus on options 2 and 4. In any event, you have increased your chances of choosing the correct answer to 50%.

6. 1. The dorsal recumbent position is contraindicated because it promotes aspiration by allowing vomitus to flow to the posterior oral pharynx and enter the trachea.
   2. A high Fowler position provides inadequate support for an unconscious client.
   3. The supine position is contraindicated because it promotes aspiration by allowing vomitus to flow to the posterior oral pharynx and enter the trachea.
   4. **The lateral position prevents aspiration because it allows vomitus to drain out of the mouth via gravity.**

TEST-TAKING TIP: The word *immediately* in the stem sets a priority. Options 1 and 3 are equally plausible because both are back-lying positions that promote aspiration of vomitus.

7. 1. Uncomplicated grief is the natural response to loss. The person experiencing uncomplicated grief may display a range of feelings, behaviors, and thoughts related to loss. Emotions are intense shortly after loss and then subside over months to years.
   2. Chronic grief continues for a longer period of time than expected. This interferes with the person's ability to return to normal life.
   3. Masked grief is a maladaptive grieving process. Examples include drinking heavily or intense arguments with others that the person may not recognize as a response to grief.
   4. **Anticipatory grief occurs before the loss occurs. In this situation, the client has already died and the spouse is not experiencing anticipatory grief.**

TEST-TAKING TIP: Option 1 is the only option that does not represent a maladaptive response.

8. 1. Although a client may awaken only once during the night, the length of sleep or the depth of sleep may be insufficient to restore or renew the body.
   2. Remembering dreams is unrelated to adequate sleep.
   3. One cannot assume that a client feels rested just because the client is ambulating. Feeling rested is subjective information that only the client can report.
   4. **Expressing renewed strength after sleeping reflects a restored mind and body and contributes to the conclusion that the client had an adequate night's sleep.**
   5. Sleeping 6 hours may or may not be enough because each person has unique needs as well as a personal biological clock for determining sleeping intervals.

TEST-TAKING TIP: The word *only* in option 1 is a specific determiner. The words *sleep* in the stem and *sleeps* in option 5 are clang associations. Use of the test-taking tip *Identify the clang association* will not help you focus on a potential correct answer in this question. In this question, option 5 is a distractor. More often than not, an option with a clang association is a correct answer, *but not always*.

9. 1. Critical thinking involves approaching problems with intellectual autonomy. This nurse should ask for clarification or look up the information using reputable resources instead of simply accepting what they are told.
   2. This is a practice commonly taught in nursing schools 5 to 10 years ago. An experienced nurse may be unaware of the change in evidence related to this practice. Critical thinking involves understanding that knowledge evolves and a willingness to change as new evidence becomes available.
   3. **Critical thinking involves recognizing the need for more information and seeking clarification when needed. This is a critical thinking skill that can be applied regardless of experience level.**
   4. **Critical thinking involves recognizing the need for more information and seeking clarification when needed. This is a critical thinking skill that can be applied regardless of experience level.**

5. This nurse recognizes the importance of understanding medications and gaps in their own knowledge. This nurse is taking the time to safely administer medications and addressing their individual knowledge gaps.

6. This represents intellectual empathy and fair-mindedness. The nurse who recognizes personal bias and how that bias might influence the way they manage a client is exercising critical thinking skills.

10. 1. Hypoglycemia is indicated by fatigue, dizziness, restlessness, hunger, sweating, palpitations, tremors, nausea, and a capillary blood glucose level less than 70 mg/dL.

2. Hyponatremia is indicated by lethargy, confusion, apprehension, muscle cramps, anorexia, nausea, vomiting, and a serum sodium level less than 135 mEq/L.

3. Hyperkalemia is indicated by muscle weakness, decreased heart rate, irregular pulse, irritability, apathy, confusion, and a serum potassium level more than 5.0 mEq/L.

4. These are signs of excess fluid volume; fluids are administered during surgery to maintain an adequate circulating blood volume. Occasionally, intraoperative IV fluids may be excessive, and this is a complication that must be monitored by the nurse in the postanesthesia care unit.

11. 1. This statement identifies the client's feelings and provides an opportunity for further discussion.

2. This statement is a generalization that may not be true; also, it cuts off communication.

3. This statement focuses on the inability to move rather than feelings of helplessness, dependence, and regression.

4. This statement is false reassurance because the nurse does not know whether things will get better.

TEST-TAKING TIP: The word *best* in the stem sets a priority. The word *most* in option 2 is a specific determiner. Option 4 is false reassurance and denies the client's feelings. Option 1 is client-centered.

12. 1. Clients who are constipated or have a fecal impaction hold their breath and bear down (Valsalva maneuver) while attempting to have a bowel movement. This maneuver increases intraabdominal pressure, which sometimes facilitates the passage of stool. The client should be taught to avoid straining on defecation (Valsalva maneuver) because it can precipitate a cardiac dysrhythmia.

2. There are no formed stools with a fecal impaction. Knowing how long ago the client had a formed stool helps to identify if the client has a fecal impaction.

3. A fecal impaction is an obstruction in the large intestine; peristalsis behind the obstruction initially increases in an attempt to move the mass, causing liquid stool to pass around the area of the impaction.

4. A bad odor to the breath is unrelated to a fecal impaction in the large intestine. A bad odor to the breath may be related to a small bowel obstruction.

5. Although foods with fiber promote intestinal peristalsis, which prevents constipation, this question is not significant at this time.

6. People with a fecal impaction may experience rectal pressure, bloating, and nausea, but rarely do they vomit; nausea and vomiting occur more frequently with small bowel obstructions.

TEST-TAKING TIP: The words *fecal impaction* are key words in the stem that direct attention to content. The words *bowel movement* and fecal in the stem and the word *stool* in options 2 and 3 are obscure clang associations.

13. 1. The client should wear a surgical mask when being transported outside the room for essential tests. The mask will contain respiratory droplets protecting the people exposed to the client.

2. A respirator mask is unnecessary. A respirator mask is used with airborne precautions.

3. The client should be encouraged to wash their hands after eating. The hands may have come in contact with contaminated respiratory secretions. The hands should be washed before eating as well.

4. Gloves will protect the nurse from the client's oral body fluids, a requirement for droplet precautions.

5. **Contaminated disposable articles can be bagged and discarded, which prevents the spread of microorganisms.**

TEST-TAKING TIP: The words *droplet precautions* are key words in the stem that direct attention to content.

14. 1. Denial involves feelings of disbelief. It is not necessarily negative and may give the grieving person time to prepare psychologically.
2. Anger is a response to situations perceived as unfair. It is the second stage of grief according to Kübler-Ross.
3. **This statement represents bargaining according to Kübler-Ross. Bargaining is often with God or a higher power to allow the person to live until a certain period of time.**
4. Depression is the fourth stage of grief, according to Kübler-Ross. It is often evidenced by sadness and the person may be withdrawn. This stage differs from clinical depression.

TEST-TAKING TIP: The word *please* draws attention to content and is associated with bargaining.

15. 1. **Clients awaiting blood cultures for suspected MRSA infection require strict adherence to contact precautions to prevent the spread of this multidrug-resistant organism. It is spread by direct contact between two people or a person and the environment.**
2. Clients with signs of infection following an orthopedic surgery, such as a hip replacement, require standard precautions to prevent the spread of infection.
3. Clients receiving chemotherapy for blood cancers such as leukemia may require reverse isolation to prevent infection. This client has a history of leukemia and is not currently receiving treatment. Therefore, this client requires standard precautions to prevent the spread of infection.
4. **The client receiving metronidazole to manage diarrhea is likely being treated for a *Clostridium difficile* infection. This is an infection that requires contact precautions to prevent the spread of disease. It is spread by direct contact between two people or a person and the environment.**
5. The client receiving antiretroviral therapy for an HIV infection requires standard precautions to prevent the spread of infection. An undetectable viral load means that the antiretroviral therapy is effective and the likelihood of disease transmission is reduced. Clients living with HIV who have a high or detectable viral load also require standard precautions.

16. 1. Hand washing is the most effective way to prevent the spread of disease. It is a priority to protect all people from the spread of disease: health-care workers, clients, caregivers, and family.
2. Although hand washing is a good habit that all nurses should practice, this is not the best answer in this situation. This is an opportunity to educate a family member about preventing the spread of disease.
3. It is recommended that clients with COVID-19 infections are placed on both droplet and contact precautions in addition to standard precautions.
4. **Droplet precautions are used in addition to standard precautions when caring for clients with COVID-19 infections. Standard precautions are used when caring for all clients and include the assumption that all body fluids contain pathogens. Standard precautions require hand washing, appropriate PPE, and safe injection practices.**

TEST-TAKING TIP: The word *only* in option 3 should lead to elimination of that option. The word *COVID-19* in the stem draws attention to content.

17. 1. In the dorsal recumbent position, pressure will still be on the sacrum because it is a back-lying position. The dorsal recumbent position is the supine position with the hips and knees flexed.
2. In the semi-Fowler position, pressure will still be on the sacrum because it is a back-lying position; with the head of the bed elevated, shearing force to the back and sacral areas may occur if the client slides down in bed.
3. **In the left- or right-lateral position, the iliac crest and greater trochanter, not the sacrum, bear the body's weight.**
4. In the supine position, pressure will still be on the sacrum because it is a back-lying position.
5. **In the left or right semi-prone position, the anterior iliac crest, not the sacrum, bears the body's weight.**

18. Answer: 3600 mg
This problem requires addition.

650 × 2 = 1300

325 × 4 = 1300

500 × 2 = 1000

1300 + 1300 + 1000 = 3600 mg

The maximum recommended dose for an adult is 4000 mg in 24 hours. The maximum dose does not indicate the safe dose for everyone. Nausea, vomiting, and abdominal pain are signs associated with acetaminophen overdose.

19. 1. Providing perineal care should eventually be done, but it is not the priority.
2. Urine is leaking around the urinary retention catheter, and a larger-size catheter is required. However, this is not the priority intervention. Although inserting a urinary catheter is a dependent function of the nurse, the selection of the size of the urinary catheter is an independent function of the nurse.
3. Changing the linen should eventually be done, but it is not the priority. Also, it may not be necessary to change the top linen.
4. Once it is determined that urine is leaking around the indwelling urinary catheter and that the catheter is patent, the catheter should be removed and replaced with a larger-size catheter.

TEST-TAKING TIP: The word *next* in the stem sets a priority. The word *catheter* in the stem and in options 2 and 4 is a clang association. The word *all* in option 3 is a specific determiner.

20. 1. This statement is objective and captures appropriate assessments related to pain.
2. This statement is objective and captures an appropriate intervention to manage pain.
3. This statement is objective and captures appropriate follow-up assessment after a pain management intervention.
4. This statement is not client-centered. The client experiencing pain should not be labeled as a client who is overusing the call bell. This statement indicates that the nurse does not believe the client's reports of pain. A more appropriate approach is to document objectively, reassess the pain management strategies for this client, and adjust the pain management plan to improve this client's experience.

21. 1. These interventions are not the first things that the nurse should do in this scenario. Although the nurse should place shoes on the client's feet, the feet should be positioned on the footrests of the wheelchair. Shoes protect feet from microbiological and physical injury. Placing the feet on the footrests of the wheelchair reduces the risk of the client accidently pushing the overbed table forward with the feet. This may alter the client's balance, which could result in the client falling out of the wheelchair.
2. Although the nurse should position pillows under the client's arms and behind the client's back for comfort, this is not the first thing the nurse should do in this scenario.
3. Although both of these interventions should be done, they are not the priority in this scenario. Draping a sheet under the client inserts a barrier between the wheelchair and the client that provides comfort and microbiological safety. Placing a sheet over the client's legs provides privacy and reduces the risk of chilling.
4. Locking the wheels of the wheelchair and securing a call bell within reach are the priority actions because they meet the safety and security needs of the client. Although overbed tables generally have locks on the wheels, they are not the most stable surface; the client's feet should be on the footrests of the wheelchair because this is the safest way to protect the feet. A call bell provides a way for the client to summon the nurse.

TEST-TAKING TIP: The word *first* in the stem sets a priority.

22. 1. Placing a padded tongue blade between the teeth before beginning will keep the mouth open throughout the procedure. Clients in a coma tend to clench the teeth when something is placed in the mouth, thus preventing access to the teeth and oral cavity during mouth care.
2. Glycerin and lemon swabs should not be used. Glycerin may moisten the oral membranes, but it will not clean them. Lemon will cause drying of the mucous membranes.
3. A suction device may be necessary during and/or after the procedure if

oral secretions and the rinsing solution do not exit the oral cavity entirely.
4. A petroleum-based lubricant is for external, not internal, use.
5. The dorsal recumbent position promotes aspiration and is contraindicated during the provision of mouth care. A side-lying position is appropriate.
6. **Hearing is the last sense to deteriorate, and the client may hear the nurse. All clients have a right to know what will be done and why.**

TEST-TAKING TIP: Option 6 is unique because it is the only option that addresses the client's emotional needs and is client-centered. The word *oral* in the stem and in option 1 is a clang association.

23. 1. As the body ages, muscle strength, body mass, and joint mobility decrease. Taking more time is an appropriate adaptation to these changes, and this client continues their routine without interference with ADLs.
2. Gastrointestinal changes that occur with aging include decreased saliva and gastric acid production and decreased gastrointestinal motility. Hard candies and peppermints are a strategy to promote salivation and prevent dry mouth. The nurse should promote the use of sugar-free candies.
3. As the body ages, changes in the senses occur, including a decline in visual acuity. This client is expressing a positive adaptation to these changes. The nurse should promote regular eye examinations and recognize that this change does not prevent this client from enjoying a hobby.
4. **This client is experiencing neuropathy. Although nerve changes occur with aging, the inability to independently perform ADLs should alert the nurse to identify causes of neuropathy in this client.**

TEST-TAKING TIP: Option 3 is unique. Option 3 is the only option that has a positive connotation (healthy). Options 1, 2, and 4 have negative connotations (frail, tired, and dependent).

24. 1. An appropriate therapeutic dose will have a serum level between 50 and 100 mcg/mL for this client.
2. A subtherapeutic dose will have a serum level below 50 mcg/mL for this client.
3. The size of the dose, not the length of time it is administered, affects the serum level of the drug.
4. **A serum level of 125 mcg/mL is higher than the therapeutic range. The client requires further assessment, including drug adherence and factors that influence the serum drug level. The drug dose should be adjusted to ensure a safe and therapeutic range is maintained.**

25. 1. **Fluid preferences should be provided. This individualizes care and makes the experience of drinking fluid more enjoyable.**
2. Liquid intake should be dispersed over the hours when the client is awake and not just ingested with meals.
3. Fluid restriction is concerned with limiting the volume of fluid, not the type of fluid.
4. Consuming equal amounts of fluids during three 8-hour periods is unrealistic because the client will be sleeping at night.
5. **The client and nurse should make a fluid schedule, taking into consideration factors such as periods of wakefulness, number of meals, oral medications, and personal preferences. An appropriate schedule might be 500 mL between 8 a.m. and 4 p.m., 400 mL between 4 p.m. and 11 p.m., and the remainder of the fluid, 100 mL, during the night.**

TEST-TAKING TIP: The words *fluid restriction* are key words in the stem that direct attention to content. The word *fluid* in the stem and the word *fluids* in options 1, 4, and 5 are clang associations. Seriously consider these options. Although options 1 and 5 are correct answers, option 4 is a distractor.

26. 1. **Rattling sounds in the pharynx indicate mucus in the airway. The nurse can apply the nursing diagnosis *Ineffective Airway Clearance,* which is a high-priority problem and poses the highest degree of threat from the options provided. Suctioning is the immediate intervention required to maintain a patent airway because an unconscious client cannot cough voluntarily.**
2. Expectorating copious amounts of mucus indicates that this client is able to clear secretions and maintain their airway. Assessment is required to identify and treat a cause of the mucus production and to support this client in maintaining their airway. This is a low to moderate priority.

3. Anxiety related to the anticipation of pain with ambulation is a low priority. Anticipation of pain does not pose an immediate threat or require immediate intervention. This should be addressed and the client's pain should be prevented, but this is not the option that requires immediate intervention.
4. A normal respiratory rate is 12 to 20 breaths per minute. While asleep, the need for oxygen declines and the respiratory rate may decrease and the depth of respirations may increase. This option represents a normal finding and does not require immediate intervention.

TEST-TAKING TIP: The word *immediate* in the stem sets a priority.

27.
1. Leaving abandons the client; a crying client needs support, not isolation.
2. Calling the client by name supports the client's need for identity, dignity, and respect, not privacy.
3. **Closing the door provides a personal, secluded environment for a confidential discussion.**
4. **Placing a bath blanket over the client during a bath prevents unnecessary exposure of the client. The bath blanket allows the nurse to expose just the areas being washed, which provides for client privacy.**
5. **Pulling a curtain closed when performing a physically invasive procedure provides privacy.**

TEST-TAKING TIP: The words *right to privacy* are key words in the stem that direct attention to content. Option 1 denies the needs of the client.

28.
1. The shoulder is a ball-and-socket joint. Flexion of the shoulder begins with the arm at the side of the body and then it is raised forward and upward to along the side of the head.
2. Inversion is turning the sole of the foot medially.
3. **Adduction of the shoulder occurs when the arm and hand are brought across the midline in the front of the body with the elbow straight.**
4. Circumduction is movement of a ball-and-socket joint in a full circle.

29.
1. **Using a circular motion from the meatus outward to clean the head of the penis follows the principle of "clean" to "dirty." The urinary meatus is considered cleaner than the rest of the head of the penis or the shaft of the penis.**
2. **Smegma collects under the foreskin, which must be retracted to permit thorough cleaning.**
3. Washing should move secretions and debris away from the urinary meatus, preventing infection.
4. A rubbing motion may injure delicate perineal tissue and be too stimulating.
5. A light touch may be too stimulating; a gentle but firm touch is more effective.

30.
1. **Safety bars provide a stationary support around the toilet; this facilitates client safety and requires less exertion to sit and stand when using the toilet.**
2. **A shower chair helps to prevent falls when taking a shower. Also, it conserves energy and minimizes the fear of falling.**
3. **A higher toilet seat facilitates sitting and rising when using the toilet, which requires less exertion.**
4. Regardless of backing, all scatter rugs should be avoided to prevent falls. A scatter rug can cause a person to trip on the edge of the rug, resulting in a fall.
5. **A walker without wheels has four legs that touch the floor, thus providing a wide base of support. This device will promote safety when ambulating.**

31.
1. A temperature of 99.2°F is within the expected range of 97.7°F to 99.2°F for an adult and is not a cause for concern.
2. **A potassium level of 3.0 mEq/L is below the expected range of 3.5 to 5.3 mEq/L and is a cause for concern. In addition, a low serum potassium level (hypokalemia) enhances the action of digoxin. Classic clinical indicators of hypokalemia include dizziness, cardiac dysrhythmias, nausea and vomiting, abdominal distention, diarrhea, muscle weakness, leg cramps, confusion, irritability, and hypotension.**
3. A pulse rate of 62 beats per minute is within the expected range of 60 to 100 beats per minute for an adult and is not a cause for concern.
4. Two hundred milligrams of ibuprofen by mouth every 4 hours is within the over-the-counter maximum daily dose of 1200 milligrams daily and is not a cause for concern.

32. 1. Although antiemetics reduce nausea, anxiolytics reduce anxiety.

2. Antiemetics block the emetogenic receptors to prevent or treat nausea or vomiting.

3. Antitussives reduce the frequency and intensity of coughing. Anxiolytics reduce anxiety.

4. Although antiemetics reduce vomiting, antitussives reduce coughing.

TEST-TAKING TIP: The words *antiemetic* and *decrease* are key words in the stem that direct attention to content. There are duplicate facts in the options. The question presents four responses: nausea, anxiety, vomiting, and coughing. If you can identify one response unrelated to an antiemetic, you can eliminate two options. If you can identify one response related to an antiemetic, you can focus on two options. You have increased your chances of selecting the correct answer to 50%.

33. 1. Weighing a client twice a day is unnecessary. Weight varies over the course of the day depending on food and fluids ingested and the weight of clothing being worn. These factors produce information that is not comparable.

2. Weighing a client 1 hour before meals is unnecessary. Meal times may vary from day to day, and the information collected will not be comparable.

3. To obtain the most accurate comparable data, clients should be weighed at the same time every day, preferably first thing in the morning, after toileting, before eating or drinking, wearing the same clothing, and using the same scale. This controls as many variables as possible in order to make the daily measurements an accurate reflection of the client's weight.

4. Weighing the client before the client urinates in the morning collects information influenced by the volume of urine in the urinary bladder. Weights should always be measured after, not before, voiding (generally in the morning) to obtain the most accurate, comparable measurements. One liter of fluid is equal to 2.2 pounds.

34. 1. Heat causes vasodilation that increases circulation to the area and results in erythema, not reactive hyperemia.

2. Effleurage, light stroking of the skin, stimulates the peripheral nerves and should not change skin coloration.

3. Pulling a client up in bed without using a pull sheet exerts a shearing force, which can injure blood vessels and tissues and result in a friction burn.

4. Compressed skin appears pale because circulation to the area is impaired. When pressure is relieved, the skin takes on a bright red flush as extra blood flows to the area to compensate for the period of impeded blood flow (reactive hyperemia).

TEST-TAKING TIP: The words *reactive hyperemia* are key words in the stem that direct attention to content.

35. **1. Inspiratory stridor is an obvious, audible, shrill, harsh sound caused by a laryngeal obstruction. Obstruction of the larynx is life threatening because it prevents the exchange of gasses between the lungs and atmospheric air.**

2. Although a pleural friction rub reflects a problem, it is not as life threatening as a condition in another option. A pleural friction rub is a grating, rubbing sound that is heard by auscultating over the base of the lung. It is caused by inflamed pleura (pleurisy) rubbing together.

3. Although expiratory wheezing reflects a problem, it is not as life threatening as a condition in another option. Expiratory wheezing is the presence of high-pitched musical sounds caused by the high-velocity movement of air through narrowed airways. It is associated with asthma, bronchitis, and pneumonia.

4. Although a nonproductive cough reflects a problem, it is not as life threatening as a condition in another option. A nonproductive cough is coughing without mobilizing or expectorating sputum.

TEST-TAKING TIP: The word *most* in the stem sets a priority. The word *inspiratory* in option 1 is opposite to the word *expiratory* in option 3. Carefully examine options that are opposites; often, one of them is the correct answer. In this question, option 1 is the correct answer.

36. 1. The Nurse Licensure Compact is an important agreement between some states that allows a nurse to practice in multiple states without having to acquire additional licenses. However, it is individual states, under the Nurse Practice Acts, that authorize licensure in the United States.

2. The Nurse Practice Acts are enacted by individual states. They are a compilation of laws that govern nursing and allow each state board of nursing to oversee and regulate nurse licensure.

3. The Accreditation Commission for Education in Nursing is one of several organizations that accredit nursing programs. It does not grant licensure.
4. The American Nurses Association (ANA) is a national professional organization for nursing in the United States. It fosters high standards of nursing practice. It does not grant licensure.

37. 1. Discharging a client is not the priority from among the options presented.

2. The headache may indicate that the client's blood pressure is too high, which may precipitate a brain attack (stroke, cerebrovascular accident). The client should be assessed immediately.

3. Orthostatic hypotension is a common occurrence when moving from a sitting to a standing position. The client is safe in bed at this time. This concern can be addressed later, after clients who need immediate attention receive care.
4. Although this needs to be done, it is not life threatening and can wait.

TEST-TAKING TIP: The words *attend to before the others* set a priority.

38. 1. With hypernatremia, the nervous system is stimulated, causing muscle twitches.

2. Hypernatremia is associated with fluid loss, which reduces the blood volume (hypovolemia). The heart rate increases to ensure enough oxygen reaches body cells until the blood volume is restored.

3. With hypernatremia, excitable tissue such as cerebral cells becomes stimulated, causing confusion.

4. With hypernatremia, excitable tissue such as cerebral cells becomes stimulated, causing agitation.

5. Marked thirst is a clinical indicator of hypernatremia because of cellular dehydration.

39. 1. A special syringe is not required for administering a medication via Z-track. The barrel of the syringe must be large enough to accommodate the volume of solution to be injected (usually 1 to 3 mL), and the needle must be long enough to enter a muscle (usually 1½-inch needle).

2. Pulling laterally and downward on the skin before inserting the needle creates a zigzag track through the various tissue layers, which prevents backflow of medication up the needle track when simultaneously removing the needle and releasing traction on the skin.

3. The use of the vastus lateralis muscle for a Z-track injection may cause discomfort for the client. Z-track injections are tolerated better when the well-developed gluteal muscles are used.

4. Waiting 5 to 10 seconds before withdrawing the needle while hand holding the skin in a lateral position allows time for the medication to disperse. This limits the risk of solution leaking up the needle track.

5. With a Z-track injection, the needle is inserted into a large muscle, not the abdomen. The Z represents the zigzag pattern of the needle track that results when the skin traction and the needle are simultaneously removed.

TEST-TAKING TIP: The word *correct* in the stem indicates positive polarity. Options 1 and 5 both have the letter "Z," which are clang associations with the letter "Z" in the stem. Consider these options carefully; however, neither of these options is the correct answer. More often than not, an option with a clang association is one of the correct answers in a multiple response item, *but not always*.

40. 1. Although clear, accurate articulation allows the client to decode the combination of vowels and consonants, it does not determine whether the message was heard.
2. Although facing the client allows the speaker's lips and facial expression to be seen, which helps the client to receive and decode the message, it does not determine whether the message was heard.

3. A client is the only person who can tell the nurse whether the message was heard and understood.

4. Raising the voice does not make the message clearer; it may actually make it more difficult to understand. In addition, shouting can be demeaning.

TEST-TAKING TIP: The word *most* in the stem sets a priority. Option 3 is unique because it is an action that occurs after

the message is sent and is the only option that seeks information on which an evaluation can be made.

41. 1. 250 mL is too little fluid; this is the recommended amount for a toddler.
2. 500 mL is too little fluid; this is the recommended amount for a large school-age child or small adolescent.
3. 700 mL is too little fluid for an adult; 700 mL is the recommended volume for an average-sized adolescent.
4. The range of 750 to 1000 mL, with an average of 900 mL, is the suggested volume of solution for a soapsuds or tap water enema administered to an adult to stimulate effective evacuation of the bowel. It provides enough fluid to fill the bowel and apply pressure to the intestinal mucosa to stimulate defecation.

TEST-TAKING TIP: The words *soapsuds enema* and *adult* are key words in the stem that direct attention to content.

42. **1. Taking the pulse for a full minute is necessary to obtain an accurate count. Taking the pulse for 15 seconds and multiplying by 4 or taking the pulse for 30 seconds and multiplying by 2 may result in an inaccurate reading and is unsafe.**
2. Ultimately, the apical and radial rates should be obtained and compared to determine whether there is a pulse deficit.
3. Taking the pulse rate using a Doppler probe is unnecessary; when a pulse rate is irregular, the apical pulse rate should be measured using a stethoscope.
4. The apical, not the carotid, pulse should be obtained when the pulse is irregular. An apical rate is most accurate, because a pulse rate at another site may be weak or low.

TEST-TAKING TIP: The word *first* in the stem sets a priority. The word *irregular* is the key word in the stem that directs attention to content.

43. **Answer: 390 mL**

One ounce equals 30 mL

4 ounces × 30 mL = 120 mL

Half of 8 = 4 ounces × 30 mL = 120 mL

120 mL + 120 mL + 150 mL = 390 mL

44. 1. Rinsing the mouth with diluted hydrogen peroxide does not provide the friction needed to remove debris that contributes to the formation of plaque.
2. A dental hygienist will use various dental instruments to remove tartar, which is hardened plaque. Also, most dentists recommend that this procedure be performed twice a year.
3. Although brushing the biting surface of the teeth using a forward and backward motion is an integral part of dental hygiene, it removes debris from the biting surface of the teeth, not plaque where the teeth and gums meet.
4. Plaque, composed of bacteria and saliva, forms on the teeth primarily at the gum line. Vibrating a toothbrush at a 45° angle where the teeth meet the gums provides friction that helps to dislodge plaque from the teeth.

TEST-TAKING TIP: The words *prevent dental plaque* are key words in the stem that direct attention to content.

45. 1. The nurse can suspect the hematological findings in this case to be related to a gastrointestinal (GI) problem, and the assessment should focus on the GI system to rule out emergencies such as a GI bleed or bowel obstruction. The hemoglobin level is below the reference range of 12 to 15 g/dL, and the hematocrit is on the low end of the reference range of 36% to 46%. The white blood cell count and temperature are elevated.
2. Although the client's blood pressure is elevated, the assessment should focus on the GI system. Abdominal pain, a low hemoglobin and hematocrit, and signs of infection should be prioritized.
3. This client has a history of diverticulitis and is currently experiencing severe abdominal pain despite receiving pain medication an hour ago. A focused GI assessment should be completed for this client.
4. Although the client's respirations of 24 breaths per minute are more than the expected range of 12 to 20 breaths per minute for an adult, they are unlabored. The increased respiratory rate most likely is a response to anxiety associated with pain.

TEST-TAKING TIP: The words *focus on* in the stem set a priority.

46. 1. Determination of a client's need for a restraint requires the knowledge and

judgment of a registered nurse. It requires an assessment of numerous systems and risk factors, a complex level of interaction with the client, problem solving, and innovation in the form of an individually designed plan of care that provides for the client's safety.

2. The skill of evaluation requires the knowledge and judgment of a registered nurse. This task has great potential for harm if the caregiver incorrectly evaluates the client's response.
3. The type of restraint used requires a primary health-care provider's prescription. The application and maintenance of restraints are dependent functions of the nurse.
4. **Restraints can be removed, the client supervised to maintain client safety, and the restraints reapplied by an unlicensed nursing assistant. The application and removal of restraints are not complex activities.**
5. **Performing range-of-motion exercises is not complex, requires simple problem-solving skills, and employs a simple level of interaction with the client. It is within the scope of practice of an unlicensed nursing assistant and does not require the more advanced competencies of a registered nurse.**

TEST-TAKING TIP: The words *delegate* and *nursing assistant* are key words in the stem that direct attention to content.

47\. 1. **Assessing the client's urinary patterns is appropriate. There are multiple types of urinary incontinence, such as urge incontinence and reflex incontinence. A major difference between these types is whether or not the client perceives an urge to void.**

2. **This is an appropriate strategy. Offering toileting before the client experiences incontinence gives the client the opportunity to void before becoming incontinent. If effective, it contributes to self-esteem and personal hygiene.**
3. Inserting a Foley catheter is not an appropriate strategy to manage incontinence in most clients. This intervention carries the risk for infection.
4. **This is an appropriate intervention. The client can be taught pelvic floor muscle strengthening exercises. Kegel exercises involve contracting the pelvic floor muscles, holding for 5 to 10 seconds, and then slowly releasing the contraction over 5 to 10 seconds.**
5. Bedside commodes, raised toilet seats, bedpans, and bedside urinals are appropriate strategies to promote independent urination and to manage urinary incontinence. If the cause is urgency, these tools may prevent incontinence by limiting the time needed to reach the toilet.

48\. 1. **The trachea is considered sterile and is suctioned before the oropharyngeal area, which is considered clean; this minimizes contamination of the sterile area.**

2. Rotating the catheter while applying suction should be done on the catheter's removal from the trachea. Rotating the catheter exposes the tip of the catheter to respiratory secretions and facilitates the removal of secretions.
3. **Intermittent suctioning prevents the catheter tip from adhering to the respiratory mucosa, preventing trauma to the mucosa.**
4. For wall suction to be effective when suctioning an adult, it should be maintained at 100 to 120 mm Hg.
5. **Lubricating the catheter with sterile normal saline limits trauma to the mucous membranes, and sterile normal saline maintains sterility of the procedure.**

TEST-TAKING TIP: The words *tracheal* in the stem and *trachea* in options 1 and 2 are clang associations. Assess these options carefully. Option 1 is one of the correct answers, but option 2 is not.

49\. 1. Avoiding a circumcision at this time may or may not be advisable. A ritual circumcision is an important ceremony in the parents' religion and should not be negated lightly.

2. Although this is true, the discussion regarding a circumcision should be conducted among the surgeon, the parents, the ritual circumciser, and the parent's religious advisor.
3. The ritual circumcision and a surgical reconstruction are both important. A ritual circumcision, a significant ceremony in the parent's religion, should not be negated lightly.
4. **Depending on the extent of the hypospadias, removing just a small portion of the foreskin may be possible.**

50. 1. **Placing food on the strong side of the mouth allows the unaffected muscles to control chewing, moves the bolus of food to the posterior oral cavity, and facilitates swallowing.**
2. **Small amounts of food allow the client to chew (masticate) a manageable mass of food (bolus) safely.**
3. Offering fluids to assist with swallowing will promote aspiration and is contraindicated. Fluids should be taken after a mouthful of food is swallowed.
4. **Allowing adequate time between bites permits the client to chew (masticate) and swallow food.**
5. **A high Fowler position allows gravity to facilitate swallowing.**

TEST-TAKING TIP: The words *feeding* in the stem and *food* in options 1 and 2 are obscure clang associations. Examine options 1 and 2 carefully.

51. Answer: 4, 3, 5, 6, 2, 1
4. **Cleaning the eyelid and eyelashes removes debris and minimizes the presence of microorganisms. Swiping from the inner to the outer canthus moves microorganisms and debris away from the lacrimal duct.**
3. **Tilting the head slightly back and toward the eye being medicated prevents the solution from flowing toward the other eye.**
5. **Placing a finger just below the lower eyelashes and exerting gentle downward pressure over the bony prominence of the cheek exposes the conjunctival sac, where the drops should be placed to avoid trauma to the cornea.**
6. **Holding the dropper close to the eye without touching the eye and administering the prescribed number of drops so they fall into the conjunctival sac prevent injury to the eyeball and contamination of the dropper.**
2. **Instructing the client to close the eyes gently prevents the medication from being squeezed out of the eye.**
1. **Applying gentle pressure over the inner canthus prevents medication from flowing into the lacrimal duct.**

52. 1. The ketogenic diet is a low-carbohydrate and high-fat diet that promotes weight loss. Although weight loss can help manage hypertension, it is not the most appropriate diet for this client.
2. The Atkins diet is a low-carbohydrate diet that promotes weight loss. Although weight loss can help manage hypertension, it is not the most appropriate diet for this client.
3. **The Dietary Approaches to Stop Hypertension, or DASH, diet is a low-sodium and high-nutrient diet designed to combat hypertension. It can also promote weight loss. This is the most appropriate dietary recommendation for this client.**
4. A vegan diet is not the most appropriate recommendation for this client based on the options provided. The focus for this client should be to reduce sodium and increase the consumption of whole grains, fresh fruits and vegetables, and low-fat dairy products and meats.

53. 1. **An intradermal injection usually involves a small volume of fluid (e.g., 0.1 mL). A 1-mL syringe, rather than a syringe that can accommodate larger volumes, permits a more precise measurement of a small volume of fluid.**
2. **A 26-gauge needle has a narrow diameter and a short bevel that are conducive to the formation of the wheal associated with an intradermal injection.**
3. An intradermal injection usually is administered with a needle that is ½ inch in length.
4. Aspiration of a syringe after needle insertion is used for intramuscular, not intradermal, injections. An intradermal injection inserts fluid into the dermis just below the epidermis and away from any obvious blood vessels. Intradermal injection sites commonly used for allergy testing are the right ventral forearm, upper chest, and upper back over the scapulae.
5. **The skin over the site of needle insertion should be stretched with the index finger and thumb. This action facilitates the insertion of the needle ⅛ inch below the surface of the skin and into the dermis, rather than the subcutaneous tissue.**

TEST-TAKING TIP: The word *intradermal* is the key word in the stem that directs attention to content.

54. 1. *Mandatory Reporting* requires anyone who suspects that a person is being abused report that abuse to the appropriate authorities. This does not apply in the given situation.

2. As long as the nurse's actions are reasonable, the nurse is protected by *Good Samaritan Laws*. These laws protect any volunteer who helps in an emergency situation.

3. The *Nurse Practice Acts* define the scope and responsibilities of nurses. They also pertain to nursing licensure regulations.

4. The *Nursing Code of Ethics* describes the ethical responsibilities of nurses to provide quality care. Although this document indicates that the nurse has a duty to help in this situation, it does not protect the nurse as a volunteer.

55. **1. The abdominal girth will increase as blood accumulates within the abdominal cavity. Abdominal girth should be measured using a centimeter tape placed around the body over the umbilicus.**

2. The respiratory rate will increase, not decrease, in an effort to bring more oxygen to body cells.

3. With hemorrhage there is a decrease in the circulating blood volume, resulting in a pulse that can easily be obliterated when using palpation to assess a peripheral pulse.

4. With hemorrhage there is a decrease in the circulating blood volume, resulting in a decrease in the systolic blood pressure less than 100 mm Hg (hypotension).

5. The skin will be cool and clammy because of the sympathetic nervous system response.

6. The respiratory rate will increase, not decrease, in an effort to deliver more oxygen to body cells.

56. 1. Providing time for the heart rate to return to its expected range is not the primary reason for sitting on the side of the bed before transfer.

2. Orthostatic hypotension is a condition that contributes to impaired stability. When a person moves to a sitting or standing position from a lying or sitting position, cerebral circulation is reduced, resulting in light-headedness and dizziness; sitting on the side of the bed allows the peripheral blood vessels to constrict in response to the vertical position.

3. Although the client may take several deep breaths, this is not the primary reason for sitting on the side of the bed before transfer.

4. Allowing the client to regain energy is not the primary reason for sitting on the side of the bed before transfer.

TEST-TAKING TIP: The word *primary* in the stem sets a priority.

57. 1. Sublingual nitroglycerin has a rapid onset and a relatively short duration of action. One dose may not be enough.

2. Doubling the dose may precipitate severe or even life-threatening hypotension.

3. Excessive administration of nitroglycerin can cause severe hypotension and death; when a therapeutic response does not occur after following the prescribed nitroglycerin protocol, medical attention is necessary because the person may be experiencing an acute cardiac event.

4. Sublingual nitroglycerin has a rapid onset and a relatively short duration of action. Three doses may be necessary to achieve a desired therapeutic response. However, if pain persists beyond 15 minutes, it may indicate the presence of an acute cardiac event that requires immediate emergency medical intervention.

TEST-TAKING TIP: The word *only* in option 1 is a specific determiner.

58. **1. Rhonchi are low-pitched gurgling sounds caused by secretions in the airways. They often resolve when the client coughs.**

2. Wheezes are high-pitched musical sounds caused by narrowing of the airways.

3. Crackles are popping or bubbling sounds caused by fluid in the alveoli.

4. Stridor is a high-pitched sound typically heard when the airway is obstructed.

59. 1. Elisabeth Kübler Ross described a framework for the process of coping with death and dying. It includes five stages: denial, anger, bargaining, depression, acceptance.

2. Mishel developed a theory describing the experience of uncertainty in illness.

3. **Jean Watson's nursing theories emphasize perception. A terminally ill client with a high level of functioning and coping can still be described as healthy.**
4. Elisabeth Kübler Ross described a framework for the process of coping with death and dying. It includes five stages: denial, anger, bargaining, depression, acceptance.

TEST-TAKING TIP: Options 3 and 4 are opposites. Options 1 and 2 are equally plausible.

60. **Answer: 3, 4, 5, 1, 2, 6**

3. **Shaking the ampule with a rapid snap of the wrist moves medication trapped in the top of the ampule into the body of the ampule. This permits all of the medication to be available for withdrawal, ensuring an accurate dose.**
4. **Using an ampule opener over the neck of the ampule protects the nurse's hand from shattered glass when the neck of the ampule is snapped off.**
5. **Snapping the head of the ampule away from the nurse propels any shattered glass away from the nurse.**
1. **Using a filtered needle when solution is withdrawn from the ampule prevents glass shards from entering the syringe.**
2. **Withdrawing the volume of solution prescribed by the primary health-care provider ensures that the client receives the desired dose.**
6. **Replacing the filtered needle ensures that a sterile needle free of glass shards is used to administer the medication.**

61.
1. **Beta blockers can mask the symptoms of hypoglycemia. Although not contraindicated in clients with diabetes, they are not the most appropriate antihypertensive in clients with poorly controlled diabetes.**
2. Beta blockers are used to treat tachycardia, hypertension, myocardial infarction, heart failure, and coronary artery disease. The client with a personal and family history of hypertension is appropriately treated with a beta blocker.
3. Beta blockers, specifically labetalol, are used to treat hypertension during pregnancy. Other antihypertensives (ACE inhibitors, ARBs, and nitroprusside) are teratogenic and contraindicated in pregnancy.
4. **Beta blockers are contraindicated in clients with bradycardia. Beta blockers block the action of hormones at beta receptors and slow the heart rate. Administering a beta blocker to a client with bradycardia can exacerbate the bradycardia.**
5. **Beta blockers are used to treat tachycardia, hypertension, myocardial infarction, heart failure, and coronary artery disease. The client with a history of myocardial infarction is appropriately treated with a beta blocker.**

62.
1. This illustration reflects the administration of medication via the sublingual route. The medication is placed under the tongue, where it dissolves quickly and is absorbed via the mucous membranes. The sublingual route is used for a systemic effect.
2. This illustration reflects the administration of medication via the rectal route. The rectum is the last 7 to 8 inches of the large intestine. The medication is inserted through the anus and anal canal to reach the rectum. The rectal route is used for either a local or a systemic effect.
3. **This illustration reflects the administration of medication via the buccal route. The medication is placed in the mouth between the cheek and gum, where it dissolves slowly and is absorbed via the mucous membranes. The buccal route is used for a local effect.**
4. This illustration reflects the administration of medication via the vaginal route. The medication is inserted through the vaginal introitus and advanced deep within the vaginal canal. The vaginal route is used for a local effect.

63.
1. **The aging adult is at increased risk for constipation due to decreased gastrointestinal motility. A low-fiber diet results in decreased bulk of stool and subsequent decreased motility. This increases the risk of constipation.**
2. The middle-aged client who consumes a high-fiber diet is not at increased risk for constipation. Fiber results in an increased bulk of stool and promotes motility. This reduces the risk for constipation.
3. The client who consumes adequate fluids is not at increased risk for constipation. Adequate hydration reduces the need to absorb fluid from the contents of the colon. This promotes stools that are soft and easier to pass.

4. The client with NPO orders is at increased risk for dehydration. Dehydration leads to increased absorption of fluid from the contents of the colon. This leads to stools that are drier and harder and more difficult to pass.
5. The client who jogs every morning is active. Activity promotes gastrointestinal motility and prevents constipation.
6. The client recovering from a fractured femur is likely experiencing impaired mobility and a decreased activity level. An important side effect of opioids is constipation. This client is at increased risk for constipation.

TEST-TAKING TIP: Identify opposites. Options 1 and 2 are opposite. Options 3 and 4 are opposite. Options 5 and 6 are opposite.

64. 1. In the analysis step of the nursing process, the nurse interprets data, determines the significance of the data, and comes to a conclusion or formulates a nursing diagnosis.
2. Evaluation involves determining client responses to nursing interventions, identifying whether goals and outcomes have been met, and revising the plan of care when necessary.
3. Observation of human responses is part of the assessment phase of the nursing process; assessment involves collecting, verifying, clustering, and documenting objective and subjective data.
4. Implementation involves carrying out the plan of care and documenting the care provided.

65. 1. Although learning more is appropriate, the nurse must understand that individuals of the same culture may not embrace all values and beliefs of that culture. Stereotyping, the assigning of a trait that exists in some members of a group to all members of the group, must be avoided in order to provide culturally competent care.
2. Ethnocentrism is the view that one's own attitudes, beliefs, customs, and culture are better than those of another. This interferes with the nurse's ability to provide culturally competent care.
3. The nurse has to clarify personal values and beliefs before understanding and nonjudgmentally accepting the cultural beliefs and practices of others.
4. Although different cultures share common elements, they may be demonstrated through different behaviors and customs. Recognizing only the similarities denies the differences that make cultures unique.

TEST-TAKING TIP: The word *first* in the stem sets a priority.

66. 1. Oral hygiene does not play a major role in the prevention of a subsequent stroke.
2. Good oral hygiene in clients who have suffered a stroke is a strategy that can prevent aspiration and lung infections.
3. This client may be at increased risk for blood clots. This risk should be managed appropriately. However, oral hygiene does not play a major role in preventing blood clots.
4. This client may be at increased risk for falls. This risk should be managed appropriately. However, oral hygiene does not play a major role in preventing blood clots.

TEST-TAKING TIP: Options 1, 3, and 4 are related to stroke. Blood clots can cause ischemic stroke and falls can cause hemorrhagic stroke. Option 2 is a unique answer. Oral hygiene limits debris in the oral cavity that can be aspirated.

67. 1. Rest, sleep, and relaxation associated with pain relief are not based on the gate control theory.
2. Activity may provide distraction, focusing attention on stimuli other than the pain. However, when in pain, clients often do not have the physical or emotional energy to concentrate on activities.
3. The gate control theory assumes that pain fibers that originate in the peripheral areas of the body have synapses in the gray matter of the dorsal horns of the spinal cord. Large nerve fibers stimulated by heat, cold, and touch transmit impulses through the same synapses as those that transmit pain. When larger fibers are stimulated, they close the gate to painful stimuli and thus reduce pain.
4. Relaxing music provides a distraction to help minimize the perception of pain. The music focuses the client's attention on a stimulus other than pain.
5. Narcotics act on the higher centers of the brain to modify the perception of pain.

68. **1. Circulatory stasis occurs after surgery because postoperative clients are not**

as active as they were before surgery; active leg exercises promote venous return and prevent the formation of thrombi and thrombophlebitis.

2. Although active leg exercises prevent muscle atrophy, this is not the primary reason for performing leg exercises postoperatively.
3. Although active or passive leg exercises may prevent contractures, this is not the primary reason for performing leg exercises postoperatively.
4. Although active leg exercises increase muscle strength, this is not the primary reason for postoperative leg exercises.

TEST-TAKING TIP: The word *primary* in the stem sets a priority.

69. **1. Brussels sprouts are an excellent source of vitamin C. One cup of Brussels sprouts contains approximately 100 mg of vitamin C.**
2. Yellow peppers are an excellent source of vitamin C (ascorbic acid). One pepper contains approximately 137 mg of vitamin C.
3. Broccoli is an excellent source of vitamin C. One cup of fresh boiled broccoli contains approximately 116 mg of vitamin C.
4. Tomato juice is an excellent source of vitamin C. One cup of tomato juice contains approximately 170 mg of vitamin C.
5. Citrus fruits, such as oranges and grapefruit, are excellent sources of vitamin C. One cup of orange juice contains approximately 124 mg of vitamin C.

70. **1. Clients receiving rosuvastatin (Crestor®), a hydroxymethylglutaryl-coenzyme A (HMG-CoA) reductase inhibitor, usually have several risk factors for cardiovascular disease, including high serum cholesterol, lactate dehydrogenase (LDH), and triglyceride levels. These clients usually are prescribed a diet low in fat and cholesterol.**
2. Clients should not drink more than 200 mL of grapefruit juice while taking this drug because it potentiates the action of the medication, which can result in toxicity.
3. It is not necessary to take rosuvastatin with food. It does not cause gastric irritation.
4. Rosuvastatin can be taken at any time of the day because it remains in the body longer than other statins. Other statins such as fluvastatin (Lescol®), pravastatin (Pravachol®), and simvastatin (Zocor®) should be taken in the evening because they are shorter acting. The body produces cholesterol mostly at night.
5. Common side effects of rosuvastatin are muscle aches, weakness, nausea, and headache. However, rhabdomyolysis, a rare serious effect, can occur. It is the accumulation of the by-products of skeletal muscle destruction in the renal tubules; it can result in renal failure and death. Rhabdomyolysis is manifested by muscle pain, weakness, fever, and dark urine.

71. **1. With urinary retention, urine is kept in the bladder and there is a lack of voiding.**
2. Urine is being passed from, not retained in, the bladder when voiding occurs. Wet undergarments may indicate urinary incontinence.
3. With urinary retention, urine accumulates in the bladder, with resulting bladder fullness. When the bladder is full, it expands and appears as suprapubic distention.
4. Painful or difficult urination is called *dysuria*, not *urinary retention*.
5. A sudden, overwhelming need to void is called *urgency*, which is not related to urinary retention.

TEST-TAKING TIP: The words *urinary retention* in the stem direct attention to content. The word *urinary* in the stem and the word *urine* in option 1 are clang associations.

72. 1. Maintenance fluids replace fluids lost during basic physiological functions (urination, passage of stool, sweat, respiration). Normal Saline at KVO means at a very slow rate to "keep vein open" or to maintain IV patency.
2. PO fluids at 30 mL/kg/day is the required amount for maintenance fluids. Maintenance fluids replace fluids lost during basic physiological functions.
3. Fluid replacement is fluids required beyond basic physiological function. For example, the client with decreased renal function requires fluid replacement beyond what is required for basic physiological function.

4. The client with diarrhea has lost more fluids than with basic physiological functions. This client requires additional fluids. Therefore, this order is classified as fluid replacement instead of fluid maintenance.
5. A bolus of normal saline to manage hypotension is a fluid requirement beyond basic physiological function. This is classified as fluid replacement instead of fluid maintenance.

73. 1. Although a good habit for the nurse to have, this does not explain the rationale to the client's spouse.
2. Some hospital beds include air mattresses designed to prevent skin breakdown. Wrinkled sheets do not interfere with the efficacy of these air mattresses. Wrinkled sheets, however, can cause skin breakdown regardless of the type of mattress used.
3. Smoothing the wrinkles of the sheets prevents skin breakdown related to shear and friction when repositioning the client.
4. There are more effective strategies for repositioning clients than using a bedsheet. Examples include repositioning pillows, sliders, or mattresses that reposition clients. Using the bedsheet to reposition the client carries the risk of damaging skin due to friction and shear.

TEST-TAKING TIP: The word *best* in the stem sets a priority.

74. 1. Headache is a physiological response to stress.
2. Irritability can be an emotional response to stress; the body is using physical and emotional energy to cope with stress.
3. Heartburn (epigastric pain associated with gastric reflux) can be a physiological response to stress.
4. Depression can be an emotional response to stress. Depression serves as an escape from stress.
5. An increase in blood pressure (hypertension) is a physiological response to stress.

TEST-TAKING TIP: The word *emotional* is the key word in the stem that directs attention to content.

75. 1. This is the vertical strip method of breast palpation. The vertical strip method is preferred because it ensures that all breast tissues are examined. The client is better able to track which areas have been examined, and the entire nipple/areolar complex is included.
2. This is the pie wedge (radial spoke) method of breast palpation. With this method, it is difficult to ensure that all breast tissues are examined, especially the areas around and under the nipple and areola, as well as the area in the upper outer quadrant into the axilla (tail of Spence).
3. This is the concentric circles method. With this method, it is difficult to ensure that all breast tissues are examined, especially the areas around and under the nipple and areola, as well as the area in the upper outer quadrant into the axilla (tail of Spence).

TEST-TAKING TIP: The word *most* in the stem sets a priority.

76. 1. The abdomen rises on inspiration as the lungs fill with air. As the lungs fill with inhaled air, they push the diaphragm down, causing the abdomen to rise.
2. A slow deep breath helps to completely inflate the lungs. Research demonstrates that breathing through the nose increases end-tidal CO_2 concentrations and overall oxygenation of all body cells versus mouth breathing.
3. These accessory muscles should not be involved consciously with diaphragmatic breathing. The abdomen should rise and fall rather than the shoulders; the chest naturally expands and recoils.
4. Diaphragmatic breathing involves a pattern of a slow deep inhalation, holding the breath for 2 to 3 seconds at the height of inhalation just before exhalation, followed by a slow exhalation with a tightening of the abdominal muscles to aid exhalation.
5. Pressure against the abdomen will interfere with the amount of air that is drawn into the lungs on inspiration.

TEST-TAKING TIP: The word *breathing* in the stem and the word *breath* in options 2 and 4 are clang associations.

77. 1. An increase in weight may indicate that the client is retaining fluid because the heart is not efficiently circulating blood to the kidneys. A decrease in renal

perfusion stimulates the renin-angiotensin response, which causes vasoconstriction and the release of aldosterone. Aldosterone causes sodium and water retention. One liter of fluid weighs 2.2 pounds.

2. Metoprolol (Lopressor®) blocks the stimulation of beta-1 (myocardial) adrenergic receptors that can result in an irregular or slow (bradycardia) heart rate.

3. Metoprolol should not be stopped abruptly because it can precipitate life-threatening dysrhythmias, hypertension, or myocardial ischemia.

4. Taking metoprolol at the same time every day maintains a therapeutic blood level of the drug.

5. Metoprolol can cause orthostatic hypotension, a vasomotor response. Therefore, the client should be cautioned to change from horizontal to vertical positions slowly to allow the cardiovascular system to adjust to the change in position.

6. Obtaining the blood pressure reading before taking each dose of metoprolol is unnecessary. It is sufficient to monitor blood pressure twice a week.

78. 1. Perfumes may not be perceived as pleasant-smelling to all clients. Perfumes can exacerbate nausea. Strong odors should be reduced and the nurse should ensure good ventilation.

2. Nausea is a subjective experience that may or may not occur with vomiting. Especially if nausea occurs with vomiting, the nurse should choose interventions that maintain fluid and electrolyte balance. The nurse should offer ice chips, sips of water, clear liquids, and other fluid replacement strategies that the client can tolerate.

3. Smaller, more frequent meals can reduce the experience of nausea. The client should avoid spicy foods and other foods known to cause nausea.

4. The nurse should keep an emesis basin nearby so the client can easily access it should they need to vomit. This promotes comfort and reduces anxiety. The basin should be kept within an arm's reach, be emptied promptly, and be kept out of eyesight of the client.

79. Answer: 2, 3, 5, 4, 1, 6

2. The port is close to the perineal area, and privacy provides for emotional comfort. Exposing the port permits adequate visualization of the port and tubing during the procedure.

3. Gloves protect the nurse from the client's body excretions. Wiping the port removes microorganisms before insertion of the syringe.

5. Inserting the syringe (via a needle or needleless system) accesses the lumen of the urinary catheter; 5 mL of urine usually is adequate for most urine specimens.

4. Wiping the port after removal of the syringe removes microorganisms from the port.

1. Removing the clamp allows urine to flow down into the collection chamber, which prevents a backflow of urine into the bladder.

6. Urine collected via a sterile procedure should be placed in a sterile specimen cup to prevent extraneous microorganisms from contaminating the specimen. Syringes should be placed into a hard-sided sharps container to prevent injury to and contamination of others. Contaminated gloves can be placed into a plastic-lined garbage container.

80. 1. Potassium chloride is used for the treatment or prevention of potassium deficiency and is unrelated to heparin therapy.

2. Protamine sulfate can chemically combine with heparin, neutralizing its anticoagulant action; it should be kept readily available for the treatment of heparin overdose.

3. Prothrombin is a plasma protein coagulation factor synthesized by the liver, not a drug that should be used as an antidote to heparin.

4. If a heparin overdose occurs, plasma may be prescribed after the antidote has been given. Packed red blood cells will more likely be prescribed than plasma.

TEST-TAKING TIP: The word *most* in the stem sets a priority.

81. 1. Covering the nose when sneezing interferes with the chain of infection at the portal of exit stage, not at the transmission stage.

2. Placing used linen in a linen hamper contains microorganisms in an

appropriate receptacle, which prevents cross contamination. This interrupts the chain of infection at the level of transmission.

3. Turning and positioning contribute to maintaining skin integrity. An intact skin interrupts the chain of infection at the portal of entry stage, not the transmission stage, of the chain of infection.
4. Limiting talking when performing a sterile procedure interferes with the chain of infection at the portal of exit stage.
5. Applying a sterile dressing over a contaminated wound interferes with the chain of infection at the reservoir or source of the infection. It interrupts the chain of infection at the portal of exit stage.

TEST-TAKING TIP: The words *level of transmission* in the stem direct attention to content.

82. **1. The nursing assistant should stand on the client's strong side when assisting with ambulation. This maximizes the client's strengths and provides firm support. If a client is extremely weak and unstable, then two health-care personnel should ambulate the client, one on each side of the client.**
2. Raising the head of the bed before moving a client up in bed requires making the move against gravity; this requires more energy to facilitate the move and places a strain on both the client and nurse. The head of the bed should be lowered when moving a client up in bed.
3. Using the strong muscles of the legs to carry a load helps prevent back strain.
4. The wider the base of support and the lower the center of gravity, the greater the stability of the individual.
5. Bending from the waist puts stress on the vertebrae and muscles of the back because it does not distribute the work among the largest and strongest muscle groups of the legs.

TEST-TAKING TIP: The word *inappropriate* in the stem indicates negative polarity. The question is asking which action violates principles of body mechanics.

83. 1. Climbing off the end of the bed at night can be addressed by interventions other than a restraint.
2. A restraint may be necessary to protect the client from self-harm. Pulling out an IV catheter can cause tissue injury and can interrupt medical therapy.
3. Wandering should be controlled by observation, not a restraint.
4. Picking at the gown and bed linens is not an unsafe behavior that requires application of a restraint.

84. **The client vomited a total of 350 mL of greenish-yellow fluid during the 11 to 7 shift. This total amount should be recorded in the first column (11-7) next to Emesis.**

Intake and Output

INTAKE	11-7	7-3	3-11	24 HR	11-
Oral/Tube					
Blood/Plasma					
I.V.					
Other					
Other					
TOTAL					
OUTPUT	**11-7**	**7-3**	**3-11**	**24 HR**	**11-**
Liquid Stool					
Urine					
G.I. Suction					
Emesis	X				
Bowel Movement					
Other					
TOTAL					
INITIALS					

85. **1. A dark and unfamiliar environment can increase the risk of falls. Clients with dementia may become confused and disoriented at this time of day and experience an increased frequency of falls during this time.**
2. The incidence of falls may increase after meals, not before, because the gastrocolic reflex increases peristalsis. When ambulating to the bathroom, the client may experience an increased risk of falls.
3. Postoperative clients should be assisted with ambulation until they are able to ambulate safely and independently. Postoperative clients should always be assisted with ambulation and the frequency of falls should be decreased.
4. An aging adult client living with dementia with visitors is directly observed by visitors, and the frequency of falls is lower when visitors are present.

86. Compressing the tragus disperses the medication throughout the external auditory canal.

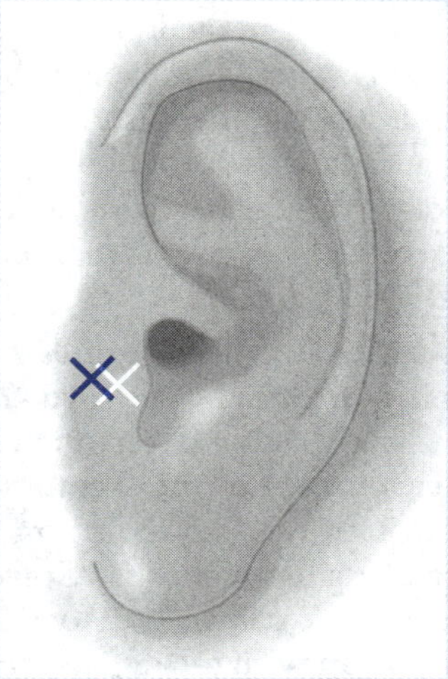

87. Answer: 27%

One gram of fat equals 9 calories; 60 grams of fat × 9 = 540 calories, and 540 ÷ 2000 = 0.27, or 27%.

88. Answer: 4, 3, 1, 2

4. This client is the priority because epigastric pain could indicate a life-threatening cardiac event. This client must be assessed first to initiate a rapid response team, if appropriate.
3. This client should be assessed for pain. This client is prioritized over the other two clients because they are either awaiting nonurgent education or currently under the care of another member of the health-care team. This client is of a lower priority than the client with epigastric pain because that client may be experiencing a cardiac emergency.
1. The client receiving passive range of motion is typically assessed every 30 minutes. This client is currently receiving care from a physical therapist and is stable. The nurse can care for two other higher priority clients before addressing this client's needs. This client is also able to alert the health-care team via the call bell system because they are alert.
2. Although it may be inconvenient for this client to wait for the teaching session to begin, the other three clients have higher priority and physiological needs that require earlier assessment.

89. 1. Recapping a sterile syringe that has not had contact with a client or a nonsterile surface supports sterile technique; the needle of a syringe and the area inside the needle cap are both sterile and pose no microbiological risk of contamination.
2. Holding sterile gloved hands below the waist during a sterile procedure is considered an unsafe practice. Hands held below the waist may not be seen and may inadvertently become contaminated; this violates sterile technique.
3. This is the correct technique. Fluids flow in the direction of gravity. When the tip is held lower than the handle, fluid remains at the level of the gauze and the tip of the forceps; this area is considered sterile.
4. When the metal protective ring and cap are removed from around the top of a multiple-dose vial, the rubber port surface is sterile until it is touched by something nonsterile. The rubber stopper does not have to be wiped with alcohol the first time the vial is accessed with a sterile syringe.
5. Although the inside of a sterile gauze wrapper is sterile, when the paper wrapper becomes wet, capillary action transfers microorganisms from the nonsterile surface of the table to the inside of the wrapper; the gauze then becomes contaminated, which violates sterile technique.

TEST-TAKING TIP: The words *surgical asepsis* in the stem direct attention to content.

90. 1. Pedal pulses are assessed to determine circulation to the feet. The dorsalis pedis (palpable just lateral to the extensor tendon of the great toe) and the posterior tibial (palpable behind and slightly below the medial malleolus of the ankle) are the most frequently assessed pedal pulses.
2. Assessment of blood pressure does not evaluate peripheral circulation in the lower extremities. It assesses the pressure within the arteries when the heart contracts (systolic blood pressure) and between heart contractions (diastolic blood pressure).
3. Lack of hair on the feet and lower extremities is associated with prolonged hypoxia. The hair follicles are denied adequate oxygen and nutrients.
4. Applying pressure to the skin at the tip of a toe causes blanching; when the pressure is released, the normal color should return quickly (within 2 to 3 seconds), indicating adequate

arterial perfusion. A toenail should not be compressed because often a client with impaired peripheral circulation will have thick, yellow toenails.

5. **Discomfort in the legs when walking that is relieved with rest (intermittent claudication) is due to inadequate oxygen at the cellular level for muscle contraction.**

91. 1. **Range-of-motion exercises maximally stretch all muscle groups; this prevents shortening of muscles, which can result in contractures.**
2. Although movement of joints experienced during activity will contribute to preventing contractures, it will not move all joints through their full range; also, prolonged sitting can cause flexion contractures of the hips and knees.
3. Although supporting joints contributes to maintaining functional alignment, which helps prevent contractures, it is not the best intervention.
4. Turning and repositioning a client every 2 hours will reduce pressure, not prevent contractures.

TEST-TAKING TIP: The word *best* in the stem sets a priority.

92. 1. Although *E. coli* is the most common bacteria responsible for UTI, these symptoms are consistent with a complicated UTI and infection of the upper urinary tract.
2. **Dysuria, frequency, hesitancy, urgency, and hematuria are seen in uncomplicated UTIs. Fever, chills, nausea, vomiting, and back pain are signs of an infection of the upper urinary tract or the kidneys.**
3. Although nausea, vomiting, and fever are associated with many gastrointestinal infections, the nurse should suspect complications related to UTI in clients diagnosed with a UTI.
4. Although a fever may be associated with a respiratory infection, this is not the most appropriate option.

93. 1. Instructing a confused client to call the nurse when incontinent of urine and stool is an unrealistic instruction; a cognitively impaired client will have difficulty with this task.
2. **When clients are incontinent, they should be checked frequently and cleaned immediately; feces contain digestive enzymes, and urine contains ammonia and other irritating substances that contribute to skin breakdown.**
3. Sheepskin and an incontinence device (the word *diaper* should be avoided because it is demeaning) hold moisture next to the skin, and their use should be avoided.
4. Although the client should be repositioned frequently, the action in another option is more significant.

TEST-TAKING TIP: The word *best* in the stem sets a priority. The word *always* in option 1 is a specific determiner. The words *incontinent* in the stem and *soiled* in option 1 and *soiling* in option 2 are obscure clang associations. Consider options 1 and 2 carefully. More often than not, an option with a clang association is the correct answer.

94. 1. **The main purpose of pain relief medication is to enable a client to comfortably engage in necessary activity.**
2. If clients remain perfectly still in the semi-Fowler position, they may be able to tolerate pain. However, being sedentary can precipitate complications such as atelectasis, venous stasis, and muscle atrophy.
3. The client is experiencing pain before the next scheduled dose, indicating that the intervention was ineffective.
4. A decrease in the respiratory rate is a side effect, not a therapeutic effect, of an opioid; opioids decrease respiration by depressing the respiratory center in the brainstem.

95. 1. Although visits by siblings are appropriate, this does not address the task of initiative versus guilt.
2. A stuffed animal is appropriate for an infant or a toddler.
3. **Completing homework is an appropriate activity for a school-age child. School-age children are interested in doing and producing.**
4. Watching television does not support the developmental tasks of a school-age child.

TEST-TAKING TIP: The words *school-age child* are key words in the stem that direct attention to content. The word *hospitalized* in the stem and the word *hospital* in option 3 are clang associations.

96. 1. A client with urge incontinence generally is unable to wait 4 hours between voidings.
2. **Toileting the client immediately on request supports continence because the person with urge incontinence must immediately void or lose control of urine.**
3. Encouraging the client to stay near the bathroom promotes isolation and should be avoided.
4. Limiting fluid intake during the early evening and night may be part of a toileting program to provide uninterrupted sleep; however, it does not address the client's need to urinate immediately when feeling the urge to void.

TEST-TAKING TIP: The word *best* in the stem sets a priority. Option 2 is client-centered.

97. **1. Holding the breath at the height of inhalation is desirable because it allows tiny drops of aerosol spray to reach deeper branches of the airway.**
2. Shaking the canister for 3 to 5 seconds before administration is an acceptable practice because it mixes the medication within the solution so that the aerosol drug concentration is even.
3. Rinsing the mouth removes remaining medication, which reduces mucosal irritation.
4. When a metered-dose inhaler is used, inhalation should be slow; this limits bronchial constriction and promotes a more even distribution of the aerosolized medication.
5. Tilting the head back slightly while using a metered-dose inhaler is desirable because it maximizes airway exposure to medication from the inhaler. Tilting the head backward moves the tongue away from the back of the throat, moves the epiglottis away from the trachea, and straightens the passage from the mouth to the trachea.

98. 1. Standing in front of the client is unsafe and does not support confidence. Corridor rails are not continuous, and standing in front does not position the nurse in a way that will protect the client.
2. Instructing the blind client to hold on to the nurse's arm allows the nurse to guide and the client to follow; it supports the client's comfort and promotes confidence.
3. Verbal directions do not provide for the client's safety; also, they do not promote comfort and confidence.
4. Walking on the side while holding the client's elbow is one method to assist a client who has a mobility, not a visual, deficit.

99. 1. The tube is in the stomach, not the lungs.
2. Placing the end of the tube in water is unsafe; if the tube is in the respiratory system rather than the stomach, a deep inhalation may cause aspiration of fluid.
3. Instilling a small amount of normal saline is unsafe; if the tube is in the wrong place (e.g., esophagus, trachea), it may result in aspiration of the fluid.
4. The tube is in the stomach, and application of negative pressure to the tube will cause gastric contents to be pulled up the tube and into the syringe.

TEST-TAKING TIP: The word *tube* in the stem and options 2 and 4 is a clang association. You should examine options 2 and 4 carefully. Option 4 is the correct answer.

100. **1. This provides an opportunity to discuss the illness; eventually, a developing awareness occurs, and the client probably will move on to other coping mechanisms.**
2. This blunt response is confrontational. It may take away the client's coping mechanism, is demeaning, and cuts off communication; the client is using denial to cope with the diagnosis.
3. This response may take away the client's coping mechanism, is demeaning, and cuts off communication; the client is using denial to cope with the diagnosis.
4. This response is demeaning and may cut off communication; the client is using denial to cope with the diagnosis.

TEST-TAKING TIP: Options 2, 3, and 4 deny the client's feelings; confronting the client with reality takes away the coping mechanism of denial that is protecting the ego. Although the word *cancer* in the stem and option 2 is a clang association, this option denies the client's feelings and can be eliminated. Option 1 is client-centered.

Bibliography

Academy of Breastfeeding Medicine (2017). ABM clinical protocol #22: Guidelines for management of jaundice in the breastfeeding infant 35 weeks or more of gestation. 12(5). DOI: 10.1089/bfm.2017.29014.vjf

Ackley BJ, Ladwig GB, Flynn Makic MB: *Nursing diagnosis handbook: An evidence-based guide to planning care.* ed. 11. Mosby Elsevier, St. Louis, 2017.

Adams AK: *The home book of humorous quotations.* Dodd, Mead & Company, New York, 1969.

Alfaro-LeFevre R: *Critical thinking and clinical judgment: A practical approach to outcome-focused thinking.* ed. 4. WB Saunders, Philadelphia, 2009.

Alfaro-LeFevre R: *Critical thinking, clinical reasoning, and clinical judgment: A practical approach.* ed. 6. Elsevier, St. Louis, 2017.

American Association of Colleges of Nursing: *AACN white paper: Distance technology in nursing education.* 2000. http://eric.ed.gov/?id=ED446494, accessed 8/5/2017.

American Hospital Association: *The patient care partnership: Understanding expectations, rights and responsibilities* [patient brochure]. Chicago, 2003. https://www.aha.org/system/files/2018-01/aha-patient-care-partnership.pdf, accessed 1/9/2019.

American Nurses Association: *Nurse's bill of rights.* n.d. http://nursingworld.org/practice-policy/work-environment/health-safety/bill-of-rights-faqs, accessed 8/28/2019.

American Nurses Association: *What is nursing?* n.d. http://www.nursingworld.org/practice-policy/workforce/what-is-nursing/, accessed 8/28/2019.

American Nurses Association: Medication errors: Best practices. n.d. *American Nurse Today.* https://www.americannursetoday.com/medication-errors-best-practices/, accessed 1/10/2019.

American Philosophical Association: *Critical thinking: A statement of expert consensus for purposes of educational assessment and instruction.* The Delphi report: Research findings and recommendations prepared for the committee on pre-college philosophy. (ERIC Document Reproduction Service No. ED 315–423). 1990.

Anderson A: Getting and giving report. *American Journal of Nursing* 118(6):56-60, 2018.

Anthony M: The aging of America. *Home Healthcare Now* 36(6):346, 2018.

Aschenbrenner DS: Promoting drug safety in older adults. *American Journal of Nursing* 118(7):23-24, 2018.

Association for Professionals in Infection Control and Epidemiology, Greene L (ed.), Felix K (lead author): *APIC releases updated guide to preventing catheter-associated urinary tract infections.* 2014. https://www.ajicjournal.org/article/S0196-6553(14)00874-8/fulltext, accessed 8/28/2019.

Barfield, W. D., & Lee, K. G. (2021). Late preterm infants, *UpToDate.* https://www.uptodate.com/contents/late-preterm-infants

Baranoski S, Ayello EA (eds.): *Wound care essentials: Practice principles.* ed. 4. Lippincott Williams & Wilkins, Philadelphia, 2016.

Bastable SB: *Essentials of patient education.* ed. 2. Jones & Bartlett, Sudbury, MA, 2017.

Black BP: *Professional nursing: Concepts & challenges.* ed. 8. Elsevier, St. Louis, 2016.

Boskabadi, H., Rakhshanizadeh, F., & Zakerihamidi, M. (2020). Evaluation of maternal risk factors in neonatal hyperbilirubinemia. *Archives of Iranian Medicine,* 23(2), 128-140

Bradshaw MJ, Hultquist BL: *Innovative teaching strategies in nursing and related health professions.* ed. 7. Jones & Bartlett Learning, Burlington, MA, 2016.

Brennan J, Fischer N, Mauk T, McKinney S, Ruiz D: Optimizing safety for the visually impaired patient. *Nursing Incredibly Easy!* 16(1):44-49, 2018.

Brewer S, Seth S: Stool characteristics explained. *Nursing Incredibly Easy*! 16(3):14-19, 2018.

Brookfield DD: *Developing critical thinkers: Challenging adults to explore alternative ways of thinking and acting*. Josey-Bass, San Francisco, 1991.

Brous E: Lessons learned from litigation: Maintaining professional boundaries. *American Journal of Nursing* 114(7):60-63, 2014.

Brown SJ: *Evidence-based nursing: The research-practice connection*. ed. 4. Jones & Bartlett Learning, Burlington, MA, 2016.

Brown T: Fixing America's health care system. *American Journal of Nursing* 118(11):62, 2018.

Bryant RA, Nix DP: *Acute and chronic wounds: Current management concepts*. ed. 5. Elsevier Mosby, St. Louis, 2015.

Burton MA, Smith D, Ludwig LJ: *Fundamentals of nursing care: Concepts, connections & skills*. ed. 3. FA Davis, Philadelphia, 2019.

Butcher H, Bulechek G, McCloskey Diochterman J, Wagner C: *Nursing interventions classification (NIC)*. ed. 7. St. Louis, Mosby, 2019.

Case B: Walking around the elephant: A critical-thinking strategy for decision making. *Journal of Continuing Education in Nursing* 25(3):101-109, 1994.

Catalano JT: *Nursing now!* ed. 7. FA Davis, Philadelphia, 2015.

Center for Nursing Classification and Clinical Effectiveness (CNC): n.d. www.nursing.uiowa.edu/center-for-nursing-classification-and-clinical-effectiveness, accessed 1/8/2019.

Centers for Disease Control and Prevention. *Clean hands count for safe healthcare*. 2017. https://www.cdc.gov/features/handhygiene/index.html, accessed 1/8/2019.

Centers for Disease Control and Prevention: *Hand hygiene saves lives*. 2010. http://www.cdc.gov/cdctv/healthyliving/hygiene/hand-hygiene-saves-lives.html, accessed 1/8/2019.

Centers for Disease Control and Prevention: *Important facts about falls*. 2017. https://www.cdc.gov/homeandrecreationalsafety/falls/adultfalls.html, accessed 1/8/2019.

Centers for Disease Control and Prevention: *Ten leading causes of death and injury*. 2017. https://www.cdc.gov/injury/wisqars/LeadingCauses.html, accessed 8/28/2019.

Chaffee J: *Thinking critically*. ed. 12. Cengage Learning, Stamford, CT, 2018.

Chancellor J: Student voices: Effective study habits for nursing students. *Nursing* 43(4): 68-69, 2013.

Cherry B, Jacob SR: *Contemporary nursing: Issues, trends, & management*. ed. 7. Elsevier, St. Louis, 2017.

Colgrove KC, Doherty C: *Pharmacology success*. ed. 3. FA Davis, Philadelphia, 2019.

Coyle R, Mazaleski A: Initiating and sustaining a fall prevention program. *Nursing* 46(5):16-21, 2016.

Dahlkemper TR: *Anderson's caring for older adults holistically*. 6th ed. FA Davis, Philadelphia, 2016.

Daly W: Critical thinking as an outcome of nursing education: What is it? Why is it important to nursing practice? *Journal of Advanced Nursing* 28(2):323-331, 1998.

Davis C: Critical thinking skills for back to school. *Nursing Made Incredibly Easy!* 12(5): 11-13, 2014.

Davis C: The importance of professional standards. *Nursing Made Incredibly Easy!* 12(5):4, 2014.

de Castillo SLM, Werner-McCullough M: *Calculating drug dosages: A patient-safe approach to nursing and math*. FA Davis, Philadelphia, 2017.

de Castillo SLM: *Strategies, techniques, & approaches to critical thinking: A clinical reasoning workbook for nurses*. ed. 6. Elsevier, St. Louis, 2017.

Delamont A: On the horizon: How to avoid the top seven nursing errors. *Nursing Made Incredibly Easy!* 11(2):8-10, 2013.

Dillon PM: *Clinical simulations for nursing education—participant volume*. ed. 2. FA Davis, Philadelphia, 2018.

Dillon PM: *Nursing health assessment: A critical thinking, case studies approach*. ed. 2. FA Davis, Philadelphia, 2007.

Dillon PM: *Nursing health assessment: Clinical pocket guide*. ed. 2. FA Davis, Philadelphia, 2006.

Dillon PM: *Nursing health assessment: The foundation of clinical practice*. ed. 3. FA Davis, Philadelphia, 2016.

Doenges ME, Moorhouse MF, Murr AC: *Nursing diagnosis manual: Planning, individualizing, and documenting client care*. ed. 5. FA Davis, Philadelphia, 2016.

Erikson EH: *Childhood and society*. Norton, New York, 1993.

Facione PA: *The executive summary: The Delphi Report.* California Academic Press, Millbrae, CA, 1990.

Ferguson R: Care coordination at end of life: The nurse's role. *Nursing* 48(2):11-13, 2018.

Finkelman A: *Leadership and management for nurses: Core competencies for quality care*. ed. 3. Pearson Education, Upper Saddle River, NJ, 2016.

Flynn J: Understanding the needs of transgender patients. *Home Healthcare Now* 36(2): 136-137, 2018.

Gerber L: Understanding the nurse's role as a patient advocate. *Nursing* 48(4):55-58, 2018.

Gibson A, VanRiel Y, Kautz D: Encourage early conversations about palliative care. *Nursing* 48(5):11-12, 2018.

Gibson M, Keeling A: Shaping family and community health: A historical perspective. *Family & Community Health* 37(3):168-169, 2014.

Glennon R: It's about quality of life, not quantity. *Nursing* 44(8):18, 2014.

Gobeyn JL: Caring for undocumented immigrants. *Nursing* 48(8):54-57, 2018.

Godshall M, Riehl M: Preventing medication errors in the information age. *Nursing* 48(9):56-58, 2018.

Gordon M: *Assess notes: Assessment and diagnostic reasoning*. FA Davis, Philadelphia, 2008.

Gordon M: *Nursing diagnosis: Process and application*. ed. 3. Mosby, St. Louis, 1994.

Gorski LA: *Phillips's manual of I.V. therapeutics*. ed. 7. FA Davis, Philadelphia, 2018.

Green YS: Safety implications for the homebound patient with dementia. *Home Healthcare Now* 36(6):386-391, 2018.

Grey JE, Enoch S, Harding KG: Wound assessment. *BMJ* 332(7536):285-288, 2006. https://www.ncbi.nlm.nih.gov/pmc/articles/PMC1360405/, accessed 1/9/2019.

Grimley-Baker K: Preventing suicide beyond psychiatric units. *Nursing* 48(3):59-61, 2018.

Grossman SC, Valiga TM: *The new leadership challenge: Creating the future of nursing*. ed. 5. FA Davis, Philadelphia, 2017.

Gulanick M, Myers JL: *Nursing care plans: Diagnoses, interventions, and outcomes*. ed. 9. Elsevier Health Sciences, St. Louis, 2016.

Hale A, Hovey J: *Fluid and electrolyte notes: Nurse's clinical pocket guide*. FA Davis, Philadelphia, 2013.

Hale D, Marshall K: Multiple health problems in older adults. *Home Healthcare Now* 37(1):50, 2019.

Hamric AB, Schwartz JK, Cohen L, Mahon M: Assisted suicide/aid in dying: What is the nurse's role? *American Journal of Nursing* 118(5):50-59, 2018.

Hargrove-Huttel RA, Colgrove KC: *Prioritization, delegation, & management of care for the NCLEX-RN®* exam. FA Davis, Philadelphia, 2014.

Hayes K, Hayes D: Best practices for unclogging feeding tubes in adults. *Nursing* 48(6):66, 2018.

Henry Ford Quotes. ps://www.goodreads.com/quotes/978-whether-you-think-you-can-or-you-think-you-can-t—you-re, accessed 7/12/19.

Holmes TH, Rahe RH: The social readjustment rating scale. *Journal of Psychosomatic Research* 11(2):213-218, 1967.

Hopp L, Rittenmeyer L: *Introduction to evidence-based practice: A practical guide for nursing.* FA Davis, Philadelphia, 2012.

Horntvedt T: *Calculating dosages safely: A dimensional analysis approach*. FA Davis, Philadelphia, 2014.

Huber D: *Leadership and nursing care management*. ed. 6. Elsevier, St. Louis, 2017.

Hurst D: Mortal distress in families. *American Journal of Nursing* 16(5):6-7, 2018.

Huston CJ: *Leadership roles and management functions in nursing: Theory and application*. ed. 9. Lippincott Williams & Wilkins, Baltimore, 2017.

Huston CJ: *Professional issues in nursing: Challenges and opportunities*. ed. 4. Lippincott Williams & Wilkins, Baltimore, 2016.

Irland, N. (2021). Comprehensive examination. In *Maternal and newborn success* (4th edition, p. 483). F. A. Davis Publishers.

Jackson SA: Rapid response teams: What's the latest? *Nursing* 47(12):34-41, 2017.

Jones J: Misread labels as a cause of medication errors. *American Journal of Nursing* 114(3): 11, 2014.

Jones SA: *Pocket anatomy and physiology*. ed. 3. FA Davis, Philadelphia, 2017.

Kaakinen JR, Coehlo DP, Steele R, Tabacco A, Harmon Hanson SM: *Family health care nursing: Theory, practice, and research*. ed. 6. FA Davis, Philadelphia, 2018.

Kirkland-Kyhn H, Generao SA, Teleten, O, Young, H: Teaching wound care to family caregivers. *American Journal of Nursing* 118(3):63-67, 2018.

Kirkland-Kyhn H, Martin S, Zaratkiewicz S, Whitmore M, Young H: Ostomy care at home. *American Journal of Nursing* 118(4):63-68, 2018.

Kirkland-Kyhn H, Zaratkiewicz S, Teleten O, Young H: Caring for aging skin. *American Journal of Nursing* 118(2):60-63, 2018.

Kübler-Ross E: *On death and dying*. Macmillan, New York, 1969.

Labriole J, MacAulay C, Williams K, Bunting D, Pettorini-D'Amico S: Implementing bedside shift report: Walking the walk and talking the talk. *Nursing* 48(3):1-4, 2018.

LaCharity LA, Kumagai CK, Bartz B. *Prioritization, delegation, and assignment: Practice exercises for the NCLEX®* examination. ed. 4. Elsevier, St. Louis, 2019.

Lange JW: *The nurse's role in promoting optimal health of older adults: Thriving in the wisdom years*. FA Davis, Philadelphia, 2012.

Laske RA, Stephens BA: Confusion states: Sorting out delirium, dementia, and depression. *Nursing Incredibility Easy!* 16(6):13-16, 2018.

Laskowski-Jones L: Communication: The good, the bad, and the ugly. *Nursing* 44(6):6, 2014.

LeBlanc K, Campbell KE, Wood E, Beeckman D: Best practice recommendations for prevention and management of skin tears in aged skin: An overview. *Journal of Wound, Ostomy and Continence Nursing* 45(6):540-542, 2018.

Lee A: The role of informatics in nursing. *Nursing Made Incredibly Easy!* 12(4):55, 2014.

Lewis M, Kohtz C, Emmerling S, Fisher M, Mcgarvey J: Pain control and nonpharmacologic interventions. *Nursing* 48(9):65-68, 2018.

Lindauer A, Sexson K, Harvath TA: Medication management for people with dementia. *American Journal of Nursing* 117(5 Suppl 1):S17-S21, 2017.

Lippincott's Nursing Center.com: Evidence-Based Practice Network. Wolters Kluwer Health/Lippincott Williams & Wilkins, Philadelphia, n.d. https://www.nursingcenter.com/evidencebasedpracticenetwork, accessed 1/9/2019.

Marquis BL, Huston CJ: *Leadership roles and management functions in nursing: Theory and application*. ed. 9. Lippincott Williams & Wilkins, Baltimore, 2017.

Marrelli TM: *Home care nursing: Surviving in an ever-changing care environment*. Sigma Theta Tau International, Indianapolis, IN, Marrelli and Associates, 2017.

Marshall KA, Hale D: Elder abuse. *Home Healthcare Now* 36(1):51-52, 2018.

Marshall KA, Hale D: Nutrition in older adults. *Home Healthcare Now* 36(3):192-193, 2018.

Maslow AH: *A theory of human motivation*. Martino Fine Books Publishers, Eastford, CT, 2013.

Maslow AH: *Motivation and personality*. ed. 2. Harper & Row, New York, 1970.

Mason J, Leavitt JK, Chaffee MW (eds.): *Policy and politics in nursing and healthcare*. ed. 7. Elsevier Saunders, St. Louis, 2015.

Mazur EE, Litch NA: *Lutz's nutrition and diet therapy*. ed. 7. FA Davis, Philadelphia, 2018.

Mazurek Melnyk B, Fineout-Overholt E: *Evidence-based practice in nursing and health care: A guide to best practice*. ed. 4. Wolters Kluwer Health/Lippincott Williams & Wilkins, Philadelphia, 2019.

McFarland MR, Wehbe-Alamah HB: *Leininger's culture care diversity and universality: A worldwide nursing theory*. ed. 3. Jones & Bartlett Learning, Burlington, MA, 2015.

McKenny LM, Teessier E, Hogan MA: *Mosby's pharmacology in nursing*. ed. 22. Elsevier, St. Louis, 2006.

Meyers E: *RNotes: Nurse's clinical pocket guide*. ed. 5. FA Davis, Philadelphia, 2008.

Meyers E, Hale A: *RN pocket procedures*. ed. 2. FA Davis, Philadelphia, 2013.

Mick J: Call to action: How to implement evidence-based nursing practice. *Nursing* 47(4):36-43, 2017.

Moorhead S, Swanson E, Johnson M, Maas ML: *Nursing outcomes classification (NOC): Measurement of health outcomes*. ed. 6. Elsevier, St. Louis, 2018.

Muntean, W., Lindsay, M., Betts, J., Kim, D., Woo, A., Dickison, P. (2016). Separating assessment of subject matter knowledge from assessment of higher-order cognitive constructs. Paper presented at American Educational Research Association Annual Meeting, Washington, D.C. https://www.ncsbn.org/NextGenNCLEX_InFocusWinter2018.pdf

National Council of State Boards of Nursing: *Innovations in education regulation report: Background and literature review*. 2009. www.ncsbn.org/Innovations_Report.pdf, accessed 1/9/2019.

National Pressure Ulcer Advisory Panel: Pressure ulcers get new terminology and staging definitions: Staff report. *Nursing Management* 48(1):46-50, 2017.

Nix S: *Williams' basic nutrition and diet therapy*. ed. 15. Elsevier Health Sciences, St Louis, MO, 2017.

Norlander L: *A nurse's guide to end-of-life care*. ed. 2. Sigma Theta Tau International, Indianapolis, IN, 2014. https://www.sigmanursing.org/connect-engage/news-detail/2014/06/18/a-nurse-s-guide-to-end-of-life-care, accessed 8/28/2019.

Nugent PM, Vitale BA: *Fundamentals: Davis essential nursing content + practice questions*. ed. 2. FA Davis, Philadelphia, 2017.

Nugent PM, Vitale BA: *Fundamentals success: A course review applying critical thinking to test taking*. ed. 6. FA Davis, Philadelphia, 2022.

O'Keeffe M, Saver C (contributors): *Communication, collaboration & you: Tools, tips, and techniques for nursing practice*. American Nurses Association, Silver Spring, MD, 2013.

Perry AG, Potter PA, Ostendorf W: *Clinical nursing skills and techniques*. ed. 9. Mosby, St. Louis, 2017.

Pless BS, Clayton GM: Clarifying the concept of critical thinking in nursing. *Journal of Nursing Education* 32(9):425-428, 1993.

Polan EU, Taylor DR: *Journey across the life span: Human development and health promotion*. ed. 6. FA Davis, Philadelphia, 2019.

Pond EE, Bradshaw MJ: Teaching strategies for critical thinking. *Nurse Educator* 16(3): 18-22, 1991.

Powell-Cope G, Thomason S, Bulat T, Pippins KM, Young H: Preventing falls and fall-related injuries at home. *American Journal of Nursing* 118(1):58-61, 2018.

Pozgar GD: *Legal and ethical issues for health professionals*. ed. 4. Jones & Bartlett Learning, Burlington, MA, 2016.

Quinlan-Colwell A: Controlling pain: Making an ethical plan for treating patients in pain. *Nursing* 43(10):64-68, 2013.

Quinn J: Five ways healthcare informatics help nurses. *EBSCO Health Notes* September 13, 2017. https://health.ebsco.com/blog/article/five-way-healthcare-informatics-help-nurses, accessed 1/10/2019.

Raines V: *Davis's basic math review for nursing and health professionals: With step-by-step solutions*. ed. 2. FA Davis, Philadelphia, 2017.

Ray MA: *Transcultural caring dynamics in nursing and health care*. ed. 2. FA Davis, Philadelphia, 2016.

Riley JB: *Communication in nursing*. ed. 8. Elsevier Health Sciences, St. Louis, 2017.

Saba VK, McCormick K: *Essentials of nursing informatics*. ed. 6. McGraw-Hill, New York, 2015.

Sabella D: Antidepressant medications. *American Journal of Nursing* 118(9):52-59, 2018.

Safire W: *Good advice*. Times Books, New York, 1982.

Salladay SA: Ethical problems. [Intimate Partner Violence]. *Nursing* 46(8):12-13, 2016.

Satorre J: Managing medication errors. *American Journal of Nursing* 117(4):13, 2017.

Savage CL, Kub JE, Groves SL: *Public health science and nursing practice: Caring for populations*. FA Davis, Philadelphia, 2016.

Scanlon V, Sanders T: *Essentials of anatomy and physiology*. ed. 8. FA Davis, Philadelphia, 2019.

Schuster PM: *Communication for nurses: How to prevent harmful events and promote patient safety*. FA Davis, Philadelphia, 2010.

Scottish Proverbs. https://ww.inspirationalstories.com/proverbs/scottish-many-brings-the-rake-but-few-the-shovel/, accessed 7/12/2019.

Selye H: *The stress of life*. Rev ed. McGraw Hill, New York, 1976.

Shastay A: Correct use of inhalers: Help patients breathe easier. *Home Healthcare Now* 35(4):262-263, 2018.

Smith DM, Kautz D: Protect older adults from polypharmacy hazards. *Nursing* 48(2): 56-59, 2018.

Sofer D: Making hospitals less threatening to patients with dementia. *American Journal of Nursing* 118(6):18-19, 2018.

Squires A: Evidence-based approaches to breaking down language barriers. *Nursing* 47(9):34-40. 2017.

Stanhope M, Lancaster J: *Foundations of nursing in the community: Community-oriented practice*. ed. 4. Elsevier Mosby, St. Louis, 2019.

Stanhope M, Lancaster J: *Public health nursing: Population centered health care in the community*. ed. 9. Elsevier Mosby, St. Louis, 2015.

Stevenson E, Purpuro T: Homeless people: Nursing care with dignity. *Nursing* 48(6): 58-62, 2018.

Taber's cyclopedic medical dictionary. ed. 20. FA Davis, Philadelphia, 2017.

Taggart, W, and Torrance, PE: *Administrator's Manual for the Human Information Processing and Survey.* Bensenville, IL: Scholastic Testing Service, 1984.

The Joint Commission: Facts about the official "do not use" list of abbreviation. 2019. https://www.jointcommission.org/facts_about_do_not_use_list/, accessed 8/28/2019.

The Leapfrog Group: *Safe practices*. n.d. http://www.leapfroggroup.org/ratings-reports/safe-practices, accessed 1/9/2019.

Thompson GS: *Understanding anatomy & physiology: A visual, auditory, interactive approach*. ed. 3. FA Davis, Philadelphia, 2019.

Thompson J: *Essential health assessment*. FA Davis, Philadelphia, 2017.

Todd B: Multidrug-resistant organisms and contact precautions. *American Journal of Nursing* 118(8):67-69, 2018.

Townsend MC, Morgan KI: *Pocket guide to psychiatric nursing*. ed. 10. FA Davis, Philadelphia, 2018.

Townsend MC, Morgan KI: *Psychiatric mental health nursing: Concepts of care in evidence-based practice*. ed. 9. FA Davis, Philadelphia, 2018.

Treas LS: *Basic nursing: Thinking, doing, and caring*. ed. 3. FA Davis, Philadelphia, 2022.

Ulbricht C: *Davis's pocket guide to herbs and supplements*. FA Davis, Philadelphia, 2011.

U.S. Department of Health and Human Services: *Healthy People 2030 framework*. 2019. https://www.healthypeople.gov/2020/About-Healthy-People/Development-Healthy-People-2030/Framework/, accessed 8/28/2019.

U.S. Department of Labor, Occupational Safety and Health Administration: *Bloodborne pathogens and needlestick prevention*. n.d. https://www.osha.gov/SLTC/bloodbornepathogens/index.html, accessed 1/9/2019.

U.S. Food and Drug Administration: *Changes to the nutrition facts label*. 2018. https://www.fda.gov/Food/GuidanceRegulation/GuidanceDocumentsRegulatoryInformation/LabelingNutrition/ucm385663.htm, accessed 1/9/2019.

U.S. Food and Drug Administration: *How to understand and use the nutrition facts label*. 2018. https://www.fda.gov/Food/LabelingNutrition/ucm274593.htm, accessed 1/9/2019.

U.S. Food and Drug Administration: *Orange book: Approved drug products with therapeutic equivalence evaluations*. 2018. http://www.accessdata.fda.gov/scripts/cder/ob/default.cfm, accessed 1/9/2019.

U.S. Food and Drug Administration: *Working to reduce medication errors*. 2019. https://www.fda.gov/drugs/drug-information-consumers/working-reduce-medication-errors, accessed 8/28/2019.

Valiga T: Leaders, managers, and followers: Working in harmony. *Nursing* 49(1):45-48, 2019.

Vallerand AH, Sanoski CA: *Davis's drug guide for nurses*. ed. 17. FA Davis, Philadelphia, 2021.

Van Leeuwen AM, Bladh ML: *Davis's comprehensive handbook of laboratory and diagnostic tests with nursing implications*. ed. 9. FA Davis, Philadelphia, 2021.

Venes D (ed.): *Taber's cyclopedic medical dictionary*. ed. 23. FA Davis, Philadelphia, 2017.

Vitale BA: *NCLEX-RN Notes: Core review and exam prep*. ed. 3. FA Davis, Philadelphia, 2017.

Vogelstein E: Questioning orders: A bioethical framework. *Nursing* 49(1):14-16, 2019.

Weiss SA, Tappen RM: *Essentials of nursing leadership & management*. ed. 7. FA Davis, Philadelphia, 2019.

Weston D, Burgess A, Roberts S: *Infection prevention and control at a glance*. Wiley Blackwell, Hoboken, NJ, 2017.

Wilkinson JM: *Nursing process and critical thinking*. ed. 5. Prentice Hall, Upper Saddle River, NJ, 2012.

Wilkinson JM, Treas LS, Barnett KL, Smith MH: *Fundamentals of nursing*. ed. 4. FA Davis, Philadelphia, 2019.

Williams LS, Hopper PD: *Understanding medical-surgical nursing*. ed. 6. FA Davis, Philadelphia, 2019.

Wilson A: Antibiotic treatment for *Clostridium difficile* infection in adults. *American Journal of Nursing* 118(7):63, 2018.

Woodruff J, Hohler SE: Taking the initiative to reduce surgical site infections. *Nursing* 48(12):62-64, 2018.

Wormer, K. C., Jamil, R. T., & Bryant, S. B. (2022). Acute postpartum hemorrhage. *StatPearls*, Treasure Island (FL). *StatPearls* Publishing. https://www.ncbi.nlm.nih.gov/books/NBK499988/

World Health Organization: *Falls.* 2018. https://www.who.int/news-room/fact-sheets/detail/falls/, accessed 8/28/2019.

Zerwekh J, Garneau AZ: *Nursing today: Transition and trends*. ed. 9. Elsevier Saunders, St. Louis, 2018.

Zolot J: First guidelines for diagnosing and managing concussion in kids. *American Journal of Nursing* 118(12):14, 2018.

Glossary of English Words Commonly Encountered on Nursing Examinations

Abnormality — defect, irregularity, anomaly, oddity, malformation

Absence — nonappearance, lack, nonattendance

Abundant — plentiful, rich, profuse, copious

Accelerate — go faster, speed up, increase, hasten

Accumulate — build up, collect, gather, multiply, assemble

Accurate — precise, correct, exact, valid

Achievement — accomplishment, success, reaching, attainment, completing

Acknowledge — admit, recognize, accept, reply, allow, realize

Activate — start, turn on, stimulate, operate, initiate

Adequate — sufficient, ample, plenty, enough, acceptable

Angle — slant, approach, direction, point of view

Application — use, treatment, request, claim

Approximately — about, around, in the region of, more or less, roughly speaking, nearly, almost

Arrange — position, place, organize, display, order, align

Associated — linked, related, connected

Attention — notice, concentration, awareness, thought

Authority — power, right, influence, clout, expert

Avoid — keep away from, evade, let alone, refrain from

Balanced — stable, neutral, steady, fair, impartial, level

Barrier — barricade, blockage, obstruction, obstacle

Best — most excellent, most important, greatest, leading, supreme, ideal, perfect

Capable — able, competent, accomplished, experienced, qualified, skilled

Capacity — ability, capability, aptitude, role, power, size

Central — middle, mid, innermost, vital, halfway, interior, nuclear

Challenge — confront, dare, dispute, test, defy, face up to

Characteristic — trait, feature, attribute, quality, typical, normal

Circular — round, spherical, globular

Collect — gather, assemble, amass, accumulate, bring together, accrue, multiply

Commitment — promise, vow, dedication, obligation, pledge, assurance, duty

Commonly — usually, normally, frequently, generally, universally, repeatedly

Compare — contrast, evaluate, match up to, weigh or judge against

Compartment — section, part, cubicle, booth, stall, pocket, pouch

Complex — difficult, multifaceted, compound, multipart, intricate

Complexity — difficulty, intricacy, complication, problem, involvement

Component — part, element, factor, section, constituent, piece, item, portion

Comprehensive — complete, inclusive, broad, thorough

Conceal — hide, cover up, obscure, mask, suppress, secrete, secret, camouflage

Conceptualize — to form an idea

Concern — worry, anxiety, fear, alarm, distress, unease, trouble

Concisely — briefly, in a few words, succinctly

Conclude — make a judgment, determine, decide

Confidence — self-assurance, certainty, poise, self-reliance

Congruent — matching, fitting, going together well, identical in form

Consequence — result, effect, outcome, end result

Constituents — elements, components, parts that make up a whole

Contain — hold, enclose, surround, include, control, limit

Continual — repeated, constant, persistent, recurrent, frequent, recurring

Continuous — constant, incessant, nonstop, unremitting, permanent

Contribute — be a factor, add, give, supply, lend

Convene — assemble, call together, summon, organize, arrange

Convenience — expediency, handiness, ease

Coordinate — organize, direct, manage, bring together, arrange

Create — make, invent, establish, generate, produce, fashion, build, construct

Creative — imaginative, original, inspired, inventive, resourceful, innovative

Critical — serious, grave, significant, dangerous, life-threatening

Cue — signal, reminder, prompt, sign, indication

Curiosity — inquisitiveness, interest, nosiness, snooping

Damage — injure, harm, hurt, break, wound, impair, disfigure, ruin

Deduct — subtract, take away, remove, withhold

Deficient — lacking, wanting, underprovided, scarce, faulty

Defining — important, crucial, major, essential, significant, central

Defuse — resolve, calm, soothe, neutralize, rescue, mollify

Delay — hold up, wait, hinder, postpone, slow down, hesitate, linger

Demand — insist, claim, require, command, stipulate, ask

Describe — explain, tell, express, illustrate, depict, portray

Design — plan, invent, intend, aim, propose, devise

Desirable — wanted, pleasing, enviable, popular, sought after, attractive, advantageous

Detail — feature, aspect, element, factor, facet, characteristic

Deteriorate — worsen, decline, weaken, decay, degrade

Determine — decide, conclude, resolve, agree on

Dexterity — skillfulness, handiness, agility, deftness

Dignity — self-respect, self-esteem, decorum, formality, poise

Dimension — aspect, measurement, feature, element, facet

Diminish — reduce, lessen, weaken, detract, moderate

Discharge — release, dismiss, set free, leak, exude, emit, dispense

Discontinue — stop, cease, halt, suspend, terminate, withdraw

Disorder — complaint, problem, confusion, chaos

Display — show, exhibit, demonstrate, present, put on view

Dispose — get rid of, arrange, order, set out, discard

Dissatisfaction — displeasure, discontent, unhappiness, disappointment

Distinguish — separate, classify, recognize differences

Distract — divert, sidetrack, disturb, confusing

Distress — suffering, trouble, anguish, misery, agony, concern, sorrow

Distribute — deliver, spread out, hand out, issue, dispense, administer

Disturbed — troubled, unstable, concerned, worried, distressed, anxious, uneasy

Diversional — serving to distract

Don — put on, dress oneself in

Dramatic — spectacular

Drape — cover, wrap, dress, swathe

Dysfunction — abnormal, impaired

Edge — perimeter, boundary, periphery, brink, border, rim, margin

Effective — successful, useful, helpful, valuable, functional

Efficient — not wasteful, effective, competent, resourceful, capable

Elasticity — stretch, spring, suppleness, flexibility

Eliminate — get rid of, eradicate, abolish, remove, purge, end, stop, terminate

Embarrass — make uncomfortable, make self-conscious, humiliate, mortify

Emerge — appear, come, materialize, become known

Emphasize — call attention to, accentuate, stress, highlight

Ensure — make certain, guarantee, secure, confirm, verify, check

Environment — setting, surroundings, location, atmosphere, milieu, situation

Episode — event, incident, occurrence, experience

Essential — necessary, fundamental, vital, important, crucial, critical, indispensable

Etiology — assigned cause, origin

Exaggerate — overstate, inflate

Excel — stand out, shine, surpass, outclass

Excessive — extreme, too much, unwarranted

Exertion — intense or prolonged physical effort, exercise, labor, activity

Exhibit — show signs of, reveal, display, present, demonstrate

Expand — get bigger, enlarge, spread out, increase, swell, inflate

Expect — wait for, anticipate, imagine

Expectation — hope, anticipation, belief, prospect, probability

Experience — knowledge, skill, occurrence, know-how

Expose — lay open, leave unprotected, allow to be seen, reveal, disclose, exhibit

External — outside, exterior, outer, surface, superficial, visible

Facilitate — make easy, make possible, help, assist, aid, promote, advance

Factor — part, feature, reason, cause, think, issue

Focus — center, focal point, hub

Fragment — piece, portion, section, part, splinter, chip, particle, sliver, flake

Function — purpose, role, job, task, use

Furnish — supply, provide, give, deliver, equip

Further — additional, more, extra, added, supplementary

Generalize — take a broad view, simplify, make inferences from particulars

Generate — make, produce, create, initiate, induce

Gentle — mild, calm, tender, peaceful, kind

Girth — circumference, bulk, weight, size

Highest — uppermost, maximum, peak, main

Hinder — hold back, delay, hamper, obstruct, impede, inhibit, arrest

Humane — caring, kind, gentle, compassionate, benevolent, civilized

Ignore — pay no attention to, disregard, overlook, discount

Imbalance — unevenness, inequality, disparity, variance
Immediate — insistent, urgent, direct, rapid, quick, sudden
Impair — damage, harm, weaken, diminish, reduce, impede
Implantation — insertion
Implement — employ, execute, carry out, administer
Impotent — powerless, weak, incapable, ineffective, unable, unsuccessful
Inadvertent — unintentional, chance, unplanned, accidental
Include — comprise, take in, contain, involve
Indicate — point out, sign of, designate, specify, show
Ineffective — unproductive, unsuccessful, useless, vain, futile
Inevitable — predictable, expected, unavoidable, foreseeable, certain
Influence — power, pressure, sway, manipulate, affect, effect
Initiate — start, begin, open, commence, instigate, launch, establish
Insert — put in, add, supplement, introduce
Inspect — look over, check, examine
Inspire — motivate, energize, encourage, enthuse
Institutionalize — place in a facility for treatment
Integrate — put together, mix, add, combine, assimilate, merge, unite, join, fuse, blend
Integrity — honesty, ethics, morals, nobility, virtue, fairness, sincerity, truthfulness
Interfere — get in the way, hinder, obstruct, impede, hamper
Interpret — explain the meaning of, make understandable
Intervention — action, activity
Intolerance — bigotry, prejudice, narrow-mindedness, bias, inequality
Involuntary — instinctive, reflex, unintentional, automatic, uncontrolled
Irreversible — permanent, irrevocable, irreparable, unalterable
Irritability — sensitivity to stimuli, fretful, quick excitability
Justify — explain in accordance with reason, rationalize, defend
Likely — probably, possible, expected
Liquefy — change into or make more fluid, dissolve, melt
Logical — using reason, thinking, intelligent, wise, sensible
Longevity — long life
Lowest — inferior in rank, common, simple, subordinate
Maintain — continue, uphold, preserve, sustain, retain
Majority — the greater part of, more than half
Mention — talk about, refer to, state, cite, declare, point out
Minimal — least, smallest, nominal, negligible, token
Minimize — reduce, diminish, lessen, curtail, decrease to smallest possible
Mobilize — activate, organize, assemble, gather together, rally
Modify — change, adapt, adjust, revise, alter, improve, reform, transform
Moist — slightly wet, damp, humid, clammy, sweaty
Multiple — many, numerous, several, various
Natural — normal, ordinary, unaffected
Negative — no, harmful, downbeat, pessimistic, adverse
Negotiate — bargain, talk, discuss, consult, cooperate, settle
Notice — become aware of, see, observe, discern, detect
Notify — inform, tell, alert, advise, warn, report, caution
Nurture — care for, raise, rear, foster, support, encourage, promote, develop
Obsess — preoccupy, consume, torment, dominate, rule, control, be fixated
Occupy — live in, inhabit, reside in, engage in, settled, dwell in
Occurrence — event, incident, happening, experience, phenomenon
Odorous — scented, stinking, aromatic, smelly, pungent
Offensive — unpleasant, distasteful, nasty, disgusting
Opportunity — chance, prospect, break
Organize — put in order, arrange, sort, categorize, classify
Origin — source, starting point, cause, beginning, derivation, etiology
Pace — speed, rate, swiftness, quickness, velocity
Parameter — limit, factor, limitation, issue
Participant — member, contributor, partaker, applicant, candidate
Perspective — viewpoint, view, perception
Position — place, location, point, spot, situation, site, setting, area
Practice — do, carry out, perform, apply, follow
Precipitate — cause to happen, bring on, hasten, abrupt, sudden
Predetermine — fix or set beforehand
Predictable — expected, knowable, foreseeable, anticipated, likely
Preference — favorite, liking, first choice
Prepare — get ready, plan, make, train, arrange, organize
Prescribe — set down, stipulate, order, recommend, impose
Previous — earlier, prior, before, preceding
Primarily — first, above all, mainly, mostly, largely, principally, predominantly
Primary — first, main, basic, chief, most important, key, prime, major, crucial

Priority — main concern, giving first attention to, order of importance, preference

Production — making, creation, construction, assembly, building

Profuse — a lot of, plentiful, copious, abundant, generous, prolific, bountiful

Prolong — extend, delay, put off, lengthen, draw out, elongate, continue

Promote — encourage, support, endorse, sponsor

Proportion — ratio, amount, quantity, part of, percentage, section of

Provide — give, offer, supply, make available, issue, furnish, dispense, yield

Rationalize — explain, reason, justify

Realistic — practical, sensible, reasonable, rational, logical

Receive — get, accept, take delivery of, obtain, secure, acquire, derive

Recognize — acknowledge, appreciate, identify, aware of

Recovery — healing, mending, improvement, recuperation, renewal

Reduce — decrease, lessen, ease, moderate, diminish, minimize, shrink, narrow

Reestablish — reinstate, restore, return, bring back

Regard — consider, look upon, relate to, respect

Regular — usual, normal, ordinary, standard, expected, conventional

Relative — comparative, family member

Relevance — importance of

Reluctant — unwilling, hesitant, disinclined, indisposed, adverse

Reminisce — recall and review remembered experiences

Remove — take away, get rid of, eliminate, eradicate, detach, separate

Reposition — move, relocate, change position

Require — need, want, necessitate

Resist — oppose, defend against, keep from, refuse to go along with, defy

Resolution — decree, solution, decision, ruling, promise

Resolve — make up your mind, solve, determine, decide, fix, rectify

Response — reply, answer, reaction, retort

Restore — reinstate, reestablish, bring back, return to, refurbish

Restrict — limit, confine, curb, control, contain, hold back, hamper

Retract — take back, draw in, withdraw, apologize

Reveal — make known, disclose, divulge, expose, tell, make public

Review — appraisal, reconsider, evaluation, assessment, examination, analysis

Ritual — custom, ceremony, formal procedure

Robust — sturdy, vigorous, strong, powerful, muscular, hardy, healthy, fit

Rotate — turn, go around, spin, swivel, revolve

Routine — usual, habit, custom, practice

Satisfaction — approval, fulfillment, pleasure, happiness, content, pride, delight

Satisfy — please, convince, fulfill, make happy, gratify

Secure — safe, protected, fixed firmly, sheltered, confident, obtain

Sequential — chronological, in order of occurrence

Significant — important, major, considerable, noteworthy, momentous

Slight — small, slim, minor, unimportant, insignificant, insult, snub

Source — basis, foundation, starting place, cause

Specific — exact, particular, detail, explicit, definite, certain, fixed, set, distinct

Stable — steady, even, constant, firm, solid, secure, sturdy, immovable

Statistics — figures, data, information

Subtract — take away, deduct, remove, withdraw

Success — achievement, victory, accomplishment

Surround — enclose, encircle, contain

Suspect — think, believe, suppose, guess, deduce, infer, distrust, doubtful

Sustain — maintain, carry on, prolong, continue, nourish, suffer

Synonymous — same as, identical, equal, tantamount

Systemic — affecting the entire organism

Thorough — careful, detailed, methodical, systematic, meticulous, comprehensive, exhaustive

Tilt — tip, slant, slope, lean, angle, incline

Translucent — see-through, transparent, clear, translucid

Unique — one and only, sole, exclusive, distinctive

Universal — general, widespread, common, worldwide

Unoccupied — vacant, not busy, empty

Unrelated — unconnected, unlinked, distinct, dissimilar, irrelevant

Unresolved — unsettled, uncertain, unsolved, unclear, in doubt

Utilize — make use of, employ

Various — numerous, variety, range of, mixture of, assortment of

Verbalize — express, voice, speak, articulate

Verify — confirm, make sure, prove, attest to, validate, substantiate, corroborate, authenticate

Vigorous — forceful, strong, brisk, energetic, healthy, hardy, tough, athletic, vibrant

Volume — quantity, amount, size

Withdraw — remove, pull out, take out, extract

Illustration Credits

Chapter 6

Figure 6-1: Maslow AH: *Motivation and personality*. ed. 2. Harper & Row, New York, 1970.

Chapter 8

Sample Item 8-41

Reproduced with permission from Merck Sharp & Dohme Corp, a subsidiary of Merck & Co., Inc., Whitehouse Station, NJ.

Chapter 11

Diversity and Spirituality

Question 21: U.S. Census Bureau, Population Division. Retrieved August 28, 2019, from http://www.census.gov/topics/population.html

Index

Page numbers followed by "f" indicate figures.

Q

R

S